Extracellular Vesicles: Biology and Potentials in Cancer Therapeutics

Extracellular Vesicles: Biology and Potentials in Cancer Therapeutics

Editor

William C. S. Cho

MDPI • Basel • Beijing • Wuhan • Barcelona • Belgrade • Manchester • Tokyo • Cluj • Tianjin

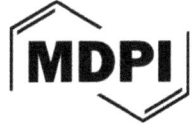

Editor
William C. S. Cho
Queen Elizabeth Hospital
China

Editorial Office
MDPI
St. Alban-Anlage 66
4052 Basel, Switzerland

This is a reprint of articles from the Special Issue published online in the open access journal *International Journal of Molecular Sciences* (ISSN 1422-0067) (available at: https://www.mdpi.com/journal/ijms/special_issues/EV_cancer).

For citation purposes, cite each article independently as indicated on the article page online and as indicated below:

LastName, A.A.; LastName, B.B.; LastName, C.C. Article Title. *Journal Name* **Year**, *Volume Number*, Page Range.

ISBN 978-3-0365-2217-3 (Hbk)
ISBN 978-3-0365-2218-0 (PDF)

© 2021 by the authors. Articles in this book are Open Access and distributed under the Creative Commons Attribution (CC BY) license, which allows users to download, copy and build upon published articles, as long as the author and publisher are properly credited, which ensures maximum dissemination and a wider impact of our publications.

The book as a whole is distributed by MDPI under the terms and conditions of the Creative Commons license CC BY-NC-ND.

Contents

About the Editor vii

William C. S. Cho
Extracellular Vesicles: Biology and Potentials in Cancer Therapeutics
Reprinted from: *Int. J. Mol. Sci.* **2021**, *22*, 9586, doi:10.3390/ijms22179586 1

Kerstin Menck, Suganja Sivaloganathan, Annalen Bleckmann and Claudia Binder
Microvesicles in Cancer: Small Size, Large Potential
Reprinted from: *Int. J. Mol. Sci.* **2020**, *21*, 5373, doi:10.3390/ijms21155373 7

Magdalena Żmigrodzka, Olga Witkowska-Piłaszewicz and Anna Winnicka
Platelets Extracellular Vesicles as Regulators of Cancer Progression—An Updated Perspective
Reprinted from: *Int. J. Mol. Sci.* **2020**, *21*, 5195, doi:10.3390/ijms21155195 35

Maria Luisa Fiani, Valeria Barreca, Massimo Sargiacomo, Flavia Ferrantelli, Francesco Manfredi and Maurizio Federico
Exploiting Manipulated Small Extracellular Vesicles to Subvert Immunosuppression at the Tumor Microenvironment through Mannose Receptor/CD206 Targeting
Reprinted from: *Int. J. Mol. Sci.* **2020**, *21*, 6318, doi:10.3390/ijms21176318 53

Seda Tuncay Cagatay, Ammar Mayah, Mariateresa Mancuso, Paola Giardullo, Simonetta Pazzaglia, Anna Saran, Amuthachelvi Daniel, Damien Traynor, Aidan D. Meade, Fiona Lyng, Soile Tapio and Munira Kadhim
Phenotypic and Functional Characteristics of Exosomes Derived from Irradiated Mouse Organs and Their Role in the Mechanisms Driving Non-Targeted Effects
Reprinted from: *Int. J. Mol. Sci.* **2020**, *21*, 8389, doi:10.3390/ijms21218389 73

Suzanne M Johnson, Antonia Banyard, Christopher Smith, Aleksandr Mironov and Martin G. McCabe
Large Extracellular Vesicles Can be Characterised by Multiplex Labelling Using Imaging Flow Cytometry
Reprinted from: *Int. J. Mol. Sci.* **2020**, *21*, 8723, doi:10.3390/ijms21228723 99

Thomas Simon, Anish Kumaran, Diana-Florentina Veselu and Georgios Giamas
Three Method-Combination Protocol for Improving Purity of Extracellular Vesicles
Reprinted from: *Int. J. Mol. Sci.* **2020**, *21*, 3071, doi:10.3390/ijms21093071 123

Marie Bordas, Géraldine Genard, Sibylle Ohl, Michelle Nessling, Karsten Richter, Tobias Roider, Sascha Dietrich, Kendra K. Maaß and Martina Seiffert
Optimized Protocol for Isolation of Small Extracellular Vesicles from Human and Murine Lymphoid Tissues
Reprinted from: *Int. J. Mol. Sci.* **2020**, *21*, 5586, doi:10.3390/ijms21155586 133

Donatella Lucchetti, Alessandra Battaglia, Claudio Ricciardi-Tenore, Filomena Colella, Luigi Perelli, Ruggero De Maria, Giovanni Scambia, Alessandro Sgambato and Andrea Fattorossi
Measuring Extracellular Vesicles by Conventional Flow Cytometry: Dream or Reality?
Reprinted from: *Int. J. Mol. Sci.* **2020**, *21*, 6257, doi:10.3390/ijms21176257 149

Ancuta Jurj, Cecilia Pop-Bica, Ondrej Slaby, Cristina D. Ştefan, William C. Cho, Schuyler S. Korban and Ioana Berindan-Neagoe
Tiny Actors in the Big Cellular World: Extracellular Vesicles Playing Critical Roles in Cancer
Reprinted from: *Int. J. Mol. Sci.* **2020**, *21*, 7688, doi:10.3390/ijms21207688 165

Tomasz Lorenc, Katarzyna Klimczyk, Izabela Michalczewska, Monika Słomka, Grażyna Kubiak-Tomaszewska and Wioletta Olejarz
Exosomes in Prostate Cancer Diagnosis, Prognosis and Therapy
Reprinted from: *Int. J. Mol. Sci.* **2020**, *21*, 2118, doi:10.3390/ijms21062118 193

Yuana Yuana, Banuja Balachandran, Kim M. G. van der Wurff-Jacobs, Raymond M. Schiffelers and Chrit T. Moonen
Potential Use of Extracellular Vesicles Generated by Microbubble-Assisted Ultrasound as Drug Nanocarriers for Cancer Treatment
Reprinted from: *Int. J. Mol. Sci.* **2020**, *21*, 3024, doi:10.3390/ijms21083024 207

Haoyao Sun, Stephanie Burrola, Jinchang Wu and Wei-Qun Ding
Extracellular Vesicles in the Development of Cancer Therapeutics
Reprinted from: *Int. J. Mol. Sci.* **2020**, *21*, 6097, doi:10.3390/ijms21176097 223

Ki-Uk Kim, Wan-Hoon Kim, Chi Hwan Jeong, Dae Yong Yi and Hyeyoung Min
More than Nutrition: Therapeutic Potential of Breast Milk-Derived Exosomes in Cancer
Reprinted from: *Int. J. Mol. Sci.* **2020**, *21*, 7327, doi:10.3390/ijms21197327 245

Jeong Uk Choi, In-Kyu Park, Yong-Kyu Lee and Seung Rim Hwang
The Biological Function and Therapeutic Potential of Exosomes in Cancer: Exosomes as Efficient Nanocommunicators for Cancer Therapy
Reprinted from: *Int. J. Mol. Sci.* **2020**, *21*, 7363, doi:10.3390/ijms21197363 263

Eliane Ebnoether and Laurent Muller
Diagnostic and Therapeutic Applications of Exosomes in Cancer with a Special Focus on Head and Neck Squamous Cell Carcinoma (HNSCC)
Reprinted from: *Int. J. Mol. Sci.* **2020**, *21*, 4344, doi:10.3390/ijms21124344 287

Aneta Zebrowska, Piotr Widlak, Theresa Whiteside and Monika Pietrowska
Signaling of Tumor-Derived sEV Impacts Melanoma Progression
Reprinted from: *Int. J. Mol. Sci.* **2020**, *21*, 5066, doi:10.3390/ijms21145066 305

Gabriella Dobra, Matyas Bukva, Zoltan Szabo, Bella Bruszel, Maria Harmati, Edina Gyukity-Sebestyen, Adrienn Jenei, Monika Szucs, Peter Horvath, Tamas Biro, Almos Klekner and Krisztina Buzas
Small Extracellular Vesicles Isolated from Serum May Serve as Signal-Enhancers for the Monitoring of CNS Tumors
Reprinted from: *Int. J. Mol. Sci.* **2020**, *21*, 5359, doi:10.3390/ijms21155359 327

Theophilos Tzaridis, Katrin S Reiners, Johannes Weller, Daniel Bachurski, Niklas Schäfer, Christina Schaub, Michael Hallek, Björn Scheffler, Martin Glas, Ulrich Herrlinger, Stefan Wild, Christoph Coch and Gunther Hartmann
Analysis of Serum miRNA in Glioblastoma Patients: CD44-Based Enrichment of Extracellular Vesicles Enhances Specificity for the Prognostic Signature
Reprinted from: *Int. J. Mol. Sci.* **2020**, *21*, 7211, doi:10.3390/ijms21197211 347

Agnieszka Szyposzynska, Aleksandra Bielawska-Pohl, Agnieszka Krawczenko, Olga Doszyn, Maria Paprocka and Aleksandra Klimczak
Suppression of Ovarian Cancer Cell Growth by AT-MSC Microvesicles
Reprinted from: *Int. J. Mol. Sci.* **2020**, *21*, 9143, doi:10.3390/ijms21239143 363

About the Editor

William C. S. Cho's main research interests focus on cancer studies to discover biomarkers for cancer diagnosis, treatment prediction, and prognostication. As a seasoned researcher, Dr Cho has conducted cancer research using molecular biology, proteomics, genomics, immunology, as well as bioinformatics; his current H-index is 60. Dr Cho has published over 400 peer-reviewed papers (e.g., *Lancet Oncology, Annals of Oncology, Journal of Extracellular Vesicles, Advanced Science, Nature Communications, PNAS, Journal of the National Cancer Institute, Clinical Cancer Research, Clinical Chemistry, Molecular Cancer, Theranostics*, etc.) covering cancer biomarkers, proteomics, non-coding RNAs, and Chinese medicine, and these papers have received over 18,000 citations. Dr Cho has also composed 30 book chapters and edited 20 academic books, including "MicroRNAs in Cancer Translational Research", "An Omics Perspective on Cancer Research", "Supportive Cancer Care with Chinese Medicine", "Drug Repurposing in Cancer Therapy: Approaches and Applications", etc.

Editorial

Extracellular Vesicles: Biology and Potentials in Cancer Therapeutics

William C. S. Cho

Department of Clinical Oncology, Queen Elizabeth Hospital, Hong Kong, China; chocs@ha.org.hk

Background

Extracellular vesicles (EVs) are particles wrapped in a lipid bilayer membrane and are naturally released from cells. This kind of cargo vessel is a nanostructure, which mainly transfers lipids, proteins, various nucleic acid fragments, and metabolic components to neighboring cells or distant parts of the body through the circulatory system. EV is of great significance to the communication mechanism between cells. This Special Issue aims to collect articles to enhance our understanding of the biological characteristics of EVs and their potential applications. It features a set of high-impact articles from leading experts in the field. Through a rigorous peer-review process, a total of nineteen articles were accepted, including eight original research articles, ten review articles, and one communication article.

Biology of EVs

Menck et al. [1] summarized the current knowledge about the biology and composition of microvesicles (MV), as well as their role in the tumor microenvironment (TME). Increasing evidence shows that although MVs are biologically different, they have the tumor-promoting properties of endosomal-derived small exosomes in TME. Due to their larger size, they can be easily collected from the patient's blood and characterized by conventional flow cytometry using excess molecules expressed on their surface.

Żmigrodzka et al. [2] reviewed the biogenesis and cargo molecules of platelet extracellular vesicles (PEV), as well as their effects on cancer progression. During platelet activation or apoptosis, PEV is formed, which presents a highly heterogeneous EV group and is the most abundant EV group in the circulatory system. Since the role of platelets in cancer development is well known, and PEV is the most abundant EV in the blood, its possible impact on cancer growth has been strongly discussed. The crosstalk of PEV can promote proliferation, change TME, and promote the formation of metastasis. In many cases, these functions are related to specific cargo molecules transferred from PEV to recipient cells.

Today, in multiple studies exploring TME, the interaction between tumors and macrophages is certainly interesting. Among them, tumor-associated macrophages include a subgroup that has a variety of tumor-promoting effects (including general immunosuppression) in tumor development, which can be identified based on the high expression of mannose receptor/CD206 [3].

Radiation affects not only target cells, but also neighboring cells that have not been exposed to radiation. This response is described as radiation-induced bystander effects (RIBE). Molecular communication between irradiated and unirradiated adjacent cells can trigger RIBE and out-of-field (distance) effects. Cagatay et al. [4] evaluated the changes in the spectrum of exosomes and the role of exosomes as possible molecular signaling mediators for radiation damage. After 24 hours and 15 days of irradiation, exosomes derived from the whole body or partial body of irradiated mouse organs were transferred to recipient mouse embryonic fibroblast (MEF) cells. The changes in cell viability, DNA damage and calcium, reactive oxygen species, and nitric oxide signals were compared with exosome-treated MEF cells from unirradiated mice. Their results showed that whole and local irradiation would increase the number of exosomes and induce changes in MEF cells treated by exosomes.

EV Isolation and Characterization

Many isolation techniques typically discard large EVs in the early stage of sEV or exosome isolation protocols. Johnson et al. [5] described the stepwise separation and characterization of large EV subsets in a medulloblastoma cell line using fluorescent light microscopy, transmission electron microscopy, and tunable resistance pulse sensing. They developed a labeling and strict gating strategy to explore the expression of EV markers (CD63, CD9, and LAMP 1) on a single EV in a wide heterogeneous population. Their data strongly support the exploration of large EVs in clinical samples to obtain potential biomarkers, which are very useful in diagnostic screening and disease monitoring.

EV concentrations often result in low final yields or severe contamination of vesicle samples, which greatly limits further applications and data reproducibility, and contamination greatly affects a wide range of functional studies. Simon et al. [6] described a new combination of three well-known methods (size exclusion chromatography (SEC), Western blotting, and transmission electron microscopy) to obtain medium to high yields of EVs while reducing protein contamination. They believe that this method may have great benefits for in vitro and in vivo functional studies.

Efforts have also been made to standardize the separation and characterization techniques of sEV. Current protocols often result in the co-separation of soluble proteins or lipid complexes with other EVs. Bordas et al. [7] reported an optimized protocol for the isolation of sEV from human and murine lymphoid tissues. To separate sEV from freshly resected human lymph nodes and mouse spleen, two different methods were compared: (1) ultracentrifugation on a sucrose density pad and (2) a combination of ultracentrifugation and SEC. The purity of sEV preparations was analyzed using Western blotting, nanoparticle tracking analysis, and electron microscopy. Their results clearly demonstrated the superiority of SEC in improving the yield and purity of sEV.

On the other hand, it is questionable whether clinical laboratories can conduct in-depth research through flow cytometry to evaluate EV surface cargo in various diseases. Lucchetti et al. [8] reported the difficulty of evaluating small and medium-sized EVs through traditional flow cytometry. Running a sample of medium EVs stained with equal amounts of Calcein-green and Calcein-violet, they found that the cluster detection produced false double positive events. This phenomenon was significantly reduced by sample dilution, but it was not completely eliminated. In addition, running highly diluted samples required a longer cytometer time. Their findings question the routine applicability of traditional flow cytometry in EV analysis.

Therapeutic Potential of EVs

It is well known that the potential use of EVs as therapeutic agents lies not only in their cell membrane-bound components but also in their cargo. Jurj et al. [9] highlighted the characteristics of EV involvement in cancer cells, paying special attention to those molecular processes that were affected by EV cargo. In addition, they explored the role of RNA types and proteins carried by EVs in triggering the drug resistance phenotype. Interestingly, in various in vivo and in vitro studies and multiple clinical trials, engineered EVs have been proposed as therapeutic agents.

The composition of exosomes and the possibility of interacting with cells make exosomes a multifaceted regulator of cancer development. Lorenc et al. [10] discussed the role of tumor-derived exosome (TEX) in the progression of prostate cancer and the potential use of exosomes in the management of prostate cancer. The biophysical properties of EVs (such as stability, biocompatibility, permeability, low toxicity, and low immunogenicity) are the key to the successful development of innovative drug delivery systems. EV has enhanced circulation stability and biological barrier permeability, so it can be used as an effective chemotherapy carrier to improve the regulation of target tissues and organs.

Exosomes can deliver different types of cargo and target specific cells. They may help deliver chemotherapy drugs, natural products, and RNA-based cancer gene therapy [11].

The combination of ultrasound and microbubbles has been shown to trigger cancer cells to release EVs. Yuana et al. [12] used microbubbles-assisted ultrasound (USMB) to load the model drug CellTracker green fluorescent dye (CTG) or bovine serum albumin coupled with fluorescein isothiocyanate (BSA FITC) into primary human endothelial cells in vitro. They found that USMB loaded CTG and BSA FITC into human endothelial cells and triggered the release of EVs containing these compounds in the cell supernatant within two hours after treatment. The amount of EV released seems to be related to the increase in ultrasound acoustic pressure. They concluded that USMB can load model drugs into endothelial cells and trigger the release of EV-carrying model drugs, highlighting the potential of EV as a drug nanocarrier for future cancer drug delivery.

Sun et al. [13] elaborated about the role of EV in the development of cancer therapeutics. They emphasized that some EVs (such as tumor exosomes) have a tumor-homing tendency, which has led to the use of EV as a drug carrier to effectively provide cancer treatment. The results of preclinical research and early clinical trials were mainly reviewed. For example, a phase I clinical trial designed to evaluate the ability of plant sEVs to prevent oral mucositis during chemotherapy and radiotherapy of head and neck cancer revealed the potential of using plant sEVs to reduce side effects during cancer treatment. It was also reported that isolating fibroblast-like mesenchymal cell-derived sEV and loading siRNA or shRNA targeting *KRAS* mutation (*KrasG12D*) could more effectively inhibit the progression of pancreatic ductal adenocarcinoma in vitro and in vivo compared with other drug carriers.

Interestingly, human breast milk (HBM) is an irreplaceable source of nutrition for early infant growth and development. Kim et al. [14] reviewed the various components of HBM (especially exosomes and miRNA) and their therapeutic potential for cancer. Milk-derived exosomes play a variety of physiological and therapeutic functions in cell proliferation, inflammation, and immune regulation, mainly due to their cargo molecules (such as proteins and miRNA). Exosomal miRNA is not affected by enzymatic digestion and acidic conditions, and it plays a key role in immune regulation and cancer. In addition, milk-derived exosomes have been developed as drug carriers for the delivery of small molecules and siRNA to tumor sites.

Although cancer treatments encounter physiological obstacles in TME, they must be delivered to their target to improve efficacy and reduce toxicity. Choi et al. [15] summarized the biological function and therapeutic potential of exosomes as diagnostic biomarkers and drug delivery vehicles for cancer treatment. They also explored whether exosomes could be used as effective nanocommunicators to promote drug design for personalized cancer immunotherapy.

Despite the tremendous technological advances in the treatment of head and neck squamous cell carcinoma (HNSCC), the overall survival rate is usually low. Ebnoether and Muller [16] summarized the diagnostic and therapeutic applications of exosomes in HNSCC. They also reviewed the impressive preliminary results obtained in recent studies.

Since TEX is involved in the crosstalk between cancer and immune cells, it plays a key role in suppressing the anti-tumor immune response to promote tumor progression. Most of the available information about the molecular composition and function of TEX was obtained using small EV (sEV) isolated from the supernatant of cancer cell lines. However, new data linking plasma TEX levels to cancer progression focuses on TEX in the peripheral circulation of patients as a potential biomarker for cancer diagnosis, development, activity, and response to treatment. Zebrowska et al. [17] published an article on the signaling of melanoma cell-derived sEV, with particular emphasis on exosome-mediated signal transduction between melanoma cells and the host immune system. They argue that the signaling of TEX may impact melanoma progression.

Dobra et al. [18] initiated the first proteomic study comparing whole-serum and serum-derived sEV. They aimed to determine the characteristic protein fingerprints associated with central nervous system (CNS) tumors. A total of 96 human serum samples were obtained from four patient groups (glioblastoma multiforme, brain metastases from non-small-cell lung cancer, meningioma, and lumbar disc herniation). Among the 311 identified proteins, 10 whole serum proteins and 17 serum-derived sEV proteins showed the highest difference between each group. A total of 65 proteins were significantly enriched in serum-derived sEV samples, while 129 proteins were significantly reduced compared with whole-serum sEV samples. Based on principal component analysis, serum-derived sEV was more suitable for distinguishing patient groups and has a greater potential for monitoring CNS tumors than whole-serum sEV.

Glioblastoma is a devastating disease, and there is an urgent need for biomarkers that can predict prognosis. Tzaridis et al. [19] analyzed a set of serum microRNAs (miRNAs) in the EV from glioblastoma patients and examined their relevance to the prognosis of these patients. Using RT-qPCR and CD44 immunoprecipitation (sinusoidal endothelial cell + CD44), the levels of 15 miRNAs in EVs separated by SEC were compared with those of glioblastoma patients and healthy volunteers. Combining miR-15b-3p in serum or miR-106a-5p in CD44 immunoprecipitation EVs with any of the other three miRNAs in CD44 immunoprecipitation EV could stratify the prognosis of glioblastoma patients.

Transporting the biologically active cargo of MVs to target cells can affect their fate and behavior and change their microenvironment. Szyposzynska et al. [20] evaluated the biological activity of MV derived from human immortalized mesenchymal stem cells of adipose tissue-origin (HATMSC2-MVs) against two ovarian cancer cell lines ES-2 and OAW-42. They prove that HATMSC2-MVs can effectively metastasize to ovarian cancer cells and inhibit cell proliferation, apoptosis, and/or necrosis through different pathways, which may be related to the presence of different anti-tumor factors secreted by ES-2 and OAW-42 cells.

Conclusions

We hope that all these efforts will improve our understanding of the EV world and provide some insights into its potential clinical applications. With its multiple encapsulated macromolecules and powerful extraction platform, we envision a more comprehensive understanding of EV biology through multi-omics approaches.

Funding: This research received no external funding.

Institutional Review Board Statement: Not applicable.

Informed Consent Statement: Not applicable.

Conflicts of Interest: The author declares no conflict of interest.

References

1. Menck, K.; Sivaloganathan, S.; Bleckmann, A.; Binder, C. Microvesicles in cancer: Small size, large potential. *Int. J. Mol. Sci.* **2020**, *21*, 5373. [CrossRef] [PubMed]
2. Żmigrodzka, M.; Witkowska-Piłaszewicz, O.; Winnicka, A. Platelets extracellular vesicles as regulators of cancer progression - An updated perspective. *Int. J. Mol. Sci.* **2020**, *21*, 5195. [CrossRef] [PubMed]
3. Fiani, M.L.; Barreca, V.; Sargiacomo, M.; Ferrantelli, F.; Manfredi, F.; Federico, M. Exploiting manipulated small extracellular vesicles to subvert immunosuppression at the tumor microenvironment through mannose receptor/CD206 targeting. *Int. J. Mol. Sci.* **2020**, *21*, 6318. [CrossRef] [PubMed]
4. Cagatay, S.T.; Mayah, A.; Mancuso, M.; Giardullo, P.; Pazzaglia, S.; Saran, A.; Daniel, A.; Traynor, D.; Meade, A.D.; Lyng, F.; et al. Phenotypic and functional characteristics of exosomes derived from irradiated mouse organs and their role in the mechanisms driving non-targeted effects. *Int. J. Mol. Sci.* **2020**, *21*, 8389. [CrossRef] [PubMed]
5. Johnson, S.M.; Banyard, A.; Smith, C.; Mironov, A.; McCabe, M.G. Large extracellular vesicles can be characterized by multiplex labelling using imaging flow cytometry. *Int. J. Mol. Sci.* **2020**, *21*, 8723. [CrossRef] [PubMed]
6. Simon, T.; Kumaran, A.; Veselu, D.F.; Giamas, G. Three method-combination protocol for improving purity of extracellular vesicles. *Int. J. Mol. Sci.* **2020**, *21*, 3071. [CrossRef] [PubMed]
7. Bordas, M.; Genard, G.; Ohl, S.; Nessling, M.; Richter, K.; Roider, T.; Dietrich, S.; Maaß, K.K.; Seiffert, M. Optimized protocol for isolation of small extracellular vesicles from human and murine lymphoid tissues. *Int. J. Mol. Sci.* **2020**, *21*, 5586. [CrossRef] [PubMed]

8. Lucchetti, D.; Battaglia, A.; Ricciardi-Tenore, C.; Colella, F.; Perelli, L.; Maria, R.D.; Scambia, G.; Sgambato, A.; Fattorossi, A. Measuring extracellular vesicles by conventional flow cytometry: Dream or reality? *Int. J. Mol. Sci.* **2020**, *21*, 6257. [CrossRef] [PubMed]
9. Jurj, A.; Pop-Bica, C.; Slaby, O.; Ştefan, C.D.; Cho, W.C.; Korban, S.S.; Berindan-Neagoe, I. Tiny actors in the big cellular world: Extracellular vesicles playing critical roles in cancer. *Int. J. Mol. Sci.* **2020**, *21*, 7688. [CrossRef] [PubMed]
10. Lorenc, T.; Klimczyk, K.; Michalczewska, I.; Słomka, M.; Kubiak-Tomaszewska, G.; Olejarz, W. Exosomes in prostate cancer diagnosis, prognosis and therapy. *Int. J. Mol. Sci.* **2020**, *21*, 2118. [CrossRef] [PubMed]
11. Xue, V.W.; Wong, S.C.C.; Song, G.; Cho, W.C.S. Promising RNA-based cancer gene therapy using extracellular vesicles for drug delivery. *Expert Opin. Biol. Ther.* **2020**, *20*, 767–777. [CrossRef] [PubMed]
12. Yuana, Y.; Balachandran, B.; Wurff-Jacobs, K.M.G.; Schiffelers, R.M.; Moonen, C.T. Potential use of extracellular vesicles generated by microbubble-assisted ultrasound as drug nanocarriers for cancer treatment. *Int. J. Mol. Sci.* **2020**, *21*, 3024. [CrossRef] [PubMed]
13. Sun, H.; Burrola, S.; Wu, J.; Ding, W.Q. Extracellular vesicles in the development of cancer therapeutics. *Int. J. Mol. Sci.* **2020**, *21*, 6097. [CrossRef] [PubMed]
14. Kim, K.U.; Kim, W.H.; Jeong, C.H.; Yi, D.Y.; Min, H. More than nutrition: Therapeutic potential of breast milk-derived exosomes in cancer. *Int. J. Mol. Sci.* **2020**, *21*, 7327. [CrossRef] [PubMed]
15. Choi, J.U.; Park, I.K.; Lee, Y.K.; Hwang, S.R. The biological function and therapeutic potential of exosomes in cancer: Exosomes as efficient nanocommunicators for cancer therapy. *Int. J. Mol. Sci.* **2020**, *21*, 7363. [CrossRef] [PubMed]
16. Ebnoether, E.; Muller, L. Diagnostic and therapeutic applications of exosomes in cancer with a special focus on head and neck squamous cell carcinoma (HNSCC). *Int. J. Mol. Sci.* **2020**, *21*, 4344. [CrossRef] [PubMed]
17. Zebrowska, A.; Widlak, P.; Whiteside, T.; Pietrowska, M. Signaling of tumor-derived sEV impacts melanoma progression. *Int. J. Mol. Sci.* **2020**, *21*, 5066. [CrossRef] [PubMed]
18. Dobra, G.; Bukva, M.; Szabo, Z.; Bruszel, B.; Harmati, M.; Gyukity-Sebestyen, E.; Jenei, A.; Szucs, M.; Horvath, P.; Biro, T.; et al. Small extracellular vesicles isolated from serum may serve as signal-enhancers for the monitoring of CNS tumors. *Int. J. Mol. Sci.* **2020**, *21*, 5359. [CrossRef] [PubMed]
19. Tzaridis, T.; Reiners, K.S.; Weller, J.; Bachurski, D.; Schäfer, N.; Schaub, C.; Hallek, M.; Scheffler, B.; Glas, M.; Herrlinger, U.; et al. Analysis of serum miRNA in glioblastoma patients: CD44-based enrichment of extracellular vesicles enhances specificity for the prognostic signature. *Int. J. Mol. Sci.* **2020**, *21*, 7211. [CrossRef] [PubMed]
20. Szyposzynska, A.; Bielawska-Pohl, A.; Krawczenko, A.; Doszyn, O.; Paprocka, M.; Klimczak, A. Suppression of ovarian cancer cell growth by AT-MSC microvesicles. *Int. J. Mol. Sci.* **2020**, *21*, 9143. [CrossRef] [PubMed]

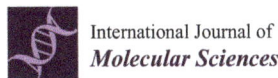 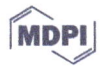

Review

Microvesicles in Cancer: Small Size, Large Potential

Kerstin Menck [1,†], Suganja Sivaloganathan [1,†], Annalen Bleckmann [1,2] and Claudia Binder [2,*]

1. Department of Medicine A, Hematology, Oncology, and Pneumology, University Hospital Münster, 48149 Münster, Germany; Kerstin.Menck@ukmuenster.de (K.M.); Suganja.Sivaloganathan@ukmuenster.de (S.S.); annalen.bleckmann@ukmuenster.de (A.B.)
2. Department of Hematology/Medical Oncology, University Medical Center Göttingen, 37075 Göttingen, Germany
* Correspondence: claudia.binder@med.uni-goettingen.de; Tel.: +49-0551-398-943
† These authors contributed equally.

Received: 30 June 2020; Accepted: 27 July 2020; Published: 28 July 2020

Abstract: Extracellular vesicles (EV) are secreted by all cell types in a tumor and its microenvironment (TME), playing an essential role in intercellular communication and the establishment of a TME favorable for tumor invasion and metastasis. They encompass a variety of vesicle populations, among them the well-known endosomal-derived small exosomes (Exo), but also larger vesicles (diameter > 100 nm) that are shed directly from the plasma membrane, the so-called microvesicles (MV). Increasing evidence suggests that MV, although biologically different, share the tumor-promoting features of Exo in the TME. Due to their larger size, they can be readily harvested from patients' blood and characterized by routine methods such as conventional flow cytometry, exploiting the plethora of molecules expressed on their surface. In this review, we summarize the current knowledge about the biology and the composition of MV, as well as their role within the TME. We highlight not only the challenges and potential of MV as novel biomarkers for cancer, but also discuss their possible use for therapeutic intervention.

Keywords: microvesicles; biomarker; cancer; tumor microenvironment; therapy

---

1. Introduction

Tumor development is a multistep process that is accompanied by various cellular reprogramming events in which cells acquire the hallmarks of cancer cells to gain and sustain abnormal growth and invasive capacity [1]. The complex process of tumor formation and spreading not only depends on the tumor cells themselves but also requires rewiring of the surrounding stromal cells. This can be induced by cell intrinsic events (genetic or epigenetic aberrations) or by external factors originating from direct cell–cell contact or from indirect cell communication. While soluble factors, such as chemokines, cytokines, and growth factors, have long been known for their role during tumor development, extracellular vesicles (EV) have recently attracted increasing attention as mediators of intercellular communication. Conserved from prokaryotes to eukaryotes, the secretion of EV is observed in all cell types [2]. The term EV encompasses all types of secreted membrane-enclosed vesicles, which are highly heterogeneous. On the basis of various characteristics, ranging from size, biogenesis, cell of origin, morphology, and content, EV are categorized into four main classes: endosomal-derived small exosomes (Exo) (50–150 nm), plasma membrane-derived middle-sized microvesicles (MV) (100–1000 nm), and large oncosomes (LO) (1000–10,000 nm), as well as apoptotic bodies (500–4000 nm) that are released from dying cells [3,4]. Although commonly used to categorize EV, this classification has been challenged by recent evidence demonstrating that, for instance, the Exo contain further subtypes with different biological and biochemical properties [5]. In order to avoid terminological ambiguities, the term "small EV" was coined for EV harvested at > 100,000 g. However, since most authors still use the term Exo, we will adhere to this nomination throughout the review.

In cancer, EV have been shown to be essential for various steps during tumor initiation and progression. By horizontal transfer of bioactive molecules between cancer cells and the neighboring stroma, EV interfere with signaling and regulation of gene expression in the recipient cell. Thus, the malignant cells can convert the phenotype of surrounding benign cells into a tumor-supporting one and create a favorable environment for cancer progression and metastatic spread. While much attention has been paid to the role of Exo in cancer, the function of the larger MV is still poorly defined. This seems surprising, since MV, in contrast to Exo, are easily accessible in patients' blood and are characterizable by routine methods that should make them ideal candidates for "liquid biopsies". Additionally, MV have long been known for their involvement in metastasis formation. This was initially attributed to their procoagulant activity, favoring the formation of microthrombi and facilitating the extravasation of the thus captured circulating tumor cells (reviewed in [6]). However, more recently, accumulating evidence points to a plethora of different ways in which MV are involved in the various steps of tumor progression.

In this review, we discuss the current knowledge about the role of MV during cancer development and shed light on how these insights can be exploited clinically for cancer diagnostics. Moreover, we highlight the divergent features of MV compared to Exo as cancer therapeutics and illustrate the various ways in which MV can either promote or counteract cancer therapy. For this purpose, we specifically included studies in which EV were harvested at 10,000–20,000 g and collectively refer to them as MV.

2. Preparation of MV

In order to decipher the role of MV in cancer development and progression, effective methods are required that allow for the stringent isolation of pure MV populations from different cell types and biological fluids. A major caveat in MV research is that the currently available isolation methods potentially co-isolate LO or Exo, yielding a mixed population of EV. This may explain many of the apparently conflicting results in the field of EV research. To address this major challenge, new technologies are under development, but they are not yet suitable for laboratory use. In an endeavor to standardize the experimental procedures and limit experimental variability in the field, scientists of the International Society of Extracellular Vesicles (ISEV) published a position paper indicating the appropriate methods for isolation of EV from cells or biological fluids and highlighting the current knowledge and major caveats of these procedures [7]. A variety of methods are available on the basis of different principles for enriching the various EV subpopulations, including density gradient centrifugation, size-exclusion chromatography, precipitation via volume-excluding polymers, immunoaffinity capture methods, high-pressure liquid chromatography, field flow fractionation, and flow cytometry [7,8].

To date, differential centrifugation is still the method of choice for isolating MV since it yields a reasonably good separation of MV from Exo with regard to protein and RNA content as well as function [9–11]. In principle, samples are spun down at 2000 g to initially pellet large EV such as LO, followed by centrifugation at 10,000–20,000 g to sediment the middle-sized MV, while ultracentrifugation at ≥100,000 g leads to a harvest of small Exo [8]. Although ultracentrifugation has been criticized for inducing vesicle aggregation and thus affecting downstream applications [12–14], these studies were conducted on the 100,000 g Exo pellet. It is unclear to what extent these problems also apply to the 10,000 g MV pellet as well. Another popular method to separate EV from contaminations with non-vesicular proteins or RNA aggregates is ultracentrifugation of EV samples on density gradients. However, the typically used sucrose gradients lack sufficient resolution to separate EV that have slightly different densities and are released by different mechanisms [15]. Since the density of MV and Exo is comparable, they cannot be separated on sucrose gradients easily [11]. Likewise, precipitation methods such as protein organic solvent precipitation (PROSPR) have been demonstrated to co-isolate MV, but the preparations were mainly enriched in smaller Exo, with MV being only a minor side population [16]. Immunoaffinity capture methods rely on antibodies for specific EV surface markers that are coupled to beads and used to isolate specific vesicle subpopulations. Due to the current lack of specific markers for MV, this method has been scarcely used for the preparation of MV. Currently, novel micro-/nano-based devices for MV isolation from clinical samples are being developed (reviewed in [17]). However, one major problem is that the thus isolated vesicle preparations have often been poorly characterized and it is unclear whether they yield MV with a purity comparable to sequential centrifugation protocols. The same applies to methods originally established for Exo isolation such as precipitation or size-exclusion chromatography. While none of the currently available isolation procedures for MV and Exo yield pure vesicle populations, but rather MV- or Exo-enriched fractions, more effective techniques that separate pure MV from Exo might help to shed light on their distinct cell biological features such as biogenesis, uptake, and cargo trafficking routes. Then again, from a clinical viewpoint, the isolation of pure MV populations might not be absolutely necessary for their use as biomarkers, since recent studies have demonstrated the potential of MV for cancer diagnostics or therapy monitoring, even when the preparations contain some smaller Exo.

No matter which method is chosen for EV isolation, the researchers of the ISEV community highly recommend validating the obtained EV by different techniques [7]. This includes the analysis of marker protein expression comprising (i) transmembrane, (GPI)-anchored, as well as cytosolic EV marker proteins (e.g., CD63, CD9, Alix, Syntenin, Rgap1, along with negative controls consisting of (ii) non-EV co-isolated proteins (e.g., ApoB, albumin), (iii) proteins typically present in non-EV subcellular structures such as the Golgi or endoplasmatic reticulum (e.g., GM130, Calreticulin, histones), and (iv) secreted proteins (e.g., collagen, epidermal growth factor (EGF), interleukins). Moreover, EV should be characterized by at least two distinct techniques including their visualization by, for instance, electron or atomic force microscopy, as well as the analysis of their biophysical properties via, for example, nanoparticle tracking analysis (NTA) or Raman spectroscopy. Nanoparticle tracking analysis (NTA) is the most suitable method for analyzing the isolated MV in terms of quantification and sizing. NTA tracks the Brownian movement of laser-illuminated particles and calculates the diameter based on the Stokes–Einstein equation [18]. While NTA remains the most commonly used method for quantitative MV analysis, other methods such as tunable resistive pulse sensing or dynamic light scattering are also available [19]. However, a major limitation of these methods is that they cannot efficiently analyze larger vesicles and that they do not yield any information on the molecular composition of the MV. They are, therefore, combined with other methods such as tunable resistive pulse sensing and Raman spectroscopy or NTA with fluorescence labelling to obtain more information about the isolated MV [19].

A major caveat in MV research is that the currently available isolation methods potentially co-isolate LO or Exo, yielding a mixed population of EV. This may explain many of the apparently conflicting results in the field of EV research. To address this major challenge, new technologies are under development, but are not yet suitable for laboratory use. In an endeavor to standardize the experimental procedures and limit experimental variability in the field, scientists of the International Society of Extracellular Vesicles (ISEV) published a position paper that indicated the appropriate methods for isolation of EV from cells or biological fluids and highlighted the current knowledge and major caveats of these procedures [7]. Furthermore, the researchers of the ISEV community highly recommend validating different techniques for various cell types and biological fluids. A crowdsourcing knowledge base was established to create further transparency with regards to experimental and methodological parameters of EV isolation (http://evtrack.org) [20]. This platform encourages researchers to upload published and unpublished experiments, thereby creating an informed dialogue among researchers about relevant experimental parameters. This represents a major step in facilitating standardization in EV, as well as MV, research.

3. Biogenesis of MV

MV directly bud off from the outer cell membrane. The shedding process comprises molecular rearrangements of the plasma membrane regarding lipid and protein composition as well as Ca^{2+} levels. Ca^{2+}-dependent aminophospholipid translocases, flippases, floppases, scramblases, and calpain drive the translocation of phosphatidylserine from the inner to the outer membrane leaflet, which is considered a typical characteristic of MV (comprehensively reviewed in [21]). Apoptotic bodies, which are larger in size, also externalize phosphatidylserine on their surface [22,23]. Therefore, the isolation of MV should be conducted solely from healthy and viable cells to avoid contamination with apoptotic bodies, which otherwise can be difficult to discriminate from MV. Ca^{2+} levels regulate membrane rigidity and curvature and maintain physical bending of the membrane, which leads to restructuring and contraction of the underlying actin cytoskeleton enabling MV formation and pinching (reviewed in [24]). MV formation and release are also affected by the lipids ceramide and cholesterol [25]. Neutral sphingomyelinase activity, which hydrolyses lipid sphingomyelin into phosphorylcholine and ceramide, was shown to be involved in Exo and MV release. Inhibition of the enzyme led to a reduction in Exo release, while simultaneously increasing MV budding [26], which suggests that the release of both EV subpopulations is interconnected, albeit on the basis of distinct biogenetic mechanisms.

In addition to lipids, enzyme machineries involved in cytoskeletal regulation play a key role in MV formation and budding. One example is the small GTPase protein ADP-ribosylation factor 6 (ARF6), which stimulates phospholipase D (PLD) that subsequently associates with extracellular signal-regulated kinase (ERK) at the plasma membrane. ERK activates a signaling cascade downstream of the myosin light chain kinase (MLCK) that results in contraction of actinomyosin and enables MV release [27]. Similar to MV, LO are thought to derive from the plasma membrane. However, in contrast to MV, the shedding of LO has been exclusively attributed to aggressive cancer cells that have acquired an amoeboid phenotype to facilitate motility and invasiveness ([4]). Other Rho family small GTPases such as RhoA and RHO-associated protein kinases are equally important regulators of actin dynamics relevant for MV formation [28]. In addition, the endosomal sorting complex required for transport (ESCRT), which is mainly known for its role in the biogenesis of Exo [29], is also involved in MV formation and the last phase of their release. Interaction of arrestin domain-containing protein 1 (ARRDC1) with the late endosomal protein tumor susceptibility gene 101 (TSG101) results in relocation of TSG101 from the endosomal to the plasma membrane, which then induces the release of MV [30].

4. Membrane Composition of MV

EV-mediated cell–cell communication requires targeting and uptake into the recipient cell to deliver the bioactive cargo, which then induces functional and phenotypical changes. These events depend on the composition of the EV membrane, as surface molecules on EV are responsible for binding and docking to recipient cells [31,32]. The molecular composition of the MV membrane closely resembles that of the parental cell [33]. It is enriched in phospholipid lysophosphatidylcholine, sphingolipid sphingomyelins, acylcarnitine, and fatty acyl esters of L-carnitine [34]. ARF6, a key regulator of MV biogenesis, was shown to mediate MV surface molecule selection by recruiting proteins such as ß1 integrin receptor, major histocompatibility complex (MHC) class I and II molecules, membrane type 1-matrix metalloproteinase (MT1-MMP), vesicular SNARE (v-SNARE), and vesicle-associated membrane protein 3 (VAMP3) to tumor MV [27]. Moreover, the bioactive cargo of MV depends on the conditions the parental cells are subjected to, such as inflammation or other stressors. An additional example is hypoxia, which induces recruitment of the RAS-related protein Rab22a to the site of MV budding in breast cancer cells, thus influencing MV formation and loading [35].

Since both LO and MV are derived from the plasma membrane, it is not surprising that some transmembrane proteins are present on either of these EV. Analysis of protein marker expression on LO and MV revealed a common signature, underlining the fact that the definition of MV-specific markers remains challenging. Of note, some of the markers initially thought to be specific for Exo, including tetraspanins (CD9, CD63, CD81, HSP60, HSP70, HSP90), membrane transporters and fusion proteins (annexin, flotillin), and multivesicular body (MVB) synthesis proteins (Alix, TSG101) were also found in varying amounts on MV and LO [9]. The fact that, despite their different routes of origin, EV share some common surface molecules and MV-specific markers are still lacking represents major challenges in EV research. It further emphasizes that to correctly characterize EV populations it is indispensable to combine a variety of parameters in addition to marker expression, such as size, sedimentation coefficient, and others.

5. Role of Cancer-Associated MV and Their Protein Cargo in Tumor Progression

EV-mediated cell–cell communication within the tumor microenvironment (TME) is highly complex and has recently been comprehensively reviewed in [36,37]. The role of EV in promoting tumor progression has mostly been elucidated in studies on mixed populations of EV without focusing on a specific subpopulation. Therefore, the specific contribution of MV in this complex process remained enigmatic for a long time. However, with increasing awareness of the presence of large MV, accumulating evidence has begun to unravel the tumor-promoting role of MV in TME communication, as described below by selected examples. The function of MV largely depends on their bioactive cargo, in particular the shuttling of tumor-specific proteins to the surrounding cells. While researchers initially concentrated on the role of nucleic acids transported via EV (e.g., DNA, mRNA, or miRNA), the focus has more recently shifted towards the analysis of the EV proteome. The protein content of MV has been found to be strikingly different from that of the Exo proteome and is enriched in proteins involved in microtubule/cortical actin and cytoskeleton networks, ARF6, its effector phospholipase D2, and parts of the ESCRT family (ESCRT-I) [27,38]. Carrying these bioactive cargo molecules, MV are able to influence either the adjacent tumor cells in an autologous way or the neighboring stromal cells in a heterologous kind of cell–cell communication.

MV-mediated autologous communication transfers oncogenic traits between tumor cells, resulting in enhanced tumor growth and progression. One example is multiple myeloma in which MV shed by the cancer cells were shown to enhance tumor cell proliferation and thereby stimulate tumor growth [39]. Interestingly, this effect was related to the enrichment of the extracellular matrix metalloproteinase inducer (EMMPRIN/CD147) on the tumor MV. This protein is known to be frequently overexpressed in solid tumors as well as in some lymphomas and leukemias [40]. In line with this finding, another study in breast cancer cells showed that the highly glycosylated isoform of EMMPRIN in particular is present in high levels on breast cancer cell-derived MV and stimulates tumor cell invasion via activation of p38/MAPK signaling [11]. Strikingly, a similar, high-EMMPRIN expression was also found on blood MV from patients with metastatic breast cancer where it was co-expressed with the tumor marker Mucin-1 (MUC1/CA 15-3) [11]. Another tumor-specific factor implicated in pro-tumorigenic tumor–tumor crosstalk via MV is the truncated oncogenic form of the epidermal growth factor receptor (EGFR), EGFRvIII, which is commonly expressed in aggressive brain tumor cells. It was shown that MV secreted by U373 glioma cells contained EGFRvIII, enabling them to transfer malignant characteristics from highly aggressive tumor cells to EGFRvIII-negative, more benign tumor cells, thereby promoting their oncogenic transformation [41]. Hence, MV are convenient communicators within the TME that can either mediate the horizontal transfer of oncogenic material or activate oncogenic signaling pathways in neighboring cancer cells, stimulating their proliferative, survival, mitogenic, and angiogenic potential and shifting them to a highly invasive phenotype.

In addition to tumor–tumor communication, MV were also found to mediate reciprocal crosstalk between the tumor and the surrounding stroma cells. Such heterologous interactions were observed, for instance, between tumor cells and surrounding immune cells, being seemingly essential for cancer immune evasion. As shown for breast cancer cells, the secretion of both tumor MV as well as Exo induced the expression of Wnt5a in tumor-associated macrophages. Macrophage Wnt5a was then, in turn, delivered to breast cancer cells via macrophage-derived MV and Exo, where it activated ß-catenin-independent Wnt signaling, leading to increased tumor invasion [42]. This example indicates that EV-based cell–cell communication can occur bidirectionally in a reciprocal loop and reprogram tumor-associated immune cells towards a tumor-supporting phenotype. The finding that MV-enriched preparations isolated at 50,000 g induced the differentiation of monocytes producing the anti-inflammatory cytokine IL-10 further supports this notion [43,44]. In line with this, early stimulation with tumor MV triggered macrophage polarization towards an anti-inflammatory phenotype with decreased anti-tumor cytotoxic potential [45].

Apart from macrophages, other immune cells can be affected by MV, such as the T cells. As T cells represent the first line of the immune defense, tumor cells seem to have established strategies to suppress T cell activity and dampen antitumoral immune response by exploiting MV-mediated cell–cell communication. For instance, leukemia-derived MV deliver miRNAs to T cells, which then interact with their targets, resulting in a T cell exhaustion phenotype [46]. Moreover, MV released by irradiated breast cancer cells were shown to carry an increased amount of immune-modulating proteins, such as programmed cell death ligand 1 (PD-L1). Via transfer of this immunosuppressive protein, tumor MV inhibited cytotoxic T cell activity and enabled tumor growth [47].

Tumor cell-derived MV were also shown to modulate fibroblasts in the tumor stroma. Stimulation of fibroblasts with prostate cancer MV converted them to an activated phenotype and triggered the release of tumor-promoting fibroblast MV [48]. Similar observations were made in oral squamous carcinoma when normal human fibroblasts were treated with tumor-derived MV [49]. In this study, the switch to cancer-associated fibroblasts (CAF) was mainly mediated via metabolic reprogramming of the fibroblasts to aerobic glycolysis, with an increase in glucose uptake and lactate secretion. Co-culturing the generated CAF with oral squamous cell carcinoma cells again led to enhanced cancer cell invasion and migration. Interestingly, MV-induced fibroblast activation and spreading seems to occur in particular in the stiff matrix environment that is typically found in the tumor periphery [50]. Tumor MV are also able to modulate angiogenesis within the primary tumor. In a study on a mixed population of MV and Exo, normal endothelial cells were found to endocytose tumor EV, which activated PI3K/Akt signaling and promoted the motility as well as the tube formation activity of the endothelial cells [51]. As the pro-angiogenic factor vascular endothelial growth factor (VEGF) has been found on MV and Exo, this might be one important factor contributing to the stimulatory effect of tumor MV on endothelial cells [52]. Of note, MV transport a unique 90 kDa form of VEGF that has only a weak affinity for bevacizumab, the clinically used monoclonal anti-VEGF antibody, which might thus be ineffective in blocking MV-mediated activation of the VEGF receptor (VEGFR) [53]. Similarly, MV derived from multiple myeloma cells were shown to transfer CD138, a myeloma cell marker, to endothelial cells. This stimulated the endothelial cells to proliferate, invade, and secrete the angiogenic factors IL-6 and VEGF to promote tube formation [54]. Taken together, these observations emphasize the important role of MV in tumor–stroma crosstalk during tumor progression.

Using the same mechanisms as discussed above, MV were found to modulate the surrounding environment beyond the primary tumor by shaping the formation of pre-metastatic niches over long distances. In pancreatic cancer, tumor MV were able to enter the liver microcirculation and extravasate through the vessel wall in a CD36-dependent manner where they were taken up by perivascular macrophages and primed the liver metastatic niche [55]. Furthermore, the highly metastatic melanoma cell line B16F10 releases large amounts of tumor MV into its surroundings. These MV were found to be able to induce metastasis formation in BALB/c mice, which are normally resistant to the B1610 tumor cell line [56]. Metastatic niche formation might be essentially influenced by tumor MV uptake into organ-specific macrophage populations, and this uptake seems to be further influenced by systemic changes such as inflammation [57]. However, further in vivo studies are required to characterize the uptake kinetics and to clarify which cells are specifically targeted by tumor MV during systemic spreading. In summary, an increasing number of studies confirms that MV play a critical role in cell–cell communication within the TME and support local tumor growth and progression as well as tumor spreading to distant sites through the priming of metastatic niches (Figure 1).

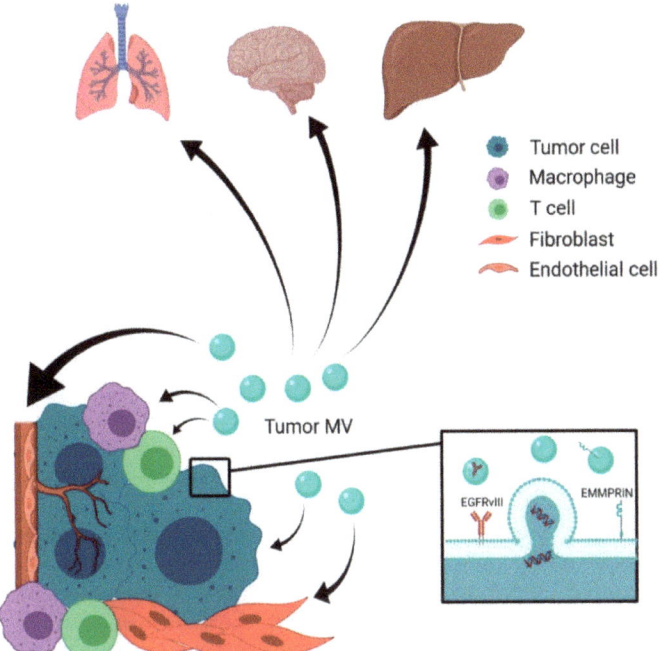

Figure 1. Microvesicles (MV) shaping the local tumor microenvironment (TME) and distant metastatic niches to promote tumor growth. On the one hand, MV shed from the plasma membrane of tumor cells act in an autologous way on other tumor cells by transferring oncogenic cargo and stimulating pro-tumorigenic signaling. On the other hand, MV are able to mediate heterologous cell–cell communication by acting on cells present within the TME, such as macrophages, T cells, fibroblasts, or endothelial cells. As a result, these cells become activated and change their phenotype to enhance tumor growth. Once the tumor has gained access to the circulation, tumor MV can be distributed throughout the body and mediate cargo transfer and cell–cell communication at distant sites. This induces the formation of pre-metastatic niches that offer a favorable environment for subsequent seeding of tumor cells in secondary organs.

6. Analysis of MV in Peripheral Blood

MV have been successfully detected in almost all body fluids, including saliva [58], urine [59], cerebrospinal fluid [60], breast milk [61], ejaculate [62], synovial fluid [63], bronchoalveolar lavages [64], and blood, wherein they were described as early as 1967 by Peter Wolf as "platelet dust" [65]. The advantage of body fluids apart from blood is that they contain MV specifically enriched for the cancers drained by them. Nevertheless, some of these liquids are either difficult to obtain or provide additional methodological problems. For instance, MV in urine are of special interest as biomarkers for urothelial cancers. However, their isolation poses two additional challenges: (1) the most abundant protein in urine, the Tamm–Horsfall protein, associates and co-precipitates with EV, and (2) standard protocols pre-clear urine samples at 17,000 g to deplete the urinary sediment, and thus also deplete the MV contained within. Therefore, the number of studies on MV in urine meeting the criteria mentioned in the introduction is very limited. Since blood is the most thoroughly studied body fluid, as well as the most likely application route for using MV with regard to diagnostic and therapeutic interventions, we chose to focus this review on MV in blood.

When isolating MV from blood, several studies have shown that the choice of anticoagulant used for blood collection has a critical influence on the obtained MV, although the results seem to be contradictory. While the use of protease inhibitors, either sodium heparin or a mix of hirudin supplemented with a factor Xa inhibitor, was initially recommended because of the high number of preserved MV [66], other reports have argued for the use of sodium citrate since the lower numbers of MV might point to less artificial MV shedding [67]. In contrast, Jamaly et al. recently used various anticoagulants to isolate MV and measure their total plasma concentrations by NTA without finding any significant differences in numbers [68]. Apart from total MV numbers, the isolation of MV from serum drawn into lithium heparin tubes seems to result in the aggregation of platelet-derived MV, with sticky vesicle pellets and a reduction in platelet MV numbers, thereby specifically affecting certain MV subpopulations [69,70]. In addition to the anticoagulant, other preanalytical factors such as centrifugation, temperature, freeze–thaw cycles, or agitation can influence MV in blood samples, which should be taken into account when setting up isolation protocols for clinical studies [66,67,71]. However, long-term storage of plasma samples without repeated freeze–thaw cycles seems feasible without significant MV loss [67,69,72]. Another important factor for the analysis of large MV in blood is the initial removal of platelets and blood cells to obtain platelet-poor plasma (PPP). Since PPP is often prepared by centrifugation at 2500–3000 × g, this step might result in a significant loss of larger MV, which already pellet at this force [9]. It has been proposed that two centrifugation steps at 1500× g might be preferable for MV isolation [70]; however, more elaborate sorting methods might be required to specifically isolate larger EV from blood.

A current study by Brennan et al. compared different EV isolation methods, including ultracentrifugation, density gradient centrifugation, and size exclusion chromatography, as well as different combinations thereof, for their potential to isolate EV from plasma [73]. While none were found to be clearly superior, the authors showed that the isolation method significantly affected the yield, size, and degree of contamination with serum (lipo)proteins [73]. This must therefore be considered carefully on the basis of the planned downstream application. Unfortunately, the study was conducted on whole EV preparations, and thus it is again unclear whether the results are also applicable for larger MV. A novel approach to specifically reduce the contamination of plasma EV preparations with lipoproteins is to use anti-apolipoprotein B (ApoB) antibody-coated magnetic beads prior to EV isolation [74]. However, the method might lead to a high loss of vesicles.

The preferred method for analyzing MV from clinical samples is flow cytometry because of its wide availability in most labs and clinical centers, its capability for rapid preparation and acquisition of a large number of samples, as well as its potential for standardization. Since the size threshold of standard flow cytometers is ~300 nm (see [75] for a current instrument comparison), this allows the quick measurement and quantification of MV protein expression in contrast to Exo, which have to be coupled prior to analysis to larger latex beads following a time-consuming protocol. Protocols exist for staining of single or multiple markers on plasma-derived MV for flow cytometry [76,77]. Even though flow cytometry might not allow the detection of very small MV <300 nm and thus not reproduce the whole spectrum of MV in blood, several studies have successfully demonstrated the potential of flow cytometry for measuring MV-associated cancer biomarkers, as discussed in detail below. However, analysis of MV samples by flow cytometry bears several pitfalls, and the settings should be chosen with care to avoid misinterpretation of the results [78]. When measuring MV by flow cytometry, their presence should be confirmed by additional methods such as NTA or electron microscopy as the correct sizing of vesicles by flow cytometry can be challenging [79]. When discriminating MV from background noise using annexin V staining, the use of saline was recommended since the routinely used PBS seemed to create artificial nano-sized vesicles and could thus lead to false positive results [80]. Another pitfall is that the insoluble fraction of immune complexes and MV have overlapping size profiles, which might interfere with their flow cytometric analysis. To confirm that MV and not immune complexes are measured, samples can be treated with low concentrations of detergents (e.g., 0.05% Triton X-100), which lyse MV, thus resulting in a loss of signal in contrast to immune complexes that keep their fluorescent signal [63]. Recently, another label-free approach called flow cytometry scatter ratio (Flow-SR) has been introduced to discriminate MV <500 nm from lipoprotein particles, which are highly abundant in plasma samples [67].

Apart from flow cytometry, there are protocols for surface profiling of plasma MV by antibody microarrays. However, this is a semiquantitative method and thus more useful for initial screening of patient samples for the expression of potential novel biomarkers [81]. In summary, the current studies have shown that isolation and analysis of MV from human biofluids, such as plasma, is feasible using standard laboratory equipment. However, it is clear that transparent reporting and standardization of protocols are highly important for implementing and translating MV as novel biomarkers and therapeutics into the clinic [82,83].

7. MV Levels in Cancer Patients

Most studies have focused on measuring total MV levels in the plasma of cancer patients. In this context, it must be kept in mind that tumors can secrete large numbers of apoptotic bodies under therapy due to the massive induction of apoptosis in the tumor tissue. Apoptotic bodies can have a similar size as MV and are equally characterized by an externalization of phosphatidylserine, a marker that is often used to identify MV by flow cytometry. Hence, care should be taken to include only patients prior to treatment into these studies. While the observed results are very contradictory, the majority of reports have documented increased MV levels in cancer patients compared with healthy controls. Augmented MV levels have been detected by flow cytometric quantification, mostly using TruCount Beads, in the plasma of patients suffering from gastric cancer [84], lung cancer [85], breast and pancreatic cancer [86,87], and colorectal cancer [88], as well as in most hematologic malignancies including chronic lymphocytic leukemia (CLL) and multiple myeloma [89–91]. The same trend has been confirmed for hepatocellular carcinoma by measuring MV protein levels by bicinchoninic acid assay (BCA) [92]. In contrast, two studies investigating heterogeneous cohorts of patients with different types of advanced cancers did not detect significant differences in total plasma MV numbers by flow cytometric quantification or analysis of MV protein content [69,93]. Similar observations were made by a novel capture/imaging approach in glioblastoma patients [94]. Another report quantified the total number of annexin V+ MV by flow cytometry and found a significant decrease of MV levels in patients with colorectal cancer and benign colorectal diseases compared with healthy controls [95]. The discrepancy between the observations might be due to the methods used for MV quantification, the composition of the patient and control cohorts, or diverging effects in different cancer subtypes. Patient selection criteria and the clinical setting of sample acquisition (before/during/after treatment) are not always conclusively reported in the studies, which could be another reason for the heterogeneous results.

While the increased levels of MV in hematologic malignancies could be explained by additional vesicle shedding from the large numbers of cancer cells in blood, the source of the elevated MV counts in solid tumor patients remains undefined. In these patients, plasma levels of tumor MV might depend on the access of the tumor to the circulation or might originate from other blood cell populations as a reaction to the growing tumor. Other limitations are that all the studies are either single center studies; include a very small number of patients; or have compared MV levels between cancer patients and younger, healthy controls. It was recently found that total MV levels were higher in healthy, untreated elderly than in younger individuals, which might have biased the results [96].

An argument for a specific increase in MV levels in cancer patients is that MV levels seem to increase with advanced tumor stages and have been found to be elevated in late stage metastatic breast cancer [86,87], colorectal cancer [88], hepatocellular carcinoma [92], or CLL [90] compared with early stage patients. Of note, a significant increase was already observed in stage I colorectal cancer patients compared with healthy controls [88]. In line with this, total MV levels decreased 1 month after surgery in hepatocellular carcinoma patients and have thus been suggested as a potential diagnostic biomarker [92]. Moreover, higher MV levels in blood might additionally serve as a prognostic biomarker since they were found to correlate with a poor clinical outcome in glioblastoma or CLL [90,97]. In contrast, in lung cancer, an increase in MV in blood was associated with better progression-free survival [85]. An interesting finding was the detection of very large vesicles (1–14 µm), measurable with the established CellSearch system used for the analysis of circulating tumor cells (CTCs) [98]. These epithelial cell adhesion molecule (EpCAM)+/cytokeratin CK+/CD45- large vesicles without nuclei were present at frequencies one order of magnitude higher than CTCs and were elevated in the plasma of prostate, breast, and colorectal, but not lung cancer patients, with high numbers correlating with shorter overall survival [99]. While these vesicles have not yet been validated to be "true EV" using the MISEV guidelines, their discovery might represent one additional opportunity of translating EV as biomarkers into the clinic using an instrument already applied in diagnostics.

8. MV as Cancer Biomarkers

The growing number of in vitro studies demonstrating that cancer cells shed large numbers of EV with tumor-specific material has fueled interest in using EV as biomarkers in the clinic. Most investigations thus far have focused on the detection of tumor-derived vesicles within the complex mixture of plasma EV. This seems to be a promising strategy for gaining information about the genetic makeup of the tumor and identifying targetable characteristics, in particular for solid tumors, which are not directly accessible without invasive procedures (e.g., pancreatic cancer, glioblastoma). In contrast to the classical soluble "tumor markers" in the serum, MV also allow for detection of non-secreted, membrane-bound, or even intracellular molecules. Thus, the MV-based liquid biopsy enlarges the spectrum of detectable tumor-associated factors that could help not only with regard to diagnosis but also with accurate patient risk stratification and therapy monitoring. Since tumors seem to gain access to the circulation quite early [100], tumor MV in blood are believed to be of potential interest as early diagnostic biomarkers. In contrast to the extremely sparse CTCs, they are present in significantly greater numbers, which might improve detection sensitivity. Recently, tumor EV, consisting of a mixture of small and large vesicles, were shown to be able to pass the intact blood–brain barrier in an orthotopic glioblastoma xenotransplant model of human cancer stem cells as well as in glioma patients [101]. In line with this finding, EV carrying tumor-specific alterations were detected in the blood of patients with low-grade glioma, most of whom still had an intact blood–brain barrier [101], thus further supporting the concept of using EV as early cancer biomarkers. Another important point is that tumors are known to be highly heterogeneous [102], a circumstance that currently gains more and more attention with the novel single cell analysis technologies. While a biopsy taken from a limited area within the tumor only partly mirrors the molecular composition of the whole tumor, EV are believed to give a more comprehensive picture. This might apply also to patients with advanced, metastatic cancer, considering that metastases often differ from the primary tumor, as well as among each other, and might thus express different markers or potential therapeutic targets [103,104]. Interestingly, an early study in glioblastoma described the detection of oncogenic EGFRvIII transcripts in plasma-derived EV in two patients who had been diagnosed as EGFRvIII-negative on the basis of a tumor tissue biopsy [105]. Thus, it may be speculated that EV might mirror tumor heterogeneity more accurately than limited biopsies.

When aiming at the specific detection of tumor-derived MV in blood, the first step is to identify cancer-specific factors that are not expressed on MV shed by other cell populations. Therefore, a thorough characterization of tumor MV is necessary, which usually has been performed on cancer cell line-derived vesicles for later translation to patient samples. A recent report has suggested that MV reflect the cellular transcriptomic landscape better than Exo and can thus give valuable information about mutation status or gene amplifications that can be used for cancer diagnostics [106]. In line with this, hallmark oncogenic fusion transcripts (e.g., BCR-ABL1, TEL-AML1, MLL-AF6) as well as other specific tumorigenic transcripts (e.g., HOXA9, MEIS1) were found in MV of leukemia cell lines [107,108]. Similarly, in a glioblastoma model, genomic DNA (gDNA) sequences of tumor-associated genes were identified with a distinct distribution in either apoptotic bodies, MV or Exo isolated from human cancer stem cells, or from the blood of xenotransplanted mice, including specific detection of PIK3CA, EGFR, AKT1, and MDM2 sequences in MV [101]. However, the question remains as to whether analysis of vesicle-associated transcripts is superior to mutation detection based on cell-free DNA. Encouraging results have been obtained in this context by the group of Krug et al., who demonstrated increased sensitivity in detecting EGFR mutations in the plasma of lung cancer patients with a combined analysis of circulating tumor and EV DNA compared to circulating tumor DNA alone [109].

MV and Exo have been shown to differ in their RNA composition [10]. While several population-specific microRNAs have been identified for both MV and Exo, there seems to be a trend that miRNAs are relatively more enriched in Exo and mRNAs in MV [106,110,111]. In addition, an enrichment compared with the whole cell has been observed as several miRNAs that were almost undetectable in colorectal cancer cell lysates (<5 transcript per million (TPM)) were found at high levels (>1000 TPM) in the respective MV and Exo from the cells [111]. However, it is currently unclear whether sufficient amounts of RNA molecules are shuttled to EV in order to functionally influence recipient cells, as several critical reports have revealed that most RNA species are present at frequencies of much less than 1 copy per EV [106,110,112]. Therefore, the focus of the rest of this review is on MV-associated proteins that have the additional benefit that they could be used not only as biomarkers, but also for specific drug delivery and targeting. The protein content of EV has been evaluated largely by Western blotting, flow cytometry, as well as different proteomic approaches. While shot-gun proteomics was initially used to thoroughly characterize the whole EV proteome, novel targeted proteomic acquisition strategies such as selected (or multiple) reaction monitoring (SRM/MRM) allow the detection of a predetermined selection of specific target peptides with high sensitivity and quantitative accuracy [113]. These methods thus facilitate the discovery and large-scale validation of biomarker pipelines in complex biological samples (e.g., blood) [114]. In a recent study, SRM/MRM was successfully employed to identify novel potential biomarkers for prostate cancer on Exo in urine [115], demonstrating its potential for future EV-related biomarker studies.

The MV proteome has been proposed to be more similar to the cellular proteome than that of Exo [35]. However, not all proteins from the cellular plasma membrane are found on MV, and some are highly enriched, which suggests specific sorting mechanisms [116]. An overview of MV-associated tumor antigens that have been successfully detected in the blood of cancer patients and used as biomarkers is presented in Table 1. In hematologic malignancies, MV carrying the respective malignancy-associated antigen (e.g., CD38 for multiple myeloma, CD30 for Hodgkin lymphoma) were detected in cancer patients but were almost undetectable in healthy controls [91]. Similar observations have been made for solid tumors. In one of the earliest studies, the oncogenic receptor human epidermal growth factor receptor 2 (Her2/Neu) was identified and significantly elevated on blood-derived MV from gastric cancer patients [84]. Meanwhile this finding has been confirmed for colorectal cancer [117]. In the largest study to date of a cohort of 330 cancer patients with advanced solid tumors and 103 healthy, non-cancer controls, the number of MV carrying the tumor antigen EMMPRIN were found to be increased with advanced tumor stage [69]. Expanding the analyses on MV co-expressing EMMPRIN together with other tumor-associated molecules, such as epithelial cell adhesion molecule (EpCAM/CD326), MUC1/CA 15-3, or EGFR1, the numbers were not only significantly elevated in cancer patients versus controls but also associated with poor overall survival, thus suggesting that MV might indeed represent valuable prognostic cancer biomarkers. EpCAM is among the most studied antigens as it is known to be overexpressed on tumors of epithelial origin and is thus a bona fide tumor marker. The combination of EpCAM with other tissue-specific markers such as, for instance, the asialoglycoprotein receptor 1 (ASGPR1), exclusively expressed in liver cells, allowed the separation of patients with liver disorders into patients with or without liver tumors (including hepatocellular or cholangiocellular carcinoma) [118]. In line with this, the EpCAM+/EMMPRIN+ MV levels correlated with tumor size in colorectal cancer patients and decreased after surgical removal of the tumor [118,119]. In yet another study performed on plasma samples from metastatic prostate cancer patients, caveolin-1 (CAV1) was found on 5–10% of large EV (1–10 μm) isolated by filtration, but with a size profile similar to the 10,000 g pellet, whereas it was barely detectable in healthy controls [120].

Table 1. Common tumor antigens detected on patient-derived MV.

Marker	Cancer Subtype	Method	Reference
CD13	Leukemia (AML/CML) Myelodysplastic syndrome	Flow cytometry	[91]
CD138	Multiple myeloma	Flow cytometry	[89]
CD19	Non-Hodgkin lymphoma Leukemia (CLL) Morbus Waldenström	Flow cytometry	[91]
CD30	Hodgkin lymphoma	Flow cytometry	[91]
CD38	Multiple myeloma	Flow cytometry	[91]
c-Met	Gastric cancer	Western blot	[84]
Caveolin-1	Prostate cancer	Flow cytometry	[120]
EGFR	Colorectal	Flow cytometry Western blot	[76] [117]
	GBM	Immunofluorescence	[94]
EGFRvIII	GBM	Immunofluorescence	[94]
EMMPRIN	Various	Flow cytometry Western blot	[11] [76]
	Colorectal cancer Lung cancer Pancreas carcinoma	Flow cytometry	[119]
	Gastric cancer	Western blot	[84]
EpCAM	Breast cancer Lung cancer Head and neck cancer Colorectal cancer Pancreatic cancer	Flow cytometry	[76] [119]
	GBM	Immunofluorescence	[94]
EpCAM/EMMPRIN	Colorectal cancer Lung cancer Pancreas carcinoma	Flow cytometry	[119]
EpCAM/ASGPR1	Hepatocellular carcinoma Cholangiocarcinoma	Flow cytometry	[118]
FAK	Breast cancer	Western blot	[87]
HepPar1	Hepatocellular carcinoma	Flow cytometry	[121]
Her2/Neu	Gastric cancer	Flow cytometry	[84]
	Colorectal cancer	Flow cytometry Western blot	[117]
MUC1	Breast cancer Pancreatic cancer	Flow cytometry	[86]
	Breast cancer	Flow cytometry Western blot	[11]
	Breast cancer Lung cancer Head and neck cancer	Flow cytometry	[76]

From the thus far published MV biomarker studies, one can deduce that the population of tumor MV carrying the respective tumor antigens constitutes up to 5–10% of the total MV in blood of advanced cancer patients [69,94,120]. A recent study has profiled MV at the single vesicle level and proposed that there is a huge heterogeneity among MV, and that not all MV, even from the same cell line, carry the respective tumor markers [94], which further hampers the detection of tumor MV in blood.

Moreover, especially low-abundance tumor MV might be concealed in the heterogeneous mixture of blood MV, which might necessitate the development of novel protocols for specific enrichment of tumor MV populations. One suggestion is to remove the platelet-derived MV prior to analysis [70] since they represent the largest MV population in blood. A protocol was recently published for isolating different subpopulations of small and large EV from solid tumor tissue, in this example from melanoma [122,123]. This is an important step that will now allow for isolation of MV from primary tumor tissues and metastases to define not only tumor-specific but even patient-specific biomarkers. The comparison of MV profiles from the tumor tissues (primary tumor/metastases) with MV present in body fluids might then provide information on clonal evolution and serve as the basis for therapy selection and monitoring.

9. MV Biomarker Signatures

The studies conducted thus far have shown that while single MV-associated biomarkers are often elevated in the blood of cancer patients, each of the antigens alone failed to reliably distinguish cancer patients from healthy controls, mainly due to low sensitivity. In contrast, combinations of several markers have proved to be of superior diagnostic value, such as the combination of EMMPRIN/EpCAM/MUC1/EGFR, which reliably separated cancer patients from healthy controls with a high AUC value of 0.85 [69]. It seems likely that more comprehensive signatures comprising cancer subtype-specific markers can even further increase sensitivity and specificity. Importantly, it has to be considered that the overexpression of certain oncogenes might impact MV protein profiles as was shown for breast cancer for the oncogene Src for Exo [124] or Her2/Neu, which was shuttled along with its associated proteins onto MV and Exo [125]. The resulting specific signatures have already been successfully used for the correct determination of breast cancer subtypes from serum EV [126]. Compared to soluble cancer biomarkers, which often suffer from low specificity and a high rate of false positive results, the strength of MV is their potential as biomarker platforms that simultaneously carry multiple markers, allowing for the recognition and detection of specific patterns.

10. The Microvesicle Reactome in Blood

Several conditions, such as hypoxia, inflammation, exercise, or nutrition, influence levels of MV subpopulations in blood (reviewed in [127]). It might thus be worth considering the fact that not only the analysis of tumor MV in blood but also changes in blood MV composition or the markers on distinct blood MV subpopulations might give information about cellular transformation (Figure 2). Although, for example, endothelial cell-derived MV were detected at elevated levels in some hematologic malignancies [91], a slight increase was observed in platelet- as well as leukocyte-derived MV in solid tumor patients [69,88,128]. An analysis of the phospho-proteome of MV and Exo isolated from plasma samples of breast cancer patients by ultracentrifugation described 156 unique phosphosites, which differed significantly between the vesiculome of healthy individuals and patients [129]. More specifically, in the blood of gastric cancer patients, the levels of MV carrying the chemokine receptor CCR6 were elevated. The cell type of origin, however, remained unclear [84].

Among the EV subpopulations, MV are considered the main source of tissue factor (TF) activity [130]. Higher amounts of MV with TF activity were detected in the plasma of metastatic cancer patients, suggesting their use as novel markers for venous thromboembolism, a common complication in advanced cancer patients [131]. In addition to TF, phosphatidylserine, whose exposure on the outer membrane is a typical feature of all MV, can further induce thrombin generation [132]. This potential side effect should therefore be carefully taken into account when considering the application of MV as therapeutics, although first studies in mice did not show an effect of the injected MV on coagulation [133].

Taken together, analysis of the whole mixture of plasma vesicles does not only detect the presence or absence of tumor EV but yields more comprehensive information since it additionally mirrors the reaction of immune and other cells against the tumor EV.

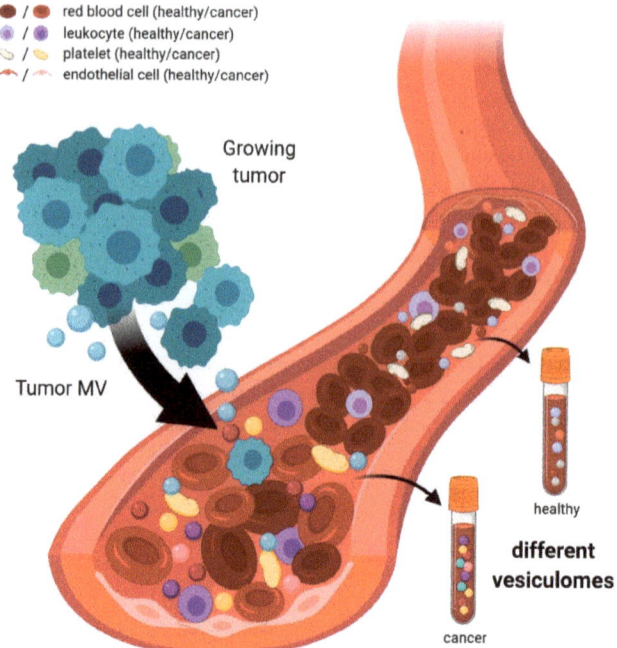

Figure 2. The microvesiculome in blood. The growth of a tumor is accompanied by secretion of circulating tumor cells (CTCs) as well as of tumor-derived soluble factors and MV. When encountering any of these components, benign blood cells can become activated and react by shedding their own, altered MV. Taken together, this results in changes in the composition as well as expression pattern of MV in the blood of cancer patients. Liquid biopsy-based MV sampling should therefore not only be focused on the detection of tumor MV, but also on alterations in non-tumor blood MV.

11. MV for Therapy Monitoring

First studies have revealed the potential of MV for monitoring therapeutic responses in cancer patients. Krishnan et al. reported that plasma levels of CD138+ MV corresponded with therapeutic response in individual multiple myeloma patients [89]. In general, total levels of MV were found to decrease after surgical removal of the tumor, which was generally associated with a better outcome [92,97]. In line with this, the number of EpCAM+ MV decreased 10 days after surgery in colorectal cancer patients, although the effect was not seen for EpCAM+/EMMPRIN+ MV [119]. This might be explained by the additional presence of EMMPRIN on platelet- and immune cell-derived MV [11], which are directly influenced by the surgery. Prolonged high levels of total EV or endothelial cell-derived CD144+ MV after chemotherapy seem to predict a poor clinical response and were found to be associated with shorter progression-free and overall survival [134,135]. The same trend was observed in glioblastoma patients showing tumor progression after radiochemotherapy who generally exhibited higher MV levels compared with patients with pseudoprogression or stable disease [136]. Moreover, an increased concentration of large and small EV prior to therapy was associated with failure of chemotherapy in breast cancer patients [134]. Taken together, these results demonstrate that MV levels not only mirror the presence of tumor, but that MV might also have a protective role against chemotherapeutic agents.

12. MV and Cancer Therapy

As discussed above, MV collected by liquid biopsies can give valuable information about targetable characteristics in the growing tumor and thus be used as an innovative read-out for targeted therapy decisions and patient stratification for personalized medicine. However, it has also become clear that MV can interfere with cancer treatment and limit therapeutic success. On the one hand, MV have been identified as transporters for P-glycoprotein (MDR1) and multidrug resistance-associated protein 1 (MRP1), two plasma membrane multidrug efflux transporters, and have thus been recognized as vehicles for spreading multidrug resistance from resistant to sensitive tumor clones [137,138]. On the other hand, cancer cells export cytotoxic agents via their MV during chemotherapy as has been shown, for instance, for doxorubicin, cisplatin, gemcitabine, or docetaxel [133,139,140]. Cancer cells seem to shed higher numbers of MV during treatment, and it has been suggested that the potential of a cell to shed MV correlates with its resistance to treatment [140]. Therefore, it seemed to be a promising strategy to inhibit MV release in order to increase treatment efficiency. Indeed, the combination of chloramine and bisindolylmaleimide-I, two inhibitors blocking the release of both MV and Exo, highly increased apoptosis in cancer cell lines treated with chemotherapeutic agents [141]. In another study, reducing MV shedding by inhibition of calpain via siRNA or the specific inhibitor calpeptin significantly elevated intracellular levels of docetaxel. This increased the susceptibility of the cell to chemotherapy, allowing for treatment with lower doses of chemotherapeutic agent at higher efficiency in vitro as well as in a xenograft mouse model in vivo [139]. Considering the toxic effects of general inhibition of EV secretion, it still remains elusive as to whether this strategy is feasible for human patients or whether it will be possible to specifically target such inhibitors to the tumor tissue.

Another mechanism as to how EV can impede cancer therapy is that cancer cells have been shown to export therapeutic targets such as CD20, Her2/Neu, or PD-L1 onto Exo [142–144] that capture the administered therapeutic antibodies and shield the tumor cells from attack, resulting in therapy failure. Moreover, Exo have been recently shown to transfer resistance-mediating cargo from stromal to cancer cells [145]. Whether the same mechanisms indeed also apply for large MV is currently unknown.

Considering the evidence for a tumor-supporting role of MV, they should also be regarded as novel targets for therapeutic approaches. This notion is supported by a study by Keklikoglou et al. showing in a mixed population of MV and Exo that chemotherapy induces the release of Annexin A6 (ANXA6+) EV from murine breast cancer cells. When these chemotherapy-induced ANXA6+ EV were injected into the tail vein of mice, they activated endothelial cells to produce the chemokine Ccl2, which led to the expansion of Ly6C+CCR2+ lung monocytes and thus pre-conditioned the lungs for the seeding of breast cancer metastases [146]. Similar observations of EV-mediated pre-metastatic niche formation have been made for melanoma [147]. In line with these findings, MV isolated from cancer patients induced a tumor-supporting phenotype in human macrophages ex vivo and highly increased the invasive potential of benign breast cancer cells, while MV isolated from healthy controls had no such effect [69].

13. MV as Cancer Vaccines

Although the studies presented thus far argue for an unfavorable role of MV in hampering cancer therapy, the final two chapters discuss how MV could also be exploited positively with regard to therapeutic interventions. In a first study, Zhang et al. reported that while the immunization of mice with PBS or tumor cell lysates failed to prevent the growth of subsequently injected tumor cells, mice treated with tumor Exo or MV developed tumors in only 87.5% or 50% of the animals, respectively [148]. These initial results suggested that tumor MV, which are enriched in a multitude of tumor-specific proteins (see Table 1), could serve as a novel, cell-free source of tumor antigens that are more immunogenic than other parts of the tumor cells, including tumor Exo. A possible explanation for their superior efficacy compared with Exo might be the presence of DNA as well as mitochondrial fragments inside MV that discriminate them from Exo and might provide an additional immunostimulatory signal for innate immune cells. However, more studies are required to confirm the differential immunogenic effect of MV and Exo and explain the potential difference.

In general, the anti-tumor immune response is believed to occur largely via cytotoxic CD8+ T cells activated by tumor antigen-presenting dendritic cells. Since immunization with tumor MV prior to tumor growth is hardly possible in human patients, strategies will have to be developed to treat already existing tumors. Indeed, in the above-mentioned study, the injection of tumor MV into mice with already growing tumors failed to induce a sufficient activation of T cells [148]. Instead, the injection of dendritic cells primed with tumor MV overcame the problem of inadequate T cell activation, enhancing T cell infiltration in the tumor tissue as well as tumor cell killing [148]. Mechanistically, incubation of dendritic cells with tumor MV induced dendritic cell maturation with concordant upregulation of the co-stimulatory molecules CD80 and CD86, increasing their homing to the tumor-draining lymph nodes [148,149]. Further evidence that the use of MV as tumor vaccines might indeed lead to successful anti-tumor immune responses has been provided by a recent study by Pineda et al. who harvested MV from C6 rat glioma cells and subsequently administered them to rats, which had been inoculated with a subcutaneous C6 glioma. MV vaccination increased the number of infiltrating T cells in the tumor tissue, induced tumor cell apoptosis, and led to a reduction of tumor growth [150]. Interestingly, it might even be possible to deliver future MV vaccines orally, as it was discovered that tumor MV injected intragastrically into mice are taken up by intestinal epithelial cells in the ileum and transferred by transcytosis to dendritic cells at the basolateral side that can subsequently induce T cell activation and anti-tumor immune responses [151]. However, this treatment was only successful with concordant anti-acidic agents, as MV are sensitive to degradation by gastric acid.

Thus far, clinical studies testing the efficiency of tumor cell- or Exo-based vaccines have shown only limited efficiency and it remains to be seen whether this trend is different for MV. The efficiency of tumor MV vaccines will critically depend on whether it will be possible, on the one hand, to find ways of boosting their efficacy in eliciting an anti-tumor immune response, while, on the other hand, limiting their immunosuppressive functions.

14. MV as Vehicles for Drug Delivery

The finding that EV transport bioactive molecules (e.g., proteins, metabolites, or nucleic acids) raised interest early on in terms of their use as a novel drug delivery system. Compared with cell-based therapeutics, EV have the advantages that they do not possess the potential for transformation or unlimited growth, they are known to cross biological barriers such as the blood–brain barrier, and as non-living material they can be stored or transported more easily and be modified with more aggressive manipulation techniques. Another positive aspect is their natural origin, which makes them more biocompatible than artificial liposomal drug carriers, with enhanced stability, less immunogenicity, and less liver toxicity [152]. In general, EV as drug carriers offer protection for their content, such as from enzymatic degradation, which enhances cargo stability in biofluids. EV can be modified with several approaches to increase their bioactive potential, including either manipulation strategies for the secreting cell, such as genetic manipulation, cell stress, or hypoxia, or post-isolation loading methods, such as electroporation, sonication, heat-shock, or EV transfection. A current overview of the techniques, their advantages, and their limitations is presented in [153,154]. Although most methods have been solely tested for Exo, the majority should be equally applicable to MV, considering the similarities in their biophysical makeup.

The first report on MV as a drug delivery system was published by Tang et al., who successfully used chemotherapy-loaded MV to inhibit tumor growth in a murine hepatocarcinoma ascites model, as well as in severe combined immunodeficient (SCID) mice injected with ovarian cancer cells [133]. Delivery was even successful to solid tumors when MV were injected intravenously [133]. In a first in vivo approach, the same group tested the therapeutic potential of intrathoracic injections of cisplatin-loaded tumor MV in six end-stage, cisplatin-resistant lung cancer patients. The injections greatly reduced the number of tumor cells (>95%) in the metastatic malignant pleural effusions in three of the six patients, suggesting an efficacy of the MV injections and also their ability to reverse drug resistance [155]. However, the treatment did not show any benefit in the other three patients, raising the question about the underlying reasons for the treatment failure. Two clinical trials are currently registered to further explore the potential of MV as therapeutic tool in cancer: a phase I/II study investigating the use of red blood cell-derived MV loaded with methotrexate in the treatment of malignant ascites (clinicaltrials.gov identifier: NCT03230708), and a phase II study aimed at generating methotrexate-loaded autologous tumor MV from malignant effusion and testing their effect on tumor growth and immune regulation (clinicaltrials.gov identifier: NCT02657460).

The majority of the conducted studies thus far has used EV from mesenchymal stem cells as native vehicles for therapeutic applications, and none of them has observed significant side effects [156]. Alternatively, red blood cell-derived EV have been suggested especially for the delivery of RNA drugs since they are easily available, do not contain DNA, and can be easily modified by electroporation [157]. However, in mouse models, their systemic administration as drug carrier was found to only be feasible for the therapy of leukemias, while successful delivery to solid tumors required intratumoral injections due to the otherwise low target organ specificity [157]. In general, EV biodistribution seems to depend on the kind of cell used for EV production, the EV delivery route, the dosage, and the uptake efficiency [158]. After systemic injection, a major part of the injected EV is trapped in the liver, spleen, or lung [158,159], which on the one hand might limit EV distribution to other organs, but on the other hand might be used for specific cargo delivery to these organs. Several engineering strategies are currently being tested to improve EV circulation kinetics and increase targeting to specific cell populations [160]. A hallmark of MV is that phosphatidylserine is exposed on their outer membrane surface, a feature which distinguishes them from Exo. Since externalized phosphatidylserine is a recognition signal for macrophages and triggers phagocytosis [161], MV might be superior for drug delivery to this specific cell population.

Interestingly, a recent report suggested that the choice of MV or Exo as drug carrier influences the intracellular delivery route of the transported cargo. While MV-loaded paclitaxel was mostly delivered by membrane fusion and endocytosis, Exo-loaded paclitaxel was predominantly taken up by endocytosis into prostate cancer cells [162]. Moreover, MV seem to promote drug entry into the nucleus, even into highly resistant tumor-repopulating cells [155]. Since the mechanism of internalization and intracellular trafficking significantly affects the functional efficiency of the delivered drug, further research aiming at elucidating the different fates of MV- and Exo-delivered cargo will help to choose the most accurate EV delivery system for a given drug.

While MV are larger and therefore allow for packaging larger amounts of drug molecules, it could be more difficult for them to penetrate into the tissue due to their size. One solution that has been presented suggests isolating MV from tumor cells grown in and adapted to soft fibrin gels, which resulted in the shedding of less stiff MV [163]. These softer MV with a higher capacity for deformation showed enhanced extravasation into the tumor with deep tissue penetration and, as a result, enhanced treatment efficacy when loaded with the chemotherapeutic agent doxorubicin [163]. Moreover, a weaker extravasation was observed in non-tumor tissue compared with MV isolated from cells cultured in 2D [163], suggesting less toxicity. A problem for both MV and Exo seems to be their limited lifespan in circulation. For fluorescently labeled pancreatic tumor MV injected into healthy mice, the signal was cleared after 60 min, while the majority of MV were already lost within 15 min after injection [164].

Taken together, while both Exo and large MV have been shown to possess the potential for drug delivery, more comparative studies are required to evaluate common as well as diverging features of both EV populations as therapeutic vehicles. Both still suffer from the lack of scalable, specific, cost-effective production and isolation methods as well as poor drug loading efficiency, problems that need to be solved for their standardized use in the clinic. Moreover, heterogeneity and batch-to-batch variability are known to strongly influence their therapeutic efficacy [165].

15. Concluding Remarks and Future Perspectives

Over the past decade, an increasing number of reports has indicated that plasma membrane-derived MV are a distinct vesicle population with some common but also several diverging features compared with the smaller Exo. While most researchers have focused on the analysis of Exo, MV offer several advantages as diagnostic and therapeutic tools. In particular, their isolation is easier and less time-consuming and does not necessarily require ultracentrifugation with its associated problems of vesicle aggregation, damage and loss, and instrument availability. Additionally, protocols are available for their rapid and thorough characterization by standard flow cytometry, a technique that is already well-established in routine clinical diagnostics. Interesting findings also include the possibility for delivery of larger amounts of drugs or distinct classes of biomolecules (e.g., mRNA) by MV compared to Exo, as well as more successful targeting of MV cargo to the nuclear or cytosolic compartment, aspects that surely require further exploration.

It has become clear that MV have a multifaceted influence on cancer therapy, as summarized in Figure 3. They can not only serve as innovative tools for targeted drug delivery but should also be considered as important therapeutic targets when developing novel treatment strategies. Therefore, it will be highly advantageous to further elucidate the molecular mechanisms underlying MV formation and secretion in order to learn how MV biogenesis, especially in cancer cells, can be specifically inhibited or modulated therapeutically. However, at present, the lack of standardization, multicenter studies, and technical challenges, such as storage, production, quality control, and targeted delivery, still hamper the use of MV as diagnostic and therapeutic tools in cancer and must be overcome for them to be exploitable in the clinic.

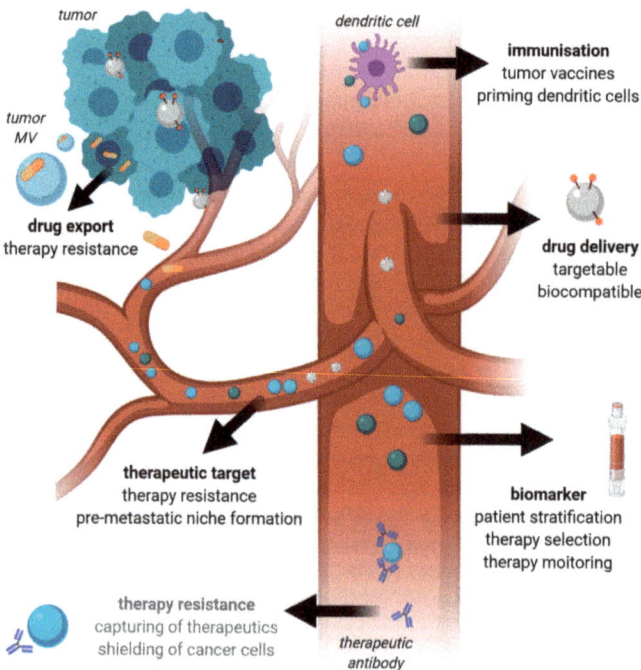

Figure 3. MV in cancer therapy. The figure summarizes the roles of MV in cancer therapy. Once a tumor has gained access to the circulation, circulating tumor MV in blood can be used as biomarkers in liquid biopsies. Moreover, they can mediate therapy resistance by capturing or exporting the administered anti-cancer drugs. Due to their role in therapy resistance and tumor microenvironment crosstalk resulting in pre-metastatic niche formation, they should be regarded as a novel therapeutic target. However, MV can also have a beneficial role in cancer therapy as they represent promising novel drug delivery systems with the benefits of high biocompatibility as well as opportunities for specific targeting and crossing of biological barriers. Vesicular functions, which have only been reported for endosomal-derived small exosomes (Exo) and lack experimental proof for MV, are highlighted in grey.

Author Contributions: Conceptualization, C.B., K.M., and A.B.; writing—original draft preparation K.M. and S.S. writing—review and editing, C.B., A.B., K.M., and S.S.; supervision, C.B., A.B., and K.M. All authors have read and agreed to the published version of the manuscript.

Funding: This work was funded by the Deutsche Forschungsgemeinschaft (DFG, German Research Foundation-project 424252458), Gerdes-Stiftung, Innovative Medizinische Forschung (IMF, project ME 1 2 19 14), and the German Ministry of Education and Research (BMBF) e:Med project MyPathSem (031L0024).

Acknowledgments: Suganja Sivaloganathan is a member of CiM-IMPRS, the joint graduate school of the Cells-in-Motion Interfaculty Centre, University of Münster, Germany, and the International Max Planck Research School-Molecular Biomedicine, Münster, Germany.

Conflicts of Interest: The authors declare no conflict of interest.

Abbreviations

Extracellular vesicle	EV
Tumor microenvironment	TME
Exosomes	Exo
Microvesicles	MV
Large oncosomes	LO
Nanoparticle tracking analysis	NTA
International society of extracellular vesicles	ISEV
ADP-ribosylation factor 6	ARF6
Phospholipase D	PLD
Myosin light chain kinase	MLCK
Endosomal sorting complex required for transport	ESCRT
Arrestin domain-containing protein 1	ARRDC1
Tumor susceptibility gene 101	TSG101
Membrane type 1-matrix metalloproteinase	MT1-MMP
Vesicular SNARE	v-SNARE
Vesicle-associated membrane protein 3	VAMP3
Extracellular matrix metalloproteinase inducer	EMMPRIN
Epidermal growth factor receptor	EGFR
Programmed cell death ligand 1	PD-L1
Cancer-associated fibroblasts	CAF
Platelet-poor plasma	PPP
Circulating tumor cells	CTCs
Chronic lymphocytic leukemia	CLL
Transcripts per million	TPM
Epithelial cell adhesion molecule	EpCAM
Asialoglycoprotein receptor 1	ASGPR1
Caveolin-1	CAV1
Tissue factor	TF
P-glycoprotein	MDR1
Multidrug resistance-associated protein 1	MRP1
Severe combined immunodeficient	SCID
Major histocompatibility complex	MHC
Vascular endothelial growth factor	VEGF
Vascular endothelial growth factor receptor	VEGFR
Transcripts per million	TPM

References

1. Hanahan, D.; Weinberg, R.A. Hallmarks of Cancer: The Next Generation. *Cell* **2011**, *144*, 646–674. [CrossRef] [PubMed]
2. Colombo, M.; Raposo, G.; Théry, C. Biogenesis, Secretion, and Intercellular Interactions of Exosomes and Other Extracellular Vesicles. *Annu. Rev. Cell Dev. Biol.* **2014**, *30*, 255–289. [CrossRef] [PubMed]

3. Yáñez-Mó, M.; Siljander, P.R.-M.; Andreu, Z.; Bedina Zavec, A.; Borràs, F.E.; Buzas, E.I.; Buzas, K.; Casal, E.; Cappello, F.; Carvalho, J.; et al. Biological properties of extracellular vesicles and their physiological functions. *J. Extracell. Vesicles* **2015**, *4*, 27066. [CrossRef] [PubMed]
4. Minciacchi, V.R.; Freeman, M.R.; Di Vizio, D. Extracellular Vesicles in Cancer: Exosomes, Microvesicles and the Emerging Role of Large Oncosomes. *Semin. Cell Dev. Biol.* **2015**, *40*, 41–51. [CrossRef] [PubMed]
5. Lee, S.-S.; Won, J.-H.; Lim, G.J.; Han, J.; Lee, J.Y.; Cho, K.-O.; Bae, Y.-K. A novel population of extracellular vesicles smaller than exosomes promotes cell proliferation. *Cell Commun. Signal.* **2019**, *17*, 95. [CrossRef]
6. Mezouar, S.; Mege, D.; Darbousset, R.; Farge, D.; Debourdeau, P.; Dignat-George, F.; Panicot-Dubois, L.; Dubois, C. Involvement of platelet-derived microparticles in tumor progression and thrombosis. *Semin. Oncol.* **2014**, *41*, 346–358. [CrossRef]
7. Théry, C.; Witwer, K.W.; Aikawa, E.; Alcaraz, M.J.; Anderson, J.D.; Andriantsitohaina, R.; Antoniou, A.; Arab, T.; Archer, F.; Atkin-Smith, G.K.; et al. Minimal information for studies of extracellular vesicles 2018 (MISEV2018): A position statement of the International Society for Extracellular Vesicles and update of the MISEV2014 guidelines. *J. Extracell. Vesicles* **2018**, *7*, 1535750. [CrossRef]
8. Mateescu, B.; Kowal, E.J.K.; van Balkom, B.W.M.; Bartel, S.; Bhattacharyya, S.N.; Buzás, E.I.; Buck, A.H.; de Candia, P.; Chow, F.W.N.; Das, S.; et al. Obstacles and opportunities in the functional analysis of extracellular vesicle RNA—An ISEV position paper. *J. Extracell. Vesicles* **2017**, *6*, 1286095. [CrossRef] [PubMed]
9. Kowal, J.; Arras, G.; Colombo, M.; Jouve, M.; Morath, J.P.; Primdal-Bengtson, B.; Dingli, F.; Loew, D.; Tkach, M.; Théry, C. Proteomic comparison defines novel markers to characterize heterogeneous populations of extracellular vesicle subtypes. *Proc. Natl. Acad. Sci. USA* **2016**, *113*, E968–E977. [CrossRef]
10. Crescitelli, R.; Lässer, C.; Szabó, T.G.; Kittel, A.; Eldh, M.; Dianzani, I.; Buzás, E.I.; Lötvall, J. Distinct RNA profiles in subpopulations of extracellular vesicles: Apoptotic bodies, microvesicles and exosomes. *J. Extracell. Vesicles* **2013**, *2*, 20677. [CrossRef] [PubMed]
11. Menck, K.; Scharf, C.; Bleckmann, A.; Dyck, L.; Rost, U.; Wenzel, D.; Dhople, V.M.; Siam, L.; Pukrop, T.; Binder, C.; et al. Tumor-derived microvesicles mediate human breast cancer invasion through differentially glycosylated EMMPRIN. *J. Mol. Cell Biol.* **2015**, *7*, 143–153. [CrossRef] [PubMed]
12. Linares, R.; Tan, S.; Gounou, C.; Arraud, N.; Brisson, A.R. High-speed centrifugation induces aggregation of extracellular vesicles. *J. Extracell. Vesicles* **2015**, *4*. [CrossRef] [PubMed]
13. Nordin, J.Z.; Lee, Y.; Vader, P.; Mäger, I.; Johansson, H.J.; Heusermann, W.; Wiklander, O.P.B.; Hällbrink, M.; Seow, Y.; Bultema, J.J.; et al. Ultrafiltration with size-exclusion liquid chromatography for high yield isolation of extracellular vesicles preserving intact biophysical and functional properties. *Nanomed. Nanotechnol. Biol. Med.* **2015**, *11*, 879–883. [CrossRef] [PubMed]
14. Mol, E.A.; Goumans, M.-J.; Doevendans, P.A.; Sluijter, J.P.G.; Vader, P. Higher functionality of extracellular vesicles isolated using size-exclusion chromatography compared to ultracentrifugation. *Nanomed. Nanotechnol. Biol. Med.* **2017**, *13*, 2061–2065. [CrossRef] [PubMed]
15. Bobrie, A.; Colombo, M.; Krumeich, S.; Raposo, G.; Théry, C. Diverse subpopulations of vesicles secreted by different intracellular mechanisms are present in exosome preparations obtained by differential ultracentrifugation. *J. Extracell. Vesicles* **2012**, *1*. [CrossRef]
16. Gallart-Palau, X.; Serra, A.; Wong, A.S.W.; Sandin, S.; Lai, M.K.P.; Chen, C.P.; Kon, O.L.; Sze, S.K. Extracellular vesicles are rapidly purified from human plasma by PRotein Organic Solvent PRecipitation (PROSPR). *Sci. Rep.* **2015**, *5*. [CrossRef]
17. Ko, J.; Carpenter, E.; Issadore, D. Detection and isolation of circulating exosomes and microvesicles for cancer monitoring and diagnostics using micro-/nano-based devices. *Analyst* **2016**, *141*, 450–460. [CrossRef]
18. Vestad, B.; Llorente, A.; Neurauter, A.; Phuyal, S.; Kierulf, B.; Kierulf, P.; Skotland, T.; Sandvig, K.; Haug, K.B.F.; Øvstebø, R. Size and concentration analyses of extracellular vesicles by nanoparticle tracking analysis: A variation study. *J. Extracell. Vesicles* **2017**, *6*, 1344087. [CrossRef]
19. Gardiner, C.; Vizio, D.D.; Sahoo, S.; Théry, C.; Witwer, K.W.; Wauben, M.; Hill, A.F. Techniques used for the isolation and characterization of extracellular vesicles: Results of a worldwide survey. *J. Extracell. Vesicles* **2016**, *5*, 32945. [CrossRef]
20. EV-TRACK Consortium; Van Deun, J.; Mestdagh, P.; Agostinis, P.; Akay, Ö.; Anand, S.; Anckaert, J.; Martinez, Z.A.; Baetens, T.; Beghein, E.; et al. EV-TRACK: Transparent reporting and centralizing knowledge in extracellular vesicle research. *Nat. Methods* **2017**, *14*, 228–232. [CrossRef]

21. Taylor, J.; Bebawy, M. Proteins Regulating Microvesicle Biogenesis and Multidrug Resistance in Cancer. *Proteomics* **2019**, *19*, 1800165. [CrossRef] [PubMed]
22. Battistelli, M.; Falcieri, E. Apoptotic Bodies: Particular Extracellular Vesicles Involved in Intercellular Communication. *Biology* **2020**, *9*, 21. [CrossRef] [PubMed]
23. Birge, R.B.; Boeltz, S.; Kumar, S.; Carlson, J.; Wanderley, J.; Calianese, D.; Barcinski, M.; Brekken, R.A.; Huang, X.; Hutchins, J.T.; et al. Phosphatidylserine is a global immunosuppressive signal in efferocytosis, infectious disease, and cancer. *Cell Death Differ.* **2016**, *23*, 962–978. [CrossRef] [PubMed]
24. van Niel, G.; D'Angelo, G.; Raposo, G. Shedding light on the cell biology of extracellular vesicles. *Nat. Rev. Mol. Cell Biol.* **2018**, *19*, 213–228. [CrossRef]
25. Sedgwick, A.E.; D'Souza-Schorey, C. The biology of extracellular microvesicles. *Traffic* **2018**, *19*, 319–327. [CrossRef]
26. Menck, K.; Sönmezer, C.; Worst, T.S.; Schulz, M.; Dihazi, G.H.; Streit, F.; Erdmann, G.; Kling, S.; Boutros, M.; Binder, C.; et al. Neutral sphingomyelinases control extracellular vesicles budding from the plasma membrane. *J. Extracell. Vesicles* **2017**, *6*, 1378056. [CrossRef]
27. Muralidharan-Chari, V.; Clancy, J.; Plou, C.; Romao, M.; Chavrier, P.; Raposo, G.; D'Souza-Schorey, C. ARF6-Regulated Shedding of Tumor Cell-Derived Plasma Membrane Microvesicles. *Curr. Biol.* **2009**, *19*, 1875–1885. [CrossRef]
28. Li, B.; Antonyak, M.A.; Zhang, J.; Cerione, R.A. RhoA triggers a specific signaling pathway that generates transforming microvesicles in cancer cells. *Oncogene* **2012**, *31*, 4740–4749. [CrossRef]
29. Colombo, M.; Moita, C.; van Niel, G.; Kowal, J.; Vigneron, J.; Benaroch, P.; Manel, N.; Moita, L.F.; Théry, C.; Raposo, G. Analysis of ESCRT functions in exosome biogenesis, composition and secretion highlights the heterogeneity of extracellular vesicles. *J. Cell Sci.* **2013**, *126*, 5553–5565. [CrossRef]
30. Nabhan, J.F.; Hu, R.; Oh, R.S.; Cohen, S.N.; Lu, Q. Formation and release of arrestin domain-containing protein 1-mediated microvesicles (ARMMs) at plasma membrane by recruitment of TSG101 protein. *Proc. Natl. Acad. Sci. USA* **2012**, *109*, 4146–4151. [CrossRef]
31. Hoshino, A.; Costa-Silva, B.; Shen, T.-L.; Rodrigues, G.; Hashimoto, A.; Tesic Mark, M.; Molina, H.; Kohsaka, S.; Di Giannatale, A.; Ceder, S.; et al. Tumour exosome integrins determine organotropic metastasis. *Nature* **2015**, *527*, 329–335. [CrossRef] [PubMed]
32. Nolte-'t Hoen, E.N.M.; Buschow, S.I.; Anderton, S.M.; Stoorvogel, W.; Wauben, M.H.M. Activated T cells recruit exosomes secreted by dendritic cells via LFA-1. *Blood* **2009**, *113*, 1977–1981. [CrossRef] [PubMed]
33. Cocucci, E.; Racchetti, G.; Meldolesi, J. Shedding microvesicles: Artefacts no more. *Trends Cell Biol.* **2009**, *19*, 43–51. [CrossRef] [PubMed]
34. Haraszti, R.A.; Didiot, M.-C.; Sapp, E.; Leszyk, J.; Shaffer, S.A.; Rockwell, H.E.; Gao, F.; Narain, N.R.; DiFiglia, M.; Kiebish, M.A.; et al. High-resolution proteomic and lipidomic analysis of exosomes and microvesicles from different cell sources. *J. Extracell. Vesicles* **2016**, *5*, 32570. [CrossRef]
35. Wang, T.; Gilkes, D.M.; Takano, N.; Xiang, L.; Luo, W.; Bishop, C.J.; Chaturvedi, P.; Green, J.J.; Semenza, G.L. Hypoxia-inducible factors and RAB22A mediate formation of microvesicles that stimulate breast cancer invasion and metastasis. *Proc. Natl. Acad. Sci. USA* **2014**, *111*, E3234–E3242. [CrossRef]
36. Maacha, S.; Bhat, A.A.; Jimenez, L.; Raza, A.; Haris, M.; Uddin, S.; Grivel, J.-C. Extracellular vesicles-mediated intercellular communication: Roles in the tumor microenvironment and anti-cancer drug resistance. *Mol. Cancer* **2019**, *18*, 55. [CrossRef]
37. Han, L.; Lam, E.W.-F.; Sun, Y. Extracellular vesicles in the tumor microenvironment: Old stories, but new tales. *Mol. Cancer* **2019**, *18*, 59. [CrossRef]
38. Xu, R.; Greening, D.W.; Zhu, H.-J.; Takahashi, N.; Simpson, R.J. Extracellular vesicle isolation and characterization: Toward clinical application. *J. Clin. Investig.* **2016**, *126*, 1152–1162. [CrossRef]
39. Arendt, B.K.; Walters, D.K.; Wu, X.; Tschumper, R.C.; Jelinek, D.F. Multiple myeloma cell-derived microvesicles are enriched in CD147 expression and enhance tumor cell proliferation. *Oncotarget* **2014**, *5*, 5686–5699. [CrossRef]
40. Riethdorf, S.; Reimers, N.; Assmann, V.; Kornfeld, J.-W.; Terracciano, L.; Sauter, G.; Pantel, K. High incidence of EMMPRIN expression in human tumors. *Int. J. Cancer* **2006**, *119*, 1800–1810. [CrossRef]
41. Al-Nedawi, K.; Meehan, B.; Micallef, J.; Lhotak, V.; May, L.; Guha, A.; Rak, J. Intercellular transfer of the oncogenic receptor EGFRvIII by microvesicles derived from tumour cells. *Nat. Cell Biol.* **2008**, *10*, 619–624. [CrossRef]

42. Menck, K.; Klemm, F.; Gross, J.C.; Pukrop, T.; Wenzel, D.; Binder, C. Induction and transport of Wnt 5a during macrophage-induced malignant invasion is mediated by two types of extracellular vesicles. *Oncotarget* **2013**, *4*, 2057–2066. [CrossRef] [PubMed]
43. Baj-Krzyworzeka, M.; Szatanek, R.; Węglarczyk, K.; Baran, J.; Zembala, M. Tumour-derived microvesicles modulate biological activity of human monocytes. *Immunol. Lett.* **2007**, *113*, 76–82. [CrossRef]
44. Lenart, M.; Rutkowska-Zapała, M.; Szatanek, R.; Węglarczyk, K.; Stec, M.; Bukowska-Strakova, K.; Gruca, A.; Czyż, J.; Siedlar, M. Alterations of TRIM21-mRNA expression during monocyte maturation. *Immunobiology* **2017**, *222*, 494–498. [CrossRef] [PubMed]
45. Baj-Krzyworzeka, M.; Mytar, B.; Szatanek, R.; Surmiak, M.; Węglarczyk, K.; Baran, J.; Siedlar, M. Colorectal cancer-derived microvesicles modulate differentiation of human monocytes to macrophages. *J. Transl. Med.* **2016**, *14*, 36. [CrossRef]
46. Timaner, M.; Kotsofruk, R.; Raviv, Z.; Magidey, K.; Shechter, D.; Kan, T.; Nevelsky, A.; Daniel, S.; de Vries, E.G.E.; Zhang, T.; et al. Microparticles from tumors exposed to radiation promote immune evasion in part by PD-L1. *Oncogene* **2020**, *39*, 187–203. [CrossRef] [PubMed]
47. Cui, J.; Li, Q.; Luo, M.; Zhong, Z.; Zhou, S.; Jiang, L.; Shen, N.; Geng, Z.; Cheng, H.; Meng, L.; et al. Leukemia cell-derived microvesicles induce T cell exhaustion via miRNA delivery. *OncoImmunology* **2018**, *7*, e1448330. [CrossRef]
48. Castellana, D.; Zobairi, F.; Martinez, M.C.; Panaro, M.A.; Mitolo, V.; Freyssinet, J.-M.; Kunzelmann, C. Membrane Microvesicles as Actors in the Establishment of a Favorable Prostatic Tumoral Niche: A Role for Activated Fibroblasts and CX3CL1-CX3CR1 Axis. *Cancer Res.* **2009**, *69*, 785–793. [CrossRef] [PubMed]
49. Jiang, E.; Xu, Z.; Wang, M.; Yan, T.; Huang, C.; Zhou, X.; Liu, Q.; Wang, L.; Chen, Y.; Wang, H.; et al. Tumoral microvesicle–activated glycometabolic reprogramming in fibroblasts promotes the progression of oral squamous cell carcinoma. *FASEB J.* **2019**, *33*, 5690–5703. [CrossRef] [PubMed]
50. Matrix Stiffness Regulates Microvesicle-Induced Fibroblast Activation|American Journal of Physiology-Cell Physiology. Available online: https://journals.physiology.org/doi/abs/10.1152/ajpcell.00418.2018 (accessed on 26 June 2020).
51. Kawamoto, T.; Ohga, N.; Akiyama, K.; Hirata, N.; Kitahara, S.; Maishi, N.; Osawa, T.; Yamamoto, K.; Kondoh, M.; Shindoh, M.; et al. Tumor-Derived Microvesicles Induce Proangiogenic Phenotype in Endothelial Cells via Endocytosis. *PLoS ONE* **2012**, *7*, e34045. [CrossRef]
52. Giusti, I.; Delle Monache, S.; Di Francesco, M.; Sanità, P.; D'Ascenzo, S.; Gravina, G.L.; Festuccia, C.; Dolo, V. From glioblastoma to endothelial cells through extracellular vesicles: Messages for angiogenesis. *Tumour Biol. J. Int. Soc. Oncodev. Biol. Med.* **2016**, *37*, 12743–12753. [CrossRef]
53. Feng, Q.; Zhang, C.; Lum, D.; Druso, J.E.; Blank, B.; Wilson, K.F.; Welm, A.; Antonyak, M.A.; Cerione, R.A. A class of extracellular vesicles from breast cancer cells activates VEGF receptors and tumour angiogenesis. *Nat. Commun.* **2017**, *8*, 14450. [CrossRef] [PubMed]
54. Liu, Y.; Zhu, X.; Zeng, C.; Wu, P.; Wang, H.; Chen, Z.; Li, Q. Microvesicles secreted from human multiple myeloma cells promote angiogenesis. *Acta Pharmacol. Sin.* **2014**, *35*, 230–238. [CrossRef] [PubMed]
55. Pfeiler, S.; Thakur, M.; Grünauer, P.; Megens, R.T.A.; Joshi, U.; Coletti, R.; Samara, V.; Müller-Stoy, G.; Ishikawa-Ankerhold, H.; Stark, K.; et al. CD36-triggered cell invasion and persistent tissue colonization by tumor microvesicles during metastasis. *FASEB J.* **2019**, *33*, 1860–1872. [CrossRef] [PubMed]
56. Lima, L.G.; Chammas, R.; Monteiro, R.Q.; Moreira, M.E.C.; Barcinski, M.A. Tumor-derived microvesicles modulate the establishment of metastatic melanoma in a phosphatidylserine-dependent manner. *Cancer Lett.* **2009**, *283*, 168–175. [CrossRef]
57. O'Dea, K.P.; Tan, Y.Y.; Shah, S.; Patel, B.V.; Tatham, K.C.; Wilson, M.R.; Soni, S.; Takata, M. Monocytes mediate homing of circulating microvesicles to the pulmonary vasculature during low-grade systemic inflammation. *J. Extracell. Vesicles* **2020**, *9*, 1706708. [CrossRef]
58. Xiao, H.; Wong, D.T.W. Proteomic analysis of microvesicles in human saliva by gel electrophoresis with liquid chromatography-mass spectrometry. *Anal. Chim. Acta* **2012**, *723*, 61–67. [CrossRef]
59. Viñuela-Berni, V.; Doníz-Padilla, L.; Figueroa-Vega, N.; Portillo-Salazar, H.; Abud-Mendoza, C.; Baranda, L.; González-Amaro, R. Proportions of several types of plasma and urine microparticles are increased in patients with rheumatoid arthritis with active disease. *Clin. Exp. Immunol.* **2015**, *180*, 442–451. [CrossRef]

60. Verderio, C.; Muzio, L.; Turola, E.; Bergami, A.; Novellino, L.; Ruffini, F.; Riganti, L.; Corradini, I.; Francolini, M.; Garzetti, L.; et al. Myeloid microvesicles are a marker and therapeutic target for neuroinflammation. *Ann. Neurol.* **2012**, *72*, 610–624. [CrossRef]
61. Zonneveld, M.I.; Brisson, A.R.; van Herwijnen, M.J.C.; Tan, S.; van de Lest, C.H.A.; Redegeld, F.A.; Garssen, J.; Wauben, M.H.M.; Hoen, E.N.M.N.-'t. Recovery of extracellular vesicles from human breast milk is influenced by sample collection and vesicle isolation procedures. *J. Extracell. Vesicles* **2014**, *3*, 24215. [CrossRef]
62. Höög, J.L.; Lötvall, J. Diversity of extracellular vesicles in human ejaculates revealed by cryo-electron microscopy. *J. Extracell. Vesicles* **2015**, *4*, 28680. [CrossRef] [PubMed]
63. György, B.; Módos, K.; Pállinger, É.; Pálóczi, K.; Pásztói, M.; Misják, P.; Deli, M.A.; Sipos, Á.; Szalai, A.; Voszka, I.; et al. Detection and isolation of cell-derived microparticles are compromised by protein complexes resulting from shared biophysical parameters. *Blood* **2011**, *117*, e39–e48. [CrossRef] [PubMed]
64. Lyberg, T.; Nakstad, B.; Hetland, O.; Boye, N.P. Procoagulant (thromboplastin) activity in human bronchoalveolar lavage fluids is derived from alveolar macrophages. *Eur. Respir. J.* **1990**, *3*, 61–67. [PubMed]
65. Wolf, P. The nature and significance of platelet products in human plasma. *Br. J. Haematol.* **1967**, *13*, 269–288. [CrossRef]
66. Jayachandran, M.; Miller, V.M.; Heit, J.A.; Owen, W.G. Methodology for Isolation, Identification and Characterization of Microvesicles in Peripheral Blood. *J. Immunol. Methods* **2012**, *375*, 207–214. [CrossRef] [PubMed]
67. Lacroix, R.; Judicone, C.; Poncelet, P.; Robert, S.; Arnaud, L.; Sampol, J.; Dignat-George, F. Impact of pre-analytical parameters on the measurement of circulating microparticles: Towards standardization of protocol. *J. Thromb. Haemost.* **2012**, *10*, 437–446. [CrossRef]
68. Jamaly, S.; Ramberg, C.; Olsen, R.; Latysheva, N.; Webster, P.; Sovershaev, T.; Brækkan, S.K.; Hansen, J.-B. Impact of preanalytical conditions on plasma concentration and size distribution of extracellular vesicles using Nanoparticle Tracking Analysis. *Sci. Rep.* **2018**, *8*, 17216. [CrossRef]
69. Menck, K.; Bleckmann, A.; Wachter, A.; Hennies, B.; Ries, L.; Schulz, M.; Balkenhol, M.; Pukrop, T.; Schatlo, B.; Rost, U.; et al. Characterisation of tumour-derived microvesicles in cancer patients' blood and correlation with clinical outcome. *J. Extracell. Vesicles* **2017**, *6*. [CrossRef]
70. Belov, L.; Hallal, S.; Matic, K.; Zhou, J.; Wissmueller, S.; Ahmed, N.; Tanjil, S.; Mulligan, S.P.; Best, O.G.; Simpson, R.J.; et al. Surface Profiling of Extracellular Vesicles from Plasma or Ascites Fluid Using DotScan Antibody Microarrays. *Methods Mol. Biol. Clifton* **2017**, *1619*, 263–301. [CrossRef]
71. Wisgrill, L.; Lamm, C.; Hartmann, J.; Preißing, F.; Dragosits, K.; Bee, A.; Hell, L.; Thaler, J.; Ay, C.; Pabinger, I.; et al. Peripheral blood microvesicles secretion is influenced by storage time, temperature, and anticoagulants. *Cytometry A* **2016**, *89*, 663–672. [CrossRef]
72. Yuana, Y.; Böing, A.N.; Grootemaat, A.E.; van der Pol, E.; Hau, C.M.; Cizmar, P.; Buhr, E.; Sturk, A.; Nieuwland, R. Handling and storage of human body fluids for analysis of extracellular vesicles. *J. Extracell. Vesicles* **2015**, *4*, 29260. [CrossRef]
73. Brennan, K.; Martin, K.; FitzGerald, S.P.; O'Sullivan, J.; Wu, Y.; Blanco, A.; Richardson, C.; Mc Gee, M.M. A comparison of methods for the isolation and separation of extracellular vesicles from protein and lipid particles in human serum. *Sci. Rep.* **2020**, *10*, 1039. [CrossRef] [PubMed]
74. Mørk, M.; Handberg, A.; Pedersen, S.; Jørgensen, M.M.; Bæk, R.; Nielsen, M.K.; Kristensen, S.R. Prospects and limitations of antibody-mediated clearing of lipoproteins from blood plasma prior to nanoparticle tracking analysis of extracellular vesicles. *J. Extracell. Vesicles* **2017**, *6*, 1308779. [CrossRef] [PubMed]
75. van der Pol, E.; Sturk, A.; van Leeuwen, T.; Nieuwland, R.; Coumans, F. Standardization of extracellular vesicle measurements by flow cytometry through vesicle diameter approximation. *J. Thromb. Haemost.* **2018**, *16*, 1236–1245. [CrossRef] [PubMed]
76. Menck, K.; Bleckmann, A.; Schulz, M.; Ries, L.; Binder, C. Isolation and Characterization of Microvesicles from Peripheral Blood. *J. Vis. Exp. JoVE* **2017**. [CrossRef]
77. Lukacs-Kornek, V.; Julich-Haertel, H.; Urban, S.K.; Kornek, M. Multi-Surface Antigen Staining of Larger Extracellular Vesicles. *Methods Mol. Biol. Clifton* **2017**, *1660*, 201–208. [CrossRef]
78. Chandler, W.L. Measurement of microvesicle levels in human blood using flow cytometry. *Cytometry B Clin. Cytom.* **2016**, *90*, 326–336. [CrossRef]
79. Erdbrügger, U.; Lannigan, J. Analytical challenges of extracellular vesicle detection: A comparison of different techniques. *Cytometry A* **2016**, *89*, 123–134. [CrossRef]

80. Xin, X.; Zhang, P.; Fu, X.; Mao, X.; Meng, F.; Tian, M.; Zhu, X.; Sun, H.; Meng, L.; Zhou, J. Saline is a more appropriate solution for microvesicles for flow cytometric analyses. *Oncotarget* **2017**, *8*, 34576–34585. [CrossRef]
81. Belov, L.; Matic, K.J.; Hallal, S.; Best, O.G.; Mulligan, S.P.; Christopherson, R.I. Extensive surface protein profiles of extracellular vesicles from cancer cells may provide diagnostic signatures from blood samples. *J. Extracell. Vesicles* **2016**, *5*. [CrossRef]
82. Witwer, K.W.; Buzás, E.I.; Bemis, L.T.; Bora, A.; Lässer, C.; Lötvall, J.; Hoen, E.N.N.-'t.; Piper, M.G.; Sivaraman, S.; Skog, J.; et al. Standardization of sample collection, isolation and analysis methods in extracellular vesicle research. *J. Extracell. Vesicles* **2013**, *2*, 20360. [CrossRef] [PubMed]
83. Clayton, A.; Boilard, E.; Buzas, E.I.; Cheng, L.; Falcón-Perez, J.M.; Gardiner, C.; Gustafson, D.; Gualerzi, A.; Hendrix, A.; Hoffman, A.; et al. Considerations towards a roadmap for collection, handling and storage of blood extracellular vesicles. *J. Extracell. Vesicles* **2019**, *8*, 1647027. [CrossRef] [PubMed]
84. Baran, J.; Baj-Krzyworzeka, M.; Weglarczyk, K.; Szatanek, R.; Zembala, M.; Barbasz, J.; Czupryna, A.; Szczepanik, A.; Zembala, M. Circulating tumour-derived microvesicles in plasma of gastric cancer patients. *Cancer Immunol. Immunother. CII* **2010**, *59*, 841–850. [CrossRef] [PubMed]
85. Fleitas, T.; Martínez-Sales, V.; Vila, V.; Reganon, E.; Mesado, D.; Martín, M.; Gómez-Codina, J.; Montalar, J.; Reynés, G. Circulating Endothelial Cells and Microparticles as Prognostic Markers in Advanced Non-Small Cell Lung Cancer. *PLoS ONE* **2012**, *7*. [CrossRef] [PubMed]
86. Tesselaar, M.E.T.; Romijn, F.P.H.T.M.; Linden, I.K.V.D.; Prins, F.A.; Bertina, R.M.; Osanto, S. Microparticle-associated tissue factor activity: A link between cancer and thrombosis? *J. Thromb. Haemost.* **2007**, *5*, 520–527. [CrossRef]
87. Galindo-Hernandez, O.; Villegas-Comonfort, S.; Candanedo, F.; González-Vázquez, M.-C.; Chavez-Ocaña, S.; Jimenez-Villanueva, X.; Sierra-Martinez, M.; Salazar, E.P. Elevated concentration of microvesicles isolated from peripheral blood in breast cancer patients. *Arch. Med. Res.* **2013**, *44*, 208–214. [CrossRef]
88. Zhao, L.; Bi, Y.; Kou, J.; Shi, J.; Piao, D. Phosphatidylserine exposing-platelets and microparticles promote procoagulant activity in colon cancer patients. *J. Exp. Clin. Cancer Res.* **2016**, *35*. [CrossRef]
89. Krishnan, S.R.; Luk, F.; Brown, R.D.; Suen, H.; Kwan, Y.; Bebawy, M. Isolation of Human CD138+ Microparticles from the Plasma of Patients with Multiple Myeloma. *Neoplasia* **2016**, *18*, 25–32. [CrossRef]
90. De Luca, L.; D'Arena, G.; Simeon, V.; Trino, S.; Laurenzana, I.; Caivano, A.; La Rocca, F.; Villani, O.; Mansueto, G.; Deaglio, S.; et al. Characterization and prognostic relevance of circulating microvesicles in chronic lymphocytic leukemia. *Leuk. Lymphoma* **2017**, *58*, 1424–1432. [CrossRef]
91. Caivano, A.; Laurenzana, I.; De Luca, L.; La Rocca, F.; Simeon, V.; Trino, S.; D'Auria, F.; Traficante, A.; Maietti, M.; Izzo, T.; et al. High serum levels of extracellular vesicles expressing malignancy-related markers are released in patients with various types of hematological neoplastic disorders. *Tumour Biol. J. Int. Soc. Oncodev. Biol. Med.* **2015**, *36*, 9739–9752. [CrossRef]
92. Wang, W.; Li, H.; Zhou, Y.; Jie, S. Peripheral blood microvesicles are potential biomarkers for hepatocellular carcinoma. *Cancer Biomark. Sect. Dis. Markers* **2013**, *13*, 351–357. [CrossRef]
93. Ender, F.; Freund, A.; Quecke, T.; Steidel, C.; Zamzow, P.; von Bubnoff, N.; Gieseler, F. Tissue factor activity on microvesicles from cancer patients. *J. Cancer Res. Clin. Oncol.* **2020**, *146*, 467–475. [CrossRef] [PubMed]
94. Fraser, K.; Jo, A.; Giedt, J.; Vinegoni, C.; Yang, K.S.; Peruzzi, P.; Chiocca, E.A.; Breakefield, X.O.; Lee, H.; Weissleder, R. Characterization of single microvesicles in plasma from glioblastoma patients. *Neuro Oncol.* **2019**, *21*, 606–615. [CrossRef] [PubMed]
95. Mege, D.; Panicot-Dubois, L.; Ouaissi, M.; Robert, S.; Sielezneff, I.; Sastre, B.; Dignat-George, F.; Dubois, C. The origin and concentration of circulating microparticles differ according to cancer type and evolution: A prospective single-center study. *Int. J. Cancer* **2016**, *138*, 939–948. [CrossRef] [PubMed]
96. Alique, M.; Ruíz-Torres, M.P.; Bodega, G.; Noci, M.V.; Troyano, N.; Bohórquez, L.; Luna, C.; Luque, R.; Carmona, A.; Carracedo, J.; et al. Microvesicles from the plasma of elderly subjects and from senescent endothelial cells promote vascular calcification. *Aging* **2017**, *9*, 778–789. [CrossRef]
97. Evans, S.M.; Putt, M.; Yang, X.-Y.; Lustig, R.A.; Martinez-Lage, M.; Williams, D.; Desai, A.; Wolf, R.; Brem, S.; Koch, C.J. Initial evidence that blood-borne microvesicles are biomarkers for recurrence and survival in newly diagnosed glioblastoma patients. *J. Neurooncol.* **2016**, *127*, 391–400. [CrossRef]

98. Coumans, F.a.W.; Doggen, C.J.M.; Attard, G.; de Bono, J.S.; Terstappen, L.W.M.M. All circulating EpCAM+CK+CD45- objects predict overall survival in castration-resistant prostate cancer. *Ann. Oncol.* **2010**, *21*, 1851–1857. [CrossRef]
99. Nanou, A.; Coumans, F.A.W.; van Dalum, G.; Zeune, L.L.; Dolling, D.; Onstenk, W.; Crespo, M.; Fontes, M.S.; Rescigno, P.; Fowler, G.; et al. Circulating tumor cells, tumor-derived extracellular vesicles and plasma cytokeratins in castration-resistant prostate cancer patients. *Oncotarget* **2018**, *9*, 19283–19293. [CrossRef]
100. Klein, C.A. Selection and adaptation during metastatic cancer progression. *Nature* **2013**, *501*, 365–372. [CrossRef]
101. García-Romero, N.; Carrión-Navarro, J.; Esteban-Rubio, S.; Lázaro-Ibáñez, E.; Peris-Celda, M.; Alonso, M.M.; Guzmán-De-Villoria, J.; Fernández-Carballal, C.; de Mendivil, A.O.; García-Duque, S.; et al. DNA sequences within glioma-derived extracellular vesicles can cross the intact blood-brain barrier and be detected in peripheral blood of patients. *Oncotarget* **2016**, *8*, 1416–1428. [CrossRef]
102. Ramón, Y.; Cajal, S.; Sesé, M.; Capdevila, C.; Aasen, T.; De Mattos-Arruda, L.; Diaz-Cano, S.J.; Hernández-Losa, J.; Castellví, J. Clinical implications of intratumor heterogeneity: Challenges and opportunities. *J. Mol. Med.* **2020**, *98*, 161–177. [CrossRef] [PubMed]
103. Ellsworth, R.E.; Blackburn, H.L.; Shriver, C.D.; Soon-Shiong, P.; Ellsworth, D.L. Molecular heterogeneity in breast cancer: State of the science and implications for patient care. *Semin. Cell Dev. Biol.* **2017**, *64*, 65–72. [CrossRef] [PubMed]
104. Ng, C.K.Y.; Bidard, F.-C.; Piscuoglio, S.; Geyer, F.C.; Lim, R.S.; de Bruijn, I.; Shen, R.; Pareja, F.; Berman, S.H.; Wang, L.; et al. Genetic Heterogeneity in Therapy-Naïve Synchronous Primary Breast Cancers and Their Metastases. *Clin. Cancer Res. Off. J. Am. Assoc. Cancer Res.* **2017**, *23*, 4402–4415. [CrossRef] [PubMed]
105. Skog, J.; Wurdinger, T.; van Rijn, S.; Meijer, D.; Gainche, L.; Sena-Esteves, M.; Curry, W.T.; Carter, R.S.; Krichevsky, A.M.; Breakefield, X.O. Glioblastoma microvesicles transport RNA and protein that promote tumor growth and provide diagnostic biomarkers. *Nat. Cell Biol.* **2008**, *10*, 1470–1476. [CrossRef]
106. Wei, Z.; Batagov, A.O.; Schinelli, S.; Wang, J.; Wang, Y.; El Fatimy, R.; Rabinovsky, R.; Balaj, L.; Chen, C.C.; Hochberg, F.; et al. Coding and noncoding landscape of extracellular RNA released by human glioma stem cells. *Nat. Commun.* **2017**, *8*. [CrossRef] [PubMed]
107. Zhu, X.; You, Y.; Li, Q.; Zeng, C.; Fu, F.; Guo, A.; Zhang, H.; Zou, P.; Zhong, Z.; Wang, H.; et al. BCR-ABL1-positive microvesicles transform normal hematopoietic transplants through genomic instability: Implications for donor cell leukemia. *Leukemia* **2014**, *28*, 1666–1675. [CrossRef]
108. Milani, G.; Lana, T.; Bresolin, S.; Aveic, S.; Pastò, A.; Frasson, C.; Kronnie, G. te Expression Profiling of Circulating Microvesicles Reveals Intercellular Transmission of Oncogenic Pathways. *Mol. Cancer Res.* **2017**, *15*, 683–695. [CrossRef]
109. Krug, A.K.; Enderle, D.; Karlovich, C.; Priewasser, T.; Bentink, S.; Spiel, A.; Brinkmann, K.; Emenegger, J.; Grimm, D.G.; Castellanos-Rizaldos, E.; et al. Improved EGFR mutation detection using combined exosomal RNA and circulating tumor DNA in NSCLC patient plasma. *Ann. Oncol.* **2018**, *29*, 700–706. [CrossRef]
110. Akers, J.C.; Ramakrishnan, V.; Kim, R.; Phillips, S.; Kaimal, V.; Mao, Y.; Hua, W.; Yang, I.; Fu, C.-C.; Nolan, J.; et al. miRNA contents of cerebrospinal fluid extracellular vesicles in glioblastoma patients. *J. Neurooncol.* **2015**, *123*, 205–216. [CrossRef]
111. Chen, M.; Xu, R.; Rai, A.; Suwakulsiri, W.; Izumikawa, K.; Ishikawa, H.; Greening, D.W.; Takahashi, N.; Simpson, R.J. Distinct shed microvesicle and exosome microRNA signatures reveal diagnostic markers for colorectal cancer. *PLoS ONE* **2019**, *14*. [CrossRef]
112. Chevillet, J.R.; Kang, Q.; Ruf, I.K.; Briggs, H.A.; Vojtech, L.N.; Hughes, S.M.; Cheng, H.H.; Arroyo, J.D.; Meredith, E.K.; Gallichotte, E.N.; et al. Quantitative and stoichiometric analysis of the microRNA content of exosomes. *Proc. Natl. Acad. Sci. USA* **2014**, *111*, 14888–14893. [CrossRef] [PubMed]
113. Rosa-Fernandes, L.; Rocha, V.B.; Carregari, V.C.; Urbani, A.; Palmisano, G. A Perspective on Extracellular Vesicles Proteomics. *Front. Chem.* **2017**, *5*. [CrossRef]
114. Whiteaker, J.R.; Lin, C.; Kennedy, J.; Hou, L.; Trute, M.; Sokal, I.; Yan, P.; Schoenherr, R.M.; Zhao, L.; Voytovich, U.J.; et al. A targeted proteomics-based pipeline for verification of biomarkers in plasma. *Nat. Biotechnol.* **2011**, *29*, 625–634. [CrossRef]
115. Fujita, K.; Kume, H.; Matsuzaki, K.; Kawashima, A.; Ujike, T.; Nagahara, A.; Uemura, M.; Miyagawa, Y.; Tomonaga, T.; Nonomura, N. Proteomic analysis of urinary extracellular vesicles from high Gleason score prostate cancer. *Sci. Rep.* **2017**, *7*, 42961. [CrossRef]

116. Crompot, E.; Van Damme, M.; Duvillier, H.; Pieters, K.; Vermeesch, M.; Perez-Morga, D.; Meuleman, N.; Mineur, P.; Bron, D.; Lagneaux, L.; et al. Avoiding False Positive Antigen Detection by Flow Cytometry on Blood Cell Derived Microparticles: The Importance of an Appropriate Negative Control. *PLoS ONE* **2015**, *10*. [CrossRef]
117. Stec, M.; Baj-Krzyworzeka, M.; Baran, J.; Węglarczyk, K.; Zembala, M.; Barbasz, J.; Szczepanik, A.; Zembala, M. Isolation and characterization of circulating micro(nano)vesicles in the plasma of colorectal cancer patients and their interactions with tumor cells. *Oncol. Rep.* **2015**, *34*, 2768–2775. [CrossRef] [PubMed]
118. Julich-Haertel, H.; Urban, S.K.; Krawczyk, M.; Willms, A.; Jankowski, K.; Patkowski, W.; Kruk, B.; Krasnodębski, M.; Ligocka, J.; Schwab, R.; et al. Cancer-associated circulating large extracellular vesicles in cholangiocarcinoma and hepatocellular carcinoma. *J. Hepatol.* **2017**, *67*, 282–292. [CrossRef] [PubMed]
119. Willms, A.; Müller, C.; Julich, H.; Klein, N.; Schwab, R.; Güsgen, C.; Richardsen, I.; Schaaf, S.; Krawczyk, M.; Krawczyk, M.; et al. Tumour-associated circulating microparticles: A novel liquid biopsy tool for screening and therapy monitoring of colorectal carcinoma and other epithelial neoplasia. *Oncotarget* **2016**, *7*, 30867–30875. [CrossRef] [PubMed]
120. Morello, M.; Minciacchi, V.R.; de Candia, P.; Yang, J.; Posadas, E.; Kim, H.; Griffiths, D.; Bhowmick, N.; Chung, L.W.; Gandellini, P.; et al. Large oncosomes mediate intercellular transfer of functional microRNA. *Cell Cycle* **2013**, *12*, 3526–3536. [CrossRef]
121. Abbate, V.; Marcantoni, M.; Giuliante, F.; Vecchio, F.; Gatto, I.; Mele, C.; Saviano, A.; Arciuolo, D.; Gaetani, E.; Ferrari, M.; et al. HepPar1-Positive Circulating Microparticles Are Increased in Subjects with Hepatocellular Carcinoma and Predict Early Recurrence after Liver Resection. *Int. J. Mol. Sci.* **2017**, *18*, 1043. [CrossRef]
122. Jang, S.C.; Crescitelli, R.; Cvjetkovic, A.; Belgrano, V.; Olofsson Bagge, R.; Sundfeldt, K.; Ochiya, T.; Kalluri, R.; Lötvall, J. Mitochondrial protein enriched extracellular vesicles discovered in human melanoma tissues can be detected in patient plasma. *J. Extracell. Vesicles* **2019**, *8*. [CrossRef] [PubMed]
123. Crescitelli, R.; Lässer, C.; Jang, S.C.; Cvjetkovic, A.; Malmhäll, C.; Karimi, N.; Höög, J.L.; Johansson, I.; Fuchs, J.; Thorsell, A.; et al. Subpopulations of extracellular vesicles from human metastatic melanoma tissue identified by quantitative proteomics after optimized isolation. *J. Extracell. Vesicles* **2020**, *9*. [CrossRef]
124. Imjeti, N.S.; Menck, K.; Egea-Jimenez, A.L.; Lecointre, C.; Lembo, F.; Bouguenina, H.; Badache, A.; Ghossoub, R.; David, G.; Roche, S.; et al. Syntenin mediates SRC function in exosomal cell-to-cell communication. *Proc. Natl. Acad. Sci. USA* **2017**, *114*, 12495–12500. [CrossRef] [PubMed]
125. Amorim, M.; Fernandes, G.; Oliveira, P.; Martins-de-Souza, D.; Dias-Neto, E.; Nunes, D. The overexpression of a single oncogene (ERBB2/HER2) alters the proteomic landscape of extracellular vesicles. *Proteomics* **2014**, *14*, 1472–1479. [CrossRef] [PubMed]
126. Rontogianni, S.; Synadaki, E.; Li, B.; Liefaard, M.C.; Lips, E.H.; Wesseling, J.; Wu, W.; Altelaar, M. Proteomic profiling of extracellular vesicles allows for human breast cancer subtyping. *Commun. Biol.* **2019**, *2*. [CrossRef] [PubMed]
127. Ayers, L.; Nieuwland, R.; Kohler, M.; Kraenkel, N.; Ferry, B.; Leeson, P. Dynamic microvesicle release and clearance within the cardiovascular system: Triggers and mechanisms. *Clin. Sci. Lond. Engl. 1979* **2015**, *129*, 915–931. [CrossRef]
128. Kim, H.K.; Song, K.S.; Park, Y.S.; Kang, Y.H.; Lee, Y.J.; Lee, K.R.; Kim, H.K.; Ryu, K.W.; Bae, J.M.; Kim, S. Elevated levels of circulating platelet microparticles, VEGF, IL-6 and RANTES in patients with gastric cancer: Possible role of a metastasis predictor. *Eur. J. Cancer* **2003**, *39*, 184–191. [CrossRef]
129. Chen, I.-H.; Xue, L.; Hsu, C.-C.; Paez, J.S.P.; Pan, L.; Andaluz, H.; Wendt, M.K.; Iliuk, A.B.; Zhu, J.-K.; Tao, W.A. Phosphoproteins in extracellular vesicles as candidate markers for breast cancer. *Proc. Natl. Acad. Sci. USA* **2017**, *114*, 3175–3180. [CrossRef]
130. Gamperl, H.; Plattfaut, C.; Freund, A.; Quecke, T.; Theophil, F.; Gieseler, F. Extracellular vesicles from malignant effusions induce tumor cell migration: Inhibitory effect of LMWH tinzaparin. *Cell Biol. Int.* **2016**, *40*, 1050–1061. [CrossRef]
131. Zwicker, J.I.; Liebman, H.A.; Neuberg, D.; Lacroix, R.; Bauer, K.A.; Furie, B.C.; Furie, B. Tumor-Derived Tissue Factor-Bearing Microparticles are Associated with Venous Thromboembolic Events in Malignancy. *Clin. Cancer Res. Off. J. Am. Assoc. Cancer Res.* **2009**, *15*, 6830–6840. [CrossRef]
132. Tripisciano, C.; Weiss, R.; Eichhorn, T.; Spittler, A.; Heuser, T.; Fischer, M.B.; Weber, V. Different Potential of Extracellular Vesicles to Support Thrombin Generation: Contributions of Phosphatidylserine, Tissue Factor, and Cellular Origin. *Sci. Rep.* **2017**, *7*. [CrossRef] [PubMed]

133. Tang, K.; Zhang, Y.; Zhang, H.; Xu, P.; Liu, J.; Ma, J.; Lv, M.; Li, D.; Katirai, F.; Shen, G.-X.; et al. Delivery of chemotherapeutic drugs in tumour cell-derived microparticles. *Nat. Commun.* **2012**, *3*, 1282. [CrossRef] [PubMed]
134. König, L.; Kasimir-Bauer, S.; Bittner, A.-K.; Hoffmann, O.; Wagner, B.; Santos Manvailer, L.F.; Kimmig, R.; Horn, P.A.; Rebmann, V. Elevated levels of extracellular vesicles are associated with therapy failure and disease progression in breast cancer patients undergoing neoadjuvant chemotherapy. *Oncoimmunology* **2017**, *7*. [CrossRef] [PubMed]
135. García Garre, E.; Luengo Gil, G.; Montoro García, S.; Gonzalez Billalabeitia, E.; Zafra Poves, M.; García Martinez, E.; Roldán Schilling, V.; Navarro Manzano, E.; Ivars Rubio, A.; Lip, G.Y.H.; et al. Circulating small-sized endothelial microparticles as predictors of clinical outcome after chemotherapy for breast cancer: An exploratory analysis. *Breast Cancer Res. Treat.* **2018**, *169*, 83–92. [CrossRef]
136. Koch, C.J.; Lustig, R.A.; Yang, X.-Y.; Jenkins, W.T.; Wolf, R.L.; Martinez-Lage, M.; Desai, A.; Williams, D.; Evans, S.M. Microvesicles as a Biomarker for Tumor Progression versus Treatment Effect in Radiation/Temozolomide-Treated Glioblastoma Patients. *Transl. Oncol.* **2014**, *7*, 752–758. [CrossRef]
137. Bebawy, M.; Combes, V.; Lee, E.; Jaiswal, R.; Gong, J.; Bonhoure, A.; Grau, G.E.R. Membrane microparticles mediate transfer of P-glycoprotein to drug sensitive cancer cells. *Leukemia* **2009**, *23*, 1643–1649. [CrossRef]
138. Lu, J.F.; Luk, F.; Gong, J.; Jaiswal, R.; Grau, G.E.R.; Bebawy, M. Microparticles mediate MRP1 intercellular transfer and the re-templating of intrinsic resistance pathways. *Pharmacol. Res.* **2013**, *76*, 77–83. [CrossRef]
139. Jorfi, S.; Ansa-Addo, E.A.; Kholia, S.; Stratton, D.; Valley, S.; Lange, S.; Inal, J. Inhibition of microvesiculation sensitizes prostate cancer cells to chemotherapy and reduces docetaxel dose required to limit tumor growth in vivo. *Sci. Rep.* **2015**, *5*. [CrossRef]
140. Muralidharan-Chari, V.; Kohan, H.G.; Asimakopoulos, A.G.; Sudha, T.; Sell, S.; Kannan, K.; Boroujerdi, M.; Davis, P.J.; Mousa, S.A. Microvesicle removal of anticancer drugs contributes to drug resistance in human pancreatic cancer cells. *Oncotarget* **2016**, *7*, 50365–50379. [CrossRef]
141. Kosgodage, U.S.; Trindade, R.P.; Thompson, P.R.; Inal, J.M.; Lange, S. Chloramidine/Bisindolylmaleimide-I-Mediated Inhibition of Exosome and Microvesicle Release and Enhanced Efficacy of Cancer Chemotherapy. *Int. J. Mol. Sci.* **2017**, *18*, 1007. [CrossRef]
142. Aung, T.; Chapuy, B.; Vogel, D.; Wenzel, D.; Oppermann, M.; Lahmann, M.; Weinhage, T.; Menck, K.; Hupfeld, T.; Koch, R.; et al. Exosomal evasion of humoral immunotherapy in aggressive B-cell lymphoma modulated by ATP-binding cassette transporter A3. *Proc. Natl. Acad. Sci. USA* **2011**, *108*, 15336–15341. [CrossRef] [PubMed]
143. Ciravolo, V.; Huber, V.; Ghedini, G.C.; Venturelli, E.; Bianchi, F.; Campiglio, M.; Morelli, D.; Villa, A.; Della Mina, P.; Menard, S.; et al. Potential role of HER2-overexpressing exosomes in countering trastuzumab-based therapy. *J. Cell. Physiol.* **2012**, *227*, 658–667. [CrossRef] [PubMed]
144. Chen, G.; Huang, A.C.; Zhang, W.; Zhang, G.; Wu, M.; Xu, W.; Yu, Z.; Yang, J.; Wang, B.; Sun, H.; et al. Exosomal PD-L1 Contributes to Immunosuppression and is Associated with anti-PD-1 Response. *Nature* **2018**, *560*, 382–386. [CrossRef] [PubMed]
145. Sansone, P.; Berishaj, M.; Rajasekhar, V.K.; Ceccarelli, C.; Chang, Q.; Strillacci, A.; Savini, C.; Shapiro, L.; Bowman, R.L.; Mastroleo, C.; et al. Evolution of cancer stem-like cells in endocrine-resistant metastatic breast cancers is mediated by stromal microvesicles. *Cancer Res.* **2017**, *77*, 1927–1941. [CrossRef]
146. Keklikoglou, I.; Cianciaruso, C.; Güç, E.; Squadrito, M.L.; Spring, L.M.; Tazzyman, S.; Lambein, L.; Poissonnier, A.; Ferraro, G.B.; Baer, C.; et al. Chemotherapy elicits pro-metastatic extracellular vesicles in breast cancer models. *Nat. Cell Biol.* **2019**, *21*, 190–202. [CrossRef]
147. Peinado, H.; Alečković, M.; Lavotshkin, S.; Matei, I.; Costa-Silva, B.; Moreno-Bueno, G.; Hergueta-Redondo, M.; Williams, C.; García-Santos, G.; Ghajar, C.; et al. Melanoma exosomes educate bone marrow progenitor cells toward a pro-metastatic phenotype through MET. *Nat. Med.* **2012**, *18*, 883–891. [CrossRef]
148. Zhang, H.; Tang, K.; Zhang, Y.; Ma, R.; Ma, J.; Li, Y.; Luo, S.; Liang, X.; Ji, T.; Gu, Z.; et al. Cell-free Tumor Microparticle Vaccines Stimulate Dendritic Cells via cGAS/STING Signaling. *Cancer Immunol. Res.* **2015**, *3*, 196–205. [CrossRef]
149. Ma, J.; Wei, K.; Zhang, H.; Tang, K.; Li, F.; Zhang, T.; Liu, J.; Xu, P.; Yu, Y.; Sun, W.; et al. Mechanisms by Which Dendritic Cells Present Tumor Microparticle Antigens to CD8+ T Cells. *Cancer Immunol. Res.* **2018**, *6*, 1057–1068. [CrossRef]

150. Pineda, B.; García, F.J.S.; Olascoaga, N.K.; de la Cruz, V.P.; Salazar, A.; Moreno-Jiménez, S.; Pedro, N.H.; Márquez-Navarro, A.; Plata, A.O.; Sotelo, J. Malignant Glioma Therapy by Vaccination with Irradiated C6 Cell-Derived Microvesicles Promotes an Antitumoral Immune Response. *Mol. Ther.* **2019**, *27*, 1612–1620. [CrossRef]
151. Dong, W.; Zhang, H.; Yin, X.; Liu, Y.; Chen, D.; Liang, X.; Jin, X.; Lv, J.; Ma, J.; Tang, K.; et al. Oral delivery of tumor microparticle vaccines activates NOD2 signaling pathway in ileac epithelium rendering potent antitumor T cell immunity. *Oncoimmunology* **2017**, *6*. [CrossRef]
152. Wu, T.; Tang, M. Review of the effects of manufactured nanoparticles on mammalian target organs. *J. Appl. Toxicol. JAT* **2018**, *38*, 25–40. [CrossRef] [PubMed]
153. Armstrong, J.P.; Holme, M.N.; Stevens, M.M. Re-Engineering Extracellular Vesicles as Smart Nanoscale Therapeutics. *ACS Nano* **2017**, *11*, 69–83. [CrossRef] [PubMed]
154. Sil, S.; Dagur, R.S.; Liao, K.; Peeples, E.S.; Hu, G.; Periyasamy, P.; Buch, S. Strategies for the use of Extracellular Vesicles for the Delivery of Therapeutics. *J. Neuroimmune Pharmacol.* **2019**. [CrossRef] [PubMed]
155. Ma, J.; Zhang, Y.; Tang, K.; Zhang, H.; Yin, X.; Li, Y.; Xu, P.; Sun, Y.; Ma, R.; Ji, T.; et al. Reversing drug resistance of soft tumor-repopulating cells by tumor cell-derived chemotherapeutic microparticles. *Cell Res.* **2016**, *26*, 713–727. [CrossRef] [PubMed]
156. Lener, T.; Gimona, M.; Aigner, L.; Börger, V.; Buzas, E.; Camussi, G.; Chaput, N.; Chatterjee, D.; Court, F.A.; del Portillo, H.A.; et al. Applying extracellular vesicles based therapeutics in clinical trials—An ISEV position paper. *J. Extracell. Vesicles* **2015**, *4*. [CrossRef]
157. Usman, W.M.; Pham, T.C.; Kwok, Y.Y.; Vu, L.T.; Ma, V.; Peng, B.; Chan, Y.S.; Wei, L.; Chin, S.M.; Azad, A.; et al. Efficient RNA drug delivery using red blood cell extracellular vesicles. *Nat. Commun.* **2018**, *9*, 2359. [CrossRef]
158. Wiklander, O.P.B.; Nordin, J.Z.; O'Loughlin, A.; Gustafsson, Y.; Corso, G.; Mäger, I.; Vader, P.; Lee, Y.; Sork, H.; Seow, Y.; et al. Extracellular vesicle in vivo biodistribution is determined by cell source, route of administration and targeting. *J. Extracell. Vesicles* **2015**, *4*. [CrossRef]
159. Gangadaran, P.; Li, X.J.; Lee, H.W.; Oh, J.M.; Kalimuthu, S.; Rajendran, R.L.; Son, S.H.; Baek, S.H.; Singh, T.D.; Zhu, L.; et al. A new bioluminescent reporter system to study the biodistribution of systematically injected tumor-derived bioluminescent extracellular vesicles in mice. *Oncotarget* **2017**, *8*, 109894–109914. [CrossRef]
160. Murphy, D.E.; de Jong, O.G.; Brouwer, M.; Wood, M.J.; Lavieu, G.; Schiffelers, R.M.; Vader, P. Extracellular vesicle-based therapeutics: Natural versus engineered targeting and trafficking. *Exp. Mol. Med.* **2019**, *51*, 1–12. [CrossRef]
161. Tanaka, Y.; Schroit, A.J. Insertion of fluorescent phosphatidylserine into the plasma membrane of red blood cells. Recognition by autologous macrophages. *J. Biol. Chem.* **1983**, *258*, 11335–11343.
162. Saari, H.; Lisitsyna, E.; Rautaniemi, K.; Rojalin, T.; Niemi, L.; Nivaro, O.; Laaksonen, T.; Yliperttula, M.; Vuorimaa-Laukkanen, E. FLIM reveals alternative EV-mediated cellular up-take pathways of paclitaxel. *J. Control. Release* **2018**, *284*, 133–143. [CrossRef] [PubMed]
163. Liang, Q.; Bie, N.; Yong, T.; Tang, K.; Shi, X.; Wei, Z.; Jia, H.; Zhang, X.; Zhao, H.; Huang, W.; et al. The softness of tumour-cell-derived microparticles regulates their drug-delivery efficiency. *Nat. Biomed. Eng.* **2019**, *3*, 729–740. [CrossRef] [PubMed]
164. Thomas, G.M.; Panicot-Dubois, L.; Lacroix, R.; Dignat-George, F.; Lombardo, D.; Dubois, C. Cancer cell-derived microparticles bearing P-selectin glycoprotein ligand 1 accelerate thrombus formation in vivo. *J. Exp. Med.* **2009**, *206*, 1913–1927. [CrossRef] [PubMed]
165. Kordelas, L.; Rebmann, V.; Ludwig, A.-K.; Radtke, S.; Ruesing, J.; Doeppner, T.R.; Epple, M.; Horn, P.A.; Beelen, D.W.; Giebel, B. MSC-derived exosomes: A novel tool to treat therapy-refractory graft-versus-host disease. *Leukemia* **2014**, *28*, 970–973. [CrossRef] [PubMed]

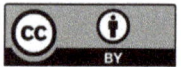

© 2020 by the authors. Licensee MDPI, Basel, Switzerland. This article is an open access article distributed under the terms and conditions of the Creative Commons Attribution (CC BY) license (http://creativecommons.org/licenses/by/4.0/).

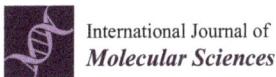

Review

Platelets Extracellular Vesicles as Regulators of Cancer Progression—An Updated Perspective

Magdalena Żmigrodzka *, Olga Witkowska-Piłaszewicz and Anna Winnicka

Department of Pathology and Veterinary Diagnostics, Institute of Veterinary Medicine, Warsaw University of Life Sciences (WULS-SGGW), Nowoursynowska 159c, 02-787 Warsaw, Poland; olga_witkowska_pilaszewicz@sggw.edu.pl (O.W.-P.); anna_winnicka@sggw.edu.pl (A.W.)
* Correspondence: magdalena_zmigrodzka@sggw.edu.pl

Received: 26 June 2020; Accepted: 20 July 2020; Published: 22 July 2020

Abstract: Extracellular vesicles (EVs) are a diverse group of membrane-bound structures secreted in physiological and pathological conditions by prokaryotic and eukaryotic cells. Their role in cell-to-cell communications has been discussed for more than two decades. More attention is paid to assess the impact of EVs in cancer. Numerous papers showed EVs as tumorigenesis regulators, by transferring their cargo molecules (miRNA, DNA, protein, cytokines, receptors, etc.) among cancer cells and cells in the tumor microenvironment. During platelet activation or apoptosis, platelet extracellular vesicles (PEVs) are formed. PEVs present a highly heterogeneous EVs population and are the most abundant EVs group in the circulatory system. The reason for the PEVs heterogeneity are their maternal activators, which is reflected on PEVs size and cargo. As PLTs role in cancer development is well-known, and PEVs are the most numerous EVs in blood, their feasible impact on cancer growth is strongly discussed. PEVs crosstalk could promote proliferation, change tumor microenvironment, favor metastasis formation. In many cases these functions were linked to the transfer into recipient cells specific cargo molecules from PEVs. The article reviews the PEVs biogenesis, cargo molecules, and their impact on the cancer progression.

Keywords: extracellular vesicles; exosomes; ectosomes; neoplasia

1. Introduction

The number of research work and scientific papers that discuss the involvement of cell-derived extracellular vesicles (EVs) in multiple physiological and pathological processes has increased rapidly during the last two decades. EVs might have an influence on target cells by delivering ligands and signaling complexes, and transferring mRNA and transcription factors that cause the epigenetic reprograming of recipient cells. EVs are submicron spherical membrane bound structures, that are generated by different prokaryotic (termed as membrane vesicles) and eukaryotic cells [1–3]. EVs nomenclature take into account their cellular origin and size. Their size ranges between 10 nm to 5 µm and comprises three heterogeneous populations of vesicles—exosomes (EXSMs), ectosomes (ECTSMs) also named microparticles (MPs), and apoptotic bodies (ABs) [4,5]. EVs actively secreted form parental cells with a diameter of 10 to 100 nm are named EXSMs, and those with a diameter ranging between 100 nm to 1 µm are ECTSMs. Lipid bilayer membrane protects their cargo from enzymes like proteases and ribonucleases [6]. The largest of EVs are ABs (with diameter 1–5 µm) represented by clumps of material generated during the late stage of cell apoptosis [5–7].

During activation, maturation, proliferation, stress, aging, or apoptosis, cells shed EVs into the extracellular space [8]. Their presence in a number of body fluids including—urine, synovial fluid, bronchoalveolar lavage fluid, saliva, and bile was confirmed [7,9–11]. In the bloodstream, EVs are released by—erythrocytes, leukocytes, platelets (PEVs), megakaryocytes, and endothelial cells [10,12].

In addition, EVs are also secreted by cancer cells known as tumor-derived extracellular vesicles (TEVs) [4,12]. In both healthy subjects and those with a variety of pathologies, peripheral blood is a rich source of EVs, where the most abundant population are PEVs. Their percentage ranges between 70 to 90% of all EVs in the plasma of healthy individuals [13–15].

In 1967, Peter Wolf described "platelet dust"—a subcellular material derived from thrombocytes in the plasma and serum of healthy individuals [16,17]. This was a milestone in medicine research, allowing further examinations evaluating PEVs involvement in physiological and pathological processes. PEVs share many functional features with PLTs. These tiny fragments smaller than platelets (PLTs) were secreted during PLT activation and were known to be crucial in coagulation and clot formation [16,18]. Despite the fact that PLTs play a crucial role in hemostasis, PEVs coagulation capacity is several dozen higher than PLTs [19]. Platelets microparticles (PMPs) are enriched in tissue factor (TF), coagulation factors, and dozens of them expose about 3-fold higher phosphatidylserine (PS) concentration on the outer membrane than PLTs [20]. The coagulation process initiated by TF connection with coagulation factor VII, activates coagulation cascade. Activated PLTs, PMPs PS + offer a catalytic surface for the coagulation and binding of consecutive clotting factors. Moreover, in healthy individuals, the presence of integrin αIIbβ3 (CD41/CD61) on PMPs supports fibrin clot formation [21]. In various bleeding disorders, abnormalities in PMPs functions and their reduced number in blood were reported [22]. On the other hand, their increased amount was presented in thrombotic state and other pathologies [23]. PLTs of patients described by Castaman are unable to shed PMPs, conversely to patients with Scott syndrome in which the PMPs number is adequate, but the incorrect translocation of PS impairs prothrombinase activity, and causes hemorrhagic diathesis [22]. Patients with immune thrombocytopenia have higher PEVs level than healthy individuals, which might be an evolutionary way to prevent blood loss and maintain tissue integrity [24]. Additionally, contemporary papers showed that PEVs might be a potential biomarker or prognostic factor in other pathologies—inflammatory, cardiovascular, and autoimmune diseases, solid tumors and hematological malignancies [14,25].

In this review, the role of PEVs in the cancerogenesis, tumor growth, and metastasis formation in distant organs is reported. Furthermore, the possible evaluation of PEVs as markers for cancer detection, and effectiveness of anticancer treatment is discussed.

2. EVs Biogenesis and Elimination

Based on the current knowledge, the mechanism of EVs formation and secretion to the extracellular space vary, depending on the EXSMs or ECTSMs descent. The EXSM definition was originally used for microparticles secreted from variety of cultured cells, thereafter, Johnstone and colleagues in 1987 explained the mechanism of transferrin receptor loss during reticulocytes maturation via secretion of nanosize vesicles; for this term EXSMs is used [26]. The latest research confirmed that the pathways of EVs biogenesis might differ between the parental cells types and EVs secretion, which does not seem to be accidental [1,27].

2.1. ECTSMs Formation

The blebbing of the plasma was documented in apoptosis during ABs formation, but it was confirmed as well in ECTSMs biogenesis. Changes in lipid components affect the rearrangement within plasma membrane. This process is initiated by an increased level of intracellular calcium ions. It causes activation of floppase and scramblase enzymes and inhibition of flippase (Figure 1) [1,8]. The membrane phospholipids—PS and phosphatidyl-ethanolamine, are vertically translocated from the inner leaflet to the outer cell membrane surface. The rearrangement breaks the bonds between cytoskeleton and cell membrane phospholipids. Partial degradation of actin filaments leads to restructuring of the cytoskeleton filaments, which favor formation of ECTSMs [1,8,10].

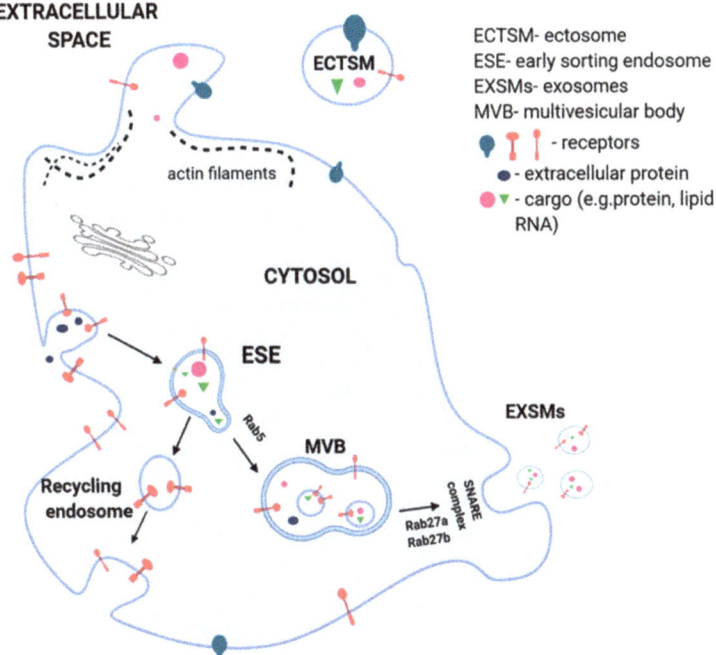

Figure 1. Extracellular vesicle biogenesis and secretion. The exosomes (EXSMs) generation begins with the membrane bulging into the lumen of the ESE. Part of them form a part of the plasma membrane (recycling endosome), others are converted into multi vesicular body (MVB). Members of the Rab family, Rab27a and Rab27b, are involved in MVB transport and fusion with cell membrane. Transmembrane protein complex SNARE enables the MVB to dock with the cell membrane that leads to release of EXSMs to extracellular space. Ectosome (ECTSM) are formed directly by cell membrane blebbing. This process is initiated with an increase in intracellular calcium that causes the activation of enzymes—floppase and scramblase and the inhibition of flippase. This causes the rearrangement of phospholipids in the cell membrane, as well as results in breaking bonds between cytoskeleton and partial degradation of actin filaments. During formation of EXSMs and ECTSMs, mRNA and miRNA that are located in cytoplasm are randomly entered.

The fast phospholipid membrane remodeling and PS exposure are relevant for PLTs physiological procoagulant response in hemostasis. PMPs formation in the circulation could result from PLTs activation via multiple agonists, high shear stress or apoptosis [20,28]. In the high shear rate, the loss of membrane integrity is initiated through the dislocated connection between the membrane glycoprotein Ib receptor (CD42b) and PLTs cytoskeleton, which began PMPs formation [20]. Natural PLTs activators, such as thrombin or collagen, induce PMPs formation via transmembrane integrin receptor gpIIb/IIIa (CD41/CD61) or tetraspanin 29 [29]. Altogether, these observations become the starting point for subsequent works assessing, how different types of PLTs activators induce PMPs formation, and how they affect the heterogeneity of PEVs population. Noticeably, a research conducted in 2017 confirmed that PS negative tubular PMPs population with structural similarities to filopodia could be formed during PLTs activation. Lack of PS expression on their surface implied that during their formation, there is no PS translocation [30].

2.2. EXSMs Formation

EXSMs generation begins with the inward bulging of the plasma membrane by endocytosis into the cytoplasm lumen. It leads to forming early sorting endosomes (ESEs) (Figure 1) [1].

Part of ESEs is returned into plasma membrane, other under the Rab5 control are changed into late endosomes or multivesicular bodies (MVBs) [1,10]. During this process, proteins and antigens are packaged into intraluminal vesicles (ILVs) and the budding of the ESEs membrane transform into MVBs [31]. Four protein subunits of the endosomal sorting complex required for transport (ESCRT) machinery are involved in this process. ESCTR-III is essential for the scission of ILVs into MVBs lumen. Cargo clustering and membrane budding can occur by ESCRT-dependent or -independent machinery [1]. ESCRT-0 recognizes ubiquitinated proteins (cargo) by the hepatocyte growth factor-regulated tyrosine kinase substrate (Hrs), in association with clathrin. This complex helps ESCRT I and II to connect with ESCRT 0 and ubiquitinated cargo, on the part of the endosomal membrane, where it will finally pullulate. ESCRT III connects with the complex and ultimately bud ILVs into the endosome [32]. The MVBs fuse with the plasma membrane to secrete the ILVs as exosomes or absorb with lysosomes for their degradation [1]. Members of Rab family, Rab27a and Rab27b, are essential mediators in transport of MVBs and its fusion with cell membrane. Transmembrane protein complex SANRE enables dock EXSMs with cell membrane that leads to the release of EXSMs to extracellular space (exocytosis). Increased concentration of calcium ions is one of the EXSMs secretion regulators [33]. Targeting selected Rabs via specific inhibitors modulates their structure or secretory function and becomes a new promising strategy of limiting EXSMs formation, both by PLTs and cancer cells. Wang et al. showed in a pre-clinical study, that elevated number of PMPs in patients with sepsis after intravenous administration of small GTPase inhibitor NSC23766, reduced PMPs secretion for about 87% [34,35].

Aatonen et al. showed that PMPs and platelet derived EXSMs (PdEXSMs) biogenesis is also observed by non-activated PLTs [36]. Examination potency of various agonists on EVs formation confirmed that Ca^{2+} ionophore is the strongest agonist, these include—thrombin, collagen, LPS, TRAP-6, and the weakest one is ADP [36]. Moreover, authors considered that Ca^{2+} ionophore causes vesiculation in unselective way or fragmentation and ABs formation, and should be advisedly used as agonist. The strongest PdEXSMs activators are thrombin and collagen or collagen-related peptide XL. Interestingly, the proteins cargo in PdEXSMs derived from stimulated PLTs was richer than from resting PLTs [36]. Nowadays, the utility of EXSMs as a new diagnostic cancer marker is extensively studied. Recent work performed by Lea et al. showed an increased number of EXSMs with PS expression in peritoneal fluid and plasma of patients with ovarian carcinoma [37]. It confirmed that, when PS is routinely used as a PMPs marker, it is also present on cancer derived EXSMs and causes a possibility to exploit these results in early diagnostic tests of women with ovarian malignancies [37].

2.3. EVs Elimination and Impact of Storage Conditions on PEVs Number

The PEVs rapid clearance from circulation varied depending on their molecular content, and the induction signal in different species [38,39]. As they have pro-coagulant and pro-inflammatory nanosize structures, their rapid turnover is essential for prevention of thrombotic diseases. PMPs turnover in rabbits is less than ten minutes, compared to people where PMPs were shown in circulation for more than 3 h [20,38,39]. Flumenhaft found that mice PMPs are eliminated from bloodstream within 30 min [40]. PEVs could be phagocytized after their opsonization with thrombospondin or complement components C3b [40]. The PS on the PMPs outer leaflet of the plasma membrane is recognized by macrophages and it originates a signal to remove them. Moreover, the role of lactadherin (LA) in clearance of EVs from circulation is discussed [41]. LA secreted by macrophages and adipocytes is also detected on the circulating PMPs. An increased PEVs level was observed in lactadherin–deficient mice, which could suggest the role of LA as a one of "eat-me" signals for phagocytosis [41]. Dasgupta et al. showed that developmental endothelial locus–1 in endothelial cells mediates PS-positive PMPs elimination via endocytosis [17,42]. Shorter half-life of ECTSMs, compared to EXSMs in blood, might arise from the higher concentration of membrane lipids in ECTSMs and activity of phospholipase A2 in serum [43]. Furthermore, EXSMs elimination via IgM immunoglobulins binding to lipid lysophosphatidylcholine was reported and liver macrophages were shown to be crucial elements of EXSMs clearance [43,44].

In EVs analysis, preanalytical steps standardization is crucial for the minimization of false results of PEVs number and their quality tests. Different anticoagulants could activate PLTs during blood collection and storage. Wisgrill et al. confirmed that the EVs number and their functionality is stable in sodium citrate for 8 h in room temperature (RT), after blood samples collection [45]. In EDTA, routinely used in clinical practice, PMPs and erythrocytes' derived EVs count is stable for 48 h in RT [45]. Thus, it could be an alternative when the collected samples are stored before analysis [45].

3. Content of Platelet Extracellular Vesicles

Physiological or pathological processes in parental cells define their EVs cargo and biological properties. As described above, the PEVs formation, membrane composition and specific markers expression on the outer membrane leaflet depends on the PLTs activators (Ca^{2+} ionophore, adenosine diphosphate, thrombin, collagen, epinephrine) [20]. Most of the EVs circulating in plasma are classified as PEVs based on their surface receptors. Nevertheless, heterogeneity of PEVs surface receptors starts discussion about EVs derived from megakaryocytes (Mk-EVs), as a part of PEVs subpopulation [46]. The EVs phenotyping conception to distinguish PEVs from Mk-EVs involves the usefulness of cluster of differentiation (CD) CD41/CD61 as a constitutive marker for both PLTs and Mks, while CD62P and CD107a act as a PLTs activation markers [47]. Flaumenhaft et al. showed that mouse and human Mk-EVs are PS/CD41/CD61 positive and CD62/CD107a negative [46]. In support of this finding, after irradiation of bone marrow, the CD61 positive EVs population largely disappears from mice circulation, whereas CD62P remains unchanged [48]. A study by Brisson et al. showed that small PMPs population—PS negative and CD41 positive, is a result of cell membrane shedding without PS redistribution. Moreover, PMPs could contain organelles like mitochondria and dense granules [30]. EVs are identified based on their size and expression of characteristic surface markers. PS expression is an a ECTSMs marker, when the presence of tetraspanin CD63 is used for EXSMs identification. During PLTs activation, both ECTSMs and EXSMs are CD63 positive but the CD63 expression is higher on EXSMs. It could be useful for determining the purity of the EXSMs population [30,49]. A characteristic of PEVs is the diversity of their surface markers and cargo. PEVs display a wide array of bioactive molecules like adhesion molecules, chemo- and cytokines, apoptosis regulators, miRNAs. They also harbor a broad spectrum of coagulation factors, enzymes, complement proteins, and bioactive lipids (Table 1). PEVs express glycoprotein (gp) IIb/IIIa, Ib, IIa, as well as P-selectin and a lysosome-associated glycoprotein-1 (LAMP-1). C-type lectin domain family 1-member B (CLEC-2) and gp VI expression was documented on Mk-EVs [17]. PdEXSMs are substantial with proteins from α granules, whereas ECTSMs are substantial with lipid mediators and mitochondrial proteins [17,50].

Molecules presented on PEVs were involved in triggering receptors on the target cells or regulating them via bioactive molecules, signaling molecules or a plethora of genetic material including miRNAs [51]. PEVs can interact with donor cells in multiple ways—(i) stimulation via signaling complex, using specific PEVs surface receptors and lipids; (ii) transfer membrane receptors and adhesion molecules; (iii) horizontal transfer of heterogeneous proteins, miRNAs, bioactive lipids, and other factors including infectious particles (prions) or even organelles (mitochondria) [3].

Table 1. Comparison of the PEVs cargo and their function. Biologically active molecules, receptors, enzymes, chemokines were categorized based on their functions of the PEVs, but there are no discrepancies detailed for some molecules.

				Function or Category Name				
	Clotting	Enzymes	Adhesion Molecules	Bioactive Lipids	Programmed Cell Death	Growth Factors	Chemokines /Cytokines	Immune Response
PEVs	TF [52–54]	12-LO [55]	CD41/61 [56–59] CD31 [49,59]	PS [60]	caspase-3 [58]	TGF β1 [50]	CXCR4-(PF-4) [57,61]	CD 154 [32,62]
	FVa, FVIII [60,63]	heparynase [64]	CD62P [57,59,65,66]	AA [67,68]	CD95 [57]	PDGF bFGF [64]	IL-1β [69]	C5b-9 [70]
Cargo (Ref)	PAR-1 [57]	PDI [71]	fibrinogen, vWF, vitronectin [65]	LPA [70]	caspase-9 [72]	VEGF [64]	CCL5, CCL23 [50,73]	CD55, CD59 [52]
	TFPI [74]	NADPH oxidase [75]	CD42a, CD42b [49,59]	TXA2 [76]			CX3CR1 [73]	Factor H [52]

PEVs are able to transfer receptors expressed on their surface (i.e., CD41, CD61, CD184, CD62P, PAR-1) to recipient cells (monocytes, myeloblasts, hematopoietic stem cells) and induce their adhesion or proliferation [3,27]. PEVs functional gpIIb/IIIa (CD41/CD61) transferred to neutrophils, activated NF-κB, in response to GM-CSF and enhanced inflammation [77]. Tang and colleagues showed that PEVs transfer arachidonate 12-lipoxygenase to mast cells, which increased synthesis of one of the negative regulator of inflammation lipoxin A4 (LXA4) [27,55]. Thus, PEVs play both positive and negative role in inflammation response, depending on the target cell.

PEVs are rich in sphingosine 1-phosphate, metalloproteinases, heparyanase, PDI, and arachidonic acid (AA) [3]. Transfer of AA by PMPs to monocytes and endothelial cells induced by prostanoids and cyclooxygenase 2 synthesis enhances these cells interactions [3]. Treatment of human umbilical vein endothelial cells (HUVECs) with PEVs showed intensification of angiogenesis and cell proliferation versus activated charcoal treated PEVs (removed nonpolar lipids), where a reduction of these effects was observed. This experiment showed that PEVs lipid components were involved in HUVECs stimulation [27,78]. The horizontal transfer of non-coding RNAs via EVs regulates gene expression by post-transcriptional repression. miRNA from parental cells encapsulated in EVs was protected from ribonuclease activity in circulation [51]. In human's, several PMPs miRNAs were detected, e.g., miR-19, miR-21, miR-22, miR-126, miR-133, miR-146, miR-185, miR-223, and miR-320b [3]. Moreover, it was confirmed that PEVs miRNA was transferred to macrophages, endothelial, and cancer cells. In macrophages, MiR-126–3p transferred from PEVs led to decreased ATF3 and ATP1B1 expression and protein synthesis [27]. Recently presented data support the notion of PEVs tumor microenvironment infiltration and interaction with cancer cells via the mechanisms described above.

4. PEVs in Cancer Progression

PEVs are highly interesting group of EVs because of their percentage participation in bloodstream, as well as their increased number in patients with cancer, such as glioblastoma, gastric, lung and skin cancer, and other diseases. This makes them potentially useful as a diagnostic marker [79]. It is known that PLTs facilitate cancer metastasis. Moreover, the number of papers that discuss PEVs contribution in cancerogenesis increased recently [51,80]. EVs as cell-to-cell messenger molecules can start phenotypic and functional changes in donor cells, by reaching the recipient cells and delivering EVs content. PEVs are also discussed as potentially early markers of disease progression.

4.1. PEVs in Tumor Angiogenesis

The cancer cells without blood circulation can grow up to 2 mm^3 in diameter, forming a tumor and then stop and undergo apoptosis or necrosis [81]. Growth of the vascular network is pivotal for the cancer cells survival, proliferation, as well as metastatic spread of cancer [81]. Angiogenesis is essential for formation of a new vascular network that supplies nutrients, oxygen, and immune cells, and also removes waste products of cellular metabolism. Therefore, angiogenesis is a critical factor in the progression of cancer. The tumor microenvironment (TME) consists of diverse cellular populations, including tumor cells, endothelial cells, fibroblasts, infiltrating immune cells (monocytes, macrophages, neutrophils, mast cells, T cells), extracellular matrix, and newly formed blood vessels [79]. The PEVs interaction with TME components could reveal their functions in cancer progression. Newly stirring blood vessels permit tumor growth, which is critical in cancer progression. Interestingly, Happonen et al. demonstrated a mechanism of PEVs transfer to human aortic endothelial cells (HAECs) and HUVECs [82]. PS-positive PEVs are taken up by phagocytosis via tyrosine kinase receptor Axl, and its ligand protein Gas6 on endothelial cells [82]. Janowska-Wieczorek et al. used lung cancer cell lines to elucidate PEVs importance in cancer angiogenesis [83]. After PEVs stimulation of IL-8 (about 35-fold), vascular endothelial growth factor (VEGF) (3-fold) and scatter factor (4-fold) mRNA expression increased in the A549 cell line [83].

PEVs delivery of bioactive molecules like cytokines or microRNA to recipient cells could regulate tumor growth [84]. miRNAs are small non-coding RNAs that regulate gene expression post-transcriptionally. Anene et al. demonstrated regulatory angiogenesis miRNAs transfer from PEVs to HUVECs cells during co-culturing on extracellular matrix gel [85]. A robust capillary-like structure formation and simultaneously decreased synthesis of anti-angiogenic thrombospondin-1 (THBS-1) was observed. miRNA Let-7 a from PEVs was delivered to HUVECs and targeted THBS-1 mRNA to induce angiogenic responses of HUVECs [85]. Blood vessel formation is controlled by a balance between localized production of pro- and anti-angiogenic molecules and changes in THBS-1 concentration is the key determinant of this "angiogenic switch" [85]. PEVs ability to bind TF and the platelet-activating factor potentiates their pro- angiogenic competence even more [86].

Pan et al. demonstrated that after incubation, PEVs with HUVECs cells miR-223 level in endothelial cells increased, which promoted glycation end-product-induced vascular endothelial cell apoptosis via targeting insulin-like growth factor 1 receptor [87]. Another work showed that HUVECs cells preferentially uptake miR-223 from PEVs generated by thrombin-activated PLTs [4,88]. This leads to the formation of functional Argonaute 2 (Ago2) miR-223 complexes. These complexes are able to regulate gene expression and protein level for ephrin A1 and F-box/WD repeat-containing protein 7 in HUVECs cells and conduces apoptosis [4].

Increased angiogenesis in TME could be a result of metalloproteinase-1 (MMP-1) transfer, as well as increased MMP-9, VEGF, and IL-8 mRNA expression in lung cancer cells lines, after co-incubation with PEVs [83]. Moreover, PEVs molecules from α granules like VEGF, platelet-derived growth factor and fibroblast growth factor are a component of their cargo with pro-angiogenic properties.

4.2. PEVs in Migration, Invasion, and Metastasis

A key for distant metastases formation is cancer cells passage through the newly formed vascular walls in primary tumor, surviving in the circulation, and finally proliferation at the distant tissue. In solid tumors, vasculature is highly permeable, allowing the possibility to PEVs infiltration to TEM and contact with cells. A great number of studies indicate the PEVs involvement in cancer progression and some discuss their anti-cancer properties. Michael et al. showed that PEVs have the ability to infiltrate murine and human tumors [84]. This ability creates conditions for the horizontal transfer of miRNA-24, which targets mitochondrial mt-Nd2, and Snora75. This entails mitochondrial dysfunction and results in an increased cancer cell apoptosis [84].

Bakewell and colleagues showed that platelets gpIIb/IIIa antagonists minimize formation of distant metastasis from B16 melanoma cells in bones, due to the inhibition of the interaction between cancer cells and PLTs [89]. Lung cancer cell line A549 increases adhesiveness to the fibrinogen and HUVECs, after receiving CD41 from PEVs. PEVs chemoattract lung cell lines from 2.5 to 7-fold more than the control [83]. Moreover, evaluation of PEVs interaction with lung cancer cell lines confirmed the activation of mitogen-activated protein kinase (MAPK) MAPK p42/44 and AKT, signaling pathways participating in proliferative responses [83]. Murine lung cells covered by PEVs injected intravenously into mince resulted in significant increase metastasis formation in lungs and bone marrow [83]. Transfer onto the surface of donor cells CD184-, a chemokine receptor type 4 from PEVs and respond to stromal cell-derived factor 1, which is rich niche in bone marrow in the murine model, confirmed their high metastatic potential [83]. Moreover, activation of cyclin D2 by PEVs in lung cancer cell lines could change the phenotype of cancer cells into a more invasive phenotype. Similar observations were made in human squamous carcinoma or breast cancer cell lines in murine in vivo model [90].

Interestingly, Gasperi and colleagues confirmed the modulatory influence of polyunsaturated fatty acids (PUFAs) diet, especially the ω3 and ω6 on cellular processes in carcinogenesis [62]. The PUFAs ω3 cancer preventive activity is well known, in contrast to high concentration of ω6 in diet, which correlates with higher risk of breast and prostate cancer [62,91]. Their role in cancerogenesis is related to changes in fatty acids compositions of membrane rafts in cells membranes. PEVs contains miR-126 and miRNA-223, which are important players in tumorigenesis. VEGF-dependent proliferation of endothelial cells is stimulated by miRNA-126, while miRNA-223 inhibit formation of new blood vessels by targeting endothelial β1 integrin [92]. Gasperi et al. examined the influence of increased level of PUFAs ω6 on both PEVs formation and their cargo [62]. The newly formed PEVs had an increased amounts of miRNA-123 and miRNA233. Breast cell line BT549 blocked its cell cycle and decreased cell migration after internalizing PEVs [62].

A Tang et al. study revealed an important PEVs role in the epithelial-to-mesenchymal transition of ovarian epithelial cancer cell line (SKOV3). miR-939 transfer leads to enhanced invasion and cancer progression [93,94]. Tropomyosin 3 (TPM3) contributes cancerogenesis in thyroid papillary carcinoma and esophageal squamous cell carcinoma by fusing neurotrophic receptor tyrosine kinase 1 and PDGF receptors [95]. Yao et al. demonstrated increased TPM3 mRNA in PLTs and revealed their transfer by PEVs into breast cancer cells and promotion of an invasion [94]. Moreover, in patients with distant metastases, compared to subjects without metastases TPM3 mRNA in PLTs was significantly increased [94].

Another interesting issue is the ability of cancer cells to educate PLTs. Zarà et al. demonstrated that breast cancer cell lines—highly aggressive MDM-MB-231 and MCF7 could educate PLTs to produce PEVs in an amount similar to that after thrombin activation [96]. Next, those PEVs were co-cultured with cancer cells to investigate if the newly formed PEVs impact cells. Only in the MDM-MB-231 cell line, authors observed cells activation and phosphorylation of p38MAPK and myosin light chain. Moreover, increased migration and invasion was noted. This experiment showed that PEVs can novel paracrine-positive feedback mechanism initiated by MDA-MB-231 to escalate their invasive phenotype [96].

PEVs formed by PLTs during apoptosis-like process show surface gpIIb/IIIa, and PS and stimulate their own phagocytic removal by monocytes, moreover, they are able to change macrophages into M2 macrophages [97,98]. In contrast to effect on endothelial cells, after PEVs miR-223 transfer into gastric cell line SGC7901, increased proliferation and invasion in vitro, as well as decreased apoptosis, was observed. This showed that horizontal miRNA transfer via PEVs could have diverse effect contingent on donor cells [4,99]. Another noteworthy experimental work showed that peripheral blood mononuclear cells (PBMCs) isolated from patients with B-precursor acute lymphoblastic leukemia had increased apoptotic markers CD95, active caspse-3, and an increased number of apoptotic cells, after two days of co-culturing with PEVs [100].

Cancer cells transmigration from circulation into the tissues is mediated likewise by tissue-specific enzymes, the majority of which belongs to the MMP family. Dashevsky et al. confirmed transfer of MMP-2 and its' increased secretion from Cl-1 cells after co-culturing with PEVs. Interesting observation was made when Cl-1 cells were incubated with PEVs lysate. Values of MMP-2 concentration and secretion were similar to that after cells co-culturing with PEVs. It suggests that the transfer of MMP-2 is not dependent only on PEVs internalization. The other possible candidates for increased MMP-2 value might be free miRNA from PEVs lysate or lysophosphatidic acid (LPA) as an MMP-2 activator presented on PLTs and in prostate cancer cells [101].

Natural killer (NK) cells efficiently recognize and kill circulating tumor cells of almost any origin, but their effectiveness in TME is discussed. PEVs miR-183 transfer into NK cells suppressed activator adapter DAP12 and suppressed their cytolytic functions in tumor-associated NK cells [102]. PEVs could also horizontally transfer functional miR-126–3p into primary human macrophages. The PEVs dose-dependent down regulation of miR-126–3p targets CCL4, CSF1, and TNF was observed. Decreased secretion of cytokines/chemokines was correlated with reprogramming into phagocytic macrophages [88,103]. The role of TF in angiogenesis and metastasis formation is well documented, therefore, the role of TF-positive PEVs in tumor growth seems clear. Another interesting aspect of PEVs as a potentially important immune checkpoint in cancer biology is a presence of PS on PEVs surface. PEVs as an abundant source of PS might be a possible ligand for PS receptor (PSR) on the immune cells. Activation of PS–PSR pathway leads to the inhibition of innate and adaptive immune response in TME, as well as in circulation [104]. The new oncotherapy strategies examined the PSR inhibitors as a new anticancer target, but only a highly selective inhibition strategy could be applied in the cancer treatment. Table 2 summarize PEVs pivotal role in crosstalk between PLTs and other cells, particularly with cancer cells (Table 2).

Table 2. The role of PEVs in cell-to-cell communication. PEVs secreted from activated PLTs transfer to target cells and their cargo promotes phenotypic changes and novel functions in donor cells.

Target Cell	PEVs Derived Factors/Molecules	Functional Changes (References)
A549, CRL 2066, CRL 2062, HTB 183, HTB 177 lung CCL; LCC * CCL	CD41, CD61 CD184	(+) adhesion to fibrinogen and HUVECs [83] (+) metastatic potential [83] (+) mRNA expression of angiogenic factors (MMP-9, VEGF, IL-8) [83] (+) proliferation and chemoinvasion [83]
HUVECs	miRNA Let-7a miRNA-223	(−) synthesis THBS-1 anti-angiogenic molecule [85] (+) apoptosis by IGF-1 [4,87]
MC-38 colon CCL, LCC * CCL	miRNA-24	(+) apoptosis [84]
BT549 breast CCL	miRNA-123 miRNA-233	(−) migration [62] (−) cell cycle [62]
SKOV3 ovarian CCL	miRNA-939	(+) invasion via TPM3 [94] (+) progression [94]
MDM-MB-231 breast CCL		(+) invasion [96] (+) migration [94]
SGC7901 gastric CCL	miRNA-223	(+) proliferation and invasion [4,105] (−) apoptosis [4,105]
PBMCs from patients with ALL	CD95 Caspase-3	(+) apoptosis [100]
Cl-1 prostate CCL	MMP-2 miRNA?	(+) migration [101]
macrophages	PS, gpIIb/IIIa miR-126-3p	polarization into macrophage M2 [97] (−)CCL4, CSF1, TNF [88]
NK cells	miR-183	(−) cytolysis [102]

Abbreviations: CCL-cancer cell line; * murine cell line; (+) increase; (−) decrease.

5. The Potential of PEVs as Diagnostics Cancer Biomarkers

PEVs number in blood was raised about twice in myeloproliferative neoplasms, compared to healthy controls, up to four times in oral cancer and colorectal subjects and more than ten times in breast cancer patients [86,106]. The highest concentration of PEVs, more than 30-fold, was noticed in patients with IV stage of gastric cancer. In each group, the highest PEVs concertation were demonstrated in advanced cancer stages and in patients with distal metastases [86,106–108].

Investigation in patients with non-small cell lung cancer (NSCLC) categorized based on disease progression, showed the significantly higher number of circulating EVs from activated or apoptotic PLTs and from endothelial apoptotic cells, compared to healthy subjects. Changes in EVs levels in different stages of NSCLC showed that serial measurements of circulating PEVs are valuable prognostic biomarkers, mainly in the advanced stages of NSCLC [109].

PEVs as source of anionic phospholipids and TF on their surface are one of the important factors of procoagulant activity. Data demonstrated by Ren et al. showed the significantly increased number of EVs and PEVs in patients with oral squamous cell carcinoma (OSCC) in peripheral blood. PEVs level was also positively correlated with clinical stage and with fibrinogen concentration and patients hypercoagulable state [107]. Mege and colleagues showed correlations between increased PEVs number and the stage of the disease in patients with pancreatic cancer and colorectal cancer. They suggested that PEVs concentration in blood could be a useful marker for evaluation of the disease progression in these types of neoplasia [110].

Yenigürbüz et al. described another aspect of increased PEVs number in patients with neoplasia. Thromboembolism is one of the complications during induction of therapy in pediatric acute lymphoblastic leukemia (ALL) patients [111]. Children with ALL have increased levels of ABs, PEVs, endothelial-derived, and tissue factor-positive microvesicles during induction therapy. Further studies are needed to confirm the PEVs contribution in thromboembolism during the induction therapy period in children with ALL [111]. Similar observations were made in adult patients with myeloproliferative neoplasia, where the number of TF positive PMPs and endothelial derived EVs was significantly increased, which might also play a role in thrombotic complications in that group of subjects [112]. Tjon-Kon-Fat et al. demonstrated that tumor educated PLTs are a source of prostate cancer biomarkers [113,114]. In this context it seems to be interesting to evaluate the presence and role of EVs generated from tumor-educated PLTs.

6. The Potential of PEVs in Cancer Therapy

The paradigm of using nanoparticulate pharmaceutics as delivery vectors was established over the past decade [56]. To use EVs as drug transporters, their pharmacokinetics should be analyzed. Mice models of EXSMs distribution showed that the route of administration, EXSMs origin, and concentration critically influenced their biodistribution [115]. In the mice model, after intraperitoneal and subcutaneous administration of EXSMs, they preferentially localized in the pancreas and gastrointestinal tract. Whereas, intravenous administrated EXSMs were detected in the spleen and the liver [116]. In addition, EXSMs loaded with therapeutic anti-miRNA could be transferred locally into tumor or systemically. Other therapeutic strategies in cancer therapy were elimination of EXSMs from blood or prevention of EXSMs fusion with target cell [117,118]. Various strategies of using EXSMs in anticancer therapy are characterized in the literature, but more research is still needed.

In an elegant study, Kailashiya et al. documented that doxorubicin-loaded PEVs (doxo-PEVs) were taken by HL60, K562 cells (leukemia cell lines), and blast cells, in whole blood harvested from patients with newly diagnosed leukemia. Doxo-PEVs were uptaken by cells via P-selectin ligands and integrins. Moreover, doxo-PEVs transfer into leukemia cells was higher, compared to free doxorubicin, which could be used to increase the effectiveness of the therapy and minimize the side effects of drugs [56]. Gasperi et al. showed that PEVs with miR-126 and with miR-223 increased sensitivity of BT549 cells to the cisplatin chemotherapy [62].

PEVs drug-loaded could be a natural vectors-targeted medications. Engineering them from autologous platelets in large quantity and storing for several days, seems to be a new biocompatible and non-immunogenic new-generation medicine. However, to make PEVs applicable and efficacious in clinical treatments, some of their underlying functions still need to be better researched and understood.

7. Summary

PEVs biogenesis depends on different signals that control their formation from PLTs. The role of PEVs in various physiological conditions, like hemostasis, or pathological like inflammation or atherosclerosis was confirmed. This review focused on the PEVs participation in cancerogenesis. A better understanding of the biology of PEVs and the mechanisms that allow them to function as mediators in cell-to-cell communication in cancer growth, could become a contribution to the development of new therapeutic strategies, which could also be applicable in cancer. Moreover, determining the number of PEVs and their cargo becomes a useful diagnostic marker or prognostic factor for the different clinical stages in a variety of neoplasia. Knowledge about the formation of distinct PEVs types dependent on PLTs activators could lead to the development of specific techniques for PEVs-mediated drug delivery to cancer cells, or to TME, to modulate their immune response or angiogenesis.

Author Contributions: Conceptualization, M.Ż. and O.W.-P., Writing-Original Draft Preparation, M.Ż., O.W.-P.; Writing-Review & Editing, M.Ż., A.W. and O.W.-P. Supervision, M.Ż. All authors have read and agreed to the published version of the manuscript.

Funding: Support for this study was provided by NCN (National Science Centre, Poland) MINIATURA grant number 2017/01/X/NZ5/01481 for (M.Z.).

Conflicts of Interest: The authors declare no conflict of interest. The funders had no role in the design of the study; in the collection, analyses, or interpretation of data; in the writing of the manuscript; or in the decision to publish the results.

Abbreviations

ABs	apoptotic bodies
ALL	acute lymphoblastic leukemia
CD	cluster of differentiation
CCL	cancer cell line
CLEC-2	C-type lectin domain family 1-member B
ECTSMs	ectosomes
ESCRT	endosomal sorting complex required for transport
ESE	early sorting endosomes
EVs	extracellular vesicles
EXSMs	exosomes
HAECs	human aortic endothelial cells
HUVECs	human umbilical vein endothelial cells
ILVs	intraluminal vesicles
LA	lactadherin
LAMP-1	lysosome-associated glycoprotein-1
LPS	lipopolysaccharide
LXA4	lipoxin A4
MAPK	mitogen-activated protein kinase
Mk-EVs	EVs derived from megakaryocytes
MMP	metalloproteinase
MVBs	multivesicular bodies
MPs	microparticles
NSCLC	non-small cell lung cancer
OSCC	oral squamous cell carcinoma
PBMCs	peripheral blood mononuclear cells
PdEXSMs	platelet derived exosomes
PEVs	platelets extracellular vesicles
PLTs	platelets
PMPs	platelets microparticles
PUFAs	polyunsaturated fatty acids
RT	room temperature
TEVs	tumor derived extracellular vesicles
TF	tissue factor
TGF-β1	transforming growth factor beta 1
THBS-1	thrombospondin-1
TLR-4	toll-like receptor 4
TME	tumor microenvironment
TPM3	tropomyosin 3
VEGF	vascular endothelial growth factor
vWf	von Willebrand factor

References

1. Van Niel, G.; D'Angelo, G.; Raposo, G. Shedding light on the cell biology of extracellular vesicles. *Nat. Rev. Mol. Cell Biol.* **2018**, *4*, 213–228. [CrossRef]
2. Dauros Singorenko, P.; Chang, V.; Whitcombe, A.; Simonov, D.; Hong, J.; Phillips, A.; Swift, S.; Blenkiron, C. Isolation of membrane vesicles from prokaryotes: A technical and biological comparison reveals heterogeneity. *J. Extracell. Vesicles* **2017**, *1*, 1324731. [CrossRef] [PubMed]

3. Dovizio, M.; Bruno, A.; Contursi, A.; Grande, R.; Patrignani, P. Platelets and extracellular vesicles in cancer: Diagnostic and therapeutic implications. *Cancer Metastasis Rev.* **2018**, *37*, 455–467. [CrossRef] [PubMed]
4. Wojtukiewicz, M.Z.; Sierko, E.; Hempel, D.; Tucker, S.C.; Honn, K. Platelets and cancer angiogenesis nexus. *Cancer Metastasis Rev.* **2017**, *2*, 249–262. [CrossRef] [PubMed]
5. Navarro-Tableros, V.; Gomez, Y.; Camussi, G.; Brizzi, M.F. Extracellular vesicles: New players in lymphomas. *Int. J. Mol. Sci.* **2018**, *21*, 41. [CrossRef] [PubMed]
6. Lorenc, T.; Klimczyk, K.; Michalczewska, I.; Słomka, M.; Kubiak-Tomaszewska, G.; Olejarz, W. Exosomes in prostate cancer diagnosis, prognosis and therapy. *Int. J. Mol. Sci.* **2020**, *21*, 2118. [CrossRef]
7. Meldolesi, J. Extracellular vesicles, news about their role in immune cells: Physiology, pathology and diseases. *Clin. Exp. Immunol.* **2019**, *13*, 318–327. [CrossRef]
8. Stahl, P.D.; Raposo, G. Extracellular vesicles: Exosomes and microvesicles, integrators of homeostasis. *Physiology* **2019**, *3*, 169–177. [CrossRef]
9. Frydrychowicz, M.; Kolecka-Bednarczyk, A.; Madejczyk, M.; Yasar, S.; Dworacki, G. Exosomes—Structure, biogenesis and biological role in non-small-cell lung cancer. *Scand. J. Immunol.* **2015**, *81*, 2–10. [CrossRef]
10. Żmigrodzka, M.; Guzera, M.; Miśkiewicz, A.; Jagielski, D.; Winnicka, A. The biology of extracellular vesicles with focus on platelet microparticles and their role in cancer development and progression. *Tumour. Biol.* **2016**, *11*, 14391–14401. [CrossRef]
11. Van der Pol, E.; Böing, A.N.; Gool, E.L.; Nieuwland, R. Recent developments in the nomenclature, presence, isolation, detection and clinical impact of extracellular vesicles. *J. Thromb. Haemost.* **2016**, *14*, 48–56. [CrossRef] [PubMed]
12. Menck, K.; Bleckmann, A.; Wachter, A.; Hennies, B.; Ries, L.; Schulz, M.; Balkenhol, M.; Pukrop, T.; Schatlo, B.; Rost, U.; et al. Characterisation of tumour-derived microvesicles in cancer patients' blood and correlation with clinical outcome. *J. Extracell. Vesicles* **2017**, *1*, 1340745. [CrossRef] [PubMed]
13. Laroche, M.; Dunois, C.; Vissac, A.M.; Amiral, J. Update on functional and genetic laboratory assays for the detection of platelet microvesicles. *Platelets* **2017**, *3*, 235–241. [CrossRef] [PubMed]
14. Italiano, J.E., Jr.; Mairuhu, A.T.; Flaumenhaft, R. Clinical relevance of microparticles from platelets and megakaryocytes. *Curr. Opin. Hematol.* **2010**, *6*, 578–584. [CrossRef] [PubMed]
15. Berckmans, R.J.; Nieuwland, R.; Böing, A.N.; Romijn, F.P.; Hack, C.E.; Sturk, A. Cell-derived microparticles circulate in healthy humans and support low grade thrombin generation. *Thromb. Haemost.* **2001**, *4*, 639–646.
16. Wolf, P. The nature and significance of platelet products in human plasma. *Br. J. Haematol.* **1967**, *3*, 269–288. [CrossRef]
17. Melki, I.; Tessandier, N.; Zufferey, A.; Boilard, E. Platelet microvesicles in health and disease. *Platelets* **2017**, *3*, 214–221. [CrossRef]
18. Van der Pol, E.; Harrison, P. From platelet dust to gold dust: Physiological importance and detection of platelet microvesicles. *Platelets* **2017**, *3*, 211–213. [CrossRef]
19. Sinauridze, E.I.; Kireev, D.A.; Popenko, N.Y.; Pichugin, A.V.; Panteleev, M.A.; Krymskaya, O.V.; Ataullakhanov, F.I. Platelet microparticle membranes have 50- to 100-fold higher specific procoagulant activity than activated platelets. *Thromb. Haemost.* **2007**, *97*, 425–434.
20. Aatonen, M.; Grönholm, M.; Siljander, P.R. Platelet-derived microvesicles: Multitalented participants in intercellular communication. *Semin. Thromb. Hemost.* **2012**, *1*, 102–113. [CrossRef]
21. Zubairova, L.D.; Nabiullina, R.M.; Nagaswami, C.; Zuev, Y.F.; Mustafin, I.G.; Litvinov, R.I.; Weisel, J.W. Circulating microparticles alter formation, structure, and properties of fibrin clots. *Sci. Rep.* **2015**, *5*, 17611. [CrossRef] [PubMed]
22. Castaman, G.; Li, Y.-F.; Battistin, E.; Rodeghiero, F. Characterization of a novel bleeding disorder with isolated prolonged bleeding time and deficiency of platelet microvesicle generation. *Br. J. Haematol.* **1997**, *96*, 458–463. [CrossRef]
23. Chen, Y.; Xiao, Y.; Lin, Z.; Xiao, X.; He, C.; Bihl, J.C.; Zhao, B.; Ma, X.; Chen, Y. The role of circulating platelets microparticles and platelet parameters in acute ischemic stroke patients. *J. Stroke Cereb. Dis.* **2015**, *10*, 2313–2320. [CrossRef] [PubMed]
24. Álvarez-Román, M.T.; Fernández-Bello, I.; Jiménez-Yuste, V.; Martín-Salces, M.; Arias-Salgado, E.G.; Rivas Pollmar, M.I.; Justo Sanz, R.; Butta, N.V. Procoagulant profile in patients with immune thrombocytopenia. *Br. J. Haematol.* **2016**, *5*, 925–934. [CrossRef] [PubMed]

25. Kim, H.K.; Song, K.S.; Park, Y.S.; Kang, Y.H.; Lee, Y.J.; Lee, K.R.; Kim, H.K.; Ryu, K.W.; Bae, J.M.; Kim, S. Elevated levels of circulating platelet microparticles, VEGF, IL-6 and RANTES in patients with gastric cancer: Possible role of a metastasis predictor. *Eur. J. Cancer* **2003**, *2*, 184–191. [CrossRef]
26. Johnstone, R.M.; Adam, M.; Hammond, J.R.; Orr, L.; Turbide, C. Vesicle formation during reticulocyte maturation. Association of plasma membrane activities with released vesicles (exosomes). *J. Biol. Chem.* **1987**, *19*, 9412–9420.
27. Edelstein, L.C. The role of platelet microvesicles in intercellular communication. *Platelets* **2017**, *3*, 222–227. [CrossRef]
28. Schoenwaelder, S.M.; Yuan, Y.; Josefsson, E.C.; White, M.J.; Yao, Y.; Mason, K.D.; O'Reilly, L.A.; Henley, K.J.; Ono, A.; Hsiao, S.; et al. Two distinct pathways regulate platelet phosphatidylserine exposure and procoagulant function. *Blood* **2009**, *3*, 663–666. [CrossRef]
29. Dale, G.L.; Remenyi, G.; Friese, P. Tetraspanin CD9 is required for microparticle release from coated-platelets. *Platelets* **2009**, *20*, 361–366. [CrossRef]
30. Brisson, A.R.; Tan, S.; Linares, R.; Gounou, C.; Arraud, N. Extracellular vesicles from activated platelets: A semiquantitative cryo-electron microscopy and immuno-gold labeling study. *Platelets* **2017**, *3*, 263–271. [CrossRef]
31. Mashouri, L.; Yousefi, H.; Aref, A.R.; Ahadi, A.M.; Molaei, F.; Alahari, S.K. Exosomes: Composition, biogenesis, and mechanisms in cancer metastasis and drug resistance. *Mol. Cancer* **2019**, *75*. [CrossRef] [PubMed]
32. Meldolesi, J. Exosomes and ectosomes in intercellular communication. *Curr. Biol.* **2018**, *8*, R435–R444. [CrossRef] [PubMed]
33. Hessvik, N.P.; Llorente, A. Current knowledge on exosome biogenesis and release. *Cell Mol. Life Sci.* **2018**, *2*, 193–208. [CrossRef] [PubMed]
34. Catalano, M.; O'Driscoll, L. Inhibiting extracellular vesicles formation and release: A review of EV inhibitors. *J. Extracell. Vesicles* **2019**, *9*, 1703244. [CrossRef]
35. Wang, Y.; Zhang, S.; Luo, L.; Norstrom, E.; Braun, O.O.; Morgelin, M.; Thorlacius, H. Platelet-derived microparticles regulates thrombin generation via phophatidylserine in abdominal sepsis. *J. Cell Physiol.* **2018**, *2*, 1051–1060. [CrossRef]
36. Aatonen, M.T.; Ohman, T.; Nyman, T.A.; Laitinen, S.; Grönholm, M.; Siljander, P.R. Isolation and characterization of platelet-derived extracellular vesicles. *J. Extracell. Vesicles* **2014**. [CrossRef]
37. Lea, J.; Sharma, R.; Yang, F.; Zhu, H.; Ward, E.S.; Schroit, A.J. Detection of phosphatidylserine-positive exosomes as a diagnostic marker for ovarian malignancies: A proof of concept study. *Oncotarget* **2017**, *9*, 14395–14407. [CrossRef]
38. Rand, M.L.; Wang, H.; Bang, K.W.; Packham, M.A.; Freedman, J. Rapid clearance of procoagulant platelet-derived microparticles from the circulation of rabbits. *J. Thromb. Haemost.* **2006**, *7*, 1621–1623. [CrossRef]
39. Rank, A.; Nieuwland, R.; Crispin, A.; Grützner, S.; Iberer, M.; Toth, B.; Pihusch, R. Clearance of platelet microparticles in vivo. *Platelets* **2011**, *2*, 111–116. [CrossRef]
40. Flaumenhaft, R. Formation and fate of platelet microparticles. *Blood Cells Mol. Dis.* **2006**, *2*, 182–187. [CrossRef]
41. Abdel-Monem, H.; Dasgupta, S.K.; Le, A.; Prakasam, A.; Thiagarajan, P. Phagocytosis of platelet microvesicles and beta2- glycoprotein I. *Thromb. Haemost.* **2010**, *2*, 335–341.
42. Dasgupta, S.K.; Le, A.; Chavakis, T.; Rumbaut, R.E.; Thiagarajan, P. Developmental endothelial locus-1 (Del-1) mediates clearance of platelet microparticles by the endothelium. *Circulation* **2012**, *13*, 1664–1672. [CrossRef] [PubMed]
43. Record, M.; Silvente-Poirot, S.; Poirot, M.; Wakelam, M.J.O. Extracellular vesicles: Lipids as key components of their biogenesis and functions. *J. Lipid. Res.* **2018**, *8*, 1316–1324. [CrossRef] [PubMed]
44. Charoenviriyakul, C.; Takahashi, Y.; Morishita, M.; Matsumoto, A.; Nishikawa, M.; Takakura, Y. Cell type-specific and common characteristics of exosomes derived from mouse cell lines: Yield, physicochemical properties, and pharmacokinetics. *Eur. J. Pharm. Sci.* **2017**, *1*, 316–322. [CrossRef]
45. Wisgrill, L.; Lamm, C.; Hartmann, J.; Preiβing, F.; Dragostis, K.; Bee, A.; Hell, L.; Thaler, J.; Ay, C.; Pabinger, I.; et al. Peripheral blood microvesicles secretion is influenced by storage time, temperature, and anticoagulants. *Cytometry A* **2016**, *7*, 663–672. [CrossRef]

46. Flaumenhaft, R.; Dilks, J.R.; Richardson, J.; Alden, E.; Patel-Hett, S.R.; Battinelli, E.; Klement, G.L.; Sola-Visner, M.; Italiano, J.E., Jr. Megakaryocyte-derived microparticles: Direct visualization and distinction from platelet-derived microparticles. *Blood* **2009**, *5*, 1112–1121. [CrossRef]
47. Vajen, T.; Mause, S.F.; Koenen, R.R. Microvesicles from platelets: Novel drivers of vascular inflammation. *Thromb. Haemost.* **2015**, *2*, 228–236. [CrossRef]
48. Rank, A.; Nieuwland, R.; Delker, R.; Kohler, A.; Toth, B.; Pihusch, V. Cellular origin of platelet-derived microparticles In Vivo. *Thromb. Res.* **2010**, *126*, e255–e259. [CrossRef]
49. Heijnen, H.F.; Schiel, A.E.; Fijnheer, R.; Geuze, H.J.; Sixma, J.J. Activated platelets release two types of membrane vesicles: Microvesicles by surface shedding and exosomes derived from exocytosis of multivesicular bodies and alpha-granules. *Blood* **1999**, *11*, 3791–3799. [CrossRef]
50. Dean, W.L.; Lee, M.J.; Cummins, T.D.; Schultz, D.J.; Powell, D.W. Proteomic and functional characterisation of platelet microparticle size classes. *Thromb. Haemost.* **2009**, *102*, 711–718. [CrossRef]
51. Menter, D.G.; Kanikarla-Marie, P.; Lam, M.; Davis, J.S.; Kopetz, S. Platelet microparticles: Small payloads with profound effects on tumor growth. *Noncoding RNA Investig.* **2017**, *15*. [CrossRef] [PubMed]
52. Sadallah, S.; Eken, C.; Martin, P.J.; Schifferli, J.A. Microparticles (ectosomes) shed by stored human platelets downregulate macrophages and modify the development of dendritic cells. *J. Immunol.* **2011**, *11*, 6543–6552. [CrossRef] [PubMed]
53. Falati, S.; Liu, Q.; Gross, P.; Merrill-Skoloff, G.; Chou, J.; Vandendries, E.; Celi, A.; Croce, K.; Furie, B.C.; Furie, B. Accumulation of tissue factor into developing thrombi in vivo is dependent upon microparticle Pselectin glycoprotein ligand 1 and platelet P-selectin. *J. Exp. Med.* **2003**, *11*, 1585–1598. [CrossRef] [PubMed]
54. Diamant, M.; Nieuwland, R.; Pablo, R.F.; Sturk, A.; Smit, J.W.; Radder, J.K. Elevated numbers of tissue-factor exposing microparticles correlate with components of the metabolic syndrome in uncomplicated type 2 diabetes mellitus. *Circulation* **2002**, *19*, 2442–2447. [CrossRef]
55. Tang, K.; Liu, J.; Yang, Z.; Zhang, B.; Zhang, H.; Huang, C.; Ma, J.; Shen, G.X.; Ye, D.; Huang, B. Microparticles mediate enzyme transfer from platelets to mast cells: A new pathway for lipoxin a4 biosynthesis. *Biochem. Biophys. Res. Commun.* **2010**, *3*, 432–436. [CrossRef]
56. Kailashiya, J.; Gupta, V.; Dash, D. Engineered human platelet-derived microparticles as natural vectors for targeted drug delivery. *Oncotarget* **2019**, *56*, 5835–5846. [CrossRef]
57. Baj-Krzyworzeka, M.; Majka, M.; Pratico, D.; Ratajczak, J.; Vilaire, G.; Kijowski, J.; Reca, R.; Janowska-Wieczorek, A.; Ratajczak, M.Z. Platelet-derived microparticles stimulate proliferation, survival, adhesion, and chemotaxis of hematopoietic cells. *Exp. Hematol.* **2002**, *5*, 450–459. [CrossRef]
58. Gelderman, M.P.; Simak, J. Flow cytometric analysis of cell membrane microparticles. *Methods Mol. Biol.* **2008**, *484*, 79–93.
59. Abid, H.M.N.; Meesters, E.W.; Osmanovic, N.; Romijn, F.P.; Nieuwland, R.; Sturk, A. Antigenic characterization of endothelial cellderived microparticles and their detection ex vivo. *J. Thromb. Haemost.* **2003**, *11*, 2434–2443. [CrossRef]
60. Thiagarajan, P.; Tait, J.F. Collagen-induced exposure of anionic phospholipid in platelets and platelet-derived microparticles. *J. Biol. Chem.* **1991**, *36*, 24302–24307.
61. Rozmyslowicz, T.; Majka, M.; Kijowski, J.; Murphy, S.L.; Conover, D.O.; Poncz, M.; Ratajczak, J.; Gaulton, G.N.; Ratajczak, M.Z. Platelet- and megakaryocyte-derived microparticles transfer CXCR4 receptor to CXCR4-null cells and make them susceptible to infection by X4-HIV. *AIDS* **2003**, *1*, 33–42. [CrossRef] [PubMed]
62. Gasperi, W.; Vangapandu, C.; Savini, I.; Ventimiglia, G.; Adoro, G.; Catani, M.V. Polyunsaturated fatty acids modulate the delivery of platelet microvesicle-derived microRNAs into human breast cancer cell lines. *J. Nutr. Biochem.* **2019**, *74*, 108242. [CrossRef] [PubMed]
63. Gilbert, G.E.; Sims, P.J.; Wiedmer, T.; Furie, B.; Furie, B.C.; Shattil, S.J. Platelet-derivedmicroparticles express high affinity receptors for factor VIII. *J. Biol. Chem.* **1991**, *26*, 17261–17268.
64. Brill, A.; Dashevsky, O.; Rivo, J.; Gozal, Y.; Varon, D. Platelet-derived microparticles induce angiogenesis and stimulate post-ischemic revascularization. *Cardiovasc. Res.* **2005**, *1*, 30–38. [CrossRef]
65. Fox, J.E.; Austin, C.D.; Boyles, J.K.; Steffen, P.K. Role of the membrane skeleton in preventing the shedding of procoagulant-rich microvesicles from the platelet plasma membrane. *J. Cell Biol.* **1990**, *2*, 483–493. [CrossRef] [PubMed]

66. Podor, T.J.; Singh, D.; Chindemi, P.; Foulon, D.M.; McKelvie, R.; Weitz, J.I.; Austin, R.; Boudreau, G.; Davies, R. Vimentin exposed on activated platelets and platelet microparticles localizes vitronectin and plasminogen activator inhibitor complexes on their surface. *J. Biol. Chem.* **2002**, *9*, 7529–7539. [CrossRef]
67. Barry, O.P.; Praticò, D.; Savani, R.C.; FitzGerald, G.A. Modulation of monocyte-endothelial cell interactions by platelet microparticles. *J. Clin. Investig.* **1998**, *1*, 136–144. [CrossRef]
68. Barry, O.P.; Kazanietz, M.G.; Praticò, D.; FitzGerald, G.A. Arachidonic acid in platelet microparticles up-regulates cyclooxygenase-2-dependent prostaglandin formation via a protein kinase C/mitogen-activated protein kinase-dependent pathway. *J. Biol. Chem.* **1999**, *11*, 7545–7556. [CrossRef]
69. Boilard, E.; Nigrovic, P.A.; Larabee, K.; Watts, G.F.M.; Coblyn, J.S.; Weinblatt, M.E.; Massarotti, E.M.; Remold-O'Donnell, E.; Farndale, R.W.; Ware, J.; et al. Platelets amplify inflammation in arthritis via collagen-dependent microparticle production. *Science* **2010**, *5965*, 580–583. [CrossRef]
70. Sims, P.J.; Faioni, E.M.; Wiedmer, T.; Shattil, S.J. Complement proteins C5b-9 cause release of membrane vesicles from the platelet surface that are enriched in the membrane receptor for coagulation factor Va and express prothrombinase activity. *J. Biol. Chem.* **1988**, *34*, 18205–18212.
71. Raturi, A.; Miersch, S.; Hudson, J.W.; Mutus, B. Platelet microparticleassociated protein disulfide isomerase promotes platelet aggregation and inactivates insulin. *Biochim. Biophys. Acta* **2008**, *12*, 2790–2796. [CrossRef] [PubMed]
72. Böing, A.N.; Hau, C.M.; Sturk, A.; Nieuwland, R. Platelet microparticles contain active caspase 3. *Platelets* **2008**, *19*, 96–103. [CrossRef] [PubMed]
73. Mause, S.F.; von Hundelshausen, P.; Zernecke, A.; Koenen, R.R.; Weber, C. Platelet microparticles: A transcellular delivery system for RANTES promoting monocyte recruitment on endothelium. *Arter. Thromb. Vasc. Biol.* **2005**, *7*, 1512–1518. [CrossRef] [PubMed]
74. Maroney, S.A.; Haberichter, S.L.; Friese, P.; Collins, M.L.; Ferrel, J.P.; Dale, G.L.; Mast, A.E. Active tissue factor pathway inhibitor is expressed on the surface of coated platelets. *Blood* **2007**, *5*, 1931–1937. [CrossRef] [PubMed]
75. Gambim, M.H.; do Carmo, A.; Marti, L.; Veríssimo-Filho, S.; Lopes, L.R.; Janiszewski, M. Platelet-derived exosomes induce endothelial cell apoptosis through peroxynitrite generation: Experimental evidence for a novel mechanism of septic vascular dysfunction. *Crit. Care* **2007**, *5*, R107. [CrossRef] [PubMed]
76. Pfister, S.L. Role of platelet microparticles in the production of thromboxane by rabbit pulmonary artery. *Hypertension* **2004**, *2*, 428–433. [CrossRef]
77. Salanova, B.; Choi, M.; Rolle, S.; Wellner, M.; Luft, F.C.; Kettritz, R. Beta2-integrins and acquired glycoprotein IIb/IIIa (GPIIb/IIIa) receptors cooperate in NF-kappaB activation of human neutrophils. *J. Biol. Chem.* **2007**, *38*, 27960–27969. [CrossRef]
78. Kim, H.K.; Song, K.S.; Chung, J.H.; Lee, K.R.; Lee, S.N. Platelet microparticles induce angiogenesis in vitro. *Br. J. Haematol.* **2004**, *3*, 376–384. [CrossRef]
79. Saber, S.H.; Ali, H.E.A.; Gaballa, R.; Gaballah, M.; Ali, H.I.; Zerfaoui, M.; Abd Elmageed, Z.Y. Exosomes are the driving force in preparing the soil for the metastatic seeds: Lessons from the prostate cancer. *Cells* **2020**, *3*, 564. [CrossRef]
80. Doyle, L.M.; Wang, M.Z. Overview of extracellular vesicles, their origin, composition, purpose, and methods for exosome isolation and analysis. *Cells* **2019**, *7*, 727. [CrossRef]
81. Nishida, N.; Yano, H.; Nishida, T.; Kamura, T.; Kojiro, M. Angiogenesis in cancer. *Vasc. Health Risk Manag.* **2006**, *3*, 213–219. [CrossRef] [PubMed]
82. Happonen, K.E.; Tran, S.; Mörgelin, M.; Prince, R.; Calzavarini, S.; Angelillo-Scherrer, A.; Dählback, B. The Gas6-Axl protein interaction mediates endothelial uptake of platelet microparticles. *J. Biol. Chem.* **2016**, *20*, 10586–10601. [CrossRef] [PubMed]
83. Janowska-Wieczorek, A.; Wysoczynski, M.; Kijowski, J.; Marquez-Curtis, L.; Machalinski, B.; Ratajczak, J.; Ratajczak, M.Z. Microvesicles derived from activated platelets induce metastasis and angiogenesis in lung cancer. *Int. J. Cancer* **2005**, *5*, 752–760. [CrossRef] [PubMed]
84. Michael, J.V.; Wurtzel, J.G.T.; Mao, G.F.; Rao, A.K.; Kolpakov, M.A.; Sabri, A.; Hoffman, N.E.; Rajan, S.; Tomar, D.; Madesh, M.; et al. Platelet microparticles infiltrating solid tumors transfer miRNAs that suppress tumor growth. *Blood* **2017**, *5*, 567–580. [CrossRef]
85. Anene, C.; Graham, A.M.; Boyne, J.; Roberts, W. Platelet microparticle delivered microRNA-Let-7a promotes the angiogenic switch. *Biochim. Biophys. Acta Mol. Basis Dis.* **2018**, *8*, 2633–2643. [CrossRef]

86. Lazar, S.; Goldfinger, L.E. Platelet microparticles and miRNA transfer in cancer progression: Many targets, modes of action, and effects across cancer stages. *Front. Cardiovasc. Med.* **2018**, *5*, 13. [CrossRef]
87. Pan, Y.; Liang, H.; Liu, H.; Li, D.; Chen, X.; Li, L.; Zhang, C.Y.; Zen, K. Platelet-secreted microRNA-223 promotes endothelial cell apoptosis induced by advanced glycation end products via targeting the insulin-like growth factor 1 receptor. *J. Immunol.* **2014**, *1*, 437–446. [CrossRef]
88. Laffont, B.; Corduan, A.; Rousseau, M.; Duchez, A.C.; Lee, C.H.C.; Boilard, E.; Provost, P. Platelet microparticles reprogram macrophage gene expression and function. *Thromb. Haemost.* **2016**, *2*, 311–323.
89. Bakewell, S.J.; Nestor, P.; Prasad, S.; Tomasson, M.H.; Dowland, N.; Mehrorta, M.; Scarborough, R.; Kanter, J.; Abe, K.; Phillips, D.; et al. Platelet and osteoclast beta3 integrins are critical for bone metastasis. *Proc. Natl. Acad. Sci. USA* **2003**, *24*, 14205–14210. [CrossRef]
90. Liu, S.C.; Bassi, D.E.; Zhang, S.Y.; Holoran, D.; Conti, C.J.; Klein-Szanto, A.J. Overexpression of cyclin D2 is associated with increased in vivo invasiveness of human squamous carcinoma cells. *Mol. Carcinog.* **2002**, *3*, 131–139. [CrossRef]
91. Shahidi, F.; Ambigaipalan, P. Omega-3 polyunsaturated fatty acids and their health benefits. *Ann. Rev. Food Sci. Technol.* **2018**, *9*, 345–381. [CrossRef] [PubMed]
92. Shi, L.; Fisslthaler, B.; Zippel, N.; Frömel, T.; Hu, J.; Elgheznawy, A.; Heide, H.; Popp, R.; Fleming, I. MicroRNA-223 antagonizes angiogenesis by targeting β1 integrin and preventing growth factor signaling in endothelial cells. *Circ. Res.* **2013**, *113*, 1320–1330. [CrossRef] [PubMed]
93. Tang, M.L.; Jiang, L.; Lin, Y.Y.; Wu, X.L.; Wang, K.; He, Q.Z.; Wang, X.P.; Li, W.P. Platelet microparticle mediated transfer of miR-939 to epithelial ovarian cancer cells promotes epithelial to mesenchymal transition. *Oncotarget* **2017**, *8*, 97464–97475. [CrossRef] [PubMed]
94. Yao, B.; Qu, S.; Hu, R.; Gao, W.; Jin, S.; Ju, J.; Zhao, Q. Delivery of platelet TPM3 mRNA into breast cancer cells via microvesicles enhances metastasis. *FEBS Open Biol.* **2019**, *12*, 2159–2169. [CrossRef] [PubMed]
95. Yu, S.B.; Gao, Q.; Lin, W.W.; Kang, M.Q. Proteomic analysis indicates the importance of TPM3 in esophageal squamous cell carcinoma invasion and metastasis. *Mol. Med. Rep.* **2017**, *15*, 1236–1242. [CrossRef] [PubMed]
96. Zarà, M.; Guidetti, G.F.; Boselli, D.; Villa, C.; Canobbio, I.; Seppi, C.; Visconte, C.; Canio, J.; Torti, M. Release of prometastatic platelet-derived microparticles induced by breast cancer cells: A novel positive feedback mechanism for metastasis. *TH Open* **2017**, *2*, e155–e163. [CrossRef]
97. Burnouf, T.; Goubran, H.A.; Chou, M.L.; Devos, D.; Radosevic, M. Platelet microparticles: Detection and assessment of their paradoxical functional roles in disease and regenerative medicine. *Blood Rev.* **2014**, *4*, 155–166. [CrossRef]
98. Vasina, E.M.; Cauwenberghs, S.; Feijge, M.A.; Heemskerk, J.W.; Weber, C.; Koenen, R.R. Microparticles from apoptotic platelets promote resident macrophage differentiation. *Cell Death Dis.* **2011**, *9*, e211. [CrossRef]
99. Li, J.; Guo, Y.; Liang, X.; Sun, M.; Wang, G.; De, W.; Wu, W. MicroRNA-223 functions as an oncogene in human gastric cancer by targeting FBXW7/hCdc4. *J. Cancer Res. Clin. Oncol.* **2012**, *5*, 763–774. [CrossRef]
100. Yaftian, M.; Yari, F.; Ghasemzadeh, M.; Fallah, A.V.; Haghighi, M. Induction of apoptosis in cancer cells of pre-B ALL patients after exposure to platelets, platelet-derived microparticles and soluble CD40 ligand. *Cell J.* **2018**, *1*, 120–126.
101. Dashevsky, O.; Varon, D.; Brill, A. Platelet-derived microparticles promote invasiveness of prostate cancer cells via upregulation of MMP-2 production. *Int. J. Cancer* **2009**, *8*, 1773–1777. [CrossRef] [PubMed]
102. Sadallah, S.; Schmied, L.; Eken, C.; Charoudeh, H.N.; Amicarella, F.; Schifferli, J.A. Platelet-derived ectosomes reduce NK cell function. *J. Immunol.* **2016**, *5*, 1663–1671. [CrossRef] [PubMed]
103. Laffont, B.; Corduan, A.; Plé, H.; Duchez, A.C.; Cloutier, N.; Boilard, E.; Provost, P. Activated platelets can deliver mRNA regulatory Ago2 microRNA complexes to endothelial cells via microparticles. *Blood* **2013**, *2*, 253–261. [CrossRef] [PubMed]
104. Park, M.; Kang, K.W. Phosphatidylserine receptor-targeting therapies for the treatment of cancer. *Arch. Pharm. Res.* **2019**, *7*, 617–628. [CrossRef] [PubMed]
105. Li, B.; Antonyak, M.A.; Zhang, J.; Cerione, R.A. RhoA triggers a specific signaling pathway that generates transforming microvesicles in cancer cells. *Oncogene* **2012**, *45*, 4740–4749. [CrossRef]
106. Zhang, W.; Qi, J.; Zhao, S.; Shen, W.; Dai, L.; Han, W.; Huang, M.; Wang, Z.; Ruan, C.; Wu, D.; et al. Clinical significance of circulating microparticles in Ph- myeloproliferative neoplasms. *Oncol. Lett.* **2017**, *2*, 2531–2536. [CrossRef]

107. Ren, J.G.; Man, Q.W.; Zhang, W.; Li, C.; Xiong, X.P.; Zhu, J.Y.; Wang, W.M.; Sun, Z.J.; Jia, J.; Zhang, W.F.; et al. Elevated level of circulating platelet-derived microparticles in oral cancer. *J. Dent. Res.* **2016**, *1*, 87–93. [CrossRef]
108. Dymicka-Piekarska, V.; Gryko, M.; Lipska, A.; Korniluk, A.; Siergiejko, E.; Kemona, H. Platelet-derived microparticles in patients with colorectal cancer. *J. Cancer Ther.* **2012**, *6*, 898–901. [CrossRef]
109. Wang, C.C.; Tseng, C.C.; Chang, H.C.; Huang, K.T.; Fang, W.F.; Chen, Y.M.; Yang, C.T.; Hsiao, C.C.; Lin, M.C.; Ho, C.K.; et al. Circulating microparticles are prognostic biomarkers in advanced non-small cell lung cancer patients. *Oncotarget* **2017**, *44*, 75952–75967. [CrossRef]
110. Mege, D.; Panicot-Dubois, L.; Ouaissi, M.; Robert, S.; Sielezneff, I.; Sastre, B.; Digant-George, F.; Dubois, C. The origin and concentration of circulating microparticles differ according to cancer type and evolution: A prospective single-center study. *Int. J. Cancer* **2016**, *4*, 939–948. [CrossRef]
111. Yenigürbüz, F.D.; Kızmazoğlu, D.; Ateş, H.; Erdem, M.; Tufekci, O.; Yilmaz, S.; Oren, H. Analysis of apoptotic, platelet-derived, endothelial-derived, and tissue factor-positive microparticles of children with acute lymphoblastic leukemia during induction therapy. *Blood Coagul. Fibrinolysis* **2019**, *4*, 149–155. [CrossRef] [PubMed]
112. Ball, S.; Nugent, K. Microparticles in Hematological Malignancies: Role in Coagulopathy and Tumor Pathogenesis. *Am. J. Med. Sci.* **2018**, *3*, 207–214. [CrossRef] [PubMed]
113. Tjon-Kon-Fat, L.A.; Lundholm, M.; Schroder, M.; Wurdinger, T.; Thellenberg-Karlsson, C.; Widmark, A.; Wikstrom, P.; Nilsson, R.J.A. Platelets harbor prostate cancer biomarkers and the ability to predict therapeutic response to abiraterone in castration resistant patients. *Prostate* **2018**, *1*, 48–53. [CrossRef] [PubMed]
114. Boerrigter, E.; Groen, L.N.; Van Erp, N.P.; Verhaegh, G.W.; Schalken, J.A. Clinical utility of emerging biomarkers in prostate cancer liquid biopsies. *Expert Rev. Mol. Diagn.* **2020**, *2*, 219–230. [CrossRef]
115. Tarasov, V.V.; Svistunov, A.A.; Chubarev, V.N. Extracellular vesicles in cancer nanomedicine. *Semin. Cancer Biol.* **2019**. [CrossRef]
116. Wiklander, O.P. Extracellular vesicle in vivo biodistribution is determined by cell source, route of administration and targeting. *J. Extracell. Vesicles* **2015**, *4*, 26316. [CrossRef]
117. Dilsiz, N. Role of exosomes and exosomal microRNAs in cancer. *Future Sci. OA* **2020**, *4*, FSO465. [CrossRef]
118. Zhao, X.; Wu, D.; Ma, X.; Wang, J.; Hou, W.; Zhang, W. Exosomes as drug carriers for cancer therapy and challenges regarding exosome uptake. *Biomed. Pharmacother.* **2020**, *128*, 110237. [CrossRef]

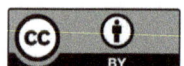

© 2020 by the authors. Licensee MDPI, Basel, Switzerland. This article is an open access article distributed under the terms and conditions of the Creative Commons Attribution (CC BY) license (http://creativecommons.org/licenses/by/4.0/).

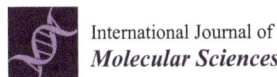

Review

Exploiting Manipulated Small Extracellular Vesicles to Subvert Immunosuppression at the Tumor Microenvironment through Mannose Receptor/CD206 Targeting

Maria Luisa Fiani *, Valeria Barreca, Massimo Sargiacomo, Flavia Ferrantelli, Francesco Manfredi and Maurizio Federico *

National Center for Global Health, Istituto Superiore di Sanità, 00161 Rome, Italy; barrecavaleria@gmail.com (V.B.); massimo.sargiacomo@iss.it (M.S.); flavia.ferrantelli@iss.it (F.F.); francesco.manfredi@iss.it (F.M.)
* Correspondence: maria.fiani@iss.it (M.L.F.); maurizio.federico@iss.it (M.F.); Tel.: +39-06-4990-2518 (M.L.F.); +39-06-4990-6016 (M.F.)

Received: 6 July 2020; Accepted: 27 August 2020; Published: 31 August 2020

Abstract: Immunosuppression at tumor microenvironment (TME) is one of the major obstacles to be overcome for an effective therapeutic intervention against solid tumors. Tumor-associated macrophages (TAMs) comprise a sub-population that plays multiple pro-tumoral roles in tumor development including general immunosuppression, which can be identified in terms of high expression of mannose receptor (MR or CD206). Immunosuppressive TAMs, like other macrophage sub-populations, display functional plasticity that allows them to be re-programmed to inflammatory macrophages. In order to mitigate immunosuppression at the TME, several efforts are ongoing to effectively re-educate pro-tumoral TAMs. Extracellular vesicles (EVs), released by both normal and tumor cells types, are emerging as key mediators of the cell to cell communication and have been shown to have a role in the modulation of immune responses in the TME. Recent studies demonstrated the enrichment of high mannose glycans on the surface of small EVs (sEVs), a subtype of EVs of endosomal origin of 30–150 nm in diameter. This characteristic renders sEVs an ideal tool for the delivery of therapeutic molecules into MR/CD206-expressing TAMs. In this review, we report the most recent literature data highlighting the critical role of TAMs in tumor development, as well as the experimental evidences that has emerged from the biochemical characterization of sEV membranes. In addition, we propose an original way to target immunosuppressive TAMs at the TME by endogenously engineered sEVs for a new therapeutic approach against solid tumors.

Keywords: tumor-associated macrophages; tumor microenvironment; macrophage polarization; mannose receptor; exosomes; extracellular vesicles; HIV-1 Nef

1. Introduction

Both immunosuppression and genetic escape are formidable weapons through which tumors can elude host immune surveillance. Solid tumors develop in a quite complex context, referred to as tumor microenvironment (TME) [1,2], which is composed of both cellular and non-cellular elements, usually resulting in an immunosuppressive behavior. Counteracting such a general effect would favor both spontaneous and therapeutic anti-tumor immunity, hence critically contributing to control tumor cell growth. Therefore, subverting TME immunosuppression represents a major goal for anticancer immunotherapies.

Both normal and tumor cells constitutively release membrane-bilayered vesicles, commonly referred to as extracellular vesicles (EVs) [3,4]. They differ in the mechanisms of biogenesis and secretion, giving rise to the generation of a heterogeneous population of vesicles with different sizes and contents [5,6], which include small EVs (sEVs) or exosomes and microvesicles or ectosomes. Exosomes are vesicles of 30–150 nm diameter generated by inward budding of endosomal membranes to form intraluminal vesicles that accumulate in intracellular organelles called multivesicular bodies (MVBs). MVBs ultimately fuse with the plasma membrane, thereby releasing intraluminal vesicles into the extracellular environment (Figure 1). On the contrary, ectosomes are 100–500 nm vesicles shed by direct budding from the plasma membrane [7,8]. Different types of EVs often show overlapping features that make difficult to obtain relatively pure preparations when purified from cell-conditioned media or biological fluids. In this review, we will use the term sEV to refer to EV types co-isolated by typical purification methods and exosomes to distinguish EV whose subcellular biogenesis strictly derives from multivesicular bodies/endosomes [8].

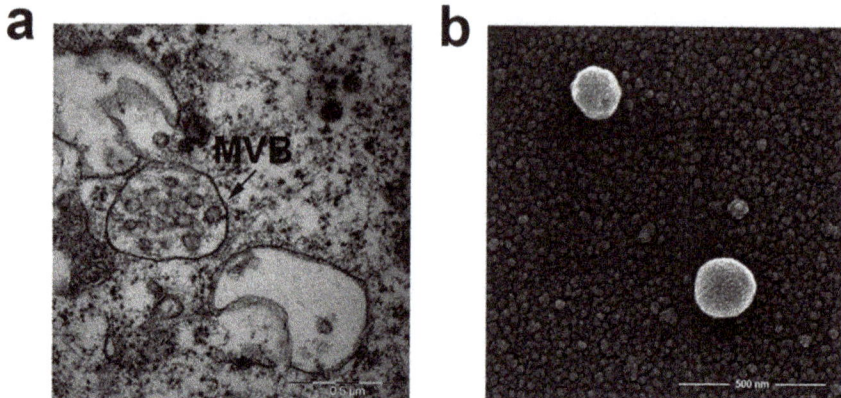

Figure 1. Electron microscopy of multivesicular bodies (MVB) and small extracellular vesicles (sEVs) (**a**) TEM micrograph of multivesicular bodies with intraluminal vesicles in Mel501, a melanoma cell line (**b**) SEM (Scanning Electron Microscope). Micrograph of sEVs purified from conditioned medium of Mel501 cells by differential centrifugations. Courtesy of Francesca Iosi and the Microscopy Area of the ISS Core Facilities.

SEVs carry a complex cargo of nucleic acids, proteins, and lipids that largely reflects the characteristics and the functional state of the cells they originate from, and that will be delivered to neighboring or distant cells [9,10]. As a result, the functions of those recipient cells will be modulated by sEVs in a manner that is strictly dependent on the nature of producer cells, making sEVs central players in intercellular communication and reprogramming of target cells [11]. Ectosomes generation is a much less known process that requires the accumulation of their cargo at the cytosolic surface of specific plasma membrane microdomains [7,12].

SEVs-mediated transfer of molecular and genetic material from one cell to another, either locally or at long distance, is a key contributor to the mechanisms of intercellular communication involved in various physiological and pathological conditions [13–15]. Moreover, for these reasons, sEVs are now considered powerful tools for clinical applications, including advanced diagnostics, therapeutics, and regenerative medicine [16–19].

The molecular composition of sEVs is determined by the cell type of origin as well as by the intracellular pathway followed en route to their release into the extracellular space [8,20,21]. This heterogeneity confers to sEVs distinct properties, such as tropism to certain organs, and uptake by specific cell types. In the case of tumor-derived sEVs, these events often lead to the impairment of immune responses at TME [22], also favoring pre-metastatic niche formation and metastasis [23,24].

In tumor cells, sEV biogenesis and ultimately sEV composition is a complex and regulated process, which involves many different molecules associated with the sEV biogenesis pathway [4,25].

Whatever the cell type of origin, sEVs can be characterized, although not exclusively, by the presence of different types of cell surface proteins, such as tetraspanins, (i.e., CD9, CD81, CD63), ESCRT (endosomal sorting complex required for transport) proteins (Alix and TSG101), integrins, RNA, DNA, lipids such as ceramide and the atypical phospholipid, lysobisphosphatidic acid (LBPA) [26], and oligosaccharides [27].

TME exerts a key influence on tumor cells, and the resulting sEVs, responsible for proteins and genetic material transfer from primary tumor cells, play a crucial role in metastatic colonization and in the formation of the pre-metastatic niche, driving recipient cells to acquire a pro-tumorigenic phenotype [23,28]. The selective conditions present in TME, such as the generation of a hypoxic [29] and acidic environment [30], strongly influence sEV secretion by tumor cells, thus contributing to the malignant tumor phenotype. Furthermore, sEV membrane composition reflects TME changes and conceivably influence and control the different mechanisms of entry or interaction of sEVs with target cells supporting tumor growth [31,32].

Interestingly, it has been described that major players of immunosuppression at the TME, i.e., immunosuppressive tumor-associated macrophages (TAMs), express on their surface high levels of mannose receptor (MR, CD206) [33]. The MR is an endocytic receptor with a high affinity for high mannose oligosaccharides, glycans highly enriched on the surface of sEVs [34]. In this review, literature data regarding both TAM functions and the molecular structure of sEVs are reviewed. In addition, we propose an original way to exploit typical molecular signatures of both TAMs and sEVs to counteract the immunosuppression at the TME.

2. The Tumor Microenvironment

In solid tumors, cancer cells are embedded within a milieu that favors their proliferation and comprises both cellular and non-cellular components. Fibroblasts, endothelial cells, and essentially all types of immune cells are part of the TME [35,36]. Among non-cellular components, tumor-derived sEVs play a key role in immune suppression. TME composition can vary among different tumors, and between primary and metastatic neo-formations in the same patient, and is tightly associated with the clinical outcome of cancer patients.

TMEs can be categorized based on different criteria. In terms of abundance of tumor-infiltrating cytotoxic CD8+ T lymphocytes (CTLs), TMEs can be distinguished in either hot/inflamed, with the highest content of CTLs, or cold/desert, with a virtual absence of infiltrated CTLs [37]. TME core infiltrated by CTLs represents a favorable condition for an effective anticancer immune response, both spontaneous and induced by immunotherapeutic interventions.

TME is populated by different kinds of immune cells having immune suppressive actions. Among these are myeloid-derived suppressor cells, neutrophils, CD4+ Treg lymphocytes, and immunosuppressive M2-like TAMs [38]. These latter cells can represent up to 50% of the tumor mass, and play a key role in the immune evasion at TME by secreting proteases, angiogenic factors, and pro-tumoral products. The functional plasticity of TAMs modifies their phenotype and activity in response to a great number of microenvironmental stimuli, although the mechanisms that determine the different polarization states are still to be elucidated [39]. These different functional states often coexist and can significantly vary between different tumors [40,41]. TAMs can also dispose at the tumor margin, where they can interact with CTLs, thus inhibiting their infiltration towards tumor cells [42]. For all these reasons, immunosuppressive TAMs have been identified as a major cell target for novel designs of cancer immunotherapies focused on improving the overall anti-tumor immune response. A schematic representation of cells populating TEM is illustrated in Figure 2.

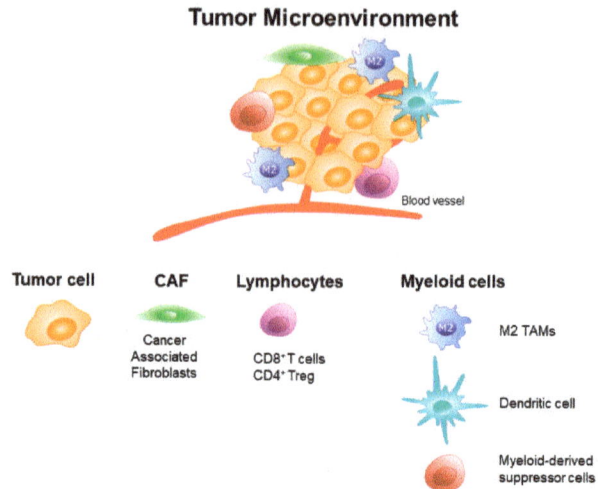

Figure 2. Schematic representation of cells populating the tumor microenvironment (TME).

3. The TAM-Mediated Immunosuppression at the TME

A large number of macrophages infiltrate solid tumors, thereby influencing several aspects of tumor development [43]. The most relevant effects include suppression of anticancer immunity, angiogenesis promotion, and support for metastasis. Macrophages are recruited at TME, in response to the secretion by tumor cells and other TME cell types, of a number of chemoattractant soluble factors, including vascular-endothelial growth factor A (VEGF-A) [44], chemokine ligand 2 (CCL2) [45], and colony-stimulating factor 1 (CSF-1) [46].

TME-populating macrophages can be schematically distinguished in M1- and M2-like macrophages. M1-like macrophages show both pro-inflammatory and immune-stimulatory properties, thus exerting an anti-tumor function. On the other hand, M2-like macrophages favor tumor angiogenesis and immunosuppression. Such a distinction, although useful from both therapeutic and diagnostic points of view, is now outdated, due to the identification of a large number of intermediate subclasses, i.e., up to 19 [47]. They have been identified through most recent transcriptomic techniques, e.g., single-cell mass cytometry and single-cell RNA sequencing [48–50], and in vivo represent a continuum of functional phenotypes with intermediates showing overlapping features.

TAMs can be characterized by the expression of different surface markers [47,51], distinct metabolic changes [52,53], and a broad transcriptional repertoire with the involvement of key transcription factors, which can be activated by the environmental signals received. In particular, members of the signal transducer and activator of transcription (STAT), peroxisome proliferator-activated receptors (PPARs), interferon regulatory factor (IRF), and nuclear transcription factor-κB (NF-κB) families are essential for macrophage polarization toward the M1 profile [41,54,55].

M2-like TAMs contribute to tumor angiogenesis by secreting soluble factors inducing endothelial cell proliferation, including VEGF-A, interleukin (IL)-1β, IL-6, tumor necrosis factor (TNF)α, CXCL8, and fibroblast growth factor (FGF)-2 [56]. In particular, the secretion of VEGF-A by perivascular TAMs can increase vascular permeability and access of tumor cells to peripheral blood circulation [57]. On the other hand, the production of proteases, e.g., matrix-metalloproteases, induces degradation of extracellular matrix and the consequent liberation of embedded soluble factors released by both cancer and stromal cells having pro-tumoral effects and favoring metastasization.

TAM-mediated immunosuppression at TME is essentially mediated by three concurrent mechanisms: (i) Release of soluble immunosuppressive factors, e.g., IL-10, CCL22, and transforming growth factor (TGF)-α as well as factors recruiting regulatory T cells (Treg) [58]; (ii) expression of ligands for lymphocyte suppressor factors PD-1 and CTLA-4, i.e., PDL-1 and CD80, as well as other checkpoint inhibitors with similar functions, including B7-H4, V-domain Ig suppressor of T cell activation (VISTA) [59], and vascular endothelial receptor (CLEVER) [60], and (iii) starving the TME of L-arginine, i.e., an essential factor for T-cell activity, through the release of arginase-1 [61]. Figure 3 illustrates the principal mechanisms of TAM mediated immunosuppression at the TME.

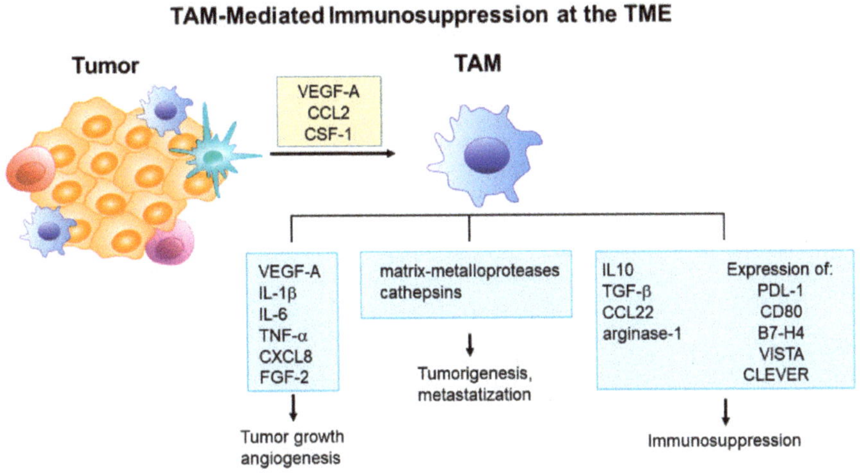

Figure 3. Principal mechanisms of tumor-associated macrophage (TAM) mediated immunosuppression at the tumor microenvironment (TME).

The multiple immunosuppressive signals at play within the TME greatly reduce the efficacy of current immunotherapies. Therefore, new strategies to effectively reprogram the various immunosuppressive cell types at the TME are urgently needed.

4. Re-Programming of TAMs

Immunosuppressive TAMs represent a privileged therapeutic target for the treatment of solid tumors, especially in the case immune checkpoint blockers (ICBs) are used. Given the enormous therapeutic value of TAMs re-education towards M1-like macrophages to promote tumor regression, much attention has focused on effective strategies aimed at targeting TAMs, including the blockade of the M2 phenotype, enhanced activation of M1 macrophages and reprogramming of TAMs toward M1-like phenotype [58,62–65]. Many of these different approaches against immunosuppressive TAMs have been summarized in Table 1 and strategies directed at TAM reprogramming illustrated in Figure 4.

Table 1. Selected strategies to target tumor-associated macrophages (TAMs).

Mechanism of Action	Active Agent	Vehicle Carrier	Target	References
Depletion of M2 TAMs	Shiga toxins	Shigella Flexneri attenuated strain	TAMs	[66]
	Immunotoxins		TAMs Receptors	[67,68]
	Bisphosphonates (e.g., clodrolip, zoledronic acid)	Liposomes	TAMs, Kupffer cells	[69,70]
	Trabectedin		TAMs	[71]
	Tyrosine Kinase Inhibitors (e.g., Dasatinib, Bosutinib)		endothelial and myeloid cells in TEM, TAMs	[72,73]
Inhibition of circulating monocyte recruitment into tumor	CCR2 inhibitors; anti-CCR2/CCL2 blocking antibodies		TAMs CCR2	[45,74–76]
	Antagonists of CXCL12/CXCR4 axis		TAMs CXCR4	[77,78]
	anti-CSF-1R antibody		TAMs CSF-1R	[79,80]
	neutralizing CD11b antibody		CD11b on Myeloid Cells	[81,82]
Blockade of M2 Phenotype	Tyrosine kinase inhibitors or drugs blocking STAT3		TAMs STAT3	[83,84]
	drugs blocking STAT6		TAMs STAT6	[85]
Enhanced Activation of M1 Macrophages	Th1 cytokines like IFN-γ		TAMs STAT1 stimulation	[86,87]
	metformin		TAMs AMPKα1 stimulation	[88]
	toll-like receptor agonists, CpG-ODNs; PI3Kγ deletion		TAMs NF-κB stimulation	[89–91]
Reprogramming TAMs Toward M1-Like Phenotype	mRNAs; miRNA	Targeted Nanocarriers	TAMs	[92,93]
	siRNA	Different types of Nanoparticles	TAMs	[94–96]
	anti-CD40 antibody		TAMs CD40	[97–99]
	anti-MARCO antibody		TAMs MARCO	[100]
	gefitinib/vorinostat	Trastuzumab-modified Mannosylated Liposomes	TAMs MR	[101]
	Drug free	Mannosylated Liposomes	TAMs MR	[102]
	RP-182 Peptide		TAMs MR	[103]

AMPKα1, AMP-activated protein kinase; CCL2, C–C chemokine ligand 2; CCR2, C–C chemokine receptor type 2; CSF-1, Colony-Stimulating Factor 1; CSF-1R, colony-stimulating factor 1 receptor; CXCL12, C–X–C motif chemokine 12; CXCR4, C-X-C chemokine receptor type 4; CpG-ODN, unmethylated cytosineguanine (CpG) oligodeoxynucleotides; IFN-γ, interferon gamma; MARCO, macrophage receptor with collagenous structure; MR, mannose receptor/CD206; NF-κB, nuclear factor kappa B; PI3Kγ, phosphoinositide 3-kinase; STAT, signal transducer and activator of transcription.

Promising results have been obtained with direct activation of M1-like macrophages by Th1 cytokines like IFN-γ [87], and by targeting toll-like receptors (TLR) and/or CD40 with agonists and monoclonal antibodies [97–99]. However, the onset of systemic inflammation limited the therapeutic efficacy of these approaches in vivo, and additional investigations are ongoing to circumvent this hurdle. In any case, considering the functional plasticity of macrophages, re-educating M2- versus an M1-like macrophage phenotype currently appears the most attractive therapeutic option.

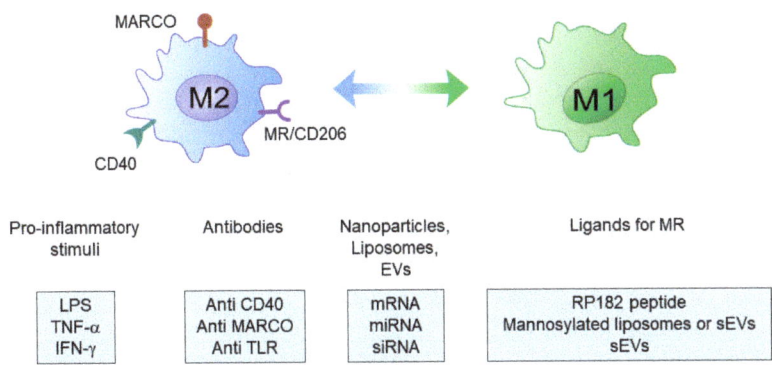

Figure 4. Scheme of current strategies for tumor-associated macrophage (TAM) reprogramming.

A major hindrance to effective targeting of immunosuppressive TAMs is represented by the scarcity of specific protein markers expressed on M2 macrophages. Some potential targets, whose expression also correlates with poor prognosis, have been investigated. Among them, the selective targeting of MARCO (macrophage receptor with collagenous structure) with monoclonal antibodies has been recently used to promote a switch to an M1-activated phenotype [100].

Increasing evidence suggests that a valuable alternative is represented by targeting the MR, which is highly expressed on M2, but not M1 macrophages [92,103–105].

5. The Mannose Receptor in M1 Polarization

MR is expressed on TAMs where is a prototypical marker of M2-type activation. It is also expressed on the surface of immature dendritic cells (DCs), liver sinusoidal endothelial cells, and other tissue macrophages. Earlier studies have demonstrated that MR expression is strongly down-regulated by IFN-γ [106], and upregulated by interleukin-4 (IL-4) [107]. The MR is a 175 kDa Type I integral membrane protein that belongs to the family of C-type lectin receptors and binds glycoconjugates terminated in mannose, fucose, or N-acetil-β-D-glucosamine (GlcNAc) in a calcium-dependent manner [108–110]. The receptor contains three distinct extracellular domains, i.e., an N-terminal cysteine-rich domain (CR) that binds sulfated carbohydrates, a fibronectin type II domain (FNII) that binds collagen, and eight tandem C-type lectin carbohydrate-recognition domains (CRDs) [111,112]. CRDs have only weak affinity affinities for single sugars, and several CRDs need to be clustered to achieve high-affinity binding to oligosaccharides. This clustering allows for the internalization of mannosylated proteins and other exogenous molecules, including allergens and microbial products.

MR is a highly effective clathrin-dependent endocytic receptor that constantly recycles between the plasma membrane and the early endosomal compartment [111]. Most part of MRs is intracellular, while only ~15% of the cellular pool can be found on the cell surface. Like other members of the C-type lectin receptor family, the MR undergoes conformational changes upon ligand binding or as pH decreases in intracellular compartments [111,113]. Once acidification takes place in the endosomal compartment, the MR dissociates from its ligands, and the empty receptor recycles back to the plasma membrane.

Several approaches have been adopted to target the MR and selectively deliver therapeutic nanoparticles. Among these, drug-free mannosylated liposomes have been shown to induce effective anti-tumor activity by enhancing the expression ratio of CD86/MR [102]. In another study, mannosylated nanoparticles suitable for intracellular delivery of drug carriers have been shown to selectively target with high specificity MR expressing macrophages [104].

MR conformational changes that occur upon ligand binding have been recently exploited to target M2 macrophages and induce reprogramming toward M1 phenotypes. For instance, precision targeting with short peptides showed some potential for the intracellular delivery of therapeutically relevant molecules [114]. In addition, a very recent report showed that direct binding of MR with a synthetic peptide (RP-182), i.e., an analogue of naturally occurring antimicrobial peptides, activates phagocytosis and autophagy in M2-like macrophages, reverting these cells into an anti-tumor M1-like phenotype with increased M1 cytokine production and phagocytosis of cancer cells [103].

On the other hand, also cell-secreted sEVs can be considered attractive candidates to specifically target M2-like macrophages via the MR, since they expose high mannose and other classes of N-linked oligosaccharides on their surface [115,116].

6. Extracellular Vesicles for Anti-Tumor Therapy

Pioneering studies have shown that sEVs secreted by DCs pulsed with cancer peptides successfully eradicate established tumors in mice [117]. Furthermore, tumor-derived EVs are a source of neoantigens that, once internalized by DCs, could cross-prime CD8+ T cells and lead to tumor rejection [118]. Since these early studies, the field of sEVs-based cancer therapeutics has attracted many efforts, and sEVs have emerged as promising tools for targeted drug delivery. Despite a growing interest in these nanovesicles as natural carriers, there are still many open questions that need further investigation. For example, specific recognition by target cells is of fundamental importance for an effective delivery of bioactive molecules. EVs uptake may occur via receptor-mediated endocytosis or phagocytosis, or direct fusion with the plasma membrane. Some studies have pointed at integrins [24] and scavenging receptors [119] as mediators of EVs targeting, but current knowledge on this matter is rapidly evolving and has been recently comprehensively reviewed [5,7,120–122].

The different modes of sEV uptake may result in distinct localization and functional effects of the sEVs components, but it is still unknown whether a specific route of entry is to be preferred for a successful transfer of EVs cargo. Thus, understanding through which mechanisms sEVs deliver their content into target cells is a central point that needs to be further elucidated. To the best of current knowledge, while either non-selective uptake or direct fusion with the plasma membrane of target cells seem to be the preferential mechanisms of bulk sEV incorporation (Figure 5) [123], alternative and more specific routes of uptake may depend on the characteristics of surface components of both sEV and target cells.

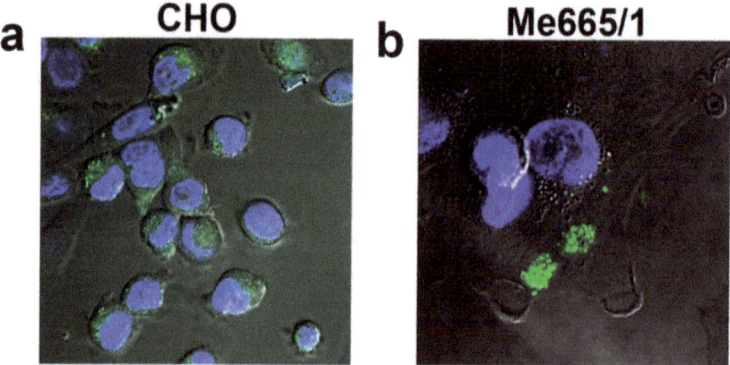

Figure 5. Fluorescent sEVs uptake by different cell lines. Confocal fluorescence microscopy images of green fluorescent sEVs derived from melanoma Me665/1 cells transferred on (**a**) CHO cells and (**b**) Me665/1 cells in nonspecific conditions [66]. Blue-fluorescent nuclei are stained with DAPI.

Tumor-derived EVs can be efficiently taken up by DCs for antigen processing and cross-presentation to tumor-specific CTLs [124]. Immature DCs (iDCs) internalize EVs more efficiently than mature DCs, whereas mature DCs retain more EVs on the cell surface [125]. The surface of iDCs harbors sugar-binding C-type lectin receptors (CLRs) [126,127], which is a characteristic shared with M2-like macrophages.

Glycomic studies conducted to date demonstrate that surface glycoprofiles of sEVs contain high amounts of mannose and other classes of N-linked oligosaccharides [27,34,128,129] making them suitable ligands for the MR. Recently, it has also been shown that mannose-modified serum sEVs display elevated uptake by murine DCs [116]. This evidence, together with a number of studies showing that mannosylation of both liposomes [102] and synthetic nanocarriers [130,131] enhance cellular uptake by M2 macrophages, inducing stimulation and polarization of macrophages toward the M1 phenotype, point to sEVs as powerful ligands of M2 macrophages. Furthermore, the affinity of EVs membrane components (i.e., proteins, lipids, and glycans) for certain tissues greatly affects biodistribution of EVs in vivo, thus, encouraging studies aimed at altering the surface of EVs to improve targeting to selected organs. Many different strategies have been adopted, but there is now accumulating evidence that carbohydrates on the vesicle surface participate in the recognition and uptake of EVs by phagocytes. Interestingly, manipulation of surface glycans on EVs either by removal of sialic acid [132] or by treatment with N-glycosidases [133,134] alters the uptake capacity of different cells. In the first case, the change also affects the in vivo biodistribution of sEVs showing accumulation of desialylated sEVs in the lungs. Altogether, these results point to the importance of N-glycosylation in cellular uptake, but since different cell types respond differently to glycosylation changes appears evident that the cell to be targeted, with its endowment of specific protein receptors, represent the cornerstone of receptor ligand recognition.

7. Molecular Basis of TAM Re-Programming by Engineered sEVs

The subversion of TAM-mediated immunosuppression at TME through macrophage transcriptional reprogramming represents a quite attractive option for anticancer combined immunotherapy. Like normal cells, tumor cells also constitutively release sEVs, which interact primarily with TME cell constituents. SEVs, as naturally occurring vesicles, have a low intrinsic immunogenic profile, are able to avoid, at least in part, the degradative pathway and possess the ability to overcome the blood-brain barrier. Consequently, they have emerged as an important means to deliver therapeutic agents. In this context, engineering tumor-derived sEVs with molecules inducing an inflammatory-like macrophage phenotype would be instrumental in alleviating the immunosuppression at TME. Over the past few years, several engineering strategies have been devised to manipulate tumor-derived sEVs in order to induce cellular and innate immunity. SEV engineering can be carried out either at the level of producer cells or directly on purified sEVs. The different approaches used mostly depend on cargo properties, such as hydrophilicity, hydrophobicity, and molecular weight, as each method has a different loading capacity. For example, chemicophysical methods like electroporation are widely used for loading relatively large molecules, such as siRNA or miRNA into sEVs [19]. Particularly for cancer research, the observation that exosomal miRNAs effectively engage target mRNA and suppress gene expression in recipient cells has been heavily favored. Due to the availability of various cellular engineering methods, different types of RNAs that are released via sEVs have also been exploited and recently reviewed [11].

During the past decade, many efforts have been devoted to transfect sEV-producing cells with plasmids encoding protein sequences that, once uploaded in the nanovesicles, are able to alter the phenotype of target cells [135–138]. However, a method to target M2 macrophages with sEVs capable of inducing their reprogramming to M1 anti-tumor phenotype is not yet available. One major hurdle in EVs research for an effective therapeutic application is represented by the lack of optimized isolation, characterization and quantification procedures. Various purification techniques, such as differential ultracentrifugation, density gradients, precipitation, filtration, size exclusion chromatography, and immunoisolation are currently used to obtain less heterogeneous sEVs preparation; however, quantification often relies on the total protein content of EVs. Fluorescent labeling techniques are more accurate and have the main advantage that track EVs in vivo [139,140]. The different approaches for TAMs reprogramming by engineered EVs are schematically illustrated in Figure 6.

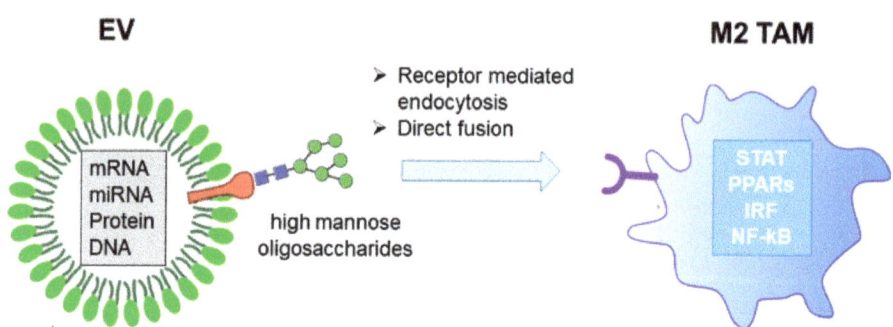

Figure 6. TAMs reprogramming by engineered EVs.

8. HIV-1 Nef Protein as Effector of TAM Reprogramming

A plausible candidate for reprogramming M2 macrophages is the Human immunodeficiency virus (HIV)-1 Negative Regulatory Factor (Nef) protein [141], a 27 kilodalton (kDa) scaffold protein, which lacks enzymatic activities. After synthesis at free ribosomes, Nef reaches both intracellular and plasma membranes with which it tightly interacts through its N-terminal myristoylation. Nef acts as a scaffold/adaptor element in triggering activation of signal transducing molecules like p21 PAK-2, NF-κB, STATs, ERK1/2, Vav, and Src family kinases. In most cases, signal activation occurs upon Nef association with lipid raft microdomains at cell membranes [142–144]. The fact that also sEV membranes are enriched in lipid raft microdomains explains why Nef can be found in EVs [145–149].

Cumulate literature data demonstrate that the presence of Nef inside macrophages induces a strong pro-inflammatory response. In particular, Nef switches on the transcription of many inflammatory genes, as well as the release of inflammatory factors like CCL3, CCL4, IL-1β, IL-6, TNF-α [150,151], and interferon gamma (IFN)-γ [152]. This potent pro-inflammatory response is mediated by the activation of several signal transduction molecules, including STAT-1, 2, and 3, NF-κB, JNK, ERK1/2, and MAPK [153,154]. The inflammatory effects of Nef on macrophages depends on four glutamate-acidic cluster domain located at 62–65 amino acid position [155].

Data from many independent investigation groups strongly support the idea that Nef associates with EVs at low levels [156,157]. Conversely, we identified a Nef mutant incorporating in sEVs/EVs at quite high levels [158]. This Nef mutant (referred to as Nef^{mut}) is defective for the most part of Nef functions, including down-regulation of cell membrane receptors, Nef-associated kinase (NAK) activation, an increase of HIV expression [159]. Nevertheless, it maintains an unaltered acidic cluster domain that correlates with the induction of cell activation in antigen-presenting cells when it is delivered by nanovesicles [160].

Considering this evidence, one may hypothesize that the delivery of Nef^{mut}-engineered EVs inside M2-TAMs would be instrumental in re-educating macrophages at TME from an M2-like to an M1-like phenotype. In the case of solid tumors, this design could be applied through a quite simple strategy, i.e., tumor cell engineering for Nef^{mut} expression through retroviral vector-mediated transduction. In this way, only actively replicating cells at the TME, hence preferably tumor cells, are expected to be transduced. Nef-engineered tumor-derived sEVs may diffuse within TME, thereby preferentially entering MR positive TAMs in view of the mannose expressed on the sEV surface. Once internalized by macrophages, Nef^{mut} might switch on intracellular signals—ultimately leading to the release of pro-inflammatory factors. These factors might act in an autocrine/paracrine loop to induce the reprogramming of macrophage transcriptional profile toward the M1-like phenotype (Figure 7).

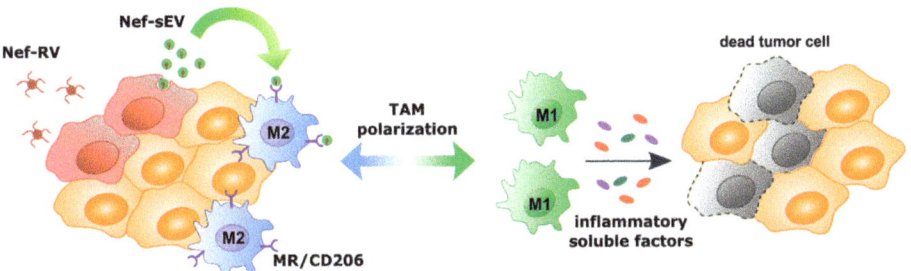

Figure 7. Scheme of the proposed mechanism for TAM reprogramming. Tumor cells are transfected with retroviral vectors expressing Nef^{mut} (Nef-RV). Nef-engineered sEVs (Nef-sEV) are then released into the TME infiltrated with M2 like macrophages expressing the mannose receptor (MR/CD206). MR mediated uptake of Nef-Sev might induce polarization of M2 into M1 like macrophages—ultimately leading to the release of pro-inflammatory factors.

Eventually, this mechanism, which essentially hijacks the sEV-mediated intercellular communication at the TME, is expected to alleviate the immune suppression at the TME, thereby favoring the action of anticancer adaptive immune responses.

Hopefully, once supported by experimental confirmation, this design would have a therapeutic utility in the battle against solid tumors.

9. Conclusions

Immunosuppression at TME protects cancer cells from both spontaneous and artificially generated host immune responses. Hence, subverting immunosuppression should be considered a priority for any anticancer immunotherapeutic strategy. Even if M2-like TAMs are major players, other cell types contribute to the general immunosuppression at TME, including CD4+ Tregs lymphocytes, myeloid-derived suppressor cells, and neutrophils [42]. Similar to macrophages, neutrophils can polarize in pro- and anti-tumor phenotypes, depending on the stimuli they receive at TME. Interestingly, it has been reported that IFN-γ can polarize neutrophils towards an anti-tumor phenotype [161]. Considering the quite high levels of IFN-γ transcripts induced by Nef in macrophages, the delivery of Nef^{mut}-engineered, tumor-derived sEVs to M2-like TAMs is expected to have paracrine anti-tumor effects also on neutrophils that populate the TME.

The strategy we propose is certainly only one of many potential new anti-tumor therapeutic approaches that the manipulation of sEVs/EVs can offer. The increase in knowledge of the sEV/EVs biology, mainly regarding the mechanisms of cell entry, will favor the implementation of new and more efficient therapeutic approaches against tumors and infectious diseases.

Funding: This work was supported by the grant PGR00810 from Ministero degli Affari Esteri e della Cooperazione Internazionale, Italy.

Conflicts of Interest: The authors declare no conflict of interest. The funders had no role in the design of the study; in the collection, analyses, or interpretation of data; in the writing of the manuscript; or in the decision to publish the results.

References

1. Fridman, W.H.; Pages, F.; Sautes-Fridman, C.; Galon, J. The immune contexture in human tumours: Impact on clinical outcome. *Nat. Rev. Cancer* **2012**, *12*, 298–306. [CrossRef] [PubMed]
2. Quail, D.F.; Joyce, J.A. Microenvironmental regulation of tumor progression and metastasis. *Nat. Med.* **2013**, *19*, 1423–1437. [CrossRef] [PubMed]
3. van Niel, G.; D'Angelo, G.; Raposo, G. Shedding light on the cell biology of extracellular vesicles. *Nat. Rev. Mol. Cell Biol.* **2018**, *19*, 213–228. [CrossRef] [PubMed]
4. Kalluri, R.; LeBleu, V.S. The biology, function, and biomedical applications of exosomes. *Science* **2020**, *367*, eaau6977. [CrossRef]
5. Raposo, G.; Stahl, P.D. Extracellular vesicles: A new communication paradigm? *Nat. Rev. Mol. Cell Biol.* **2019**, *20*, 509–510. [CrossRef] [PubMed]
6. Colombo, M.; Raposo, G.; Théry, C. Biogenesis, Secretion, and Intercellular Interactions of Exosomes and Other Extracellular Vesicles. *Annu. Rev. Cell Dev. Biol.* **2014**, *30*, 255–289. [CrossRef]
7. Meldolesi, J. Exosomes and Ectosomes in Intercellular Communication. *Curr. Biol. CB* **2018**, *28*, R435–R444. [CrossRef]
8. Thery, C.; Witwer, K.W.; Aikawa, E.; Alcaraz, M.J.; Anderson, J.D.; Andriantsitohaina, R.; Antoniou, A.; Arab, T.; Archer, F.; Atkin-Smith, G.K.; et al. Minimal information for studies of extracellular vesicles 2018 (MISEV2018): A position statement of the International Society for Extracellular Vesicles and update of the MISEV2014 guidelines. *J. Extracell Vesicles* **2018**, *7*, 1535750. [CrossRef]
9. Jeppesen, D.K.; Fenix, A.M.; Franklin, J.L.; Higginbotham, J.N.; Zhang, Q.; Zimmerman, L.J.; Liebler, D.C.; Ping, J.; Liu, Q.; Evans, R.; et al. Reassessment of Exosome Composition. *Cell* **2019**, *177*, 428–445. [CrossRef]
10. Kowal, J.; Arras, G.; Colombo, M.; Jouve, M.; Morath, J.P.; Primdal-Bengtson, B.; Dingli, F.; Loew, D.; Tkach, M.; Théry, C. Proteomic comparison defines novel markers to characterize heterogeneous populations of extracellular vesicle subtypes. *Proc. Natl. Acad. Sci. USA* **2016**, *113*, E968–E977. [CrossRef]
11. O'Brien, K.; Breyne, K.; Ughetto, S.; Laurent, L.C.; Breakefield, X.O. RNA delivery by extracellular vesicles in mammalian cells and its applications. *Nat. Rev. Mol. Cell Biol.* **2020**. [CrossRef] [PubMed]
12. Cocucci, E.; Meldolesi, J. Ectosomes and exosomes: Shedding the confusion between extracellular vesicles. *Trends Cell Biol.* **2015**, *25*, 364–372. [CrossRef] [PubMed]
13. Mathivanan, S.; Ji, H.; Simpson, R.J. Exosomes: Extracellular organelles important in intercellular communication. *J. Proteom.* **2010**, *73*, 1907–1920. [CrossRef]
14. Maia, J.; Caja, S.; Strano Moraes, M.C.; Couto, N.; Costa-Silva, B. Exosome-Based Cell-Cell Communication in the Tumor Microenvironment. *Front. Cell Dev. Biol.* **2018**, *6*, 18. [CrossRef]
15. Andaloussi, S.E.L.; Mager, I.; Breakefield, X.O.; Wood, M.J. Extracellular vesicles: Biology and emerging therapeutic opportunities. *Nat. Rev. Drug Discov.* **2013**, *12*, 347–357. [CrossRef]
16. Tkach, M.; Thery, C. Communication by Extracellular Vesicles: Where We are and Where We Need to Go. *Cell* **2016**, *164*, 1226–1232. [CrossRef] [PubMed]
17. Xu, R.; Greening, D.W.; Zhu, H.J.; Takahashi, N.; Simpson, R.J. Extracellular vesicle isolation and characterization: Toward clinical application. *J. Clin. Investig.* **2016**, *126*, 1152–1162. [CrossRef]
18. Ratajczak, M.Z.; Kucia, M.; Jadczyk, T.; Greco, N.J.; Wojakowski, W.; Tendera, M.; Ratajczak, J. Pivotal role of paracrine effects in stem cell therapies in regenerative medicine: Can we translate stem cell-secreted paracrine factors and microvesicles into better therapeutic strategies? *Leukemia* **2012**, *26*, 1166–1173. [CrossRef]
19. Luan, X.; Sansanaphongpricha, K.; Myers, I.; Chen, H.; Yuan, H.; Sun, D. Engineering exosomes as refined biological nanoplatforms for drug delivery. *Acta Pharmacol. Sin.* **2017**, *38*, 754–763. [CrossRef]
20. Nogues, L.; Benito-Martin, A.; Hergueta-Redondo, M.; Peinado, H. The influence of tumour-derived extracellular vesicles on local and distal metastatic dissemination. *Mol. Asp. Med.* **2017**. [CrossRef]
21. Maas, S.L.N.; Breakefield, X.O.; Weaver, A.M. Extracellular Vesicles: Unique Intercellular Delivery Vehicles. *Trends Cell Biol.* **2017**, *27*, 172–188. [CrossRef] [PubMed]
22. Clayton, A.; Mitchell, J.P.; Court, J.; Mason, M.D.; Tabi, Z. Human tumor-derived exosomes selectively impair lymphocyte responses to interleukin-2. *Cancer Res.* **2007**, *67*, 7458–7466. [CrossRef]

23. Peinado, H.; Aleckovic, M.; Lavotshkin, S.; Matei, I.; Costa-Silva, B.; Moreno-Bueno, G.; Hergueta-Redondo, M.; Williams, C.; Garcia-Santos, G.; Ghajar, C.; et al. Melanoma exosomes educate bone marrow progenitor cells toward a pro-metastatic phenotype through MET. *Nat. Med.* **2012**, *18*, 883–891. [CrossRef] [PubMed]
24. Hoshino, A.; Costa-Silva, B.; Shen, T.L.; Rodrigues, G.; Hashimoto, A.; Tesic Mark, M.; Molina, H.; Kohsaka, S.; Di Giannatale, A.; Ceder, S.; et al. Tumour exosome integrins determine organotropic metastasis. *Nature* **2015**. [CrossRef] [PubMed]
25. Hessvik, N.P.; Llorente, A. Current knowledge on exosome biogenesis and release. *Cell. Mol. Life Sci.* **2017**. [CrossRef] [PubMed]
26. Gruenberg, J. Life in the lumen: The multivesicular endosome. *Traffic* **2020**, *21*, 76–93. [CrossRef]
27. Williams, C.; Royo, F.; Aizpurua-Olaizola, O.; Pazos, R.; Boons, G.J.; Reichardt, N.C.; Falcon-Perez, J.M. Glycosylation of extracellular vesicles: Current knowledge, tools and clinical perspectives. *J. Extracell Vesicles* **2018**, *7*, 1442985. [CrossRef]
28. Costa-Silva, B.; Aiello, N.M.; Ocean, A.J.; Singh, S.; Zhang, H.; Thakur, B.K.; Becker, A.; Hoshino, A.; Mark, M.T.; Molina, H.; et al. Pancreatic cancer exosomes initiate pre-metastatic niche formation in the liver. *Nat. Cell Biol.* **2015**, *17*, 816–826. [CrossRef]
29. Laoui, D.; Van Overmeire, E.; Di Conza, G.; Aldeni, C.; Keirsse, J.; Morias, Y.; Movahedi, K.; Houbracken, I.; Schouppe, E.; Elkrim, Y.; et al. Tumor hypoxia does not drive differentiation of tumor-associated macrophages but rather fine-tunes the M2-like macrophage population. *Cancer Res.* **2014**, *74*, 24–30. [CrossRef]
30. Colegio, O.R.; Chu, N.Q.; Szabo, A.L.; Chu, T.; Rhebergen, A.M.; Jairam, V.; Cyrus, N.; Brokowski, C.E.; Eisenbarth, S.C.; Phillips, G.M.; et al. Functional polarization of tumour-associated macrophages by tumour-derived lactic acid. *Nature* **2014**, *513*, 559–563. [CrossRef]
31. Whiteside, T.L. Tumor-Derived Exosomes and Their Role in Cancer Progression. *Adv. Clin. Chem.* **2016**, *74*, 103–141. [CrossRef] [PubMed]
32. Han, L.; Lam, E.W.; Sun, Y. Extracellular vesicles in the tumor microenvironment: Old stories, but new tales. *Mol. Cancer* **2019**, *18*, 59. [CrossRef] [PubMed]
33. Murray, P.J.; Allen, J.E.; Biswas, S.K.; Fisher, E.A.; Gilroy, D.W.; Goerdt, S.; Gordon, S.; Hamilton, J.A.; Ivashkiv, L.B.; Lawrence, T.; et al. Macrophage activation and polarization: Nomenclature and experimental guidelines. *Immunity* **2014**, *41*, 14–20. [CrossRef] [PubMed]
34. Gerlach, J.Q.; Griffin, M.D. Getting to know the extracellular vesicle glycome. *Mol. Biosyst.* **2016**, *12*, 1071–1081. [CrossRef]
35. Nistico, P.; Ciliberto, G. Biological mechanisms linked to inflammation in cancer: Discovery of tumor microenvironment-related biomarkers and their clinical application in solid tumors. *Int. J. Biol. Markers* **2020**, *35*, 8–11. [CrossRef]
36. Hinshaw, D.C.; Shevde, L.A. The Tumor Microenvironment Innately Modulates Cancer Progression. *Cancer Res.* **2019**, *79*, 4557–4566. [CrossRef]
37. Binnewies, M.; Roberts, E.W.; Kersten, K.; Chan, V.; Fearon, D.F.; Merad, M.; Coussens, L.M.; Gabrilovich, D.I.; Ostrand-Rosenberg, S.; Hedrick, C.C.; et al. Understanding the tumor immune microenvironment (TIME) for effective therapy. *Nat. Med.* **2018**, *24*, 541–550. [CrossRef]
38. Beatty, G.L.; Winograd, R.; Evans, R.A.; Long, K.B.; Luque, S.L.; Lee, J.W.; Clendenin, C.; Gladney, W.L.; Knoblock, D.M.; Guirnalda, P.D.; et al. Exclusion of T Cells From Pancreatic Carcinomas in Mice Is Regulated by Ly6Clow F4/80+ Extratumoral Macrophages. *Gastroenterology* **2015**, *149*, 201–210. [CrossRef]
39. Mosser, D.M.; Edwards, J.P. Exploring the full spectrum of macrophage activation. *Nat. Rev. Immunol.* **2008**, *8*, 958–969. [CrossRef]
40. Yang, M.; McKay, D.; Pollard, J.W.; Lewis, C.E. Diverse Functions of Macrophages in Different Tumor Microenvironments. *Cancer Res.* **2018**, *78*, 5492–5503. [CrossRef]
41. Martinez, F.O.; Gordon, S. The M1 and M2 paradigm of macrophage activation: Time for reassessment. *F1000prime Rep.* **2014**, *6*, 13. [CrossRef] [PubMed]
42. Galdiero, M.R.; Marone, G.; Mantovani, A. Cancer Inflammation and Cytokines. *Cold Spring Harb. Perspect. Biol.* **2018**, *10*. [CrossRef] [PubMed]
43. Hanahan, D.; Coussens, L.M. Accessories to the crime: Functions of cells recruited to the tumor microenvironment. *Cancer Cell* **2012**, *21*, 309–322. [CrossRef]

44. Pollard, J.W. Tumour-educated macrophages promote tumour progression and metastasis. *Nat. Rev. Cancer* **2004**, *4*, 71–78. [CrossRef]
45. Qian, B.Z.; Li, J.; Zhang, H.; Kitamura, T.; Zhang, J.; Campion, L.R.; Kaiser, E.A.; Snyder, L.A.; Pollard, J.W. CCL2 recruits inflammatory monocytes to facilitate breast-tumour metastasis. *Nature* **2011**, *475*, 222–225. [CrossRef] [PubMed]
46. Lin, E.Y.; Nguyen, A.V.; Russell, R.G.; Pollard, J.W. Colony-stimulating factor 1 promotes progression of mammary tumors to malignancy. *J. Exp. Med.* **2001**, *193*, 727–740. [CrossRef] [PubMed]
47. Aras, S.; Zaidi, M.R. TAMeless traitors: Macrophages in cancer progression and metastasis. *Br. J. Cancer* **2017**, *117*, 1583–1591. [CrossRef]
48. Cuccarese, M.F.; Dubach, J.M.; Pfirschke, C.; Engblom, C.; Garris, C.; Miller, M.A.; Pittet, M.J.; Weissleder, R. Heterogeneity of macrophage infiltration and therapeutic response in lung carcinoma revealed by 3D organ imaging. *Nat. Commun.* **2017**, *8*, 14293. [CrossRef]
49. Huang, Y.K.; Wang, M.; Sun, Y.; Di Costanzo, N.; Mitchell, C.; Achuthan, A.; Hamilton, J.A.; Busuttil, R.A.; Boussioutas, A. Macrophage spatial heterogeneity in gastric cancer defined by multiplex immunohistochemistry. *Nat. Commun.* **2019**, *10*, 3928. [CrossRef]
50. Azizi, E.; Carr, A.J.; Plitas, G.; Cornish, A.E.; Konopacki, C.; Prabhakaran, S.; Nainys, J.; Wu, K.; Kiseliovas, V.; Setty, M.; et al. Single-Cell Map of Diverse Immune Phenotypes in the Breast Tumor Microenvironment. *Cell* **2018**, *174*, 1293–1308. [CrossRef]
51. Gordon, S.; Pluddemann, A.; Mukhopadhyay, S. Plasma membrane receptors of tissue macrophages: Functions and role in pathology. *J. Pathol.* **2020**, *250*, 656–666. [CrossRef]
52. Langston, P.K.; Shibata, M.; Horng, T. Metabolism Supports Macrophage Activation. *Front. Immunol.* **2017**, *8*, 61. [CrossRef]
53. O'Neill, L.A.; Pearce, E.J. Immunometabolism governs dendritic cell and macrophage function. *J. Exp. Med.* **2016**, *213*, 15–23. [CrossRef]
54. Xue, J.; Schmidt, S.V.; Sander, J.; Draffehn, A.; Krebs, W.; Quester, I.; De Nardo, D.; Gohel, T.D.; Emde, M.; Schmidleithner, L.; et al. Transcriptome-based network analysis reveals a spectrum model of human macrophage activation. *Immunity* **2014**, *40*, 274–288. [CrossRef]
55. Lawrence, T.; Natoli, G. Transcriptional regulation of macrophage polarization: Enabling diversity with identity. *Nat. Rev. Immunol.* **2011**, *11*, 750–761. [CrossRef]
56. Chanmee, T.; Ontong, P.; Konno, K.; Itano, N. Tumor-associated macrophages as major players in the tumor microenvironment. *Cancers* **2014**, *6*, 1670–1690. [CrossRef]
57. De Palma, M.; Biziato, D.; Petrova, T.V. Microenvironmental regulation of tumour angiogenesis. *Nat. Rev. Cancer* **2017**, *17*, 457–474. [CrossRef]
58. Beltraminelli, T.; De Palma, M. Biology and therapeutic targeting of tumour-associated macrophages. *J. Pathol.* **2020**, *250*, 573–592. [CrossRef]
59. Blando, J.; Sharma, A.; Higa, M.G.; Zhao, H.; Vence, L.; Yadav, S.S.; Kim, J.; Sepulveda, A.M.; Sharp, M.; Maitra, A.; et al. Comparison of immune infiltrates in melanoma and pancreatic cancer highlights VISTA as a potential target in pancreatic cancer. *Proc. Natl. Acad. Sci. USA* **2019**, *116*, 1692–1697. [CrossRef]
60. Mantovani, A.; Bonecchi, R. One Clever Macrophage Checkpoint. *Clin. Cancer Res. Off. J. Am. Assoc. Cancer Res.* **2019**, *25*, 3202–3204. [CrossRef]
61. Rodriguez, P.C.; Quiceno, D.G.; Zabaleta, J.; Ortiz, B.; Zea, A.H.; Piazuelo, M.B.; Delgado, A.; Correa, P.; Brayer, J.; Sotomayor, E.M.; et al. Arginase I production in the tumor microenvironment by mature myeloid cells inhibits T-cell receptor expression and antigen-specific T-cell responses. *Cancer Res.* **2004**, *64*, 5839–5849. [CrossRef]
62. Cassetta, L.; Pollard, J.W. Targeting macrophages: Therapeutic approaches in cancer. *Nat. Rev. Drug Discov.* **2018**, *17*, 887–904. [CrossRef]
63. Mantovani, A.; Marchesi, F.; Malesci, A.; Laghi, L.; Allavena, P. Tumour-associated macrophages as treatment targets in oncology. *Nat. Rev. Clin. Oncol.* **2017**, *14*, 399–416. [CrossRef]
64. Genard, G.; Lucas, S.; Michiels, C. Reprogramming of Tumor-Associated Macrophages with Anticancer Therapies: Radiotherapy versus Chemo- and Immunotherapies. *Front. Immunol.* **2017**, *8*, 828. [CrossRef]
65. Anfray, C.; Ummarino, A.; Andon, F.T.; Allavena, P. Current Strategies to Target Tumor-Associated-Macrophages to Improve Anti-Tumor Immune Responses. *Cells* **2019**, *9*, 46. [CrossRef]

66. Galmbacher, K.; Heisig, M.; Hotz, C.; Wischhusen, J.; Galmiche, A.; Bergmann, B.; Gentschev, I.; Goebel, W.; Rapp, U.R.; Fensterle, J. Shigella mediated depletion of macrophages in a murine breast cancer model is associated with tumor regression. *PLoS ONE* **2010**, *5*, e9572. [CrossRef]
67. Bak, S.P.; Walters, J.J.; Takeya, M.; Conejo-Garcia, J.R.; Berwin, B.L. Scavenger Receptor-A–Targeted Leukocyte Depletion Inhibits Peritoneal Ovarian Tumor Progression. *Cancer Res.* **2007**, *67*, 4783. [CrossRef]
68. Nagai, T.; Tanaka, M.; Tsuneyoshi, Y.; Xu, B.; Michie, S.A.; Hasui, K.; Hirano, H.; Arita, K.; Matsuyama, T. Targeting tumor-associated macrophages in an experimental glioma model with a recombinant immunotoxin to folate receptor beta. *Cancer Immunol. Immunother.* **2009**, *58*, 1577–1586. [CrossRef]
69. Lehenkari, P.P.; Kellinsalmi, M.; Näpänkangas, J.P.; Ylitalo, K.V.; Mönkkönen, J.; Rogers, M.J.; Azhayev, A.; Väänänen, H.K.; Hassinen, I.E. Further insight into mechanism of action of clodronate: Inhibition of mitochondrial ADP/ATP translocase by a nonhydrolyzable, adenine-containing metabolite. *Mol. Pharmacol.* **2002**, *61*, 1255–1262. [CrossRef]
70. Zhang, W.; Zhu, X.D.; Sun, H.C.; Xiong, Y.Q.; Zhuang, P.Y.; Xu, H.X.; Kong, L.Q.; Wang, L.; Wu, W.Z.; Tang, Z.Y. Depletion of tumor-associated macrophages enhances the effect of sorafenib in metastatic liver cancer models by antimetastatic and antiangiogenic effects. *Clin. Cancer Res. Off. J. Am. Assoc. Cancer Res.* **2010**, *16*, 3420–3430. [CrossRef]
71. Allavena, P.; Signorelli, M.; Chieppa, M.; Erba, E.; Bianchi, G.; Marchesi, F.; Olimpio, C.O.; Bonardi, C.; Garbi, A.; Lissoni, A.; et al. Anti-inflammatory properties of the novel antitumor agent yondelis (trabectedin): Inhibition of macrophage differentiation and cytokine production. *Cancer Res.* **2005**, *65*, 2964–2971. [CrossRef] [PubMed]
72. Liang, W.; Kujawski, M.; Wu, J.; Lu, J.; Herrmann, A.; Loera, S.; Yen, Y.; Lee, F.; Yu, H.; Wen, W.; et al. Antitumor activity of targeting SRC kinases in endothelial and myeloid cell compartments of the tumor microenvironment. *Clin. Cancer Res. Off. J. Am. Assoc. Cancer Res.* **2010**, *16*, 924–935. [CrossRef]
73. Ozanne, J.; Prescott, A.R.; Clark, K. The clinically approved drugs dasatinib and bosutinib induce anti-inflammatory macrophages by inhibiting the salt-inducible kinases. *Biochem. J.* **2015**, *465*, 271–279. [CrossRef]
74. Brana, I.; Calles, A.; LoRusso, P.M.; Yee, L.K.; Puchalski, T.A.; Seetharam, S.; Zhong, B.; de Boer, C.J.; Tabernero, J.; Calvo, E. Carlumab, an anti-C-C chemokine ligand 2 monoclonal antibody, in combination with four chemotherapy regimens for the treatment of patients with solid tumors: An open-label, multicenter phase 1b study. *Target. Oncol.* **2015**, *10*, 111–123. [CrossRef] [PubMed]
75. Kitamura, T.; Qian, B.-Z.; Soong, D.; Cassetta, L.; Noy, R.; Sugano, G.; Kato, Y.; Li, J.; Pollard, J.W. CCL2-induced chemokine cascade promotes breast cancer metastasis by enhancing retention of metastasis-associated macrophages. *J. Exp. Med.* **2015**, *212*, 1043–1059. [CrossRef] [PubMed]
76. Bonapace, L.; Coissieux, M.M.; Wyckoff, J.; Mertz, K.D.; Varga, Z.; Junt, T.; Bentires-Alj, M. Cessation of CCL2 inhibition accelerates breast cancer metastasis by promoting angiogenesis. *Nature* **2014**, *515*, 130–133. [CrossRef] [PubMed]
77. Sánchez-Martín, L.; Estecha, A.; Samaniego, R.; Sánchez-Ramón, S.; Vega, M.Á.; Sánchez-Mateos, P. The chemokine CXCL12 regulates monocyte-macrophage differentiation and RUNX3 expression. *Blood* **2011**, *117*, 88–97. [CrossRef] [PubMed]
78. Hughes, R.; Qian, B.Z.; Rowan, C.; Muthana, M.; Keklikoglou, I.; Olson, O.C.; Tazzyman, S.; Danson, S.; Addison, C.; Clemons, M.; et al. Perivascular M2 Macrophages Stimulate Tumor Relapse after Chemotherapy. *Cancer Res.* **2015**, *75*, 3479–3491. [CrossRef]
79. Ao, J.Y.; Zhu, X.D.; Chai, Z.T.; Cai, H.; Zhang, Y.Y.; Zhang, K.Z.; Kong, L.Q.; Zhang, N.; Ye, B.G.; Ma, D.N.; et al. Colony-Stimulating Factor 1 Receptor Blockade Inhibits Tumor Growth by Altering the Polarization of Tumor-Associated Macrophages in Hepatocellular Carcinoma. *Mol. Cancer Ther.* **2017**, *16*, 1544–1554. [CrossRef]
80. Zhu, Y.; Knolhoff, B.L.; Meyer, M.A.; Nywening, T.M.; West, B.L.; Luo, J.; Wang-Gillam, A.; Goedegebuure, S.P.; Linehan, D.C.; De Nardo, D.G. CSF1/CSF1R Blockade Reprograms Tumor-Infiltrating Macrophages and Improves Response to T-cell Checkpoint Immunotherapy in Pancreatic Cancer Models. *Cancer Res.* **2014**, *74*, 5057. [CrossRef]
81. Zhang, Q.-Q.; Hu, X.-W.; Liu, Y.-L.; Ye, Z.-J.; Gui, Y.-H.; Zhou, D.-L.; Qi, C.-L.; He, X.-D.; Wang, H.; Wang, L.-J. CD11b deficiency suppresses intestinal tumor growth by reducing myeloid cell recruitment. *Sci. Rep.* **2015**, *5*, 15948. [CrossRef]

82. Ahn, G.O.; Tseng, D.; Liao, C.H.; Dorie, M.J.; Czechowicz, A.; Brown, J.M. Inhibition of Mac-1 (CD11b/CD18) enhances tumor response to radiation by reducing myeloid cell recruitment. *Proc. Natl. Acad. Sci. USA* **2010**, *107*, 8363–8368. [CrossRef]
83. Sun, L.; Chen, B.; Jiang, R.; Li, J.; Wang, B. Resveratrol inhibits lung cancer growth by suppressing M2-like polarization of tumor associated macrophages. *Cell. Immunol.* **2017**, *311*, 86–93. [CrossRef]
84. Edwards, J.P.; Emens, L.A. The multikinase inhibitor sorafenib reverses the suppression of IL-12 and enhancement of IL-10 by PGE_2 in murine macrophages. *Int. Immunopharmacol.* **2010**, *10*, 1220–1228. [CrossRef]
85. Dong, R.; Gong, Y.; Meng, W.; Yuan, M.; Zhu, H.; Ying, M.; He, Q.; Cao, J.; Yang, B. The involvement of M2 macrophage polarization inhibition in fenretinide-mediated chemopreventive effects on colon cancer. *Cancer Lett.* **2017**, *388*, 43–53. [CrossRef]
86. Dunn, G.P.; Koebel, C.M.; Schreiber, R.D. Interferons, immunity and cancer immunoediting. *Nat. Rev. Immunol.* **2006**, *6*, 836–848. [CrossRef]
87. Parker, B.S.; Rautela, J.; Hertzog, P.J. Antitumour actions of interferons: Implications for cancer therapy. *Nat. Rev. Cancer* **2016**, *16*, 131–144. [CrossRef]
88. Ding, L.; Liang, G.; Yao, Z.; Zhang, J.; Liu, R.; Chen, H.; Zhou, Y.; Wu, H.; Yang, B.; He, Q. Metformin prevents cancer metastasis by inhibiting M2-like polarization of tumor associated macrophages. *Oncotarget* **2015**, *6*, 36441–36455. [CrossRef]
89. Huang, L.; Xu, H.; Peng, G. TLR-mediated metabolic reprogramming in the tumor microenvironment: Potential novel strategies for cancer immunotherapy. *Cell. Mol. Immunol.* **2018**, *15*, 428–437. [CrossRef]
90. Chen, N.; Wei, M.; Sun, Y.; Li, F.; Pei, H.; Li, X.; Su, S.; He, Y.; Wang, L.; Shi, J.; et al. Self-assembly of poly-adenine-tailed CpG oligonucleotide-gold nanoparticle nanoconjugates with immunostimulatory activity. *Small* **2014**, *10*, 368–375. [CrossRef]
91. Kaneda, M.M.; Messer, K.S.; Ralainirina, N.; Li, H.; Leem, C.J.; Gorjestani, S.; Woo, G.; Nguyen, A.V.; Figueiredo, C.C.; Foubert, P.; et al. PI3Kγ is a molecular switch that controls immune suppression. *Nature* **2016**, *539*, 437–442. [CrossRef] [PubMed]
92. Zhang, F.; Parayath, N.N.; Ene, C.I.; Stephan, S.B.; Koehne, A.L.; Coon, M.E.; Holland, E.C.; Stephan, M.T. Genetic programming of macrophages to perform anti-tumor functions using targeted mRNA nanocarriers. *Nat. Commun.* **2019**, *10*, 3974. [CrossRef]
93. Cai, X.; Yin, Y.; Li, N.; Zhu, D.; Zhang, J.; Zhang, C.-Y.; Zen, K. Re-polarization of tumor-associated macrophages to pro-inflammatory M1 macrophages by microRNA-155. *J. Mol. Cell Biol.* **2012**, *4*, 341–343. [CrossRef]
94. Zhang, M.; Gao, Y.; Caja, K.; Zhao, B.; Kim, J.A. Non-viral nanoparticle delivers small interfering RNA to macrophages in vitro and in vivo. *PLoS ONE* **2015**, *10*, e0118472. [CrossRef] [PubMed]
95. Jia, N.; Wu, H.; Duan, J.; Wei, C.; Wang, K.; Zhang, Y.; Mao, X. Polyethyleneimine-coated Iron Oxide Nanoparticles as a Vehicle for the Delivery of Small Interfering RNA to Macrophages In Vitro and In Vivo. *JoVE* **2019**, e58660. [CrossRef]
96. Liang, S.; Zheng, J.; Wu, W.; Li, Q.; Saw, P.E.; Chen, J.; Xu, X.; Yao, H.; Yao, Y. A Robust Nanoparticle Platform for RNA Interference in Macrophages to Suppress Tumor Cell Migration. *Front. Pharm.* **2018**, *9*, 1465. [CrossRef]
97. Zippelius, A.; Schreiner, J.; Herzig, P.; Muller, P. Induced PD-L1 expression mediates acquired resistance to agonistic anti-CD40 treatment. *Cancer Immunol. Res.* **2015**, *3*, 236–244. [CrossRef] [PubMed]
98. Rodell, C.B.; Arlauckas, S.P.; Cuccarese, M.F.; Garris, C.S.; Li, R.; Ahmed, M.S.; Kohler, R.H.; Pittet, M.J.; Weissleder, R. TLR7/8-agonist-loaded nanoparticles promote the polarization of tumour-associated macrophages to enhance cancer immunotherapy. *Nat. Biomed. Eng.* **2018**, *2*, 578–588. [CrossRef]
99. Vogel, D.Y.; Glim, J.E.; Stavenuiter, A.W.; Breur, M.; Heijnen, P.; Amor, S.; Dijkstra, C.D.; Beelen, R.H. Human macrophage polarization in vitro: Maturation and activation methods compared. *Immunobiology* **2014**, *219*, 695–703. [CrossRef]
100. Georgoudaki, A.M.; Prokopec, K.E.; Boura, V.F.; Hellqvist, E.; Sohn, S.; Ostling, J.; Dahan, R.; Harris, R.A.; Rantalainen, M.; Klevebring, D.; et al. Reprogramming Tumor-Associated Macrophages by Antibody Targeting Inhibits Cancer Progression and Metastasis. *Cell Rep.* **2016**, *15*, 2000–2011. [CrossRef]

101. Peng, H.; Chen, B.; Huang, W.; Tang, Y.; Jiang, Y.; Zhang, W.; Huang, Y. Reprogramming Tumor-Associated Macrophages To Reverse EGFRT790M Resistance by Dual-Targeting Codelivery of Gefitinib/Vorinostat. *Nano Lett.* **2017**, *17*, 7684–7690. [CrossRef] [PubMed]
102. Ye, J.; Yang, Y.; Dong, W.; Gao, Y.; Meng, Y.; Wang, H.; Li, L.; Jin, J.; Ji, M.; Xia, X.; et al. Drug-free mannosylated liposomes inhibit tumor growth by promoting the polarization of tumor-associated macrophages. *Int. J. Nanomed.* **2019**, *14*, 3203–3220. [CrossRef]
103. Jaynes, J.M.; Sable, R.; Ronzetti, M.; Bautista, W.; Knotts, Z.; Abisoye-Ogunniyan, A.; Li, D.; Calvo, R.; Dashnyam, M.; Singh, A.; et al. Mannose receptor (CD206) activation in tumor-associated macrophages enhances adaptive and innate antitumor immune responses. *Sci. Transl. Med.* **2020**, *12*. [CrossRef] [PubMed]
104. Chen, P.; Zhang, X.; Venosa, A.; Lee, I.H.; Myers, D.; Holloway, J.A.; Prud'homme, R.K.; Gao, D.; Szekely, Z.; Laskin, J.D.; et al. A Novel Bivalent Mannosylated Targeting Ligand Displayed on Nanoparticles Selectively Targets Anti-Inflammatory M2 Macrophages. *Pharmaceutics* **2020**, *12*, 243. [CrossRef] [PubMed]
105. Irache, J.M.; Salman, H.H.; Gamazo, C.; Espuelas, S. Mannose-targeted systems for the delivery of therapeutics. *Expert Opin. Drug Deliv.* **2008**, *5*, 703–724. [CrossRef]
106. Harris, N.; Super, M.; Rits, M.; Chang, G.; Ezekowitz, R.A. Characterization of the murine macrophage mannose receptor: Demonstration that the downregulation of receptor expression mediated by interferon-gamma occurs at the level of transcription. *Blood* **1992**, *80*, 2363–2373. [CrossRef]
107. Stein, M.; Keshav, S.; Harris, N.; Gordon, S. Interleukin 4 potently enhances murine macrophage mannose receptor activity: A marker of alternative immunologic macrophage activation. *J. Exp. Med.* **1992**, *176*, 287–292. [CrossRef]
108. Taylor, M.E.; Drickamer, K. Mammalian sugar-binding receptors: Known functions and unexplored roles. *FEBS J.* **2019**, *286*, 1800–1814. [CrossRef]
109. Pontow, S.E.; Kery, V.; Stahl, P.D. Mannose receptor. *Int. Rev. Cytol.* **1992**, *137b*, 221–244. [CrossRef]
110. Blum, J.S.; Stahl, P.D.; Diaz, R.; Fiani, M.L. Purification and characterization of the D-mannose receptor from J774 mouse macrophage cells. *Carbohydr. Res.* **1991**, *213*, 145–153. [CrossRef]
111. Martinez-Pomares, L. The mannose receptor. *J. Leukoc. Biol.* **2012**, *92*, 1177–1186. [CrossRef]
112. Stahl, P.D.; Ezekowitz, R.A. The mannose receptor is a pattern recognition receptor involved in host defense. *Curr. Opin. Immunol.* **1998**, *10*, 50–55. [CrossRef]
113. Hu, Z.; Shi, X.; Yu, B.; Li, N.; Huang, Y.; He, Y. Structural Insights into the pH-Dependent Conformational Change and Collagen Recognition of the Human Mannose Receptor. *Structure* **2018**, *26*, 60–71. [CrossRef]
114. Scodeller, P.; Simon-Gracia, L.; Kopanchuk, S.; Tobi, A.; Kilk, K.; Saalik, P.; Kurm, K.; Squadrito, M.L.; Kotamraju, V.R.; Rinken, A.; et al. Precision Targeting of Tumor Macrophages with a CD206 Binding Peptide. *Sci. Rep.* **2017**, *7*, 14655. [CrossRef] [PubMed]
115. Costa, J. Glycoconjugates from extracellular vesicles: Structures, functions and emerging potential as cancer biomarkers. *Biochim. Biophys. Acta* **2017**, *1868*, 157–166. [CrossRef] [PubMed]
116. Choi, E.S.; Song, J.; Kang, Y.Y.; Mok, H. Mannose-Modified Serum Exosomes for the Elevated Uptake to Murine Dendritic Cells and Lymphatic Accumulation. *Macromol. Biosci.* **2019**, *19*, e1900042. [CrossRef] [PubMed]
117. Zitvogel, L.; Regnault, A.; Lozier, A.; Wolfers, J.; Flament, C.; Tenza, D.; Ricciardi-Castagnoli, P.; Raposo, G.; Amigorena, S. Eradication of established murine tumors using a novel cell-free vaccine: Dendritic cell derived exosomes. *Nat. Med.* **1998**, *4*, 594–600. [CrossRef]
118. Wolfers, J.; Lozier, A.; Raposo, G.; Regnault, A.; Théry, C.; Masurier, C.; Flament, C.; Pouzieux, S.; Faure, F.; Tursz, T.; et al. Tumor-derived exosomes are a source of shared tumor rejection antigens for CTL cross-priming. *Nat. Med.* **2001**, *7*, 297–303. [CrossRef]
119. Plebanek, M.P.; Mutharasan, R.K.; Volpert, O.; Matov, A.; Gatlin, J.C.; Thaxton, C.S. Nanoparticle Targeting and Cholesterol Flux Through Scavenger Receptor Type B-1 Inhibits Cellular Exosome Uptake. *Sci. Rep.* **2015**, *5*, 15724. [CrossRef]
120. Mulcahy, L.A.; Pink, R.C.; Carter, D.R. Routes and mechanisms of extracellular vesicle uptake. *J. Extracell Vesicles* **2014**, *3*. [CrossRef]
121. Mathieu, M.; Martin-Jaular, L.; Lavieu, G.; Thery, C. Specificities of secretion and uptake of exosomes and other extracellular vesicles for cell-to-cell communication. *Nat. Cell Biol.* **2019**, *21*, 9–17. [CrossRef]
122. Gonda, A.; Kabagwira, J.; Senthil, G.N.; Wall, N.R. Internalization of Exosomes through Receptor-Mediated Endocytosis. *Mol. Cancer Res.* **2019**, *17*, 337–347. [CrossRef]

123. Zanetti, C.; Gallina, A.; Fabbri, A.; Parisi, S.; Palermo, A.; Fecchi, K.; Boussadia, Z.; Carollo, M.; Falchi, M.; Pasquini, L.; et al. Cell Propagation of Cholera Toxin CTA ADP-Ribosylating Factor by Exosome Mediated Transfer. *Int. J. Mol. Sci.* **2018**, *19*, 1521. [CrossRef] [PubMed]
124. Andre, F.; Schartz, N.E.C.; Movassagh, M.; Flament, C.; Pautier, P.; Morice, P.; Pomel, C.; Lhomme, C.; Escudier, B.; Le Chevalier, T.; et al. Malignant effusions and immunogenic tumour-derived exosomes. *Lancet* **2002**, *360*, 295–305. [CrossRef]
125. Montecalvo, A.; Shufesky, W.J.; Beer Stolz, D.; Sullivan, M.G.; Wang, Z.; Divito, S.J.; Papworth, G.D.; Watkins, S.C.; Robbins, P.D.; Larregina, A.T.; et al. Exosomes As a Short-Range Mechanism to Spread Alloantigen between Dendritic Cells during T Cell Allorecognition. *J. Immunol.* **2008**, *180*, 3081. [CrossRef] [PubMed]
126. Lee, R.T.; Hsu, T.L.; Huang, S.K.; Hsieh, S.L.; Wong, C.H.; Lee, Y.C. Survey of immune-related, mannose/fucose-binding C-type lectin receptors reveals widely divergent sugar-binding specificities. *Glycobiology* **2011**, *21*, 512–520. [CrossRef]
127. Robinson, M.J.; Sancho, D.; Slack, E.C.; LeibundGut-Landmann, S.; Reis e Sousa, C. Myeloid C-type lectins in innate immunity. *Nat. Immunol.* **2006**, *7*, 1258–1265. [CrossRef]
128. Krishnamoorthy, L.; Bess, J.W., Jr.; Preston, A.B.; Nagashima, K.; Mahal, L.K. HIV-1 and microvesicles from T cells share a common glycome, arguing for a common origin. *Nat. Chem. Biol.* **2009**, *5*, 244–250. [CrossRef]
129. Shimoda, A.; Sawada, S.I.; Sasaki, Y.; Akiyoshi, K. Exosome surface glycans reflect osteogenic differentiation of mesenchymal stem cells: Profiling by an evanescent field fluorescence-assisted lectin array system. *Sci. Rep.* **2019**, *9*, 11497. [CrossRef]
130. Chen, P.; Zhang, X.; Jia, L.; Prud'homme, R.K.; Szekely, Z.; Sinko, P.J. Optimal structural design of mannosylated nanocarriers for macrophage targeting. *J. Control. Release Off. J. Control. Release Soc.* **2014**, *194*, 341–349. [CrossRef]
131. Ahowesso, C.; Black, P.N.; Saini, N.; Montefusco, D.; Chekal, J.; Malosh, C.; Lindsley, C.W.; Stauffer, S.R.; Di Russo, C.C. Chemical inhibition of fatty acid absorption and cellular uptake limits lipotoxic cell death. *Biochem. Pharmacol.* **2015**, *98*, 167–181. [CrossRef]
132. Royo, F.; Cossío, U.; de Angulo, A.R.; Llop, J.; Falcon-Perez, J.M. Modification of the glycosylation of extracellular vesicles alters their biodistribution in mice. *Nanoscale* **2019**, *11*, 1531–1537. [CrossRef]
133. Williams, C.; Pazos, R.; Royo, F.; Gonzalez, E.; Roura-Ferrer, M.; Martinez, A.; Gamiz, J.; Reichardt, N.C.; Falcon-Perez, J.M. Assessing the role of surface glycans of extracellular vesicles on cellular uptake. *Sci. Rep.* **2019**, *9*, 11920. [CrossRef] [PubMed]
134. Lucchetti, D.; Colella, F.; Perelli, L.; Ricciardi-Tenore, C.; Calapà, F.; Fiori, M.E.; Carbone, F.; De Maria, R.; Sgambato, A. CD147 Promotes Cell Small Extracellular Vesicles Release during Colon Cancer Stem Cells Differentiation and Triggers Cellular Changes in Recipient Cells. *Cancers* **2020**, *12*, 260. [CrossRef] [PubMed]
135. Yuan, Z.; Kolluri, K.K.; Gowers, K.H.; Janes, S.M. TRAIL delivery by MSC-derived extracellular vesicles is an effective anticancer therapy. *J. Extracell Vesicles* **2017**, *6*, 1265291. [CrossRef] [PubMed]
136. Sterzenbach, U.; Putz, U.; Low, L.-H.; Silke, J.; Tan, S.-S.; Howitt, J. Engineered Exosomes as Vehicles for Biologically Active Proteins. *Mol. Ther. J. Am. Soc. Gene Ther.* **2017**, *25*, 1269–1278. [CrossRef] [PubMed]
137. Cooks, T.; Pateras, I.S.; Jenkins, L.M.; Patel, K.M.; Robles, A.I.; Morris, J.; Forshew, T.; Appella, E.; Gorgoulis, V.G.; Harris, C.C. Mutant p53 cancers reprogram macrophages to tumor supporting macrophages via exosomal miR-1246. *Nat. Commun.* **2018**, *9*, 771. [CrossRef] [PubMed]
138. Zhang, Z.; Dombroski, J.A.; King, M.R. Engineering of Exosomes to Target Cancer Metastasis. *Cell Mol. Bioeng.* **2020**, *13*, 1–16. [CrossRef]
139. Maas, S.L.N.; de Vrij, J.; van der Vlist, E.J.; Geragousian, B.; van Bloois, L.; Mastrobattista, E.; Schiffelers, R.M.; Wauben, M.H.M.; Broekman, M.L.D.; Nolte-'t Hoen, E.N.M. Possibilities and limitations of current technologies for quantification of biological extracellular vesicles and synthetic mimics. *J. Control. Release Off. J. Control. Release Soc.* **2015**, *200*, 87–96. [CrossRef]
140. Coscia, C.; Parolini, I.; Sanchez, M.; Biffoni, M.; Boussadia, Z.; Zanetti, C.; Fiani, M.L.; Sargiacomo, M. Generation, quantification, and tracing of metabolically labeled fluorescent exosomes. In *Lentiviral Vectors and Exosomes as Gene and Protein Delivery Tools*; Federico, M., Ed.; Springer: New York, NY, USA, 2016; pp. 217–235.
141. Pereira, E.A.; daSilva, L.L. HIV-1 Nef: Taking Control of Protein Trafficking. *Traffic* **2016**, *17*, 976–996. [CrossRef]

142. Mukhamedova, N.; Hoang, A.; Dragoljevic, D.; Dubrovsky, L.; Pushkarsky, T.; Low, H.; Ditiatkovski, M.; Fu, Y.; Ohkawa, R.; Meikle, P.J.; et al. Exosomes containing HIV protein Nef reorganize lipid rafts potentiating inflammatory response in bystander cells. *PLoS Pathog.* **2019**, *15*, e1007907. [CrossRef]
143. Zheng, Y.H.; Plemenitas, A.; Linnemann, T.; Fackler, O.T.; Peterlin, B.M. Nef increases infectivity of HIV via lipid rafts. *Curr. Biol. CB* **2001**, *11*, 875–879. [CrossRef]
144. Zheng, Y.H.; Plemenitas, A.; Fielding, C.J.; Peterlin, B.M. Nef increases the synthesis of and transports cholesterol to lipid rafts and HIV-1 progeny virions. *Proc. Natl. Acad. Sci. USA* **2003**, *100*, 8460–8465. [CrossRef] [PubMed]
145. Sami Saribas, A.; Cicalese, S.; Ahooyi, T.M.; Khalili, K.; Amini, S.; Sariyer, I.K. HIV-1 Nef is released in extracellular vesicles derived from astrocytes: Evidence for Nef-mediated neurotoxicity. *Cell Death Dis.* **2017**, *8*, e2542. [CrossRef]
146. Pužar Dominkuš, P.; Ferdin, J.; Plemenitaš, A.; Peterlin, B.M.; Lenassi, M. Nef is secreted in exosomes from Nef.GFP-expressing and HIV-1-infected human astrocytes. *J. Neurovirology* **2017**, *23*, 713–724. [CrossRef]
147. McNamara, R.P.; Costantini, L.M.; Myers, T.A.; Schouest, B.; Maness, N.J.; Griffith, J.D.; Damania, B.A.; MacLean, A.G.; Dittmer, D.P. Nef Secretion into Extracellular Vesicles or Exosomes Is Conserved across Human and Simian Immunodeficiency Viruses. *mBio* **2018**, *9*. [CrossRef] [PubMed]
148. Lee, J.H.; Wittki, S.; Brau, T.; Dreyer, F.S.; Kratzel, K.; Dindorf, J.; Johnston, I.C.; Gross, S.; Kremmer, E.; Zeidler, R.; et al. HIV Nef, paxillin, and Pak1/2 regulate activation and secretion of TACE/ADAM10 proteases. *Mol. Cell* **2013**, *49*, 668–679. [CrossRef] [PubMed]
149. Arenaccio, C.; Chiozzini, C.; Columba-Cabezas, S.; Manfredi, F.; Affabris, E.; Baur, A.; Federico, M. Exosomes from human immunodeficiency virus type 1 (HIV-1)-infected cells license quiescent CD4+ T lymphocytes to replicate HIV-1 through a Nef- and ADAM17-dependent mechanism. *J. Virol.* **2014**, *88*, 11529–11539. [CrossRef]
150. Swingler, S.; Brichacek, B.; Jacque, J.M.; Ulich, C.; Zhou, J.; Stevenson, M. HIV-1 Nef intersects the macrophage CD40L signalling pathway to promote resting-cell infection. *Nature* **2003**, *424*, 213–219. [CrossRef]
151. Olivetta, E.; Percario, Z.; Fiorucci, G.; Mattia, G.; Schiavoni, I.; Dennis, C.; Jager, J.; Harris, M.; Romeo, G.; Affabris, E.; et al. HIV-1 Nef induces the release of inflammatory factors from human monocyte/macrophages: Involvement of Nef endocytotic signals and NF-kappa B activation. *J. Immunol.* **2003**, *170*, 1716–1727. [CrossRef] [PubMed]
152. Mangino, G.; Percario, Z.A.; Fiorucci, G.; Vaccari, G.; Manrique, S.; Romeo, G.; Federico, M.; Geyer, M.; Affabris, E. In vitro treatment of human monocytes/macrophages with myristoylated recombinant Nef of human immunodeficiency virus type 1 leads to the activation of mitogen-activated protein kinases, IkappaB kinases, and interferon regulatory factor 3 and to the release of beta interferon. *J. Virol.* **2007**, *81*, 2777–2791. [CrossRef]
153. Federico, M.; Percario, Z.; Olivetta, E.; Fiorucci, G.; Muratori, C.; Micheli, A.; Romeo, G.; Affabris, E. HIV-1 Nef activates STAT1 in human monocytes/macrophages through the release of soluble factors. *Blood* **2001**, *98*, 2752–2761. [CrossRef]
154. Percario, Z.; Olivetta, E.; Fiorucci, G.; Mangino, G.; Peretti, S.; Romeo, G.; Affabris, E.; Federico, M. Human immunodeficiency virus type 1 (HIV-1) Nef activates STAT3 in primary human monocyte/macrophages through the release of soluble factors: Involvement of Nef domains interacting with the cell endocytotic machinery. *J. Leukoc. Biol.* **2003**, *74*, 821–832. [CrossRef]
155. Mangino, G.; Percario, Z.A.; Fiorucci, G.; Vaccari, G.; Acconcia, F.; Chiarabelli, C.; Leone, S.; Noto, A.; Horenkamp, F.A.; Manrique, S.; et al. HIV-1 Nef induces proinflammatory state in macrophages through its acidic cluster domain: Involvement of TNF alpha receptor associated factor 2. *PLoS ONE* **2011**, *6*, e22982. [CrossRef] [PubMed]
156. Luo, X.; Fan, Y.; Park, I.W.; He, J.J. Exosomes are unlikely involved in intercellular nef transfer. *PLoS ONE* **2015**, *10*, e0124436. [CrossRef]
157. Olivetta, E.; Arenaccio, C.; Manfredi, F.; Anticoli, S.; Federico, M. The Contribution of Extracellular Nef to HIV-Induced Pathogenesis. *Curr. Drug Targets* **2016**, *17*, 46–53. [CrossRef] [PubMed]
158. Lattanzi, L.; Federico, M. A strategy of antigen incorporation into exosomes: Comparing cross-presentation levels of antigens delivered by engineered exosomes and by lentiviral virus-like particles. *Vaccine* **2012**, *30*, 7229–7237. [CrossRef]

159. D'Aloja, P.; Santarcangelo, A.C.; Arold, S.; Baur, A.; Federico, M. Genetic and functional analysis of the human immunodeficiency virus (HIV) type 1-inhibiting F12-HIVnef allele. *J. Gen. Virol.* **2001**, *82*, 2735–2745. [CrossRef] [PubMed]
160. Sistigu, A.; Bracci, L.; Valentini, M.; Proietti, E.; Bona, R.; Negri, D.R.; Ciccaglione, A.R.; Tritarelli, E.; Nisini, R.; Equestre, M.; et al. Strong CD8+ T cell antigenicity and immunogenicity of large foreign proteins incorporated in HIV-1 VLPs able to induce a Nef-dependent activation/maturation of dendritic cells. *Vaccine* **2011**, *29*, 3465–3475. [CrossRef]
161. Andzinski, L.; Kasnitz, N.; Stahnke, S.; Wu, C.F.; Gereke, M.; von Kockritz-Blickwede, M.; Schilling, B.; Brandau, S.; Weiss, S.; Jablonska, J. Type I IFNs induce anti-tumor polarization of tumor associated neutrophils in mice and human. *Int. J. Cancer.* **2016**, *138*, 1982–1993. [CrossRef]

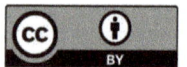

© 2020 by the authors. Licensee MDPI, Basel, Switzerland. This article is an open access article distributed under the terms and conditions of the Creative Commons Attribution (CC BY) license (http://creativecommons.org/licenses/by/4.0/).

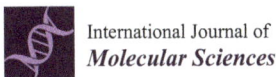

Article

Phenotypic and Functional Characteristics of Exosomes Derived from Irradiated Mouse Organs and Their Role in the Mechanisms Driving Non-Targeted Effects

Seda Tuncay Cagatay [1], Ammar Mayah [1], Mariateresa Mancuso [2], Paola Giardullo [2,3], Simonetta Pazzaglia [2], Anna Saran [2], Amuthachelvi Daniel [4], Damien Traynor [4], Aidan D. Meade [4], Fiona Lyng [4], Soile Tapio [5] and Munira Kadhim [1,*]

[1] Department of Biological and Medical Sciences, Oxford Brookes University, Oxford OX3 0BP, UK; stuncay-cagatay@brookes.ac.uk (S.T.C.); amayah@brookes.ac.uk (A.M.)
[2] Laboratory of Biomedical Technologies, Italian National Agency for New Technologies, Energy and Sustainable Economic Development (ENEA), 00123 Rome, Italy; mariateresa.mancuso@enea.it (M.M.); paola.giardullo@enea.it (P.G.); simonetta.pazzaglia@enea.it (S.P.); annasaran60@gmail.com (A.S.)
[3] Department of Radiation Physics, Guglielmo Marconi University, 00193 Rome, Italy
[4] Centre for Radiation and Environmental Science, FOCAS Research Institute, Technological University Dublin, D08 NF82 Dublin, Ireland; amuthachelvi.daniel@dit.ie (A.D.); damien.traynor@tudublin.ie (D.T.); aidan.meade@tudublin.ie (A.D.M.); fiona.lyng@tudublin.ie (F.L.)
[5] Institute of Radiation Biology, Helmholtz Zentrum München, 85764 Munich, Germany; soile.tapio@helmholtz-muenchen.de
* Correspondence: mkadhim@brookes.ac.uk

Received: 29 September 2020; Accepted: 5 November 2020; Published: 9 November 2020

Abstract: Molecular communication between irradiated and unirradiated neighbouring cells initiates radiation-induced bystander effects (RIBE) and out-of-field (abscopal) effects which are both an example of the non-targeted effects (NTE) of ionising radiation (IR). Exosomes are small membrane vesicles of endosomal origin and newly identified mediators of NTE. Although exosome-mediated changes are well documented in radiation therapy and oncology, there is a lack of knowledge regarding the role of exosomes derived from inside and outside the radiation field in the early and delayed induction of NTE following IR. Therefore, here we investigated the changes in exosome profile and the role of exosomes as possible molecular signalling mediators of radiation damage. Exosomes derived from organs of whole body irradiated (WBI) or partial body irradiated (PBI) mice after 24 h and 15 days post-irradiation were transferred to recipient mouse embryonic fibroblast (MEF) cells and changes in cellular viability, DNA damage and calcium, reactive oxygen species and nitric oxide signalling were evaluated compared to that of MEF cells treated with exosomes derived from unirradiated mice. Taken together, our results show that whole and partial-body irradiation increases the number of exosomes, instigating changes in exosome-treated MEF cells, depending on the source organ and time after exposure.

Keywords: exosomes; ionising radiation; non-targeted effects; signalling

1. Introduction

Radiation affects not only targeted cells but also non-irradiated neighbouring cells, a response described as radiation-induced bystander effects (RIBE). Molecular communication between irradiated and unirradiated neighbouring cells initiates RIBE and out-of-field (abscopal) effects [1]. Abscopal effects are not always categorised as completely separate from RIBE, and both are examples of non-targeted effects of ionising radiation (NTE) [2]. NTE, particularly RIBE, represents a plethora of other biological effects such as DNA damage, epigenetic changes, changes in proliferation, and apoptosis observed in non-targeted cells and tissues that have received molecular signals produced by irradiated cells via intercellular communication through cell gap junctions or through soluble secreted factors [3–8]. A relatively new mechanism that has been identified for mediating RIBE by soluble secreted factors is intercellular communication via exosomes.

Exosomes, which are one type of cell-derived vesicle, exist in different biological conditions and serve as an important additional pathway for signal exchange between cells. They are small (30–120 nm of diameter) membrane vesicles of endosomal origin that are secreted by normal or pathological cells into the microenvironment [9–12]. Exosomes carry a variety of bioactive molecules including proteins, mRNA, microRNA, DNA, and lipids [13–17]. Exosomes can serve as mediators of cell–cell communication. Upon internalisation, they can release their bioactive cargo molecules, which can change molecular profile, signalling pathways, and gene regulation in the recipient cells [18]. Although functions of exosomes have been extensively studied in many fields, including neurodegenerative diseases [19–21] and cancer [22–27], their roles in radiobiology have not been recognised until recently. Exosomes secreted by irradiated cells are likely to engage in various aspects of the systemic response to ionising radiation (IR), including RIBE, as well as abscopal effects. Recent studies have shown that exosomes derived from irradiated cells can cause ionising radiation-induced effects in unirradiated recipient cells [28–31]. Moreover, studies have also shown that exosomes play a role in RIBE in cancer cells and resistance to radiotherapy [32–36]. Mechanistically, IR causes changes in exosomal secretion patterns and content of exosomal cargo of the target cells, which can cause RIBE in the bystander cells as shown in several in vitro studies. [30,32,37–39].

In vivo partial body irradiation (PBI) constitutes a major problem in radiation protection, with contradictory evidence suggesting that PBI may contribute to and/or protect against detrimental health effects. PBI exposures are the norm in diagnostic radiology, radiation therapy and occupational exposures and may have significant implications for systemic consequences and human health effects at low and intermediate doses of ionising radiation [40–43]. However, to date, only limited mechanistic studies are available in understanding the consequences of PBI effects.

Diagnostic X-rays are the primary human-made source of radiation exposure to the general population, accounting for 14% of the total annual exposure worldwide from all sources. Estimates of risk of cancer from these exposures are ranged from 0.6% to 3.0% based on the annual number of diagnostic X-rays undertaken in developed countries [44]. For a better understanding of the underlying processes, epidemiological evidence mounting this risk should be augmented with radiobiological justifications. Moreover, radiation is the mainstay of cancer therapy, as radiotherapy is used in more than 50% of localised patients and is an indispensable component of comprehensive cancer treatment and care [45,46]. Therefore, it is vital to elucidate key mechanisms that could increase the risk of secondary malignancies, which could be developed as a result of non-targeted effects.

The risks posed by partial body as well as whole body exposures after both low, and therapeutic doses for cancer and non-cancer endpoints can be evaluated for radiation protection purposes if there is a plausible and consistent mechanism for detriment, a dose–response relationship that allows risk assessment, and biomarkers of response available for molecular epidemiological analysis. Exosomes can be ideal candidates as both prognostic and predictive biomarkers to monitor the radiation response and risk assessment given that radiation affects not only the production of exosomes but also their composition.

Growing evidence has suggested that radiation therapy can result in an increase in the release of exosomes and increase in oncogenic materials within the exosomes. Studies with glioblastoma multiforme cell lines have shown that radiation can elevate exosome release with a molecular profile containing an abundance of molecules essential for cell motility such as connective tissue growth factor (CTGF) mRNA and insulin-like growth factor binding protein 2 (IGFBP2) protein [32]. Evidence also showed that head and neck squamous cell carcinoma (HNSCC) FaDu cells release exosomes with a different proteome profile compared to the unirradiated control cells [47]. Other studies carried out with irradiated HNSCC cells demonstrated that exosomes carry pro-survival signals following ionising radiation [34]. Exosome transfer from stromal to breast cancer cells can regulate therapy resistance pathways including the STAT1 pathway. It has been recently reported that in glioblastoma, exosomes increase the cancer cell's ability to survive radiation by increasing oncogenic cargo and decreasing tumour-suppressive cargo [48].

Despite the extensive range of studies that have been carried out in exosome-mediated functions in radiation therapy and oncology, there is a lack of knowledge regarding the role of exosomes derived from inside and outside of the radiation field in the initial and delayed induction of non-targeted effects of ionising radiation. We have therefore investigated the role of exosomes as possible molecular signalling mediators of radiation induced out-of-target effects/RIBE. Exosomal characteristics were investigated by qNano analysis, TEM, Western blot and Raman spectroscopy. In vitro functional effects were investigated by transferring exosomes derived from whole body irradiated (WBI) or partial body irradiated (PBI) mice after 24 h and 15 days post-irradiation to recipient mouse embryonic fibroblast (MEF) cells and evaluating their effect on cellular viability, DNA damage and calcium, reactive oxygen species and nitric oxide signalling compared to that of exosomes derived from unirradiated mice. Taken together, our results show that whole and partial-body irradiation increases the number of exosomes, instigating changes in exosome-treated MEF cells, depending on the source organ and time after exposure.

2. Results

2.1. Characterisation of Exosomes

Exosomes were extracted from plasma at 24 h and from organ samples (brain, liver, and heart) at 24 h and 15 days post different IR exposure conditions by the ultracentrifugation method. Exosome concentration and their size distribution, presence of exosome markers and the biochemical profile of exosomes were evaluated by qNano analysis, TEM, Western blot and Raman spectroscopy. Significant differences were particularly observed in exosome number between samples, as fully described below.

2.1.1. Characterisation of Exosomes by qNano

Exosome size and concentration of 2 Gy WBI and PBI mice organs (brain, liver, and heart) and plasma samples were assessed by using a tunable resistance pulse sensing (TRPS) system via qNano after 24 h and 15 days after irradiation (Figure 1).

Although exosome concentration levels varied for all organs and plasma, they were increased in the brain, liver, heart, and plasma of both 2 Gy X-ray irradiated WBI and PBI mice compared to the 0 Gy control groups after 24 h post-IR. Exosome concentrations in PBI mice organs showed a more dramatic increase compared to the WBI organs, while plasma obtained from WBI irradiated mice showed a higher level of exosomes compared to the plasma obtained from PBI mice.

For 15 days post-IR samples, exosome concentrations increased in the brain, liver, and heart of both 2 Gy WBI and PBI mice compared to the 0 Gy control groups. Taken together, the results show that ionising radiation can increase the yield of exosomes derived from 2 Gy mice organs after 24 h (Figure 1a–d) and 15 days (Figure 1e–g) following irradiation.

qNano analysis also showed that the exosome suspensions had a relatively narrow size distribution (70–130 nm) for all samples. Differences in the mean diameter of exosomes were significant for 2 Gy WBI and PBI brain samples compared to the unirradiated controls, whereas no significant difference in exosome size was observed between liver, heart, and plasma samples and their controls [30], indicating that ionising radiation can also alter the size distribution of exosomes in an organ-specific manner.

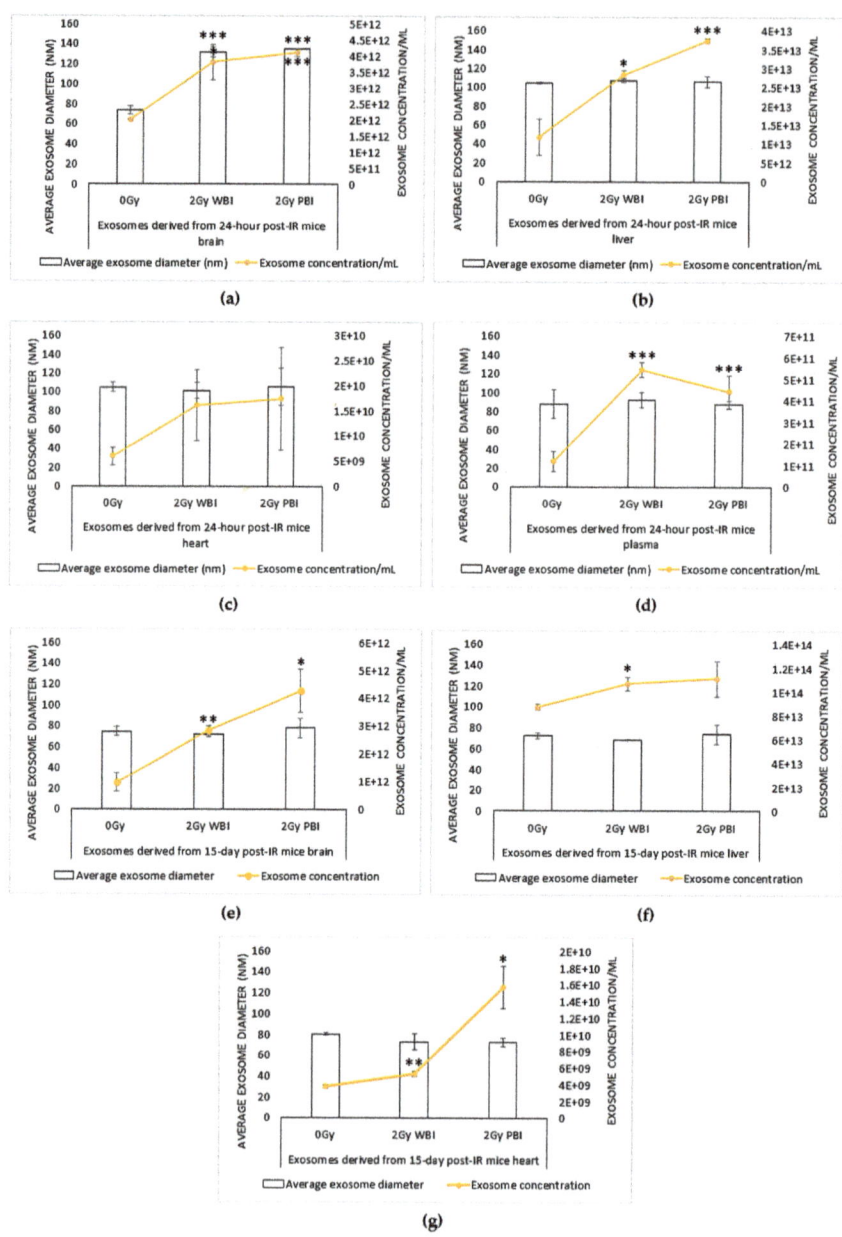

Figure 1. Concentration (exosome/mL) and size (nm) distribution of exosome suspensions obtained from (**a**–**d**) 24 h post ionising radiation (IR) and (**e**–**g**) 15 days post-IR 2 Gy whole body irradiated (WBI) and 2 Gy partial body irradiated (PBI) mouse compared to unirradiated mouse organs (brain, liver, heart) and plasma. Bars represent mean ± SD; significance was tested by Student's *t*-test (* $p < 0.05$, ** $p < 0.01$, *** $p < 0.001$).

Int. J. Mol. Sci. **2020**, *21*, 8389

2.1.2. Characterisation of Exosomes by Transmission Electron Microscopy (TEM)

Exosome suspensions were investigated by transmission electron microscopy for size. Negative staining of exosome suspensions showed vesicular structures in the anticipated size range and classical exosome morphology, as shown in Figure 2a.

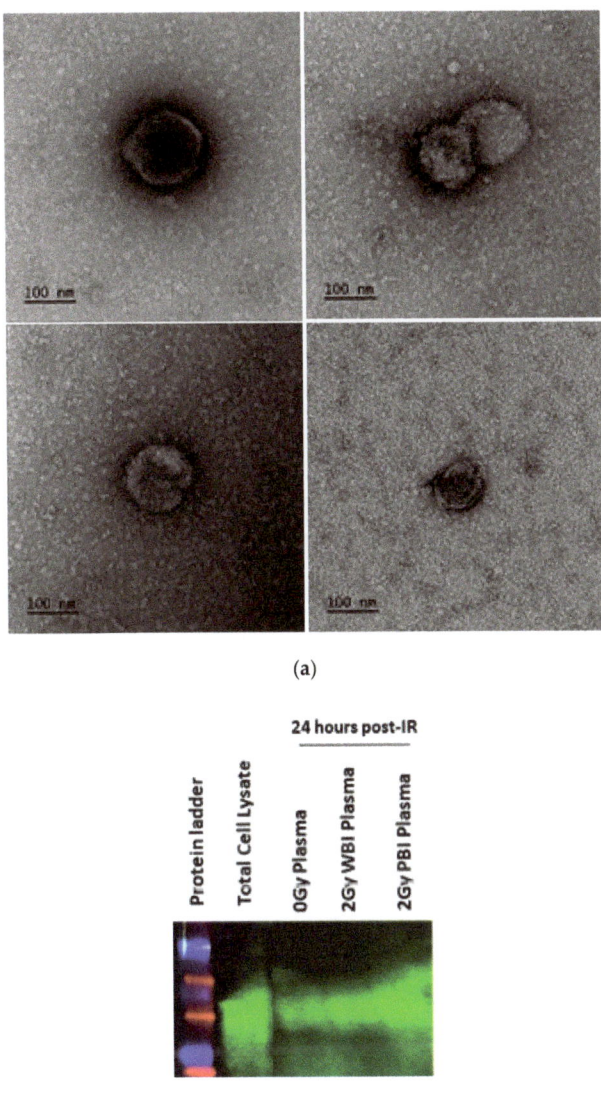

Figure 2. Confirmation of presence of exosomes. (**a**) TEM micrographs of exosomes. Representative images 1:10 or 1:100 diluted plasma exosome samples. (**b**) Western blot analysis of exosomes for CD63. Lane 1 protein ladder, lane 2: total cell lysate, lane 3: unirradiated (0 Gy) plasma sample, lane 4:2 Gy WBI plasma protein and lane 5:2 Gy PBI plasma protein sample.

2.1.3. Characterisation of Exosomes by Western Blot

The presence of exosomes in extracted samples was confirmed by Western blot analysis against exosome marker CD63. A representative Western blot analysis for plasma exosome samples is shown in Figure 2b. CD63 bands of samples were observed in the predicted molecular weight (26 kDa), which further confirms the presence of exosomes together with findings from qNano analysis and electron microscopy.

2.1.4. Characterisation of Exosomes by Raman Spectroscopy

Exosomes were also analysed by Raman spectroscopy, a label-free method based on light scattering which provides a biochemical profile of the sample [49,50]. Partial least squares discriminant analysis (PLSDA) showed good separation of the Raman spectral data from exosomes from brain, heart, and liver into control, PBI and WBI groups at 24 h and 15 days post-irradiation (Figure 3a,b). The spectral differences were based on changes in nucleic acid and protein features and these will be analysed in more detail in future work.

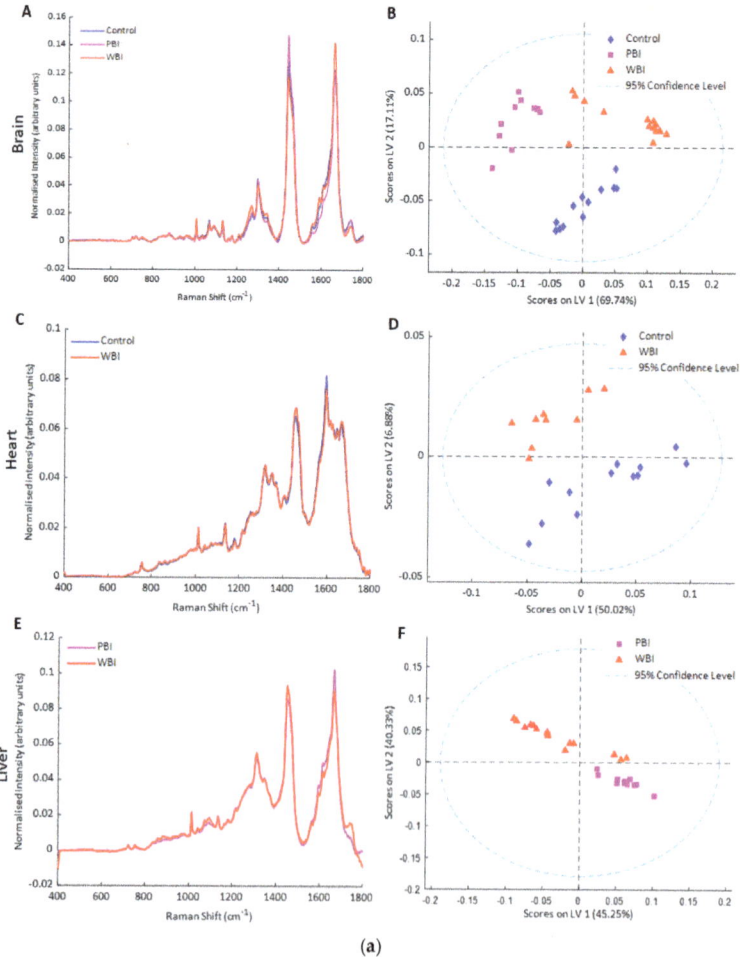

(a)

Figure 3. *Cont.*

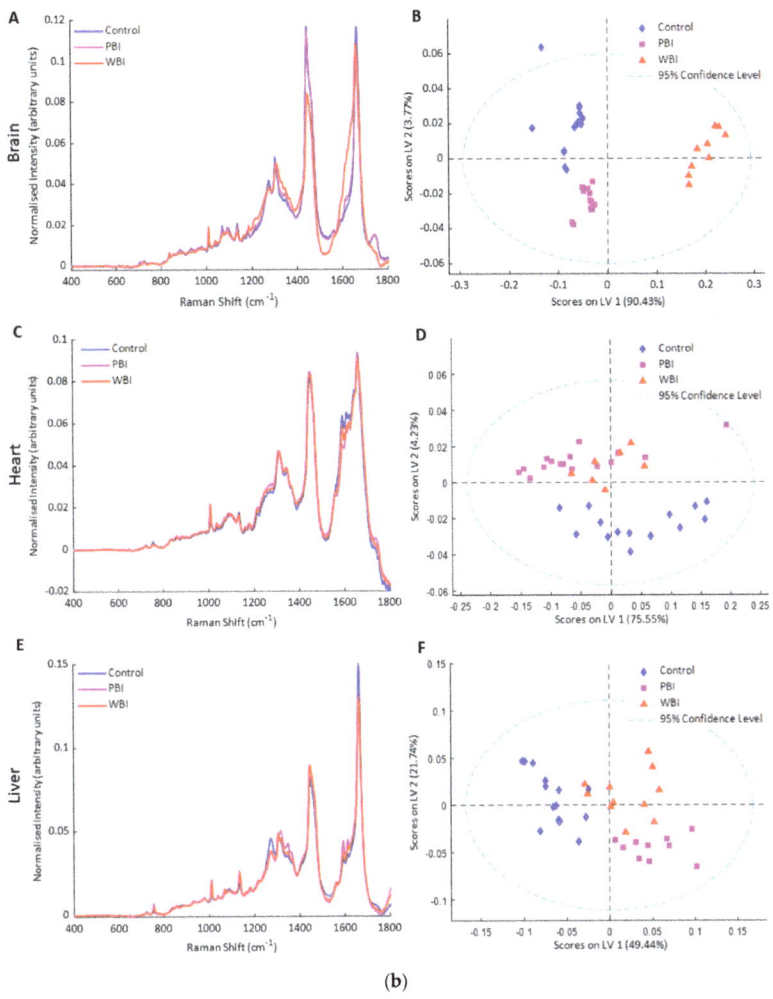

(b)

Figure 3. Raman spectroscopy of exosomes (a) 24 h post-IR. (**A**) mean Raman spectra from exosomes from brain of control, PBI and WBI mice at 24 h post irradiation, (**B**) PLSDA scatterplot of Raman spectral data from exosomes from control (blue), PBI (pink) and WBI (red) brain, (**C**) mean Raman spectra from exosomes from heart of control and WBI mice at 24 h post irradiation, (**D**) PLSDA scatterplot of Raman spectral data from exosomes from control (blue) and WBI (red) heart, (**E**) mean Raman spectra from exosomes from liver of PBI and WBI mice at 24 h post irradiation, (**F**) PLSDA scatterplot of Raman spectral data from exosomes from PBI (pink) and WBI (red) liver. (**b**) Fifteen days post-IR: (**A**) mean Raman spectra from exosomes from brain of control, PBI and WBI mice at 15 days post irradiation, (**B**) PLSDA scatterplot of Raman spectral data from exosomes from control (blue), PBI (pink) and WBI (red) brain, (**C**) mean Raman spectra from exosomes from heart of control and WBI mice at 15 days post irradiation, (**D**) PLSDA scatterplot of Raman spectral data from exosomes from control (blue) and WBI (red), (**E**) mean Raman spectra from exosomes from liver of control, PBI and WBI mice at 15 days post irradiation, (**F**) PLSDA scatterplot of Raman spectral data from exosomes from control (blue), PBI (pink) and WBI (red) liver.

2.2. Effects of Exosomes from WBI and PBI Mice on Bystander MEF Cells

2.2.1. Effects of Exosomes on Cell Viability

The effects of exosomes on cell viability were evaluated by using the MUSE Cell analyser. The results in Figure 4a show that 24 h post-IR, 2 Gy WBI brain, 2 Gy WBI liver, 2 Gy PBI liver and 2 Gy PBI heart exosomes significantly reduced the viability/survival of MEF cells. However, cells that received plasma exosomes did not show a significant change in the cell viability levels. High levels of cell death responses were observed in cells that received 15 days post-IR exosomes derived from organ samples, particularly the brain and liver, suggesting that exosomes can transfer long-lived signal-inducing radiation-induced genomic instability, as shown in Figure 4b. Moreover, a significant decrease in cell viability was also observed in cells treated with 15-day WBI and PBI exosomes compared to those that received 24-h WBI and PBI exosomes. Surprisingly, cells that received 0 Gy liver exosomes showed a high level of cell death compared to those that received WBI and PBI exosomes at the delayed time point (15-day exosomes), suggesting that delayed cell death can also be induced by exosomes derived from unirradiated liver cells. More investigations are needed to confirm this.

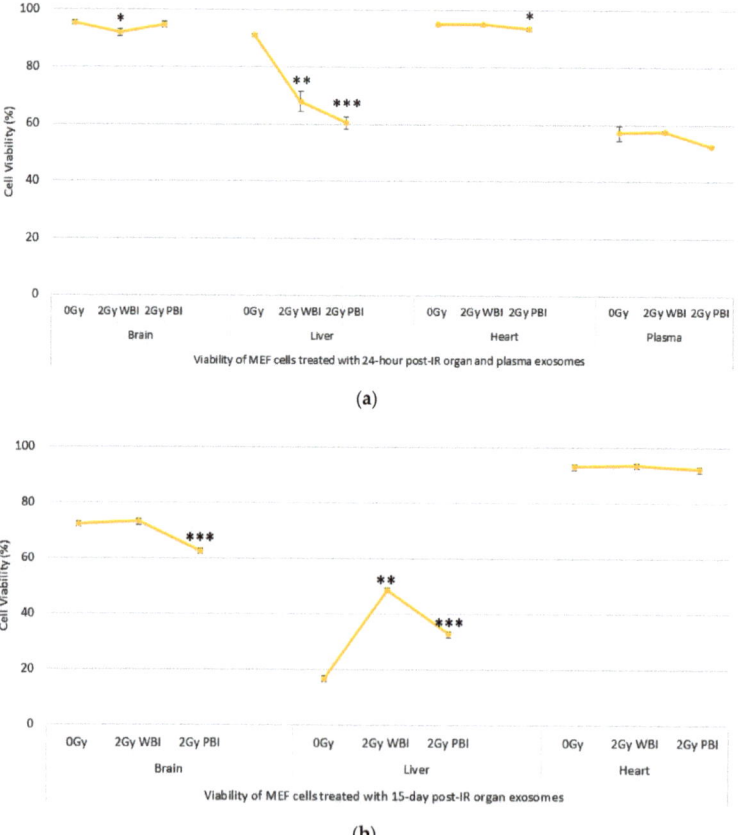

Figure 4. Viability of mouse embryonic fibroblast (MEF) cells treated with (a) 24 h post-IR and (b) 15 day post-IR exosomes obtained from organs and plasma of 2 Gy WBI or PBI mouse compared to unirradiated mouse organ and plasma exosomes. Data groups were obtained by triplicate measurements (* $p < 0.05$, ** $p < 0.01$, *** $p < 0.001$).

2.2.2. Effects of Exosomes on DNA Damage

DNA Damage in Comet Tail

Total DNA damage in the comet tail was measured in order to assess the role of exosomes obtained from 2 Gy WBI or PBI organs and plasma on the induction of DNA damage on the MEF recipient cells. As shown in Figure 5b–e, an increase in DNA damage was observed in 24 h post-IR brain, liver, heart, and plasma exosome-treated cells compared to unirradiated control groups. For brain and heart samples, significantly higher DNA damage was observed in MEF cells treated with 24 h 2 Gy WBI mice exosomes, while treatment with plasma exosomes from both 2 Gy WBI and PBI mice caused significantly higher DNA damage in MEF cells compared to unirradiated control treated MEF cells.

Similarly, as shown in Figure 5f–h, a significant increase in DNA damage was also observed in MEF cells treated with 15 days post-IR 2 Gy WBI and PBI brain, 2 Gy PBI liver, and 2 Gy WBI and PBI heart exosomes compared to their corresponding controls treated with unirradiated exosomes. In addition to the immediate bystander signal effects transferred by exosomes, exosome-transferred long-lived signals also have an ability to induce DNA damage responses in the treated cells.

γH2AX Immunostaining

In order to further evaluate DNA damage in terms of Double-strand breaks (DSBs) γH2AX immunostaining was carried out in MEF cells treated with 2 Gy PBI or WBI mice organ and plasma exosomes and unirradiated organ exosomes for both 24 h and 15 day time points. DSBs were significantly higher in MEF cells treated with all 24 h post-IR organ exosomes and plasma exosomes, as shown in Figure 6b–e, while the highest levels of DSBs were observed in MEF cells treated with 24 h post-IR brain exosomes, as shown in Figure 6a,b. The foci count was not significant for 15 days post-IR exosome-treated MEF cells (Figure 6f–h), suggesting that 15 day post-IR exosome-induced DNA DSBs could be faithfully or unfaithfully repaired. Alternatively, severely DSB damaged cells may have been removed from culture, as significantly delayed cell death was observed in the treated cells, so the γH2AX method was unable to detect the breaks in the 15 days post-IR exosome-treated samples.

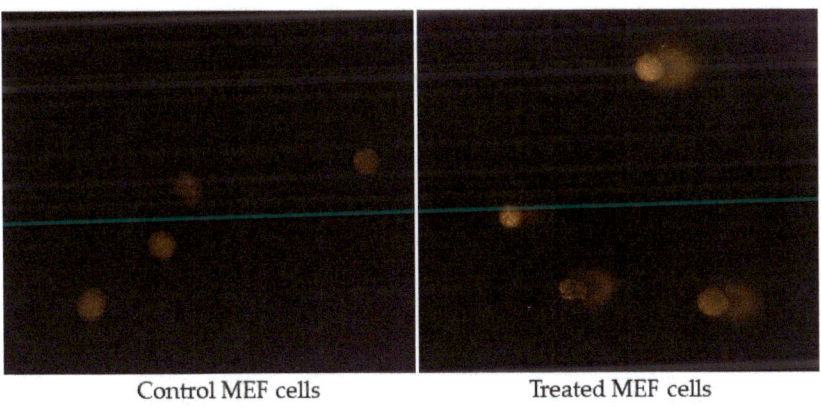

Control MEF cells   Treated MEF cells

(a)

Figure 5. *Cont.*

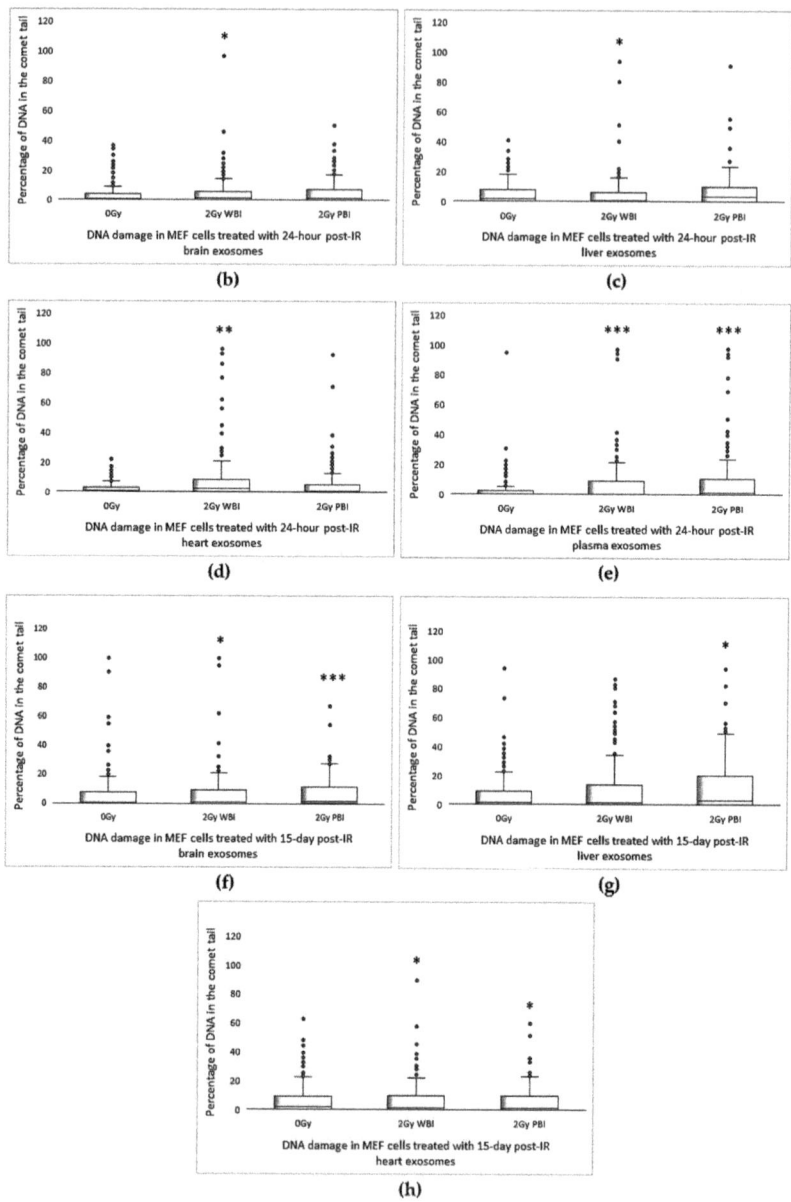

Figure 5. Comet assay showing the induction of DNA damage in MEF cells. (**a**) Representative fluorescent microscope images of untreated MEF cells and comet tails in treated MEF cells. (**b**–**e**) Induction of DNA damage in MEF cells treated with 24 h post-IR exosomes, (**f**–**h**) 15 day post-IR exosomes obtained from organs, and plasma of 2 Gy WBI or PBI mouse compared DNA damage in MEF cells treated with exosomes obtained from unirradiated mouse organ exosomes. Percentage of DNA in the comet tail was scored in 200 cells treated for each group. Statistical analysis was performed using the Mann–Whitney U Test (* $p < 0.05$, ** $p < 0.01$, *** $p < 0.001$).

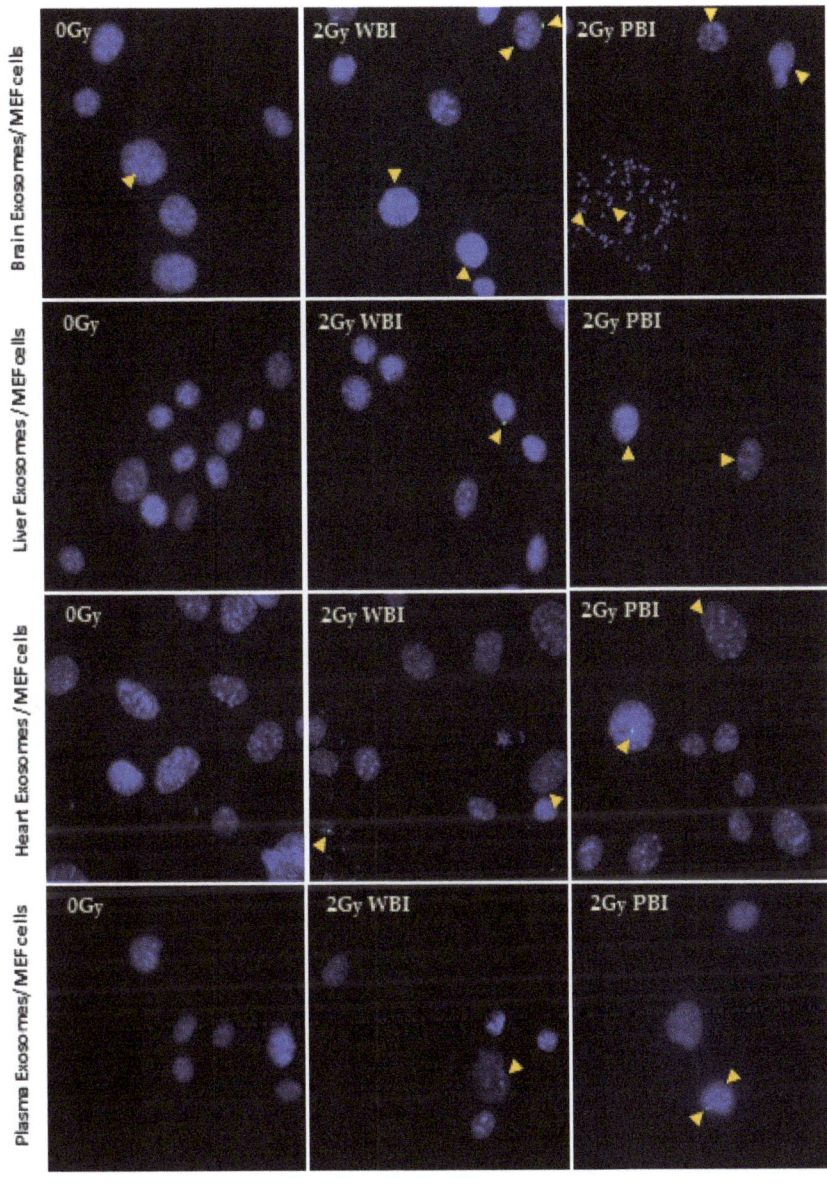

(a)

Figure 6. Cont.

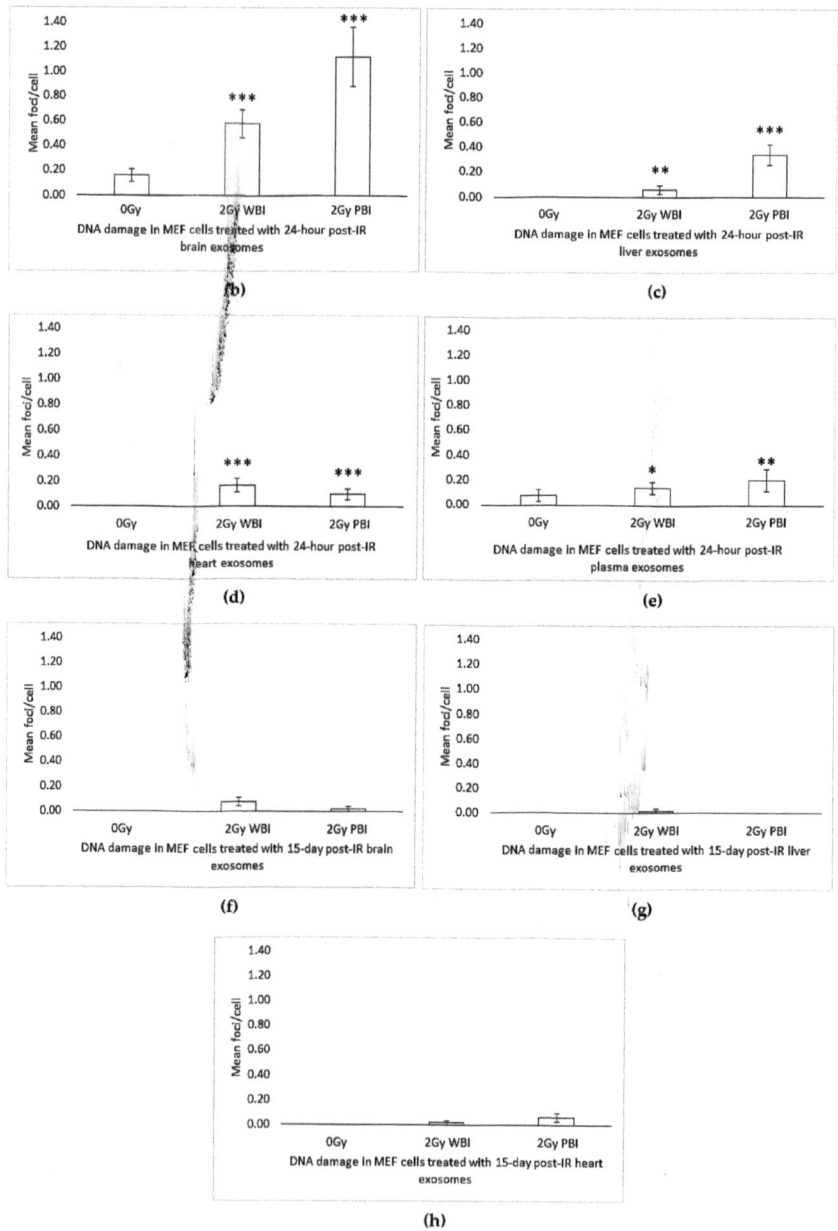

Figure 6. γH2AX foci formation in MEF cells after 24 h treatment with 24 h and 15 days post-IR organ and plasma of 2 Gy WBI or PBI mouse compared to unirradiated mouse organ exosomes treated cells. (**a**) Representative 63X fluorescent microscope images of MEF cells. Arrows indicate the location of γH2AX foci (Alexa488), cells were counterstained with 4′,6-Diamidine-2-phenylindole dihydrochloride (DAPI). (**b–e**) Bars represent the mean γH2AX foci formed per cell ± SEM after treatment with 24 h post-IR exosomes and (**f–h**) 15 day post-IR exosomes obtained from organs and plasma of 2 Gy WBI or PBI mouse compared to corresponding unirradiated mouse organ and plasma exosomes (* $p < 0.05$, ** $p < 0.01$, *** $p < 0.001$).

Chromosomal Aberrations

Chromosomal damage was assessed in metaphase chromosomes of MEF cells treated with 24 h post-IR exosomes and 15 day 2 Gy WBI and PBI mice post-IR exosomes. As shown in Figure 7b–e, chromosomal aberrations were increased significantly in MEF cells treated with 24 h post-IR WBI brain, heart, and plasma and PBI liver exosomes compared to the MEF cells treated with control organs and plasma exosomes. However, chromosomal aberrations do not show significant differences between treatment groups for MEF cells treated with 15 days post-IR exosomes, as shown in Figure 7f–h. The findings suggest that exosomes derived from organs and plasma are able to induce chromosome aberrations in the MEF cells only at early time point, while the exosomes' role in inducing chromosomal damage was reduced to the control level at the late time point post-exposure. This could be due to the ability of the cells to repair the damage at this time point of analysis.

2.2.3. Role of Exosomes as Signalling Mediators

To further investigate the role of exosomes as mediators of radiation induced damage, calcium, reactive oxygen species (ROS), and nitric oxide (NO) were monitored in real time in MEF cells exposed to media containing exosomes from organs and plasma as well as from unirradiated, WBI, and PBI mice.

Calcium Signalling

Increases in intracellular calcium were measured using the calcium-sensitive dyes Fluo 3 and Fura Red. Rapid calcium fluxes were induced in MEF recipient cells following addition of exosomes from brain, heart and liver from WBI and PBI mice but not from sham irradiated mice at 24 h (Figure 8a–c) and 15 days (Figure 8d–f) post-irradiation. Similarly, rapid calcium fluxes were induced in MEF recipient cells following addition of exosomes from plasma from WBI and PBI mice but not from sham irradiated mice at 24 h post irradiation (Figure 8g).

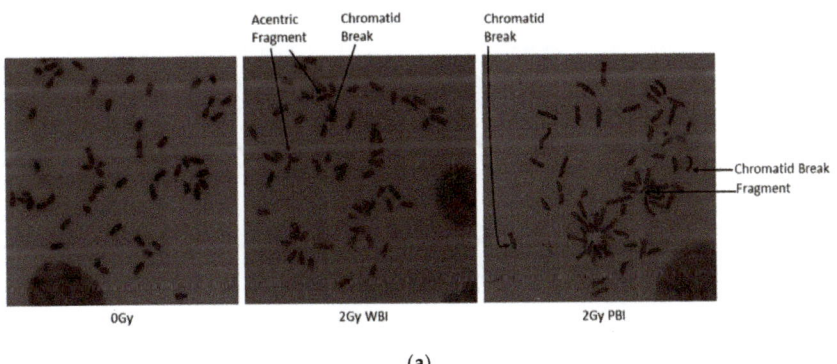

(a)

Figure 7. *Cont.*

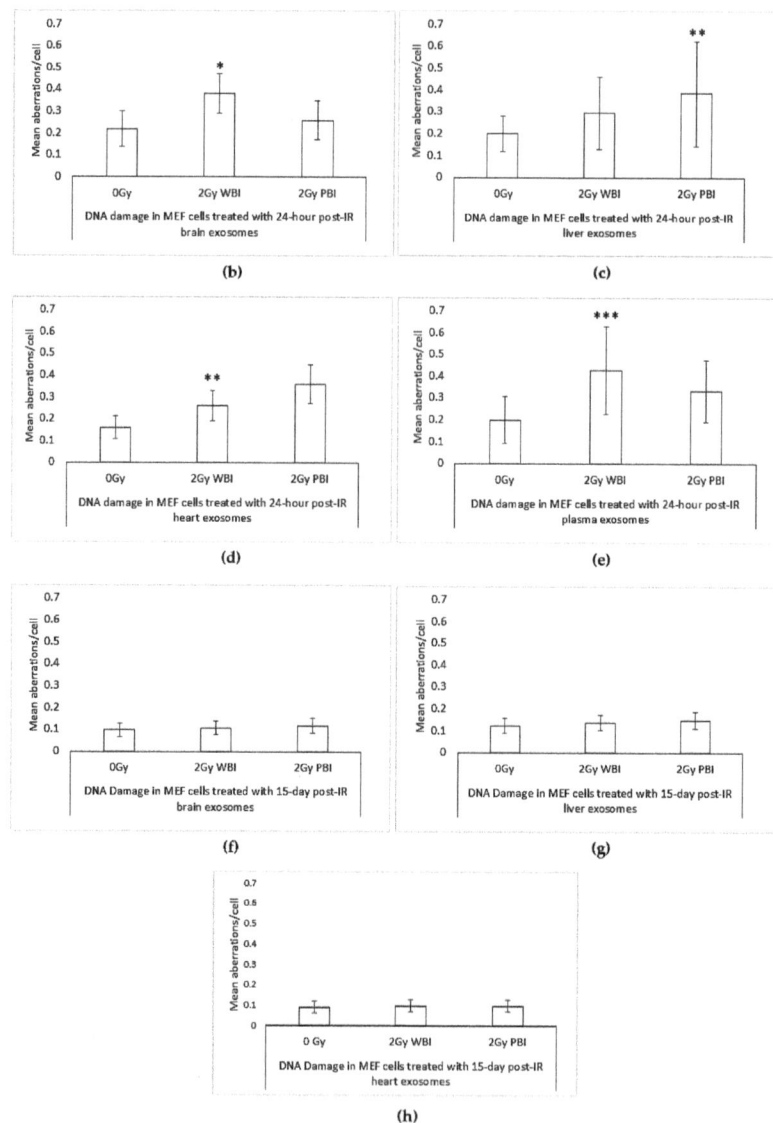

Figure 7. Chromosome analysis of MEF cells treated with 24 h and 15 days post-IR organ and plasma of 2 Gy WBI or PBI mouse compared to unirradiated mouse organ exosomes treated cells. (**a**) Normal and aberrant metaphase of MEF cells treated with exosomes derived from 24-h post-IR brain exosomes isolated from control (0 Gy), 2 Gy WBI and PBI mouse. Mean chromosomal aberrations/cell in MEF cells treated with (**b–e**) 24-h and (**f–h**) 15-day post-IR exosomes obtained from organs and plasma of 2 Gy WBI or PBI mouse compared to corresponding unirradiated mouse organ exosomes. Chromosomal aberrations (total) were scored in 100 metaphase spreads in cells treated with corresponding exosomes for 24 h. Bars represent mean chromosomal aberrations per cell ± SEM, significance was tested by Fisher's exact test. (* $p < 0.05$, ** $p < 0.01$, *** $p < 0.001$).

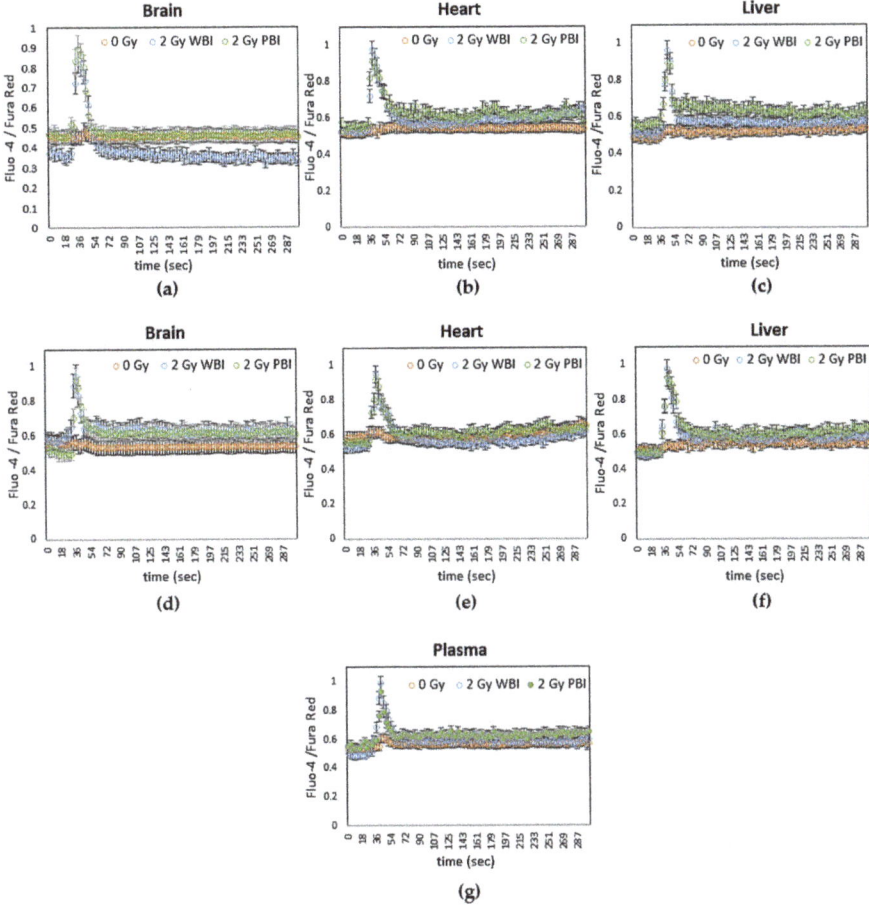

Figure 8. Intracellular calcium levels in MEF cells as indicated by the ratio of fluorescence emissions from the calcium sensitive dyes Fluo-4 and Fura Red after addition of media containing exosomes from (a–c) 24 h post-IR organs (d–f) 15 days post-IR organs and (g) 24 h post-IR plasma of 2 Gy WBI or PBI mice compared to corresponding unirradiated mouse organ and plasma exosomes.

ROS and NO Signaling

Production of ROS in MEF cells was measured using a fluorescent dye, CM-H2 DCFDA. The data were expressed as mean fluorescence intensity normalised to each respective control. Significant ROS production was observed within 5 min of addition of exosomes from brain, heart and liver from WBI and PBI mice at 24 h and 15 days post irradiation and within 5 min of addition of exosomes from plasma from WBI and PBI mice at 24 h post irradiation as shown in Figure 9a.

Similarly, NO levels were measured using a fluorescent dye, 4-amino-5-methylamino-2,7-ifluorofluorescein diacetate (DAF-FM). Again, the data were expressed as mean fluorescence intensity normalised to each respective control. Significant NO production was observed within 5 min of addition of exosomes from brain, heart and liver from WBI and PBI mice at 24 h and 15 days post-irradiation and within 5 min of addition of exosomes from plasma from WBI and PBI mice at 24 h post-irradiation (Figure 9b).

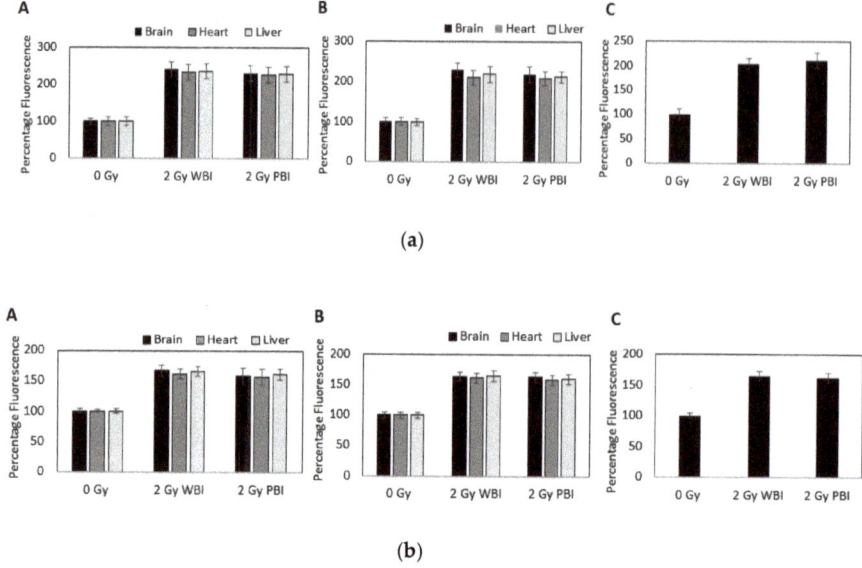

Figure 9. (**a**) Intracellular reactive oxygen species (ROS) levels in MEF cells as measured using CM-H2 DCFDA fluorescence after addition of media containing exosomes from brain, heart and liver from mice (**A**) 24 h and (**B**) 15 days after whole or partial body irradiation and (**C**) from plasma from mice 24 h after whole or partial body irradiation. Data are presented as mean ± SD after each sample was normalised to its respective control. (**b**) Intracellular NO levels in MEF cells as measured using DAF fluorescence after addition of media containing exosomes from brain, heart, and liver from mice (**A**) 24 h and (**B**) 15 days after whole or partial body irradiation and (**C**) from plasma from mice 24 h after whole or partial body irradiation. Data are presented as mean ± SD after each sample was normalised to its respective control.

3. Discussion

Exosome research is a new and growing field in radiobiology. To date, growing evidence supports the observation that ionising radiation can induce increased exosome release as well as changes in exosome content in in vitro models [32,34,51,52]. However, there is a lack of knowledge regarding the profile of exosomes released from directly irradiated versus abscopal organs and the systemic non-targeted effects of IR caused by those exosomes. Therefore, in the present study, we first investigated the organ responses to 2 Gy X-ray, a radiotherapeutic dose of ionising radiation, in terms of exosome profile including exosome concentration and size. Subsequently, we explored the role of these radiation-derived exosomes in the induction of cell death and DNA damaging effects in recipient MEF cells. Finally, the role of exosomes as mediators of radiation-induced damage was investigated by measuring calcium, ROS, and NO in exosome-exposed MEF cells.

Our data suggested that exosome yield can vary according to the organ type and whether exosomes were derived from directly irradiated organs (obtained from whole body irradiated animals) or abscopal organs (obtained from partial body irradiated animals). Differences in exosome concentrations between organs were also observed upon early (24 h post-IR) and delayed time (15 days post-IR) points.

Only significant change for size distribution of exosomes was observed in 24 h post-IR mice brain where WBI and PBI mice organs had an increased size distribution of exosomes compared to the unirradiated samples.

Although all three organs, the brain, liver, and heart, showed organ-specific exosome secretion levels, they exhibited a highly similar pattern of secretion when whole body and partial body irradiated sample organs were compared to their unirradiated counterparts at 24 h of post irradiation (Figure 1a–c). Both WBI and PBI organs showed a significantly increased level of exosome concentrations, particularly in the brain and liver, while exosome concentration levels were highest in PBI organs. One of the well-explained mechanisms of exosome release is linked to radiation-induced DNA damage and induction of the p53-related additional pathway of exosome biogenesis and secretion, which in turn leads to a significant increase in exosome release [52]. The same pattern of exosome secretion was also observed for all three organs at the delayed time point (Figure 1e–g).

Analysis of plasma samples from WBI and PBI mice, on the other hand, also showed significantly higher yield of exosomes for irradiated mice, albeit showing higher levels for WBI mice compared to PBI mice (Figure 1d). In addition, there was no alteration in size distribution between plasma samples.

Several studies support the involvement of exosomes in mediating RIBE in vivo and in vitro [29,30,37,53–55]. Bystander signals can be communicated through exosomes that can result in functional changes in target cells either by receptor-mediated interactions or by transfer of various bioactive molecules such as proteins, mRNA, miRNA or bioactive lipids carried by exosomes [56,57]. Therefore, in subsequent steps of our study, we interrogated whether WBI and PBI mice organ and plasma exosomes have an impact on the survival and DNA stability of recipient MEF cells.

It is evident from the literature that radiotherapeutic doses of X-ray can induce cell survival in cancer cell line models [34,48]. However, there has been a lack of information regarding impact of exosomes derived from both directly irradiated and abscopal organs on normal cells such as MEF cells, which was our model system in this study. Data showed that those exosomes from both early and delayed time points have an ability to reduce recipient MEF cell viability (Figure 4a,b). Albanese and co-authors showed that levels of TNFSF6 exfoliated on extracellular vesicles were increased following IR, suggesting a mechanism for abscopal and bystander effects after irradiation [58] which can also be one possible explanation for our findings.

Finally, we attempted to explore DNA damaging effects of exosomes in our model system as another aspect of bystander effects. Our findings show that both WBI and PBI organs and plasma induce DNA damage and chromosomal aberrations in the recipient MEF cells, where the extent of DNA damage was found to be organ and time specific. The amount of DNA in the comet tail showed significant results for both WBI and PBI organs when compared to MEF cells that received unirradiated organ and plasma exosomes as both early and delayed effects of IR, as depicted in Figure 5. Conversely, only early effects were significant when DSB foci (Figure 6b–e) or chromosomal aberrations (Figure 7b–e) were investigated. An absence of significant DNA DSBs or chromosomal aberrations in MEF cells that received delayed time point exosomes can be explained by the repair of DNA DSBs or removal of cells from the population (Figures 6f–h and 7f–h) as a delayed time point response to IR. It has been shown that the phosphorylation status of critical DNA damage repair proteins can be changed by exosomes released from breast cancer cells [59]. Moreover, exosomes from irradiated HNSCC cells were shown to enhance DNA repair in unirradiated recipient cells [34].

In addition, our study showed the involvement of exosomes in mediating radiation damage by increasing calcium levels (within 30 s) and inducing ROS and NO (within 5 min) following addition of exosomes from brain, heart and liver from WBI and PBI mice at 24 h and 15 days post-irradiation and from plasma from WBI and PBI mice at 24 h post irradiation. Calcium, ROS, and NO signalling has been shown previously in bystander cells exposed to media from irradiated cells [60–64], and to exosomes from irradiated cells [29].

4. Materials and Methods

4.1. Animal Breeding, Irradiation and Sample Collection

Animal studies were performed according to the European Community Council Directive 2010/63/EU, approved by the local Ethical Committee for Animal Experiments of the ENEA on 01/10/2017 with the project identification code No.004/2017- SEPARATE, and authorized by the Italian

Ministry of Health (n° 539/2018-PR). Eighty days of age C57 BL/6 female mice were either whole body irradiated (WBI) or partial body irradiated (PBI) with 2 Gy X-rays or sham irradiated (0 Gy).

For partial body exposure, the upper two-thirds of the adult mouse body was shielded, whilst exposing the lower one-third. At two different time points (24 h and 15 days) post-irradiation, animals were sacrificed by perfusion, washing out the blood and running physiological saline through the vascular system. The brains, livers and hearts were collected, snap frozen in liquid nitrogen, and stored at −80 °C for later exosome collection. Furthermore, at 24 h post-irradiation, animals were sacrificed, blood was collected and blood plasma were separated and snap frozen for later exosome extraction. All the samples were shipped to Oxford Brookes University (OBU) for exosome isolations as described below.

4.2. Exosome Isolation

The procedure of exosomes isolation from mouse organs (brain, liver and heart) were adapted from a protocol that has previously been established by Polanco et al. [65]. Briefly, organs (brain, liver and heart) were slowly defrosted, dissected and gently homogenised before being incubated in 7 mL of 20 units/mL papain (LS003119, Worthington, Lakewood, NJ, USA) in RPMI-1640 (R7388, Sigma, St Louis, MO, USA) for 20 min at 37 °C. Similarly, the reaction was stopped with 14 mL of ice-cold RPMI. The homogenised samples were then gently disrupted by pipetting with a 10 mL pipette, which was followed by a series of differential 4 °C centrifugations at $300\times g$ for 10 min, $2000\times g$ for 10 min, and $10,000\times g$ for 30 min. However, the plasma samples were slowly defrosted, collected in falcon tubes and then similarly subjected to serial centrifugations at $300\times g$ for 10 min, $2000\times g$ for 10 min, and $10,000\times g$ for 30 min. The supernatants from the $10,000\times g$ centrifugations were passed through 0.45 µm and then 0.22 µm syringe filters, and then centrifuged at $120,000\times g$ for 90 min at 4 °C to pellet exosomes. Exosome pellets were resuspended either in PBS or in exosome resuspension buffer (4478545, Invitrogen, Carlsbad, CA, USA) for downstream experiments.

4.3. Tunable Resistance Pulse Sensing (TRPS) via qNano

Exosome size and concentration were measured using TRPS via qNano machine (Izon Science™, Lyon, France), as described by Al-Mayah et al. [30], in which sample particles are driven through the nanopore (NP100 mm) by applying a combination of pressure and voltage.

Each particle causes a resistive pulse or blockade signal, which is detected and measured by the application software. Blockade magnitude is directly proportional to the volume of each particle [66], while blockade frequency is used to determine particle concentration [67]. Finally, magnitude and frequency values are converted to respective particle properties as size and concentration by normalizing against a known particle standard such as carboxylated polystyrene calibration nanoparticles.

4.4. Transmission Electron Microscopy (TEM): Morphological Analysis

In addition to qNano analysis and Western blotting to confirm existence of exosomes derived from organs and plasma, samples were morphologically analysed by electron microscopy [68]. In brief, 1:10 or 1:100 diluted exosome suspensions in PBS were incubated on formvar-coated and charged nickel grids (200 mesh) for 2 min. They were then fixed in 2.5% glutaraldehyde for 10 min, and then washed three times in 0.1 M phosphate buffer by dipping onto the surface of a water droplet and then stained with 8 µL of 2% aqueous uranyl acetate for 2 min. The stain was drawn off with cartridge paper to leave a thin negative stain. The grids were then examined and photographed under Jeol JEM-1400 Flash transmission electron microscope, with a Gatan OneView 16 Megapixel camera.

4.5. Western Blot

Western blotting has frequently been used for identifying and determining proteins, as one of the most commonly used methods in laboratories. It has also been utilised as a semi-quantitative technique in order to compare the expression of proteins in the cells and tissues [69].

Exosome proteins were extracted by using Total Exosome RNA and Protein Isolation kit (4478545, Invitrogen, Carlsbad, CA, USA). The protein content was measured using the modified Bradford assay using a Coomassie solution and Pre-Diluted Protein Assay Standards (23208, Thermo Scientific, Waltham, MA, USA). Exosome proteins were mixed with LDS sample buffer (NP0007, NuPAGE, Invitrogen, Carlsbad, CA, USA), and 30 µg from each sample were separated in a 4–20% polyacrylamide Mini-PROTEAN®TGX Stain-Free™ gels (456-8095, Bio-Rad, Hercules, CA, USA) and transferred onto Amersham™ Hybond™ PVDF membrane (10600090, GE Healthcare, Little Chalfont, UK). The membranes were blocked in 5% BSA and were incubated with the primary antibodies CD63 (ab 217345, Abcam, Cambridge, UK), in 5% BSA for 2 h at 1:1000 dilution. Membranes were washed three times with PBS-T which was followed by incubation with Goat Anti-Rabbit IgG H&L Alexa Fluor® 488 (ab150077, Abcam, Cambridge, UK) at 1:10,000 dilution for 1 h.

4.6. Raman Spectroscopy

A LabRam HR confocal Raman instrument (HORIBA, Northampton, UK) was used for spectral acquisition. Manual calibration of the grating was carried out using the 520.7 cm^{-1} Raman line of crystalline silicon. Dark current measurement and recording of the substrate and optics signal was also performed, for data correction. As a source, a 532 nm laser of ~12 mW power was focused by a 100 X (MPlanN, Olympus, NA = 0.9) objective onto the sample; and the resultant Raman signals were detected using a spectrograph with a 1200 g/mm grating coupled with a CCD. Raman spectra were acquired in the 400 to 1800 cm^{-1} region. Multiple calibration spectra of 1,4-bis(2-methylstyryl) benzene were recorded along with each sample acquisition. All spectra were subsequently wavenumber calibrated using in-house developed procedures in Matlab v.9.3 (Mathworks Inc., Natick, MA, USA). The instrument response correction was performed using the spectrum of NIST Standard Reference Material (SRM) no.2242.

Raman spectroscopic data were pre-processed (normalization, baseline subtraction, etc.) using in-house developed protocols within the Matlab (The Mathworks Inc.) environment and corrected spectra were subjected to Partial Least Squares Discriminant Analysis (PLSDA).

4.7. Cell Culture and Exosome Treatments

Mouse embryonic fibroblast (C57 BL/6) (ATCC®SCRC-1008™) cells (MEF-BL/6-1) were grown in ATCC-formulated Dulbecco's modified Eagle's medium (30-2002, ATCC, Manassas, VA, USA) in the presence of 15% Fetal Bovine Serum (FBS) and 1% penicillin (P4333, Sigma, St Louis, MO, USA) and 5% CO_2. A total of 1.5×10^6 MEF cells were treated with exosomes obtained from tissue corresponding to the 1:5 of the organ mass in15 mL for 24 h prior to experiments.

4.8. Cell Count and Viability

Cell count and viability were measured by using Muse™ Count and Viability Cell Dispersal Reagent (MCH100107, Merck, Millipore, Kenilworth, NJ, USA) and Muse™ Cell Analyzer (0500-3115, Merck, Millipore, Kenilworth, NJ, USA) as described by Laka et al. [70]. Briefly, 380 µL Muse™ Count and Viability reagent was added to 20 µL cell suspensions in PBS, and incubated for 5 min. Then, cell viability was measured in Muse™ Cell Analyzer according to the dilution factor, 20. Viability percentages were evaluated. Each sample was analysed in triplicates.

4.9. Alkaline Single Cell Gel Electrophoresis (Comet Assay)

Single-cell gel electrophoresis, or the comet assay, is a sensitive method to quantify total DNA damage (double-strand breaks, single-strand breaks and base damage) in individual cells [71,72]. The comet assay was carried out as described by Al-Mayah et al. [28]. Briefly, microscope slides were coated with 1% normal melting point agarose (NMPA) (A9539, Sigma, St Louis, MO, USA), and were allowed to dry overnight. The coated slides were then placed on a metal tray on ice. Twenty thousand cells were resuspended with 200 µL of 0.6% low melting point agarose (LMPA)

(BP165-25, Fisher Scientific, Pittsburgh, PA, USA) and placed immediately onto chilled pre-coated slides. The slides were then transferred to a Coplin jar, which was filled with cold alkaline lysis buffer (2.5 M NaCl, 100 mM EDTA pH 8.0, 10 mM Tris-HCl pH 7.6, and 1% Triton X-100, pH 10), and the jar was kept at 4 °C overnight.

The slides were then moved to a horizontal electrophoresis tank filled with electrophoresis buffer (0.3 M NaOH and 1 mM EDTA, (pH 13) at 4 °C for 40 min. The electrophoresis was run for 30 min, at 19 V, 300 A. Slides were neutralized with neutralizing buffer (0.4 M Tris-HCl, pH 7.5), washed with distilled water, and immediately stained with a 1:10,000 dilution of Diamond Nucleic Acid Dye (H1181, Promega, Madison, MA, USA). The slides were analysed using fluorescent microscopy and Comet Assay IV Image Analysis Software (Perceptive Instruments, Bury St Edmunds, UK). Tail intensities were evaluated for comparisons.

4.10. γH2AX Immunostaining

To investigate DNA damage in the exosome-treated cells, γH2AX Immunostaining assay was adapted from Zhang et al. [73]. Briefly, cells, fixed with 25% acetic acid in methanol, were dropped on slides and air-dried. Then cells were permeabilised with 0.2% Triton X-100 in PBS for 10 min. The cells were then blocked with 3% BSA in PBS for 1 h at room temperature (RT). Cells were incubated with γH2AX monoclonal antibody (ab26350, Abcam, Cambridge, UK) at 1:500 dilution overnight at 4 °C. Then, cells were washed three times with PBS-T and incubated with the secondary antibody conjugated with Alexa Fluor 488 (ab150113, Abcam, Cambridge, UK) for 1 h at RT at 1:1000 dilution. Cells were washed again three times with PBS-T and then mounted with anti-fade reagent containing DAPI.

4.11. Chromosome Analysis

Chromosomal preparation for Giemsa solid staining technique was carried out as described by [30]. Briefly, exosome-treated cells were incubated with 20 ng/mL demecolcine (D1925, Sigma, St Louis, MO, USA) for 1.5 h in a humidified 5% CO_2 incubator at 37 °C. Cells were collected and centrifuged 300× g for 10 min at RT. Cell pellet was re-suspended with 0.075 M KCL as hypotonic solution for 20 min at 37 °C. The hypotonic cell suspensions were centrifuged at 200× g for 10 min at RT after addition of few drops of 25% acetic acid in methanol 3:1 fixative. Next, the cell pellet was fixed twice with 25% acetic acid in methanol. Fixed cells were dropped onto clean slides, and stained using the Giemsa solid staining technique. Slides were mounted and at least 100 metaphases were analysed per group.

4.12. Live Cell Imaging

Intracellular calcium levels were determined using Fluo 3 and Fura Red (Invitrogen/Molecular Probes, BioSciences, Dublin, Ireland) and ROS and NO were followed in real time using the fluorescent probes 5-(and 6-)chloromethyl 2,7 dichlorodihydrofluorescein diacetate, acetyl ester (CM-H2 DCFDA) (Invitrogen/Molecular Probes) and 4-amino-5-methylamino-2,7-ifluorofluorescein diacetate (DAF-FM) (Invitrogen/Molecular Probes) respectively, as previously described (Lyng et al., 2006).

Briefly, MEF recipient cells were grown on 35 mm glass bottom culture dishes (Mat Tek Corporation, Ashland, MA, USA; # P35 G-0-20-C). Twenty-four hours after plating, cells were washed twice with a buffer containing 130 mM NaCl, 5 mM KCl, 1 mM $Na_2\ HPO_4$, 1 mM $CaCl_2$ and 1 mM $MgCl_2$ (pH 7.4) and incubated with 3 μM Fluo 3 and 3 μM Fura Red acetoxymethyl esters for 1 h and with 5 μM CM-H2 DCFDA or DAF-FM for 30 min in the buffer at 37 °C. Subsequently, the cultures were washed three times with buffer. All dyes were excited at 488 nm and fluorescence emissions at 525 (Fluo 3, CM-H2 DCFDA and DAF-FM) and 660 nm (Fura Red) were recorded using a Zeiss LSM 510 confocal microscope. Exosomes were added after 60 s when a stable baseline had been established. All measurements were performed at room temperature.

4.13. Statistical Analysis

For exosome size, diameter and viability data, significance was tested by Student's *t*-test using raw data. Each experiment was carried out in triplicate. Analysis showed no significant inter-experimental variation; therefore, data from these experiments were pooled. For analysis of comet assays, statistical analysis was performed using the Mann–Whitney test, utilising the median of the raw data. Meanwhile, chromosomal analysis and γH2AX immunostaining data were subjected to Fisher's exact test. Data were considered statistically significant if *p*-value was lower than 0.05 (* $p < 0.05$, ** $p < 0.01$, *** $p < 0.001$).

5. Conclusions

In this study, we provide the first insights into the in vivo systemic effects of early and delayed effects of X-ray irradiation in terms of exosome profile and bystander effects. Taken together, the findings show that exosome yield is organ-specific and can be significantly increased in both directly irradiated and abscopal organs. On the other hand, changes in the levels of survival and DNA damage in MEF cells, receiving PBI or WBI exosomes, were not necessarily correlated with the increase in exosome yield in different radiation conditions or time points. Those manifested bystander effects in MEF cells also differed as early and delayed responses to ionizing radiation. The role of exosomes in mediating radiation damage was shown by rapid calcium fluxes and induction of ROS and NO in MEF recipient cells following addition of exosomes from WBI and PBI mice, but not from unirradiated mice. Altogether, these results draw attention to the content of those exosomes, which can be the key to understand the observed effects. Further studies such as miRNA expression profiles and proteomics will help to discover the molecules that are responsible for the observation of bystander effects in recipient cells.

Author Contributions: Conceptualization, M.K., F.L., S.T. and M.M.; methodology, S.T.C., A.M., S.P., M.M. and M.K.; software, A.M. and S.T.C.; validation, A.M., S.T.C. and M.K.; formal analysis, A.M., S.T.C., D.T., A.D., F.L. and M.K.; investigation, S.T.C., A.M., P.G., S.P., M.M., D.T., A.D., F.L. and M.K.; resources, A.S., M.M., F.L. and M.K.; data curation, S.T.C., A.M., F.L. and M.K.; writing—original draft preparation, S.T.C., A.M., D.T., A.D., A.D.M., F.L. and M.K.; writing—review and editing, S.T.C., A.M., D.T., A.D., A.D.M., F.L. and M.K.; visualization, S.T.C., A.M., F.L. and M.K.; supervision, M.K.; project administration, M.K., F.L., S.T., A.S. and M.M. All authors have read and agreed to the published version of the manuscript.

Funding: This research was funded by the European Union's Horizon 2020 research and innovation programme under grant agreement No 662287.

Acknowledgments: We confirm there was no any support given other than was covered by the author contribution and the funding sections.

Conflicts of Interest: The authors declare no conflict of interest. The funders had no role in the design of the study; in the collection, analyses, or interpretation of data; in the writing of the manuscript; or in the decision to publish the results.

Abbreviations

NTE	Non-targeted effects
RIBE	Radiation induced bystander effects
IR	Ionizing radiation
MEF	Mouse Embryonic Fibroblast
DSB	Doublestrand break
WBI	Whole body irradiation/irradiated
PBI	Partial body irradiation/irradiated

References

1. Kadhim, M.; Salomaa, S.; Wright, E.; Hildebrandt, G.; Belyakov, O.V.; Prise, K.M.; Little, M.P. Non-targeted effects of ionising radiation—Implications for low dose risk. *Mutat. Res.* **2013**, *752*, 84–98. [CrossRef] [PubMed]

2. Mothersill, C.; Rusin, A.; Seymour, C. Relevance of Non-Targeted Effects for Radiotherapy and Diagnostic Radiology; A Historical and Conceptual Analysis of Key Players. *Cancers* **2019**, *11*, 1236. [CrossRef] [PubMed]
3. Morgan, W.F. Non-targeted and delayed effects of exposure to ionizing radiation: I. Radiation-induced genomic instability and bystander effects in vitro. *Radiat. Res.* **2003**, *159*, 567–580. [CrossRef]
4. Azzam, E.I.; Little, J.B. The radiation-induced bystander effect: Evidence and significance. *Hum. Exp. Toxicol.* **2004**, *23*, 61–65. [CrossRef]
5. Kadhim, M.A.; Moore, S.R.; Goodwin, E.H. Interrelationships amongst radiation-induced genomic instability, bystander effects, and the adaptive response. *Mutat. Res.* **2004**, *568*, 21–32. [CrossRef]
6. Boyd, M.; Ross, S.C.; Dorrens, J.; Fullerton, N.E.; Tan, K.W.; Zalutsky, M.R.; Mairs, R.J. Radiation-induced biologic bystander effect elicited in vitro by targeted radiopharmaceuticals labeled with alpha-, beta-, and auger electron-emitting radionuclides. *J. Nucl. Med.* **2006**, *47*, 1007–1015.
7. Morgan, W.F.; Sowa, M.B. Non-targeted bystander effects induced by ionizing radiation. *Mutat. Res.* **2007**, *616*, 159–164. [CrossRef]
8. Ilnytskyy, Y.; Kovalchuk, O. Non-targeted radiation effects-an epigenetic connection. *Mutat. Res.* **2011**, *714*, 113–125. [CrossRef]
9. Pan, B.T.; Johnstone, R.M. Fate of the transferrin receptor during maturation of sheep reticulocytes in vitro: Selective externalization of the receptor. *Cell* **1983**, *33*, 967–978. [CrossRef]
10. Simpson, R.J.; Lim, J.W.; Moritz, R.L.; Mathivanan, S. Exosomes: Proteomic insights and diagnostic potential. *Expert Rev. Proteom.* **2009**, *6*, 267–283. [CrossRef]
11. Vlassov, A.V.; Magdaleno, S.; Setterquist, R.; Conrad, R. Exosomes: Current knowledge of their composition, biological functions, and diagnostic and therapeutic potentials. *Biochim. Biophys. Acta* **2012**, *1820*, 940–948. [CrossRef]
12. Klein-Scory, S.; Tehrani, M.M.; Eilert-Micus, C.; Adamczyk, K.A.; Wojtalewicz, N.; Schnölzer, M.; Hahn, S.A.; Schmiegel, W.; Schwarte-Waldhoff, I. New insights in the composition of extracellular vesicles from pancreatic cancer cells: Implications for biomarkers and functions. *Proteome Sci.* **2014**, *12*. [CrossRef]
13. Thery, C.; Boussac, M.; Veron, P.; Ricciardi-Castagnoli, P.; Raposo, G.; Garin, J.; Amigorena, S. Proteomic analysis of dendritic cell-derived exosomes: A secreted subcellular compartment distinct from apoptotic vesicles. *J. Immunol.* **2001**, *166*, 7309–7318. [CrossRef]
14. Gibbings, D.J.; Ciaudo, C.; Erhardt, M.; Voinnet, O. Multivesicular bodies associate with components of miRNA effector complexes and modulate miRNA activity. *Nat. Cell Biol.* **2009**, *11*, 1143–1149. [CrossRef]
15. Taylor, D.D.; Gercel-Taylor, C. MicroRNA signatures of tumor-derived exosomes as diagnostic biomarkers of ovarian cancer. *Gynecol. Oncol.* **2008**, *110*, 13–21. [CrossRef] [PubMed]
16. Balaj, L.; Lessard, R.; Dai, L.; Cho, Y.J.; Pomeroy, S.L.; Breakefield, X.O.; Skog, J. Tumour microvesicles contain retrotransposon elements and amplified oncogene sequences. *Nat. Commun.* **2011**, *2*, 180. [CrossRef] [PubMed]
17. Subra, C.; Laulagnier, K.; Perret, B.; Record, M. Exosome lipidomics unravels lipid sorting at the level of multivesicular bodies. *Biochimie* **2007**, *89*, 205–212. [CrossRef]
18. Stoorvogel, W.; Kleijmeer, M.J.; Geuze, H.J.; Raposo, G. The biogenesis and functions of exosomes. *Traffic* **2002**, *3*, 321–330. [CrossRef]
19. Gotz, J.; Chen, F.; van Dorpe, J.; Nitsch, R.M. Formation of neurofibrillary tangles in P301l tau transgenic mice induced by Aβ42 fibrils. *Science* **2001**, *293*, 1491–1495. [CrossRef]
20. Bolmont, T.; Clavaguera, F.; Meyer-Luehmann, M.; Herzig, M.C.; Radde, R.; Staufenbiel, M.; Lewis, J.; Hutton, M.; Tolnay, M.; Jucker, M. Induction of tau pathology by intracerebral infusion of amyloid-beta -containing brain extract and by amyloid-beta deposition in APP x Tau transgenic mice. *Am. J. Pathol.* **2007**, *171*, 2012–2020. [CrossRef]
21. Simons, M.; Raposo, G. Exosomes—vesicular carriers for intercellular communication. *Curr. Opin. Cell Biol.* **2009**, *21*, 575–581. [CrossRef] [PubMed]
22. Kucharzewska, P.; Christianson, H.C.; Welch, J.E.; Svensson, K.J.; Fredlund, E.; Ringner, M.; Morgelin, M.; Bourseau-Guilmain, E.; Bengzon, J.; Belting, M. Exosomes reflect the hypoxic status of glioma cells and mediate hypoxia-dependent activation of vascular cells during tumor development. *Proc. Natl. Acad. Sci. USA* **2013**, *110*, 7312–7317. [CrossRef]
23. Webber, J.; Steadman, R.; Mason, M.D.; Tabi, Z.; Clayton, A. Cancer exosomes trigger fibroblast to myofibroblast differentiation. *Cancer Res.* **2010**, *70*, 9621–9630. [CrossRef] [PubMed]

24. Rana, S.; Malinowska, K.; Zoller, M. Exosomal tumor microRNA modulates premetastatic organ cells. *Neoplasia* **2013**, *15*, 281–295. [CrossRef]
25. Montecalvo, A.; Larregina, A.T.; Shufesky, W.J.; Stolz, D.B.; Sullivan, M.L.; Karlsson, J.M.; Baty, C.J.; Gibson, G.A.; Erdos, G.; Wang, Z.; et al. Mechanism of transfer of functional microRNAs between mouse dendritic cells via exosomes. *Blood* **2012**, *119*, 756–766. [CrossRef]
26. Peinado, H.; Aleckovic, M.; Lavotshkin, S.; Matei, I.; Costa-Silva, B.; Moreno-Bueno, G.; Hergueta-Redondo, M.; Williams, C.; Garcia-Santos, G.; Ghajar, C.; et al. Melanoma exosomes educate bone marrow progenitor cells toward a pro-metastatic phenotype through MET. *Nat. Med.* **2012**, *18*, 883–891. [CrossRef]
27. Kosaka, N.; Takeshita, F.; Yoshioka, Y.; Hagiwara, K.; Katsuda, T.; Ono, M.; Ochiya, T. Exosomal tumor-suppressive microRNAs as novel cancer therapy: "exocure" is another choice for cancer treatment. *Adv. Drug Deliv. Rev.* **2013**, *65*, 376–382. [CrossRef]
28. Al-Mayah, A.H.; Irons, S.L.; Pink, R.C.; Carter, D.R.; Kadhim, M.A. Possible role of exosomes containing RNA in mediating nontargeted effect of ionizing radiation. *Radiat. Res.* **2012**, *177*, 539–545. [CrossRef]
29. Kumar Jella, K.; Rani, S.; O'Driscoll, L.; McClean, B.; Byrne, H.J.; Lyng, F.M. Exosomes Are Involved in Mediating Radiation Induced Bystander Signaling in Human Keratinocyte Cells. *Radiat. Res.* **2014**, *181*, 138–145. [CrossRef]
30. Al-Mayah, A.; Bright, S.; Chapman, K.; Irons, S.; Luo, P.; Carter, D.; Goodwin, E.; Kadhim, M. The non-targeted effects of radiation are perpetuated by exosomes. *Mutat. Res.* **2015**, *772*, 38–45. [CrossRef]
31. Diamond, J.M.; Vanpouille-Box, C.; Spada, S.; Rudqvist, N.P.; Chapman, J.R.; Ueberheide, B.M.; Pilones, K.A.; Sarfraz, Y.; Formenti, S.C.; Demaria, S. Exosomes Shuttle TREX1-Sensitive IFN-Stimulatory dsDNA from Irradiated Cancer Cells to DCs. *Cancer Immunol. Res.* **2018**, *6*, 910–920. [CrossRef] [PubMed]
32. Arscott, W.T.; Tandle, A.T.; Zhao, S.; Shabason, J.E.; Gordon, I.K.; Schlaff, C.D.; Zhang, G.; Tofilon, P.J.; Camphausen, K.A. Ionizing radiation and glioblastoma exosomes: Implications in tumor biology and cell migration. *Transl. Oncol.* **2013**, *6*, 638–648. [CrossRef]
33. Mutschelknaus, L.; Azimzadeh, O.; Heider, T.; Winkler, K.; Vetter, M.; Kell, R.; Tapio, S.; Merl-Pham, J.; Huber, S.M.; Edalat, L.; et al. Radiation alters the cargo of exosomes released from squamous head and neck cancer cells to promote migration of recipient cells. *Sci. Rep.* **2017**, *7*, 12423. [CrossRef]
34. Mutschelknaus, L.; Peters, C.; Winkler, K.; Yentrapalli, R.; Heider, T.; Atkinson, M.J.; Moertl, S. Exosomes Derived from Squamous Head and Neck Cancer Promote Cell Survival after Ionizing Radiation. *PLoS ONE* **2016**, *11*, e0152213. [CrossRef]
35. Boelens, M.C.; Wu, T.J.; Nabet, B.Y.; Xu, B.; Qiu, Y.; Yoon, T.; Azzam, D.J.; Twyman-Saint Victor, C.; Wiemann, B.Z.; Ishwaran, H.; et al. Exosome transfer from stromal to breast cancer cells regulates therapy resistance pathways. *Cell* **2014**, *159*, 499–513. [CrossRef]
36. Tang, Y.; Cui, Y.; Li, Z.; Jiao, Z.; Zhang, Y.; He, Y.; Chen, G.; Zhou, Q.; Wang, W.; Zhou, X.; et al. Radiation-induced miR-208a increases the proliferation and radioresistance by targeting p21 in human lung cancer cells. *J. Exp. Clin. Cancer Res.* **2016**, *35*, 7. [CrossRef]
37. Xu, S.; Wang, J.; Ding, N.; Hu, W.; Zhang, X.; Wang, B.; Hua, J.; Wei, W.; Zhu, Q. Exosome-mediated microRNA transfer plays a role in radiation-induced bystander effect. *RNA Biol.* **2015**, *12*, 1355–1363. [CrossRef]
38. Le, M.; Fernandez-Palomo, C.; McNeill, F.E.; Seymour, C.B.; Rainbow, A.J.; Mothersill, C.E. Exosomes are released by bystander cells exposed to radiation-induced biophoton signals: Reconciling the mechanisms mediating the bystander effect. *PLoS ONE* **2017**, *12*, e0173685. [CrossRef]
39. Ariyoshi, K.; Miura, T.; Kasai, K.; Fujishima, Y.; Nakata, A.; Yoshida, M. Radiation-Induced Bystander Effect is Mediated by Mitochondrial DNA in Exosome-Like Vesicles. *Sci. Rep.* **2019**, *9*, 9103. [CrossRef]
40. Frenz, M.B.; Mee, A.S. Diagnostic radiation exposure and cancer risk. *Gut* **2005**, *54*, 889–890. [CrossRef]
41. Shi, F.; Wang, X.; Teng, F.; Kong, L.; Yu, J. Abscopal effect of metastatic pancreatic cancer after local radiotherapy and granulocyte-macrophage colony-stimulating factor therapy. *Cancer Biol. Ther.* **2017**, *18*, 137–141. [CrossRef]
42. Wood, J.; Yasmin-Karim, S.; Mueller, R.; Viswanathan, A.N.; Ngwa, W. Single Radiotherapy Fraction with Local Anti-CD40 Therapy Generates Effective Abscopal Responses in Mouse Models of Cervical Cancer. *Cancers* **2020**, *12*, 1026. [CrossRef]

43. Pouget, J.P.; Georgakilas, A.G.; Ravanat, J.L. Targeted and Off-Target (Bystander and Abscopal) Effects of Radiation Therapy: Redox Mechanisms and Risk/Benefit Analysis. *Antioxid. Redox Signal.* **2018**, *29*, 1447–1487. [CrossRef] [PubMed]
44. Berrington de Gonzalez, A.; Darby, S. Risk of cancer from diagnostic X-rays: Estimates for the UK and 14 other countries. *Lancet* **2004**, *363*, 345–351. [CrossRef]
45. Barton, M.B.; Jacob, S.; Shafiq, J.; Wong, K.; Thompson, S.R.; Hanna, T.P.; Delaney, G.P. Estimating the demand for radiotherapy from the evidence: A review of changes from 2003 to 2012. *Radiother. Oncol.* **2014**, *112*, 140–144. [CrossRef]
46. Atun, R.; Jaffray, D.A.; Barton, M.B.; Bray, F.; Baumann, M.; Vikram, B.; Hanna, T.P.; Knaul, F.M.; Lievens, Y.; Lui, T.Y.; et al. Expanding global access to radiotherapy. *Lancet Oncol.* **2015**, *16*, 1153–1186. [CrossRef]
47. Jelonek, K.; Wojakowska, A.; Marczak, L.; Muer, A.; Tinhofer-Keilholz, I.; Lysek-Gladysinska, M.; Widlak, P.; Pietrowska, M. Ionizing radiation affects protein composition of exosomes secreted in vitro from head and neck squamous cell carcinoma. *Acta Biochim. Pol.* **2015**, *62*, 265–272. [CrossRef]
48. Mrowczynski, O.D.; Madhankumar, A.B.; Sundstrom, J.M.; Zhao, Y.; Kawasawa, Y.I.; Slagle-Webb, B.; Mau, C.; Payne, R.A.; Rizk, E.B.; Zacharia, B.E.; et al. Exosomes impact survival to radiation exposure in cell line models of nervous system cancer. *Oncotarget* **2018**, *9*, 36083–36101. [CrossRef] [PubMed]
49. Tatischeff, I.; Larquet, E.; Falcon-Perez, J.M.; Turpin, P.Y.; Kruglik, S.G. Fast characterisation of cell-derived extracellular vesicles by nanoparticles tracking analysis, cryo-electron microscopy, and Raman tweezers microspectroscopy. *J. Extracell. Vesicles* **2012**, *1*. [CrossRef]
50. Lee, W.; Nanou, A.; Rikkert, L.; Coumans, F.A.W.; Otto, C.; Terstappen, L.; Offerhaus, H.L. Label-Free Prostate Cancer Detection by Characterization of Extracellular Vesicles Using Raman Spectroscopy. *Anal. Chem.* **2018**, *90*, 11290–11296. [CrossRef]
51. Jabbari, N.; Nawaz, M.; Rezaie, J. Ionizing Radiation Increases the Activity of Exosomal Secretory Pathway in MCF-7 Human Breast Cancer Cells: A Possible Way to Communicate Resistance against Radiotherapy. *Int. J. Mol. Sci.* **2019**, *20*, 3649. [CrossRef]
52. Yu, X.; Harris, S.L.; Levine, A.J. The regulation of exosome secretion: A novel function of the p53 protein. *Cancer Res.* **2006**, *66*, 4795–4801. [CrossRef]
53. Jelonek, K.; Widlak, P.; Pietrowska, M. The Influence of Ionizing Radiation on Exosome Composition, Secretion and Intercellular Communication. *Protein Pept. Lett.* **2016**, *23*, 656–663. [CrossRef]
54. Szatmari, T.; Kis, D.; Bogdandi, E.N.; Benedek, A.; Bright, S.; Bowler, D.; Persa, E.; Kis, E.; Balogh, A.; Naszalyi, L.N.; et al. Extracellular Vesicles Mediate Radiation-Induced Systemic Bystander Signals in the Bone Marrow and Spleen. *Front. Immunol.* **2017**, *8*, 347. [CrossRef]
55. Szatmari, T.; Persa, E.; Kis, E.; Benedek, A.; Hargitai, R.; Safrany, G.; Lumniczky, K. Extracellular vesicles mediate low dose ionizing radiation-induced immune and inflammatory responses in the blood. *Int. J. Radiat. Biol.* **2019**, *95*, 12–22. [CrossRef]
56. Camussi, G.; Deregibus, M.C.; Bruno, S.; Cantaluppi, V.; Biancone, L. Exosomes/microvesicles as a mechanism of cell-to-cell communication. *Kidney Int.* **2010**, *78*, 838–848. [CrossRef]
57. Valadi, H.; Ekstrom, K.; Bossios, A.; Sjostrand, M.; Lee, J.J.; Lotvall, J.O. Exosome-mediated transfer of mRNAs and microRNAs is a novel mechanism of genetic exchange between cells. *Nat. Cell Biol.* **2007**, *9*, 654–659. [CrossRef] [PubMed]
58. Albanese, J.; Dainiak, N. Regulation of TNFRSF6 (Fas) expression in ataxia telangiectasia cells by ionizing radiation. *Radiat. Res.* **2000**, *154*, 616–624. [CrossRef]
59. Dutta, S.; Warshall, C.; Bandyopadhyay, C.; Dutta, D.; Chandran, B. Interactions between exosomes from breast cancer cells and primary mammary epithelial cells leads to generation of reactive oxygen species which induce DNA damage response, stabilization of p53 and autophagy in epithelial cells. *PLoS ONE* **2014**, *9*, e97580. [CrossRef]
60. Lyng, F.M.; Seymour, C.B.; Mothersill, C. Production of a signal by irradiated cells which leads to a response in unirradiated cells characteristic of initiation of apoptosis. *Br. J. Cancer* **2000**, *83*, 1223–1230. [CrossRef]
61. Lyng, F.M.; Seymour, C.B.; Mothersill, C. Initiation of apoptosis in cells exposed to medium from the progeny of irradiated cells: A possible mechanism for bystander-induced genomic instability? *Radiat. Res.* **2002**, *157*, 365–370. [CrossRef]

62. Lyng, F.M.; Maguire, P.; McClean, B.; Seymour, C.; Mothersill, C. The involvement of calcium and MAP kinase signaling pathways in the production of radiation-induced bystander effects. *Radiat. Res.* **2006**, *165*, 400–409. [CrossRef]
63. Lyng, F.M.; Howe, O.L.; McClean, B. Reactive oxygen species-induced release of signalling factors in irradiated cells triggers membrane signalling and calcium influx in bystander cells. *Int. J. Radiat. Biol.* **2011**, *87*, 683–695. [CrossRef]
64. Jella, K.K.; Moriarty, R.; McClean, B.; Byrne, H.J.; Lyng, F.M. Reactive oxygen species and nitric oxide signaling in bystander cells. *PLoS ONE* **2018**, *13*, e0195371. [CrossRef]
65. Polanco, J.C.; Scicluna, B.J.; Hill, A.F.; Gotz, J. Extracellular Vesicles Isolated from the Brains of rTg4510 Mice Seed Tau Protein Aggregation in a Threshold-dependent Manner. *J. Biol. Chem.* **2016**, *291*, 12445–12466. [CrossRef]
66. Vogel, R.; Willmott, G.; Kozak, D.; Roberts, G.S.; Anderson, W.; Groenewegen, L.; Glossop, B.; Barnett, A.; Turner, A.; Trau, M. Quantitative sizing of nano/microparticles with a tunable elastomeric pore sensor. *Anal. Chem.* **2011**, *83*, 3499–3506. [CrossRef]
67. Roberts, G.S.; Yu, S.; Zeng, Q.; Chan, L.C.; Anderson, W.; Colby, A.H.; Grinstaff, M.W.; Reid, S.; Vogel, R. Tunable pores for measuring concentrations of synthetic and biological nanoparticle dispersions. *Biosens. Bioelectron.* **2012**, *31*, 17–25. [CrossRef]
68. Grigor'eva, A.E.; Dyrkheeva, N.S.; Bryzgunova, O.E.; Tamkovich, S.N.; Chelobanov, B.P.; Ryabchikova, E.I. Contamination of exosome preparations, isolated from biological fluids. *Biomed. Khim.* **2017**, *63*, 91–96. [CrossRef]
69. Kurien, B.T.; Scofield, R.H. Western blotting. *Methods* **2006**, *38*, 283–293. [CrossRef]
70. Laka, K.; Makgoo, L.; Mbita, Z. Survivin Splice Variants in Arsenic Trioxide (As(2)O(3))-Induced Deactivation of PI3K and MAPK Cell Signalling Pathways in MCF-7 Cells. *Genes* **2019**, *10*, 41. [CrossRef]
71. Chandna, S. Single-cell gel electrophoresis assay monitors precise kinetics of DNA fragmentation induced during programmed cell death. *Cytom. A* **2004**, *61*, 127–133. [CrossRef] [PubMed]
72. Collins, A.R. The comet assay for DNA damage and repair: Principles, applications, and limitations. *Mol. Biotechnol.* **2004**, *26*, 249–261. [CrossRef]
73. Zhang, X.; Kluz, T.; Gesumaria, L.; Matsui, M.S.; Costa, M.; Sun, H. Solar Simulated Ultraviolet Radiation Induces Global Histone Hypoacetylation in Human Keratinocytes. *PLoS ONE* **2016**, *11*, e0150175. [CrossRef]

Publisher's Note: MDPI stays neutral with regard to jurisdictional claims in published maps and institutional affiliations.

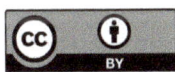

© 2020 by the authors. Licensee MDPI, Basel, Switzerland. This article is an open access article distributed under the terms and conditions of the Creative Commons Attribution (CC BY) license (http://creativecommons.org/licenses/by/4.0/).

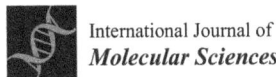

Article

Large Extracellular Vesicles Can be Characterised by Multiplex Labelling Using Imaging Flow Cytometry

Suzanne M Johnson [1,*], Antonia Banyard [2], Christopher Smith [1], Aleksandr Mironov [3] and Martin G. McCabe [1,4]

1. Children's Cancer Group, Division of Cancer Sciences, School of Medical Sciences, Faculty of Biology Medicine and Health, University of Manchester, Oglesby Cancer Research Building, Manchester Academic Health Science Centre, Manchester Cancer Research Centre, Manchester M20 4GJ, UK; Christopher.Smith-5@manchester.ac.uk (C.S.); Martin.McCabe@manchester.ac.uk (M.G.M.)
2. Flow Cytometry Core Facility, Cancer Research UK Manchester Institute, University of Manchester, Alderley Park, Macclesfield, UK; Antonia.Banyard@manchester.ac.uk
3. Electron Microscopy Core Facility, School of Biological Sciences, Faculty of Biology Medicine and Health, University of Manchester, Manchester M13 9PT, UK; Aleksandr.Mironov@manchester.ac.uk
4. Manchester Children's Brain Tumour Research Network Royal Manchester Children's Hospital, Manchester M13 9WL, UK
* Correspondence: suzanne.johnson@manchester.ac.uk

Received: 23 September 2020; Accepted: 16 November 2020; Published: 18 November 2020

Abstract: Extracellular vesicles (EVs) are heterogeneous in size (30 nm–10 µm), content (lipid, RNA, DNA, protein), and potential function(s). Many isolation techniques routinely discard the large EVs at the early stages of small EV or exosome isolation protocols. We describe here a standardised method to isolate large EVs from medulloblastoma cells and examine EV marker expression and diameter using imaging flow cytometry. Our approach permits the characterisation of each large EVs as an individual event, decorated with multiple fluorescently conjugated markers with the added advantage of visualising each event to ensure robust gating strategies are applied. Methods: We describe step-wise isolation and characterisation of a subset of large EVs from the medulloblastoma cell line UW228-2 assessed by fluorescent light microscopy, transmission electron microscopy (TEM) and tunable resistance pulse sensing (TRPS). Viability of parent cells was assessed by Annexin V exposure by flow cytometry. Imaging flow cytometry (Imagestream Mark II) identified EVs by direct fluorescent membrane labelling with Cell Mask Orange (CMO) in conjunction with EV markers. A stringent gating algorithm based on side scatter and fluorescence intensity was applied and expression of EV markers CD63, CD9 and LAMP 1 assessed. Results: UW228-2 cells prolifically release EVs of up to 6 µm. We show that the Imagestream Mark II imaging flow cytometer allows robust and reproducible analysis of large EVs, including assessment of diameter. We also demonstrate a correlation between increasing EV size and co-expression of markers screened. Conclusions: We have developed a labelling and stringent gating strategy which is able to explore EV marker expression (CD63, CD9, and LAMP1) on individual EVs within a widely heterogeneous population. Taken together, data presented here strongly support the value of exploring large EVs in clinical samples for potential biomarkers, useful in diagnostic screening and disease monitoring.

Keywords: extracellular vesicles; imaging flow cytometry; biomarker reservoirs; cancer diagnostics; disease monitoring; large EVs

1. Introduction

The term extracellular vesicle (EV) refers to particles released from cells which are delimited by a lipid bilayer, but do not contain a nucleus [1]. EVs are heterogeneous in biogenesis [2], size, and content.

They range in size from 30 nm exosomes [3] to oncosomes up to 10 μM [4], and contain cargo of all biomolecule categories [5]. Attempts to categorise EVs primarily by surface marker expression have been confounded by the recognition that many of the markers previously considered to be subset- or derivation-specific, are actually present on multiple or even all classes of EVs [6]. Delineation and characterisation of specific EV subsets is an essential goal to achieve a better understanding of EV biology [7], yet there are no techniques that accurately quantify EVs across the full EV size range, or combine quantification with the ability to screen for EV marker expression or EV content.

Small EVs are characteristically isolated by high-speed centrifugation at $100,000 \times g$ [8], and include both EVs derived intracellularly from late endosomes and released by exocytosis (exosomes), and other small EVs not derived from endosomes (3). Multiple commercial solutions exist for the isolation of exosomes from a variety of biological fluids including tissue culture supernatant, plasma, and urine. In contrast, there are no commercially available solutions for the isolation of large EVs. As a result, isolation methods vary, and knowledge of large EV content and function in biological samples is relatively lacking. Large EVs, defined as >200 nm by recent guidelines set out by the International Society of Extracellular Vesicles [1], include cancer cell-derived oncosomes, dead cell-derived apoptotic bodies and platelets, and are visible by light microscopy [9]. In published literature, EVs larger than 1 μm have historically been assumed to be apoptotic bodies [10]. However, we and others [4] have demonstrated that viable cell cultures produce large EVs which do not have the ultrastructural features reminiscent of fragments of apoptotic cells.

EVs are released by all cells providing an efficient mechanism of cell to cell communication [11]. Increasing evidence points to key roles for EVs in cancer diagnosis, prognostication, and surveillance of cancer [12]. Large EVs from prostate cancer cells were shown to contain tumour-specific biomarkers [4,13] and mediate intercellular transfer of bioactive molecules including miRNA [14]. We previously reported a population of large EVs released by leukaemic cells which were actin-rich and contained intact organelles [15]. These large EVs could be internalised by normal stromal cells and induced a switch in the preferred metabolic pathway of the recipient cells [9]. Additionally, we found that leukaemia-derived EVs expressed a surface marker indicative of their parent cell (CD19) and could be detected in the peripheral blood of murine models and patient bone marrow plasma [9]. Taken together, our previous work and existing large EV literature suggest that large EVs, often discarded in techniques to isolate smaller EVs and exosomes, could be considered as extensive reservoirs of biomolecules useful to study EV biogenesis and function, and to identify clinically relevant biomarkers for disease detection and treatment monitoring [16,17].

The principle advantage of characterising large EVs as single events by imaging flow cytometry is the potential for simultaneously identifying parent cell, EV, and tumour markers. We report for the first time a characterisation of size distribution and EV marker expression in this heterogeneous EV population, undertaken in accordance with the most recent international consensus guidelines for EV research from the International Society of Extracellular Vesicles [1].

In this proof of concept study, we set out to: (1) highlight the abundance of large EVs produced by cells derived from the malignant brain tumour medulloblastoma in vitro; (2) describe variations in the expression of established EV markers in the large EV population; (3) describe how the Imagestream (ISX) can address sample heterogeneity by facilitating high throughput, single event EV analyses. We describe a protocol to isolate intact large EVs without cell contamination, from cells growing in serum-free medium, using gravity flow filtration combined with low-speed centrifugation. Our data show the breadth of heterogeneity in the size and marker expression of large EVs isolated from a single cell line and serves to highlight the importance of sample purity, isolation techniques and experimental controls as we seek to identify tumour-specific EV markers for use in the clinic.

2. Results

Large EVs from the medulloblastoma cell line UW228-2 are visible with light microscopy, can be isolated from viable, serum-free cell culture supernatant with intact membranes, and contain a polymerised actin cytoskeleton. A proportion of these large EVs express reported EV markers.

In this study the large EV isolation SOP was applied to the SHH-driven medulloblastoma cell line UW228-2. In accordance with the recently published international consensus MISEV2018 guidelines [1], we demonstrated the existence and membrane integrity of large EVs using both light and electron microscopy (Figure 1A,B). The pan-EV marker CD63 was expressed by parent medulloblastoma cells and a proportion of large EVs in viable cultures (Figure 1A). Large EVs also exhibited an active cytoskeleton indicated by the polymerised actin marker Phalloidin, but did not stain for DAPI, indicating that they did not contain nuclear double-stranded DNA. EV membrane integrity, size, and intra-vesicle content was examined by transmission electron microscopy (TEM) (Figure 1B). Isolated EVs were spiked with medulloblastoma parent cells for comparison and adhered to ACLAR film coated with CellTak prior to TEM. Serial sections demonstrated that the EVs had a limiting membrane, internal organelles but no nucleus, and were independent from cells. By contrast, cells had internal organelles including a nucleus and cytoplasmic protrusions indicative of filopodia.

Cells were grown in serum-free medium for 24 h prior to EV isolation, staining, and analysis. Experimental conditions were optimised to eliminate false positive membrane labelling or bovine EV contamination [18]. To assess whether growth in serum-free medium resulted in increased cell apoptosis, phosphatidyl serine exposure on the surface of cells was examined. Figure 1C indicates the quadrant gating strategy applied using positive controls and the comparison of cells grown in standard culture versus serum-free conditions. Imaging flow cytometry was also performed to visualise Annexin V/PI staining on parent cells (Figure 1D). In triplicate experiments, there was no significant difference between the viability of cells cultured in complete or serum-free media (Figure 1E). Figure 1F provides a workflow for the isolation and characterisation of large EVs used in this study. At the time of each EV isolation, total parent cell count and viability was assessed using trypan blue exclusion and found to be 7.9×10^6 cells (98% viable), 8.3×10^6 cells (99% viable), and 6.8×10^6 cells (98% viable).

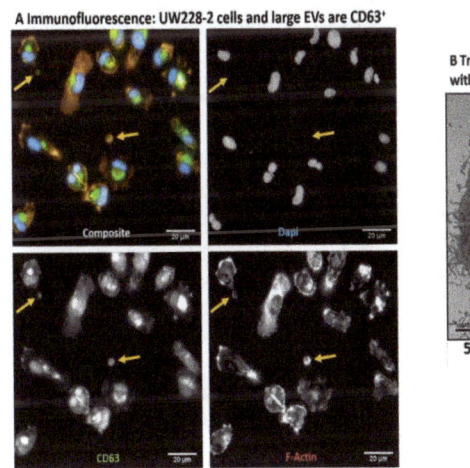
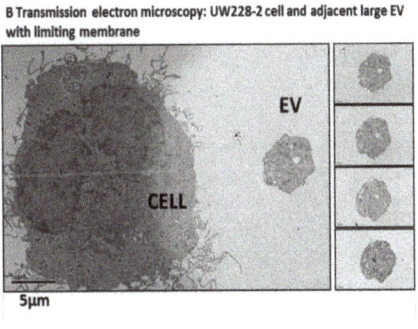

Figure 1. *Cont.*

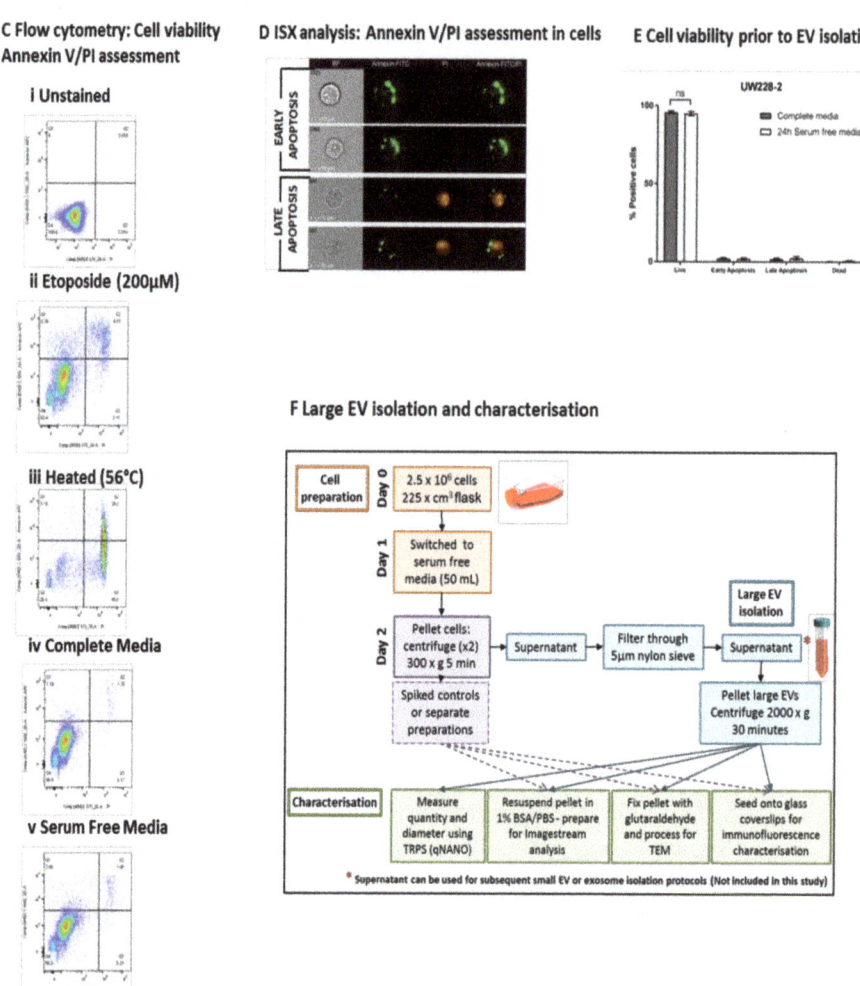

Figure 1. Immunofluorescence: UW228-2 cells and large extracellular vesicles (EVs) are CD63[+]. Medulloblastoma cell lines produce large extracellular vesicles (EVs) which can be harvested from serum-free conditioned media after 24 h. (**A**) Medulloblastoma cells produce EVs in vitro which contain polymerised actin and CD63, but no nucleus. The medulloblastoma cell line UW228-2 was cultured on glass bottom plates for 24 h; fixed and probed for the tetraspanin and EV marker CD63 (FITC—green). Polymerised actin was labelled using Alexa Fluor 555 phalloidin (f-ACTIN—red). Nuclei were counterstained with DAPI (DAPI—blue). Images of large EVs (yellow arrows) and cells were captured using the Perkin Elmer Operetta system at ×40 magnification. The individual images were captured in black and white using the appropriate emission filters and a coloured composite image created using Columbus software. Scale bar represents 20 μM. (**B**) Transmission electron microscopy: UW228-2 cell and adjacent large EV with limiting membrane. Large EVs have a limiting membrane, contain organelles but no nucleus and are < 6 μm in size. Cells and EVs were applied to Poly-D-lysine coated ACLAR film and fixed with glutaraldehyde before processing for Transmission Electron

Microscopy. Serial sections were taken to assess sample purity, EV membrane integrity, size, and content comparative to the parent cell. Images were captured using a Biotwin Philips TECNAI G2 microscope at ×1900 magnification. Scale bar represents 5 µM. Left panel shows a cell and a large EV. Right panel: serial sections taken through the entire EV (4 images shown). The wide-field image shows an EV of 5.5 µM diameter at its central plane of focus, alongside a parent medulloblastoma cell of 18 µM. (**C**) Flow cytometry: Cell viability Annexin V/PI assessment. Cell apoptosis was assessed by flow cytometry. Unstained cells (i) and cells treated with 200 µM Etoposide (ii; Annexin V positive gate) or heated (iii; PI positive gate) provided positive controls which were used to assign accurate quadrant gates to bivariate scatter plots showing PI versus Annexin V APC. Live cells appear in Q4, Annexin only in Q2 (Early apoptosis), dual labelled in Q3 (Late apoptosis) and PI only (Dead cells). UW228-2 cells were cultured for 24 h in complete media (iv; DMEM with 10% FBS) or serum-free media (v; DMEM only). Representative plots of triplicate experiments shown. (**D**) Imagestream (ISX) analysis: Annexin V/PI assessment in cells. Imaging flow cytometry allows visual distinction between early and late stages of apoptosis. Cells in standard culture conditions were labelled using an Annexin FITC/PI kit and examined using the Imagestream (ISX) Mark II. Images were captured at x60 magnification and representative gallery images demonstrate Annexin V FITC only membrane labelling, indicating early apoptosis (upper panels) and dual Annexin V FITC/PI labelling, indicating late apoptosis (lower panels). (**E**) Cell viability prior to EV isolation. UW228-2 cells can be cultured in serum-free conditions for 24 h with no loss in viability. No difference in viability could be seen between culture conditions: Percentage unlabelled cells (live), Annexin V positive only (Early apoptosis), Annexin V and PI positive (Late Apoptosis) or PI positive only (DEAD) after 24 h in complete (grey bars) or serum-free medium (open bars). (**F**) Large EV isolation and characterisation. EV isolation protocol from cultured cells was optimised to harvest large EVs with minimal processing. Cells were seeded into large flasks (225 cm^3) and allowed to adhere. Media was changed after 24 h for 50 mL serum-free DMEM and cells cultured at 37 °C for a further 24 h. Trypsinised cells were collected by 2 successive centrifugation steps at 300× g 5 min keeping the supernatant each time. EV containing supernatant was filtered using a double layered 5 µm pore nylon membrane by gravity. Filtered, cell-free supernatant was centrifuged at 2000× g for 30 min using a bench top centrifuge with swing out buckets. The resulting cell and EV pellets were processed appropriately for the downstream technique: For flow cytometry cells were processed and analysed separately, whilst cells were spiked into wells for direct comparison by microscopy.

2.1. EVs are Highly Heterogeneous and Differentially Express EV Markers

A reliable fluorescence marker was essential to demarcate EVs from background scatter events. Cell mask orange (CMO) is a fluorescent plasma membrane label composed of amphipathic molecules comprising a lipophilic moiety for membrane loading and a negatively charged hydrophilic dye for anchoring of the probe in the plasma membrane. We performed a titration using the parent cells with serial dilutions of the dye in serum-free media ranging from 1 in 1000 (5 µg/mL) to 1 in 100,000 (50 ng/mL) (Figure 2A) and found that 2.5 µg/mL (1 in 2000) was an optimal concentration providing high median fluorescence intensity without saturation. Using the Imagestream Mark II (ISX) we confirmed that the final concentration of CMO labelled EVs in a typical preparation did not result in coincidence events or swarm which could lead to false positive results when looking at multi-colour labelling. Serial dilutions of CMO labelled EVs showed a linear decrease in objects per mL (Figure 2B(i)) with an increasing dilution factor, whilst the fluorescence intensity remained stable across the dilutions (Figure 2B(ii)). To facilitate reproducible reporting across experiments and to offer a means to standardise EV measurements, we determined the minimum MESF value for CMO+ events which would distinguish between unstained and CMO labelled EVs using our staining protocol, as described elsewhere [19]. Figure 2C shows a representative bivariate plot (i) of the low, medium-low, medium-high, and high fluorescence bead populations. The histogram (ii) was used to determine the MFI of each peak and log fluorescence intensities were converted to MESF values using information supplied by the manufacturer (iii). Linear regression of log MFI versus log MESF

(iv) was used to calculate the MESF corresponding to the minimum fluorescence intensity of events within the designated CMO+ gate as follows. The maximum MESF values of the unstained EVs in each experiment were: Replicate 1: 271.42 = MESF 48.23; Replicate 2: 271.0 = MESF 49.27; Replicate 3: 272.88 = MESF 42.48. Therefore, to set a standardised lower threshold of detection which could be used across replicate experiments we assigned a lower MESF threshold for CMO$^+$ events of 50 (Example shown in Figure 2C(v)). We therefore report here CMO$^+$ events as number of events >MESF 50.

Previous reports have identified that lipid dye aggregates can mimic EVs when using fluorescence lipid markers [20]. We used Triton-X 100 treatment [21] of fully labeled EVs to disrupt EV signals demonstrated by a loss of CMO + events (Figure 2D(i)). Figure 2D(ii) shows an overlay of unstained EVs, fully stained EVs and fully stained EVs treated with Triton-X 100. The MFI of the post-Triton-X 100 treated sample is reduced to the level of the US-EVs.

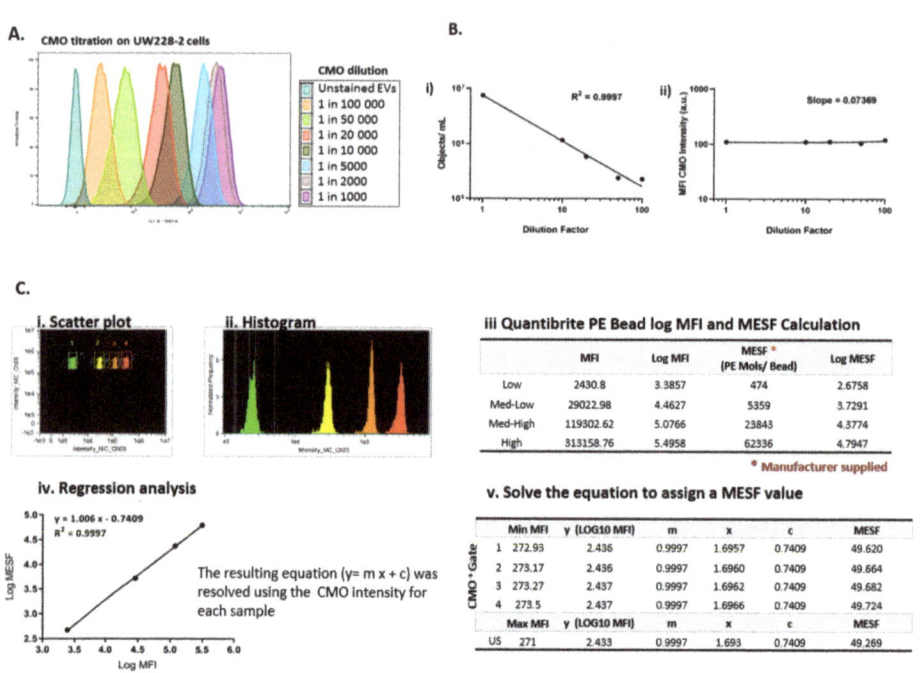

Figure 2. Cont.

D. i) Loss of CMO labelling following the addition of Triton-X confirms EV membrane labelling

ii) Overlay showing CMO intensity of unstained and fully stained EVs pre and post Triton-X treatment

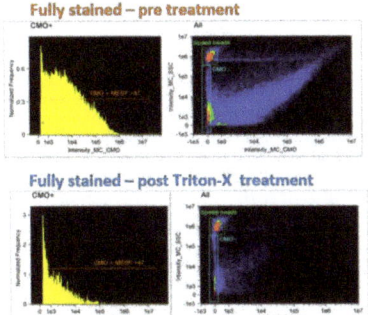

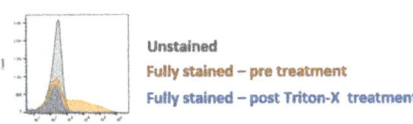

Unstained
Fully stained – pre treatment
Fully stained – post Triton-X treatment

Figure 2. Cell Mask Orange can label EVs to enable standardisation across experiments. (**A**) Cell Mask Orange (CMO) labelling was optimised by titration using parent cells. Serial dilutions from 1 in 1000–100,000 were used to label parent UW228-2 cells and analysed by flow cytometry. A clear relationship between CMO concentration and fluorescence intensity is shown. (**B**) ISX: Objects/mL reduce with increased sample dilution (i) whilst CMO intensity remains constant (ii). Sample dilution was used to validate EV staining protocol. Using a CMO dilution of 1 in 2000 (2.5 μg/mL), the Imagestream acquired fewer CMO positive objects per ml with increasing dilution of CMO labelled EVs (i), whilst the CMO fluorescence intensity in channel 03 was maintained (ii). (**C**) Quantibrite PE Beads were run at the time of each experiment and used to assign molecules of equivalent soluble fluorochrome (MESF) values to the CMO intensity of labelled EVs. (Representative example from a single experiment shown) Quantibrite PE beads were acquired at the time of each experiment to assign MESF value. Quantibrite PE beads were separated on a bivariate plot of intensity against side scatter (i). The fluorescence intensity of each bead set was gated on the histogram (ii) and assigned a MESF value according to the number of PE molecules per bead as provided by the manufacturer (iii). Log MFI against Log MESF provided a standard curve for each acquisition (iv). Regression analysis was used to extrapolate the equivalent MESF value for CMO intensity for unstained and labelled samples (v) which enabled lower threshold for CMO intensity to be set to distinguish between unstained and CMO labelled EVs. Representative experiment shown. MESF 50 was subsequently used to set the lower CMO+ threshold to standardise across experiments. (**D**) CMO labelling was diminished following the addition of detergent. CMO positive (CMO+) EVs could be distinguished from unstained EVs by ISX (i). Treatment of the same sample with Triton-X 100 diminished the CMO labelling (ii). Exported .fcs files from the same acquisition were overlaid using FlowJo 10.6 (Ashland). The fully stained sample (orange) shows increased fluorescence intensity in channel 3. The same sample post Triton–X treatment (blue) showed a reduction in fluorescence intensity to a similar level of the unstained sample (grey).

2.2. Large EVs Size Distribution and Quantity was Assessed Using Tunable Resistance Pulse Sensing (TRPS)

At the time of each preparation, an aliquot of freshly isolated EVs was assessed using the qNano GOLD particle counter to ascertain EV size distribution (diameter) in terms of percentage population (%) and concentration (particles/mL) prior to labelling for ISX analysis. Using a series of 3 overlapping Nanopores (Figure 3A(i)), each with an optimal size range which spans a total size of approximately 275 nm to 5.7 μm, we assessed the size range of particles in the EV preparations. Representative profiles of diameter against percentage population are shown for a single sample using NP600, NP1000, and NP2000 Nanopores (Figure 3A(ii–iv)). By selecting overlapping Nanopore sizes, the same calibrator beads (1000 nm) could be used and therefore it was possible to overlay the resulting profiles to visualise the total large EV population within each sample (Figure 3A(v)). As expected, the EVs present in each biological replicate were heterogeneous in size. However, the size range of EVs across biological replicates was consistent (250 nm to 6 μm); with some variation in the median diameter per sample. Size is presented with a bin of 100 (nm) and in each case the most prevalent large EVs were detected using the NP600. The median size across the replicates using the NP600 for comparison were 250–350 nm 5.15×10^7; 450–550 nm 1.7×10^7, and 250–350 nm 2.8×10^8. The starting volume of EV-containing media used per replicate was 100 mL. The resulting pellet was re-suspended in a total of 700 µL PBS (prior to labelling). As an example, applying this dilution factor (142.86) to the first replicate equates to 7.4×10^9 EVs specifically of the 250–350 nm size range that were released by 7.9×10^6 UW228-2 cells (NB cell count at harvest) in 24 h into 100 mL serum-free media. It should be noted that due to the number of washes and centrifugation steps during the isolation, this can only be considered as an illustration of the quantity of EVs produced. The total larger EVs as counted using the NP2000 (935 nm – 5.7 µm) were less common but are nevertheless abundantly present in concentrations of 2.3×10^8, 6.9×10^8 and 2.1×10^9 in the 100 mL harvested media from this particular cell line. The total particle count for each Nanopore size, across 3 biological replicates is shown in Table 1. It should be noted that the counts shown are not cumulative as they represent the same sample analysed across 3 Nanopore sizes.

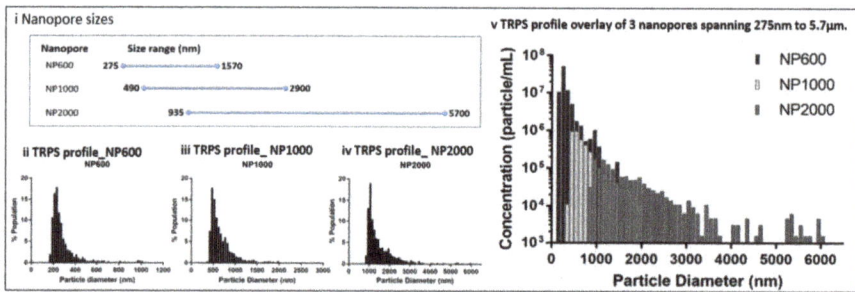

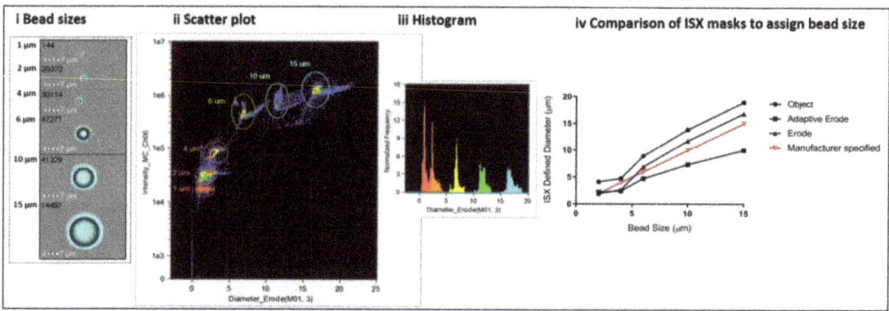

Figure 3. EV size and quantity was assessed by Tunable Resistance Pulse Sensing (TRPS) using the qNANO instrument (iZON Science) and compared to diameter masks in the ISX IDEAS software. (**A**) Three Nanopores of over-lapping size ranges were used to determine the particle diameter and concentration in each EV preparation (i). Size profiles were established for each individual Nanopore (ii NP600; iii NP1000; iv NP2000). The overlaid profiles of diameter by concentration provided by the 3 Nanopores show a size range of 250 nm and 6µm against a common calibrator bead of 1000 nm (representative sample shown) (v). (**B**) Calibration beads of known size were used to determine the most accurate diameter mask. The masks available within the ISX IDEAS software for diameter analysis were compared. The 3 which assigned the most accurate sizes according to manufacturer specified beads sizes were the Object, Erode and Adaptive Erode masks. These were compared across bead size by applying the mask (ii) visualising a scatter plot (iii) and histogram for each mask type. For the size range within our EV preparations, we found the Erode mask to be the most accurate (iv).

Table 1. Total particle count using different Nanopore sizes (qNANO) in biological replicates.

-	NP600	NP1000	NP2000
1	8.4×10^8	3.8×10^6	1.6×10^6
2	4.9×10^7	1.4×10^7	4.8×10^6
3	5.0×10^8	4.4×10^7	1.5×10^7

Size calibration beads were used to determine the most appropriate diameter mask to use for ISX analysis of EV diameter. The bead sizes provided by the manufacturer were 1, 2, 4, 6, 10, and 15 µm. We used the feature tool in IDEAS to apply a range of different diameter masks to the bright field image of the beads (Figure 3B(i)). We selected bright field for this using non-labelled beads because the Quantibrite beads showed over exaggeration of EV size, possibly due to saturation and flare of fluorescence. The beads were visualised on bivariate plots of diameter versus side scatter (channel 06). Density plots (Figure 3B(ii)) allowed the bead populations to be gated individually and subsequent histograms (Figure 3B(iii)) to be viewed. We compared the diameters for each bead population assigned using the Object, Adaptive Erode and Erode Masks against the manufacturer specified size (Figure 3B(iv)) and found the Erode mask on the bright field image, using 3 pixel reduction to be the most comparable.

2.3. Fluorescence Membrane Labelling Can Be Used to Distinguish EVs from Background and Speed Beads

We devised an analysis template within IDEAS which comprised a hierarchical gating strategy aimed at characterising heterogeneous large EVs (Figure 4A). All buffers were filtered using a 0.2 µm filter and samples were acquired for 5 min to avoid recording different amounts of background per acquisition. Speed beads were included. The speed beads and CMO⁻ events were defined using density plots of channel 03 (CMO) versus channel 06 (side scatter) intensity (Gate i). Running acquisition buffer only (left side) and unstained EVs (centre) showed the instrument detected a high level of background with low to medium side scatter. Labelling with the cell membrane dye (CMO) therefore helped to distinguish between the low CMO intensity/low side scatter EVs and background detected in both the acquisition buffer and unstained sample (right side). Applying a gate to capture low Raw Max Pixel events (channel 06—SSC: Gate ii) eliminated those events with saturated side scatter, including the speed beads. Outliers in the side scatter versus CMO intensity plots were individually inspected and found to be dual events comprising a speed bead (CMO⁻, high SSC) and an EV (CMO+, low SSC) which occupied the flow chamber at the same time. This resulted in aberrant events with both high CMO intensity and high SSC and was therefore excluded from further analysis.

Events classed as CMO+ at this point were included in the initial CMO+ gate (Gate iii). Within the same acquisition, we ran the Quantibrite PE beads which enabled a minimum threshold for CMO+ events to be calculated and converted to MESF units, as described. The lower MESF cut off for this experiment was defined at >50 and a further gate on the CMO intensity histogram (Gate iv) captured all CMO+ events with an MESF >50 for downstream analysis. The proportion of CMO+ events as a percentage of all events acquired over the 5 min period varied across 10 replicates (mean 18.73% ± 1.2 SEM) CMO+ MESF > 50; Figure 4B). A final gate was included to eliminate outliers which were either high CMO intensity but appeared on the bright field image to be membrane fragments (Gate v) or were not assigned a diameter due to lack of bright field image focus. This stringent gating strategy was designed to eliminate any events which could not be further analysed for EV marker expression or diameter.

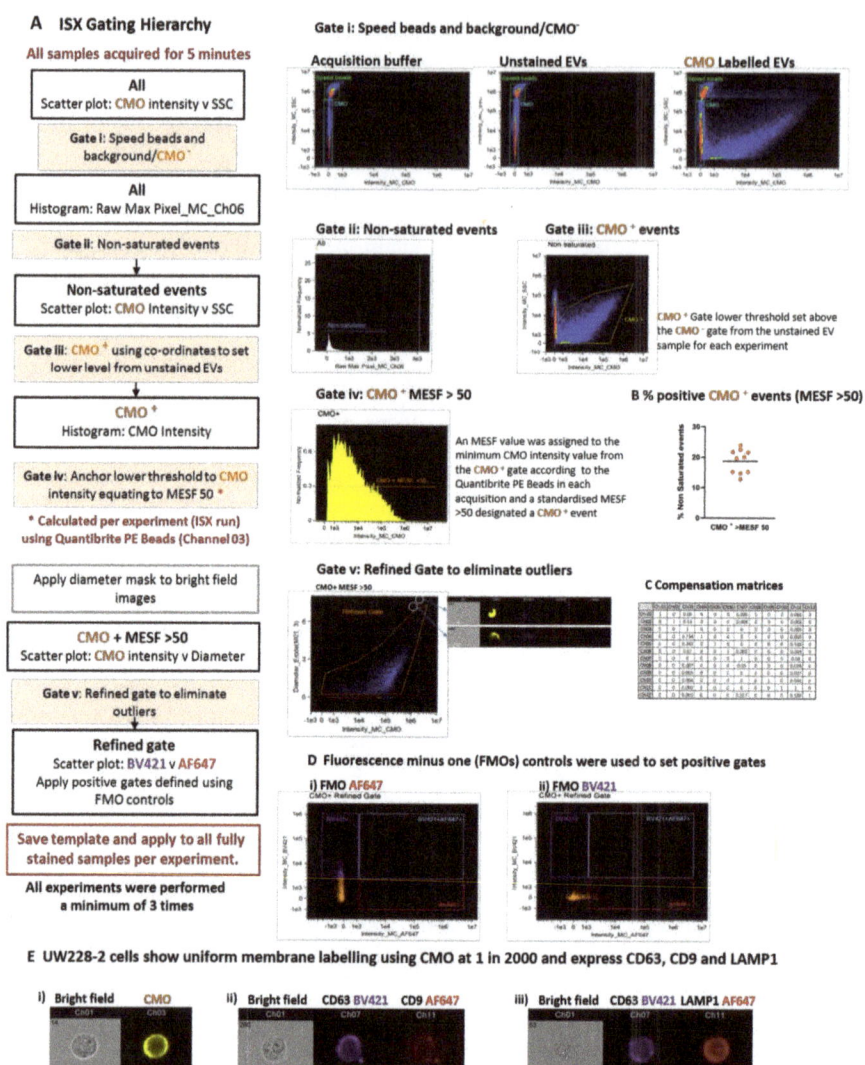

Figure 4. Optimised acquisition by Imaging flow cytometry and florescence membrane labelling can distinguish large extracellular vesicles from background and enable multiplex labelling. (**A**) Hierarchical gating can confidently refine the EV population for characterisation. Samples were acquired for 5 min using the ISX INSPIRE software and all events visualised using bivariate plots for fluorescence intensity in channel 03 (CMO) and channel 06 (side scatter). Initial gates for speed beads and CMO− events were set using the Acquisition buffer only and unstained EV samples included in each run (Gate i). These gates were applied to the labelled samples. Saturated events were excluded from the analysis by gating on the histogram plot: Raw Max Pixel for Channel 06 (Gate ii) thus removing the speed beads and very high side scatter events. An initial CMO + gate was placed (Gate iii). A lower fluorescence threshold of MESF > 50 in channel 3 (CMO) was set in each experiment using the regression analysis of Quantibrite PE Beads as described. The CMO + gate was anchored using co-ordinates for the equivalent fluorescence intensity and a further CMO + MESF > 50 gate applied to the histogram (Gate iv). Finally, a refined gate was used to eliminate outliers (Gate v). The analysis template was set for each experiment

and applied to all samples. (**B**) Percentage positive CMO+ events (MESF > 50). The percentage of CMO+ events (MESF > 50) is represented by an orange dot for 10 replicate experiments. Black bar represents mean 18.73% (± 1.2 SEM). (**C**) A compensation matrix was applied to all samples. The compensation wizard was used to create a matrix which was applied to all samples. (**D**) Single, double, and triple labelling protocols were used for compensation and accurate gating. Dual labelled EVs provided Fluorescence minus one (FMO) controls for (i) AF647; EVs labelled with CMO and CD63 BV421) or (ii) BV421; (EVs labelled with CMO and LAMP1 AF647) and used to set positive gates. (**E**) UW228-2 cells were used to optimise multiplex labelling. Cell mask orange (CMO) provides a general membrane label (i) and could be used to co-label with EV markers CD63 BV421 and CD9 AF647 (ii) or CD63 BV421 and LAMP1 AF647 (iii). Representative gallery images from IDEAS software are shown.

We tested a number of approaches to apply compensation to our data in consultation with the manufacturer's specialists. Initially, we attempted to construct a matrix using single stained EVs; however, the single pixel fluorescence was insufficient for the in-built compensation Wizard to assign a matrix. Next, we tried single stained parent cells, but the compensation matrix formulated by the wizard resulted in over-compensation and negative fluorescence intensity events. Over-compensation was thought to be due to the imbalance between the strong fluorescence signal resulting from cell mask orange, a membrane marker which indiscriminately labels lipids, and relatively weak fluorescence signal from target specific antibodies. These experiments were originally performed using a FITC conjugated CD63 antibody, however we found the level of adjustment required between channel 02 (FITC) and channel 03 (CMO) contributed to the negative populations. We re-optimised using the same CD63 antibody clone (HSC6) conjugated to BV421 (channel 07) which is spectrally more distinct from CMO. Finally, we found that using commercially available compensation beads labelled with our antibodies and acquired in the channels used for our study, in conjunction with assisted manual adjustment, provided the most reproducible compensation matrix.

We combined CMO with BV421 and AF647 and Fluorescence Minus One (FMO) controls for each fluorophore were used to set positive gates (Figure 4D). The parent UW228-2 cells were screened for expression of the EV markers chosen for this study: CD63, CD9, and LAMP1 as defined in the latest MISEV guidelines [1]. Multiplex labelling was performed using the following combinations: CMO with CD63 BV421 and CD9 AF647; or CMO with CD63 BV421 and LAMP1 AF647.

2.4. Multiplex Labelling Reveals Heterogeneity in EV Marker Expression

The proportion of CMO+ only events varied across the 10 replicates (Figure 5A). The mean percentage positive CMO+ (MESF > 50) events (63.3% ± 4.6 SEM) which did not demonstrate expression of any EV markers included in this study were designated CMO only. Considering the single EV markers, the proportion of EVs positive for each EV marker varied CD63 19.0%, (± 2.2 SEM), CD9 mean 10.3% (± 0.5 SEM); LAMP1 47.6% (± 3.8 SEM). These data shown LAMP1 to be the most prevalent EV marker screened in this study.

A Within the CMO⁺ (MESF >50) gate: The percentage positive CMO only events which did not express the EV markers screened in this study varied across replicates. The proportion of CMO⁺ events expressing a single EV marker also varied across replicate experiments with LAMP1 being the most prevalent.

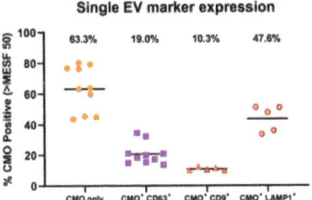

Figure 5. *Cont.*

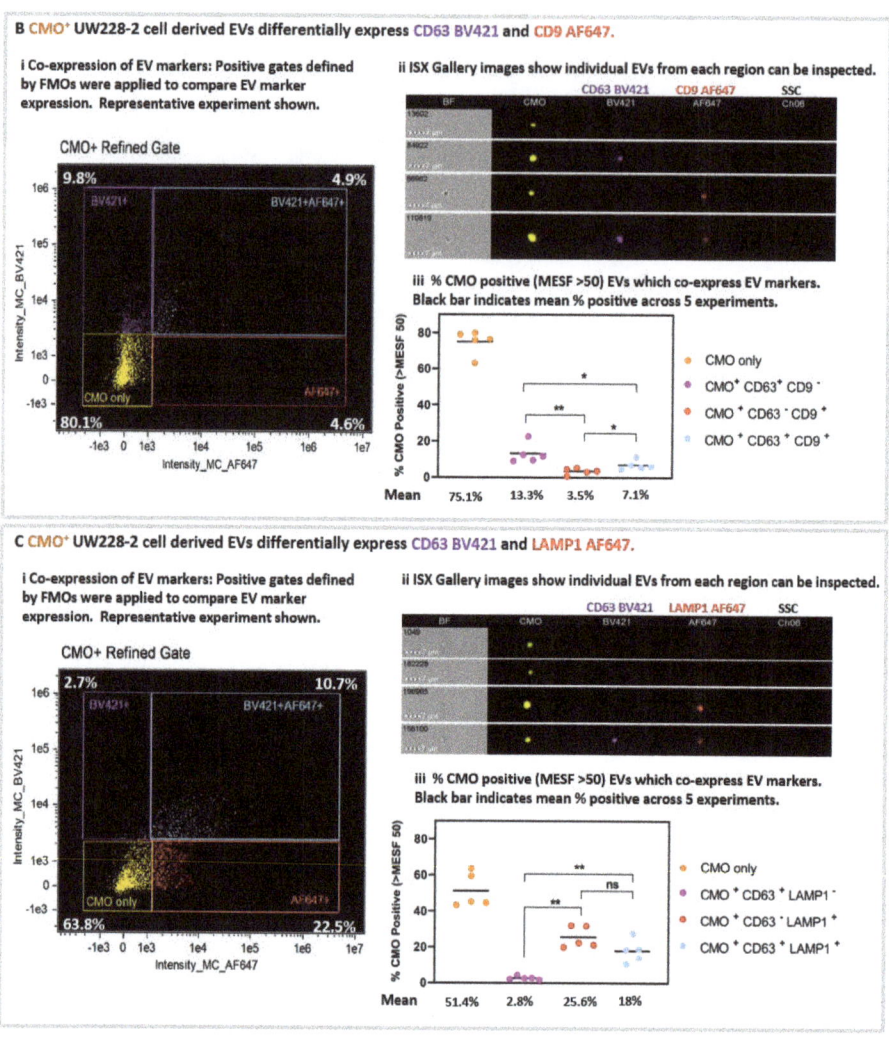

Figure 5. Isolated large EVs can be triple-labelled and individual events can be scrutinised post-acquisition. (**A**) The proportion of CMO+ events expressing a single EV marker varied across replicates. The percentage positive events within the CMO+ MESF > 50 gate which expressed either no EV marker (CMO only), CD63, CD9, or LAMP1 varied across replicates. Black bar represents the mean across 10 (CMO or CD63) or 5 (CD9 or LAMP1) replicates. CMO only 63.3% (± 4.6 SEM), CD63 only 19% (± 2.2 SEM), CD9 (± 0.5 SEM) only 10.3% and LAMP1 only 47.6% (± 3.8 SEM). (**B**) UW228-2 cell derived EVs differentially express EV markers CD63 and CD9, or both. EVs were labelled with CMO, CD63 BV421 and CD9 AF647. CMO $^+$ events (MESF > 50) were analysed for co-expression with CD63, CD9 or both. Quadrant gating of bivariate plots for fluorescence intensity in channel 07 (BV421) and channel 11 (AF647) demonstrated single labelled (CMO$^+$ only), dual and triple labelled EV populations (i). Percentage positive in each quadrant is shown. Representative experiment. Gallery images display examples of individual events from each of the 4 quadrants (ii). Bright Field (BF) and side scatter (SSC) channels are shown alongside CMO, CD63 BV421 and CD9 AF647. Of the CMO+ MESF >50: 75.1% (± 3.0 SEM) were CMO $^+$ only; 13.3% (± 2.4 SEM) expressed CD63 BV421 and 3.5% (± 0.8 SEM)

expressed CD9 AF647. 7.1% (± 1.1 SEM) of the CMO$^+$ events expressed both CD63 and CD9. (C) UW228-2 cell derived EVs differentially express EV markers CD63 and LAMP1, or both. EVs were labelled with CMO, CD63 BV421 and LAMP1 AF647. CMO$^+$ events were analysed for co-expression with CD63, LAMP1 or both. Quadrant gating of bivariate plots for fluorescence intensity in channel 07 (BV421) and channel 11 (AF647) demonstrated single labelled (CMO$^+$ only), dual and triple labelled EV populations (i). Percentage positive in each quadrant is shown. Representative experiment. Gallery images display examples of individual events from each of the 4 quadrants (ii). Bright Field (BF) and side scatter (SSC) channels are shown alongside CMO, CD63 BV421 and LAMP1 AF647. Of the CMO+ MESF >50: 54.1% (± 4.3 SEM) were CMO$^+$ only; 2.8% (± 0.4 SEM) expressed CD63 BV421 and 25.6% (± 2.7 SEM) expressed LAMP1 AF647 whilst 18.0% (± 2.8 SEM) of the CMO$^+$ events expressed both CD63 and LAMP1. (* $p = 0.0159$ or 0.0317; ** $p = 0.0079$). Mann Whitney U test.

Differential expression and co-expression of EV markers was examined between five replicate experiments. Representative bivariate plots of AF647 intensity against BV421 intensity (Figure 5B(i) and Figure 5C(i) for CD63/CD9 and CD63/LAMP1, respectively), and representative galleries (Figure 5B(ii) and Figure 5C(ii)) of EVs displaying each labelling combination taken from the quadrant plots are shown. The proportion of EVs which co-express EV markers within each gate for the five replicates is shown in Figure 5B(iii) and Figure 5C(iii). Where the EVs were labelled for CMO, CD63 BV421, and CD9 AF647 (Figure 5B(iii)): 75.1% (± 3.0 SEM; yellow) were CMO only, 13.3% (± 2.4 SEM; purple) were CMO$^+$ CD63$^+$ CD9$^-$; 3.5% (± 0.8 SEM; red) were CMO$^+$ CD63$^-$ CD9$^+$ and 7.1% (± 1.1 SEM; blue) were CMO$^+$ CD63$^+$ CD9$^+$. There were significantly fewer CD63$^-$ CD9$^+$ EVs compared with CD63$^+$ ($p = 0.0079$) only or CD63$^+$ CD9$^+$ EVs ($p = 0.0159$). Similarly, there were fewer EV co-expressing CD63 and CD9 compared with CD63$^+$ alone ($p = 0.0317$). (Mann Whitney U test). Considering the EVs labelled with CMO, CD63 BV421 and LAMP1 AF647 (Figure 5C(iii)). 51.4% (+/− 4.3 SEM; yellow) were CMO+ only, a comparatively low 2.8% (± 0.4 SEM; purple) were CMO$^+$ CD63$^+$ LAMP1$^-$; whilst 25.6% (± 2.7 SEM; red) were CMO$^+$ CD63$^-$ LAMP1$^+$ and 18% (± 2.8 SEM; blue) co-expressed both CD63 and LAMP1. There were significantly more EVs which expressed LAMP1 compared with CD63 alone ($p = 0.0079$) and more expressing both CD63 and LAMP1 compared with CD63 alone ($p = 0.0079$).

2.5. ISX Allow Correlative Analyses of Diameter with EV Marker Expression for Phenotyping

We applied the Diameter Mask; Erode (M01, 3) in IDEAS software to all fully labelled replicates using the Batch analysis function and compared the range of diameters present within the CMO+ MESF> 50 gate. Figure 6A shows single event diameters within the 10 replicates. This median diameter (indicated with the black line) varied significantly across the replicates (922–1129 nm: Kruskal-Wallis; $p > 0.0001$). However, these data represent EVs isolated as 3 biological replicates and when each replicate is analysed using ANOVA there was no significant difference between the median diameters of each EV preparation. There was a clear correlation between EV diameter and CMO intensity as shown in Figure 6B. Regression analysis was performed on the individual exported feature values from each replicate (2 representative plots are shown from different biological replicates) ($p < 0.0001$).

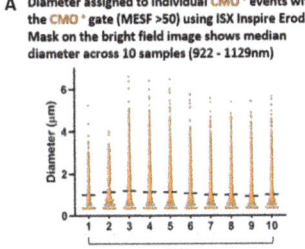
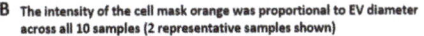
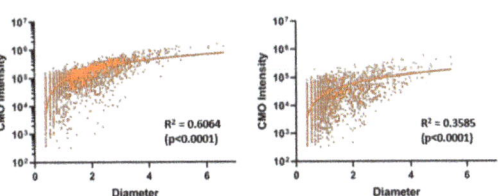

Figure 6. *Cont.*

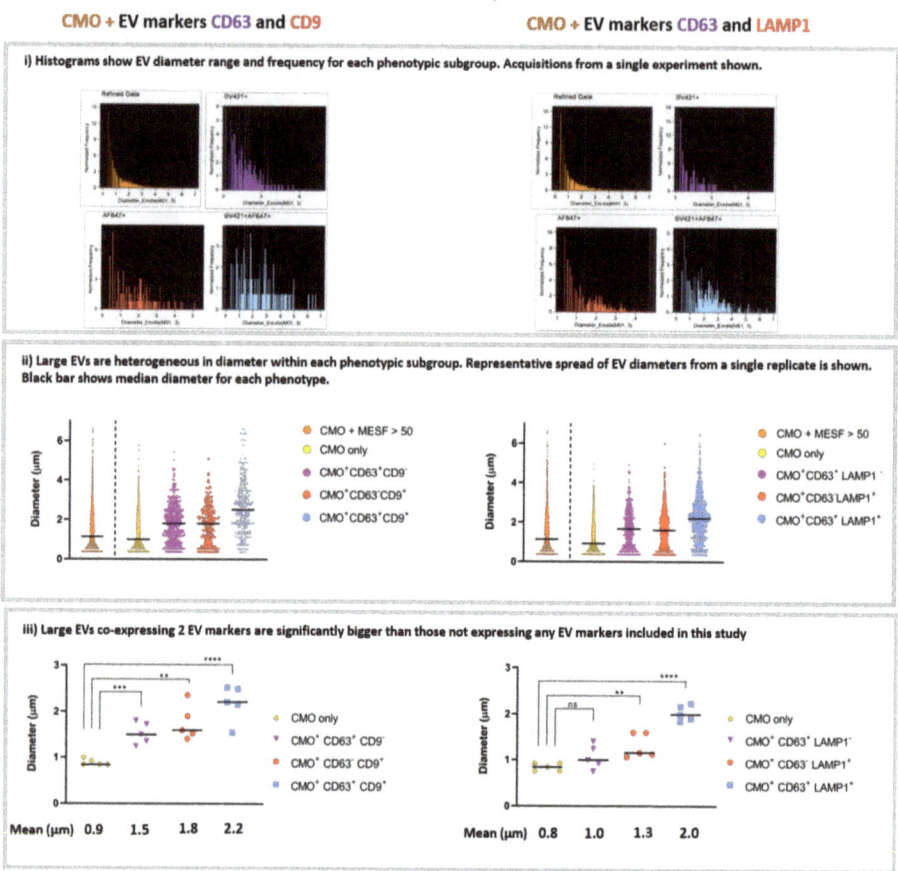

Figure 6. The ISX can accurately assign diameter to large EVs and facilitate individual event analyses to phenotype heterogeneous EV populations. (**A**) The median diameter of CMO $^+$ EVs from UW228-2 cells was comparable across 10 samples. The erode mask was applied to the bright field images of those EVs which were included in the CMO$^+$ >MESF 50 gate. The diameter of individual events within this gate was exported from IDEAS into PRISM for analysis. This figure shows a median diameter (represented by the black bar) of 922–1129 nm across the 10 samples and visualises the broad size range within each sample. (**** $p > 0.0001$ Kruskal-Wallis test). (**B**) The fluorescence intensity of the CMO was proportional to EV diameter. Bivariate plots showing CMO intensity against diameter consistently demonstrates a proportional relationship between EV size and intensity of the membrane label across samples run in triplicate experiments. 2 representative samples shown. (Regression analysis $p < 0.0001$). (**C**) Comparison of EV phenotypes across triplicate experiments. Individual histograms displaying EV diameter for each phenotype demonstrated differential size ranges according to EV marker(s) expression (i a and i b). In each case, those labelled with CMO only and not expressing either CD63, CD9 or LAMP1 have a smaller median diameter compared with EVs expressing CD63 and/or CD9 or LAMP1 (ii a and ii b). In both cases, those EVs co-expressing both CD63 with CD9 (iii a) or CD63 with LAMP1 (iii b) are significantly larger than CMO only. (** $p < 0.005$, *** $p < 0.0004$, **** $p < 0.0001$).

We found that large EVs are heterogeneous in both diameter and EV marker expression. Histogram plots of individual events exported from the quadrant positive gates show the different diameter range and frequency within each phenotypic subgroup (Figure 6C(i)). Representative acquisitions from a single replicate are shown. ISX analysis facilitates the comparison of individual EV diameters from within each phenotype (Figure 6C(ii)). A representative plot for all CMO $^+$ (MESF > 50) in a single replicate of each phenotype is shown and the black bars represent the median diameter for each subgroup. Within this typical replicate, the median diameter and range for each subgroup was as follows: All CMO >MESF 50 1.1 µm (362 nm–6.2 µm), CMO only 1.0 µm (362 nm–5.4 µm), CMO+ CD63$^+$ CD9$^-$ 1.8 µm (362 nm–5.1 µm), CMO+ CD63$^-$ CD9$^+$ 1.8 µm (362 nm–4.7 µm), and CMO+ CD63$^+$ CD9$^+$ 2.5 µm (362 nm–6.2 µm). When considering the second phenotype: All CMO >MESF 50 1.4 µm (362 nm–6.2 µm), CMO only 1.1 µm (362 nm–4.6 µm), CMO+ CD63$^+$ CD9$^-$ 1.7 µm (362 nm–4.5 µm), CMO+ CD63$^-$ CD9$^+$ 1.6 µm (362 nm–5.6 µm), and CMO+ CD63$^+$ CD9$^+$ 2.2 µm (362 nm–6.1 µm). In each case the median diameter increases in size with accumulating EV marker expression.

When considering all 5 replicates; we compared the mean diameter for each subgroup (Figure 6C(iii)). For the first group (left panel): CMO only 0.89 µm (±0.03 SEM), CMO+ CD63$^+$ CD9$^-$ 1.53 µm (± 0.1 SEM), CMO+ CD63$^-$ CD9$^+$ 1.76 µm (±0.17 SEM) and CMO+ CD63$^+$ CD9$^+$ 2.19 µm (±0.18 SEM). Those EVs expressing either CD63 ($p < 0.0004$) or CD9 ($p < 0.0010$) were significantly larger than EV which did not (CMO only). For the second subgroup (right panel) the mean diameters were as follows: CMO only 0.84 µm (±0.04 SEM), CMO+ CD63$^+$ CD9$^-$ 1.06 µm (±0.12 SEM), CMO+ CD63$^-$ CD9$^+$ 1.31 µm (±0.12 SEM), and CMO+ CD63$^+$ CD9$^+$ 2.02 µm (±0.07 SEM). In this group, those EVs expressing CD63 only were not significantly larger than those which did not. However, EVs expressing LAMP1 were larger ($p < 0.005$). In both cases, those CMO $^+$ EVs co-expressing 2 EVs markers: either CD63 and CD9, or CD63 and LAMP1 (blue) were significantly larger than those which do not carry the markers screened in this study. (**** $p < 0.0001$. Un-paired t-test).

3. Materials and Methods

3.1. Cell Line

UW228-2 cells were kindly provided by DTW Jones (DKFZ, Heidelberg, Germany). Cells were grown in DMEM with L-glutamine (Lonza, Manchester, UK; cat: R8758) supplemented with 10% FCS (SIGMA, Gillingham, UK; cat: F9665) in Corning 225 cm^2 Angled Neck Cell Culture Flask with Vent Cap (Fisher Scientific, Leicestershire, UK; cat: 431082) at 37 °C with 5% CO$_2$ in normoxia. Cell lines were passaged with 1 × Trypsin-EDTA (Lonza, UK; cat: T3924). All cell lines tested negative for Mycoplasma and all were authenticated in-house (CRUK-Manchester Institute) by examination of a total of 21 loci across the genome using the Powerplex 21 System (Promega, Southampton, UK).

3.2. Cell Culture

For each experiment, cells were seeded at 2.5 × 10^6 cells in 50 mL DMEM 10% FBS (complete media) per 225 cm^3 tissue culture flask and allowed to adhere overnight. On day 2 media was switched to 50 mL serum-free DMEM for 24 h prior to EV isolation and cell preparation. Conditioned media (containing EVs) was removed, and the cells washed x2 with PBS before trypsinisation using 1 × Trypsin-EDTA (Lonza, Manchester, UK; cat: T3924). Cell counts and viability were checked at the time of EV harvest using the trypan blue exclusion assay (0.4% Trypan blue solution; SIGMA; Gillingham, UK; cat T8154).

3.3. Vesicle Isolation

Large EVs were harvested using a standard operating procedure (SOP) as previously reported (Figure 1F) [15]. For each experiment, EVs were isolated from the serum-free, conditioned media from 2 × 225 cm^2 flasks (pooled; total 100 mL). Cell culture supernatant (conditioned media: CM) was centrifuged in 2 tubes to remove cells (300× g 5 min, ×2) and filtered using a double layered 5 µm pore nylon Sieve (Fisher Scientific, Leicestershire, UK; cat 12994257). The supernatant was collected and centrifuged at 2000× g for 30 min and prepared for ISX analysis. Centrifugation steps were performed using an Eppendorf 5702 bench top centrifuge with an A-4-38 rotor. All EV preparations were performed on the day of analysis and not stored. Experimental procedures for EV isolation have been submitted to the EV-TRACK database (EV TRACK ID: EV190013) [22].

3.4. Chemicals and Reagents Including Antibodies

3.4.1. Apoptosis Assay

UW228-2 cells were seeded at 1×10^{5}/well into 6 well plates (Corning; Fisher Scientific, Leicestershire, UK; cat CL S3516) and incubated at 37 °C overnight in DMEM containing 10% FBS. Triplicate wells were cultured in complete media or switched to serum-free DMEM for 24 h before screening with Annexin V APC/PI using the Apoptosis detection kit (Biolegend UK, London, UK; cat 640932) according to the manufacturer's instructions. 30,000 events were acquired using the LSR II flow cytometer with lasers for APC (640 nm laser, emission captured at 660 nm) and PI (488 nm laser with emission captured at 575 nm). Positive controls were generated to inform accurate gating: cells were treated with 200 µM (UW228-2) Etoposide (SIGMA; Gillingham, UK; cat E1383) for 24 h (Apoptotic cells: Annexin V), or heated at 56 °C for 10 min prior to labelling (Dead cells: PI).

3.4.2. Immunofluorescence Microscopy

Cells and EVs were immobilised onto CellCarrier 96 well plates (Perkin Elmer; Bucks, UK; Cat 6005550), fixed with 3.7% paraformaldehyde, permeabilised with 0.2% Triton X in PBS and probed using anti-human CD63 antibody (Clone: H5C6, Biolegend UK, London, UK; Cat: 353005) directly conjugated to FITC and counterstained for polymerised actin using $0.2 \times$ Alexa Fluor 555 Phalloidin (Fisher Scientific, Leicestershire, UK; cat A34055) and 300 nM DAPI (Biolegend UK, London, UK, 422801). Images were captured using the Perkin Elmer Operetta system (Perkin Elmer; Bucks, UK) at ×40 magnification.

3.4.3. Transmission Electron Microscopy (TEM)

EVs were immobilised onto ACLAR (poly-chloro-tri-fluoro-ethylene (PCTFE) film) coated with Corning CellTak (Fisher Scientific, Leicestershire, UK; cat 354240) and fixed with glutaraldehyde in sodium cacodylate buffer (pH 7.2) followed by post-fix staining with osmium tetroxide and uranyl acetate (supplied in-house by the FBMH Core Facility). Preparations were dehydrated and embedded in resin to allow serial 60–200 µm sections to be taken. Images were captured using a Biotwin Philips TECNAI G2 transmission electron microscope.

3.4.4. Tunable Resistance Pulse Sensing (TRPS)

Size and quantity were determined by Tunable Resistance Pulse Sensing (TRPS) using the qNano GOLD instrument (iZON Science, Christchurch, New Zealand) as per manufacturer's instructions. The principles are discussed elsewhere [23]. We analysed an aliquot of isolated EVs alongside downstream analyses using overlapping sizes of Nanopores (NP600, NP1000, and NP2000) to provide a full picture of EV size distribution and quantity.

3.4.5. Cell Mask Orange Labelling

100 mL (2×50 mL) EV containing media was used to harvest large EVs for each experiment as described and the $2000 \times g$ pellets re-suspended in either (1) 2 mL serum-free DMEM or (2) 2 mL Cell Mask Orange (CMO: 2.5 µg/mL in serum-free DMEM) (Fisher Scientific, Leicestershire, UK; cat C10045) and both were incubated at 37 °C for 10 min.

3.5. Antibody Labelling

See Table 2 for antibody details and manufacturer information. Antibody titrations were performed for each antibody using parent cells and EVs. In all cases, the maximum recommended volume (5 µL) provided the greatest fluorescence signal from the EVs. Antibody only controls (no EVs) were included in the ISX analysis and showed no fluorescence events above the unstained gate in each case. Both CMO labelled and unlabelled EVs preparations were washed by addition of 5 mL 1% BSA/PBS and centrifuged at 2000× g for 30 min. The pellets were re-suspended in 700 µL 0.2 µm filtered 1% BSA/PBS and split into 7 × 100 µL aliquots. For each labelling combination, 5 µL directly conjugated primary antibodies were added simultaneously as follows: Non-CMO labelled EVs were used for unstained, single labelled CD63 BV421, CD9 AF647, or LAMP1 AF647 and CMO FMO controls (×2) (BV421 + AF647: both antibodies were screened). The final aliquot was used to establish EV concentration and diameter range using TRPS analysis on the qNANO. The CMO labelled EV pellet was re-suspended in 700 µL 0.2 µm filtered 1% BSA/PBS and split into 7 × 100 µL aliquots. CMO labelled EVs were used as single stained (CMO+ only), AF647 FMO (CMO + BV421), BV421 FMO (CMO + AF647), and multiplexed CMO + CD63 BV421 + either CD9 AF647 or LAMP1 AF647. Antibodies were incubated for 1 h on ice in the dark. EVs were washed by addition of 500 µL 0.2 µm filtered 1% BSA/PBS and centrifuged at 2000× g for 30 min. Resulting pellets were re-suspended in 75 µL 0.2 µm filtered 1% BSA/PBS for ISX analysis. Fully labelled EV preparations were treated post-acquisition with 0.1% Triton-X 100 and acquired again to demonstrate loss of fluorescence due to antigen degradation.

Table 2. Chemicals and Reagents Including Antibodies.

Reagent		Manufacturer		Catalogue No.	
Cell mask orange: plasma membrane marker		Thermo Fisher Scientific		C10045	
Annexin V APC/PI: Apoptosis assay		Biolegend		640932	
Alexa Fluor 555 phalloidin: Polymerised actin cytoskeleton		Thermo Fisher Scientific		A34055	
Speed beads: Imagestream flow calibration		Amnis		400041	
Quantibrite PE Beads		Beckton Dickinson UK		340495	
Antibody	Clone	Fluorophore	Isotype	Manufacturer	Catalogue No.
Anti-human CD 63	H5C6	BV421	Mouse IgG1, k	Biolegend	353030
Anti-human CD9	MEM-61	AF647	Mouse IgG1	Fisher Scientific	15317424
Anti-human LAMP 1	H4A3	AF647	Mouse IgG1, k	Biolegend	328611

3.6. Imagestream Acquisition

Sheath buffer (PBS without calcium and magnesium: SIGMA, Gillingham, UK; Cat D5652) was filtered using 0.2 µm bottle top filters (SIGMA, Gillingham, UK, Nalgene: FIL8184) to minimise background signal. Internal instrument calibrations were performed before every run according to manufacturer's guidelines using the ASSIST Calibrations to include: camera synchronisation, spatial offsets, dark current, bright field crosstalk coefficient, core stage position, horizontal laser, side scatter, and a retro illumination scheme to maximise the amount of light incident. This was followed by a series of internal operations designed to measure performance including excitation laser power, bright field uniformity, and focus. Specific laser powers used for this study are detailed in Table 3.

Table 3. Settings used for Imagestream.

Laser	Channel/Filter	Power mW	Parameter
405	Ch07/435–80 nm	120	BV421
561	Ch03/577–35 nm	200	CMO
785	Ch06/762–35 nm	70	SSC
642	Ch11/702–85	150	AF647

Speed beads with an exaggerated irregular surface were incorporated into every analysis for internal calibration. A dedicated laser was assigned to assess side scatter (CH 06; SSC: 785 nm laser). For each experiment, a separate readout was obtained from 0.2 µm filtered 1% BSA/PBS acquisition buffer alone. All events were acquired for 5 min and visualised using bivariate plots of side scatter against fluorescence intensity.

For cells, 10,000–30,000 total events were acquired. EVs were acquired for 5 min at ×60 magnification using lasers as described (Table 3) (Image stream, Amnis, Seattle, WA, USA). The ×60 objective provides a Numerical Aperture of 0.9 enabling resolution of 0.3 µm^2/pixel [19].

4. Compensation

Antibody labelled compensation beads (anti-mouse compensation beads: BD Biosciences, San Jose, CA, USA; cat 552843) were used to acquire single colour controls within the channels used for this study. The final compensation matrices were constructed by the wizard (INSPIRE) with manual adjustment in consultation with the manufacturer's specialist adviser and applied to the .rif files of all controls, dual and triple labelled EVs. Data were analysed using the IDEAS software (v. 6.2, Amnis, Seattle, WA, USA). The compensation matrices and analysis template were applied using the batch processing tool to all .rif files to produce .daf files for each sample. FCS files were exported and uploaded onto the Flow Repository according to the requirements.

5. Mask Selection for Assessment of EV Diameter

We investigated which of the diameter masks available within the IDEAS software would be most accurate for EVs. We used non-fluorescence size calibration beads (Fisher Scientific—UK Ltd., Loughborough, UK; cat F13838) to validate the masks. The beads were acquired using the same laser powers and settings as the EV preparations and analysis templates were constructed to identify which mask fitted most closely to the bead diameter according to the manufacturer's instructions. We found that applying the diameter mask Erode (03; indicating 3 pixel erosion) to the bright field channel most closely assigned the correct diameter. This mask formed part of an analysis template which was applied to all samples using the batch analysis tool.

6. Molecules of Equivalent Soluble Fluorochrome (MESF) Calculation

To enable comparisons between experiments, Molecules of Equivalent Soluble Fluorochrome (MESF) values were calculated as previously described [19,24]. Quantibrite PE beads (BD Biosciences, San Jose, CA, USA; Cat: 340495. Lot: 90926) were the closest available calibration beads for the fluorescent channel used to detect Cell Mask Orange labelled EVs. A fresh aliquot of lyophilised Quantibrite beads was reconstituted for each run, and 5000 events were acquired using the identical laser settings for each fluorophore as described. The SSC laser (channel 06) was adjusted to ensure the beads could be visualised on the bivariate plots and therefore each bead could be gated as a separate population and the median fluorescence intensity recorded. The CMO+ events were then analysed for expression of the EV markers included in this study: CD63, CD9 and LAMP1.

7. Discussion

Our principal aim was to develop a standardised method for the isolation and characterisation of individual large EVs, which could be further developed for phenotyping large EVs from clinical samples. The value of the Imagestream to the field of EV characterisation has been explored elsewhere [19,24,25]. However, reports focussing on the large EV populations, frequently discarded during small EV isolation protocols, are rarely present in the current literature.

By using in vitro cultures, we were able to use the ideal conditions to generate EVs and optimise experiments. Specifically, by culturing in serum-free media, we eliminated contamination from bovine EVs present in FBS [18] and subsequent false positive fluorescence signals from serum lipoproteins [20]. Nevertheless, harvesting large EVs from any source presents challenges as cells or cell debris, including intracellular vesicles released due to parent cell membrane rupture from early centrifugation steps, can contaminate the subsequent EV pellets. For the EVs to be truly extracellular prior to isolation, the outer membrane of accompanying cells must not be ruptured by mechanical or chemical means during initial harvest. The centrifugation speeds we have used here are low compared to some commonly reported EV isolation protocols [26] to specifically preserve large EV membrane integrity. Electron microscopy remains the sole technique that can examine individual EVs and EV preparations for sheared cell fragments, but it is neither quantitative nor high throughput. In addition, whilst TEM is widely used for EV investigation, it cannot perhaps distinguish between bone fide EVs and other particles. In this case, cryoEM or CLEM (correlative light and electron microscopy) which facilitates overlaid fluorescence or gold labelled antibody binding and EM would prove more informative. It is necessary to use a combination of techniques to explore the quantity, quality, and biology of EVs. All techniques, many originally designed for analysing cells, have technical challenges when applied to considerably smaller entities. For flow cytometry, background scatter events due to particles in the sheath fluid are an anticipated phenomenon which is rarely reported. In the work we report here, a high level of background appeared within the same gate as unstained EVs and persisted despite 0.2 µm filtration of sheath fluid. Our protocol is therefore reliant on strong and uniform, membrane-bound fluorescence labelling in order to assign an initial gate that separates potential EVs from speed beads or background scatter events. However, we found that the lower fluorescence intensity threshold to define CMO positive events was not clearly distinct from the instrument background. This was likely due to a combination of EV size and relative fluorescence intensity. As recommended elsewhere [19] we used commercially available fluorescent beads of known intensity (Quantibrite) to provide a means to assign standardised units (MESF) and therefore a mathematical cut-off for our CMO+ gate. We acknowledge that calibration beads differ in the physical properties of EVs, in particular the refractive index, which can affect the intensity of scattered light, a particularly important consideration for the study of smaller EVs. PE was the closest available fluorophore to CMO and used as a standard for channel 03 on the ISX. CMO is a membrane label incorporated into the plasma membrane, and emits a greater fluorescence compared with a target-specific, conjugated antibody. This hampered the use of FITC alongside CMO as the spectrally close fluorophores led to overcompensation between channels 02 (FITC) and channel 03 (CMO). BV421 was a successful alternative but the difficulties encountered raised concerns about trying to further multiplex with additional fluorophores using this platform.

The challenges for choosing the correct technique(s) to analyse EVs have been well described elsewhere [27]. For detailed advice on considerations for EV separation or enrichment methodologies and recommended steps for EV characterisation, we recommend referring to the MISEV guidelines; a position paper prepared by the international EV community to support EV research [1]. A major challenge now is to adapt the protocol we describe for the analysis of large EVs from biological fluids. Clinical samples are more complex: EVs from a single cell type as described here offer the ideal model for characterisation, however clinical samples contain heterogeneous EVs from numerous cells [10]. EV isolation has been reported from peripheral blood with some correlations to clinical outcome in other cancers [28,29]. We have previously identified leukaemic EVs in patients' bone marrow plasma. This was possible using a marker which identified the cell of origin (B cell marker CD19) and understanding that the bone marrow of a leukemia patient is primarily composed of malignant B cells [9]. However, surface markers for Medulloblastoma cells are less well known, rather molecular signatures define subgroups in this cancer type [30]. Investigating surface marker expression on medulloblastoma cell-derived EVs would help to develop a more rapid screening tools. The value of a liquid biopsy to diagnose brain tumours in the clinic is clear and some suitable candidates have been identified in Glioblastoma [31,32]. A next step could be to investigate EVs released by primary medulloblastoma cells although the requirements for optimal culture conditions to generate sufficient material will add additional complexity. In the case of medulloblastoma, ideally, EVs circulating in either the cerebrospinal fluid or peripheral blood for comparison to matched primary tumour-derived EVs would be of considerable interest.

Our SOP is likely to exclude most small EVs and exosomes, expected to be present in the supernatant discarded at the final step (2000× *g*). Experiments to isolate these for comparison are on-going. One classification we examined in this study was the distinction from apoptotic bodies. Demonstration of intact EV membranes, a lack of fragmented nuclei staining (DAPI) and evidence that EVs were derived from viable cells supported our assertion that the EVs analysed were not apoptotic bodies or cell debris [33]. It might be possible to further distinguish these populations using molecular profiling. Other studies suggest that these EV subgroups display distinct RNA profiles [34] an approach which is reliant on pure populations and therefore robust and meticulous isolation protocols.

Our data show that large EVs are ubiquitous and whilst absolute quantification is not yet within reach, we demonstrated similar size profiles using two independent techniques: TRPS and ISX. We have previously identified EVs of up to 6 µM using immunofluorescence, ISX and TEM [15]. However, validating the quantity and size range has only been possible using the qNANO instrument. The qNANO employs TRPS technology to quantify EV count in a given sample and assign a size relative to a calibration bead of known diameter. It is currently the only instrument which can provide this information across the large EV population which spans 250 nm up to 6 µm (from our cells). Other platforms are restricted to small EVs (<1 µM) due to the measurements being reliant on Brownian movement (e.g., Nanosight and Zetaview). We found the most prevalent EV populations to be around 250–450 nm; however, we consistently detect EVs with a much larger diameter range in every cell line we have screened to date. We remain cautious not to define these as oncosomes; as although derived from cancer cells, we have not yet demonstrated their oncogenic potential [4].

Whilst fluorescence intensity alone cannot be used to quantify protein expression levels due to low level antigen expression on EVs, we did observe patterns of differential expression. In EV literature, 3 principle markers are used to define EVs: CD63, CD9, and CD81. CD63, however, has been identified as a pan-EV marker, present in all defined EV subgroups to date [6] and therefore CD63 was our preferred initial marker. However, large EVs are as yet poorly characterised and we found that CD63 was not the most abundant EV marker in our study. CD63 is a tetraspanin which has been used as a selection tool for immuno-capture experiments and also for tracking EV release [35,36]. Based on our observations, if a full EV repertoire was of interest, then a cocktail of multiple markers should be considered as screening with CD63 alone will likely fail to capture a significant proportion of EVs. We found LAMP1, previously identified on exosomes and EVs from a variety our cell types and biological fluids [37], was significantly more prevalent.

We also show here that the majority of large EVs did not express any of the three markers screened. We did observe a significant increase in the median diameter of individual EVs which expressed 1 or more markers compared to none (CMO only), in each of the experiments performed. Further, across all replicates, those EVs which co-expressed 2 markers (CD63 + CD9, or CD63 + LAMP1) were significantly larger than those without. Others have suggested that larger EVs are likely to accommodate a greater number of tumour-derived molecules than exosomes [13] and data presented here would support that hypothesis. Further investigations to define a broader panel of large EV markers followed by more comprehensive techniques, such as proteomic profiling, would help to fully phenotype the large EVs population. From a clinical perspective, it is likely that large EVs will be a rich source of biomarkers of benefit to the study of human disease. Standardised protocols and instruments capable of measuring multiple markers are key to moving the field forward and expanding the interest from exosomes only.

The research we report here demonstrates that high resolution, high throughput imaging flow cytometry is an exceptional tool offering the unique ability to quantify and analyse individual events within heterogeneous EV populations. We set out to develop an isolation protocol consisting of minimal manipulation and processing which may abrogate, mask, or indeed elicit changes in EV structure or biology, which could impact on any functional read outs in downstream experiments. Indeed, fully understanding the biological consequence(s) of EV release or uptake by recipient cells is an essential part of the field and will advance with new technologies and innovation.

Author Contributions: Conceptualization, S.M.J. and A.B.; Data curation, S.M.J., A.B., C.S. and A.M.; Formal analysis, S.M.J., A.B. and M.G.M.; Funding acquisition, S.M.J. and M.G.M.; Investigation, S.M.J. and C.S.; Methodology, C.S. and A.M.; Resources, A.B. and A.M.; Validation, S.M.J.; Writing—original draft, S.M.J. Writing—review & editing, A.B. and M.G.M. All authors have read and agreed to the published version of the manuscript.

Funding: This research was funded by CRUK grant number C68251/A28065.

Conflicts of Interest: The authors declare no conflict of interest.

References

1. Thery, C.; Witwer, K.W.; Aikawa, E.; Alcaraz, M.J.; Anderson, J.D.; Andriantsitohaina, R.; Antoniou, A.; Arab, T.; Archer, F.; Atkin-Smith, G.K.; et al. Minimal information for studies of extracellular vesicles 2018 (MISEV2018): A position statement of the International Society for Extracellular Vesicles and update of the MISEV2014 guidelines. *J. Extracell. Vesicles* **2018**, *7*, 1535750. [CrossRef]
2. Cocucci, E.; Meldolesi, J. Ectosomes and exosomes: Shedding the confusion between extracellular vesicles. *Trends Cell Biol.* **2015**, *25*, 364–372. [CrossRef] [PubMed]
3. Van Niel, G.; Porto-Carreiro, I.; Simoes, S.; Raposo, G. Exosomes: A common pathway for a specialized function. *J. Biochem.* **2006**, *140*, 13–21. [CrossRef] [PubMed]
4. Meehan, B.; Rak, J.; Di Vizio, D. Oncosomes—Large and small: What are they, where they came from? *J. Extracell. Vesicles* **2016**, *5*, 33109. [CrossRef] [PubMed]
5. Yanez-Mo, M.; Siljander, P.; Andreu, Z.; Zavec, A.B.; Borràs, F.E.; Buzas, E.I.; Buzas, K.; Casal, E.; Cappello, F.; Carvalho, J.; et al. Biological properties of extracellular vesicles and their physiological functions. *J. Extracell. Vesicles* **2015**, *4*, 27066. [CrossRef]
6. Kowal, J.; Arras, G.; Colombo, M.; Jouve, M.; Morath, J.P.; Primdal-Bengtson, B.; Dingli, F.; Loew, D.; Tkach, M.; Théry, C. Proteomic comparison defines novel markers to characterize heterogeneous populations of extracellular vesicle subtypes. *Proc. Natl. Acad. Sci. USA* **2016**, *113*, E968–E977. [CrossRef]
7. Simpson, R.J.; Mathivanan, S. Extracellular Microvesicles: The Need for Internationally Recognised Nomenclature and Stringent Purification Criteria. *J. Proteomics Bioinform.* **2012**, *5*. [CrossRef]
8. Tkach, M.; Thery, C. Communication by Extracellular Vesicles: Where We are and Where We Need to Go. *Cell* **2016**, *164*, 1226–1232. [CrossRef]
9. Johnson, S.M.; Dempsey, C.; Chadwick, A.; Harrison, S.; Liu, J.; Di, Y.; McGinn, O.J.; Fiorillo, M.; Sotgia, F.; Lisanti, M.P.; et al. Metabolic reprogramming of bone marrow stromal cells by leukemic extracellular vesicles in acute lymphoblastic leukemia. *Blood* **2016**, *128*, 453–456. [CrossRef]
10. Gyorgy, B.; Szabó, T.G.; Pásztói, M.; Pál, Z.; Misják, P.; Aradi, B.; László, V.; Pállinger, É; Pap, E.; Kittel, Á.; et al. Membrane vesicles, current state-of-the-art: Emerging role of extracellular vesicles. *Cell. Mol. Life Sci.* **2011**, *68*, 2667–2688. [CrossRef]
11. Colombo, M.; Raposo, G.; Thery, C. Biogenesis, secretion, and intercellular interactions of exosomes and other extracellular vesicles. *Annu. Rev. Cell Dev. Biol.* **2014**, *30*, 255–289. [CrossRef] [PubMed]
12. Xu, R.; Rai, A.; Chen, M.; Suwakulsiri, W.; Greening, D.W.; Simpson, R.J. Extracellular vesicles in cancer—Implications for future improvements in cancer care. *Nat. Rev. Clin. Oncol.* **2018**, *15*, 617–638. [CrossRef] [PubMed]
13. Minciacchi, V.R.; Freeman, M.R.; di Vizio, D. Extracellular vesicles in cancer: Exosomes, microvesicles and the emerging role of large oncosomes. *Semin. Cell Dev. Biol.* **2015**, *40*, 41–51. [CrossRef] [PubMed]
14. Morello, M.; Minciacchi, V.R.; De Candia, P.; Yang, J.; Posadas, E.; Kim, H.; Griffiths, D.; Bhowmick, N.; Chung, L.W.K.; Gandellini, P.; et al. Large oncosomes mediate intercellular transfer of functional microRNA. *Cell Cycle* **2013**, *12*, 3526–3536. [CrossRef] [PubMed]
15. Johnson, S.M.; Dempsey, C.; Parker, C.; Mironov, A.; Bradley, H.; Saha, V. Acute lymphoblastic leukaemia cells produce large extracellular vesicles containing organelles and an active cytoskeleton. *J. Extracell. Vesicles* **2017**, *6*, 1294339. [CrossRef]
16. Vagner, T.; Spinelli, C.; Minciacchi, V.R.; Balaj, L.; Zandian, M.; Conley, A.; Zijlstra, A.; Freeman, M.R.; Demichelis, F.; De, S.; et al. Large extracellular vesicles carry most of the tumour DNA circulating in prostate cancer patient plasma. *J. Extracell. Vesicles* **2018**, *7*, 1505403. [CrossRef]

17. Pezzicoli, G.; Tucci, M.; Lovero, D.; Silvestris, F.; Porta, C.; Mannavola, F. Large Extracellular Vesicles—A New Frontier of Liquid Biopsy in Oncology. *Int. J. Mol. Sci.* **2020**, *21*, 6543. [CrossRef]
18. Lehrich, B.M.; Liang, Y.; Khosravi, P.; Federoff, H.J.; Fiandaca, M.S. Fetal Bovine Serum-Derived Extracellular Vesicles Persist within Vesicle-Depleted Culture Media. *Int. J. Mol. Sci.* **2018**, *19*, 3538. [CrossRef]
19. Lannigan, J.; Erdbruegger, U. Imaging flow cytometry for the characterization of extracellular vesicles. *Methods* **2017**, *112*, 55–67. [CrossRef]
20. Simonsen, J.B. Pitfalls associated with lipophilic fluorophore staining of extracellular vesicles for uptake studies. *J. Extracell. Vesicles* **2019**, *8*, 1582237. [CrossRef]
21. Osteikoetxea, X.; Benke, M.; Rodriguez, M.; Pálóczi, K.; Sódar, B.W.; Szvicsek, Z.; Szabó-Taylor, K.; Vukman, K.V.; Kittel, Á.; Wiener, Z.; et al. Detection and proteomic characterization of extracellular vesicles in human pancreatic juice. *Biochem. Biophys. Res. Commun.* **2018**, *499*, 37–43. [CrossRef] [PubMed]
22. Consortium, E.-T.; Van Deun, J.; Mestdagh, P.; Agostinis, P.; Akay, Ö.; Anand, S.; Anckaert, J.; Martinez, Z.A.; Baetens, T.; Beghein, E.; et al. EV-TRACK: Transparent reporting and centralizing knowledge in extracellular vesicle research. *Nat. Methods* **2017**, *14*, 228–232.
23. Vogel, R.; Coumans, F.A.W.; Maltesen, R.G.; Böing, A.N.; Bonnington, K.E.; Broekman, M.L.; Broom, M.F.; Buzás, E.I.; Christiansen, G.; Hajji, N.; et al. A standardized method to determine the concentration of extracellular vesicles using tunable resistive pulse sensing. *J. Extracell. Vesicles* **2016**, *5*, 31242. [CrossRef] [PubMed]
24. Gorgens, A.; Bremer, M.; Ferrer-Tur, R.; Murke, F.; Tertel, T.; Horn, P.A.; Thalmann, S.; Welsh, J.A.; Probst, C.; Guerin, C.; et al. Optimisation of imaging flow cytometry for the analysis of single extracellular vesicles by using fluorescence-tagged vesicles as biological reference material. *J. Extracell. Vesicles* **2019**, *8*, 1587567. [CrossRef] [PubMed]
25. Headland, S.E.; Jones, H.R.; D'Sa, A.S.V.; Perretti, M.; Norling, L.V. Cutting-edge analysis of extracellular microparticles using Image Stream (X) imaging flow cytometry. *Sci. Rep.* **2014**, *4*, 5237. [CrossRef] [PubMed]
26. Witwer, K.W.; Buzás, E.I.; Bemis, L.T.; Bora, A.; Lässer, C.; Lötvall, J.; Hoen, E.N.N.T.; Piper, M.G.; Sivaraman, S.; Skog, J.; et al. Standardization of sample collection, isolation and analysis methods in extracellular vesicle research. *J. Extracell. Vesicles* **2013**, *2*, 2. [CrossRef] [PubMed]
27. Erdbrugger, U.; Lannigan, J. Analytical challenges of extracellular vesicle detection: A comparison of different techniques. *Cytom. Part A* **2016**, *89*, 123–134. [CrossRef]
28. Menck, K.; Bleckmann, A.; Wachter, A.; Hennies, B.; Ries, L.; Schulz, M.; Balkenhol, M.; Pukrop, T.; Schatlo, B.; Rost, U.; et al. Characterisation of tumour-derived microvesicles in cancer patients' blood and correlation with clinical outcome. *J. Extracell. Vesicles* **2017**, *6*, 1340745. [CrossRef]
29. Taylor, D.D.; Gercel-Taylor, C. MicroRNA signatures of tumor-derived exosomes as diagnostic biomarkers of ovarian cancer. *Gynecol. Oncol.* **2008**, *110*, 13–21. [CrossRef]
30. Juraschka, K.; Taylor, M.D. Medulloblastoma in the age of molecular subgroups: A review. *J. Neurosurg. Pediatr.* **2019**, *24*, 353–363. [CrossRef]
31. Santiago-Dieppa, D.R.; Steinberg, J.; Gonda, D.; Cheung, V.J.; Carter, B.S.; Chen, C.C. Extracellular vesicles as a platform for 'liquid biopsy' in glioblastoma patients. *Expert Rev. Mol. Diagn.* **2014**, *14*, 819–825. [CrossRef] [PubMed]
32. Saenz-Antonanzas, A.; Auzmendi-Iriarte, J.; Carrasco-Garcia, E.; Moreno-Cugnon, L.; Ruiz, I.; Villanua, J.; Egaña, L.; Otaegui, D.; Samprón, N.; Matheu, A. Liquid Biopsy in Glioblastoma: Opportunities, Applications and Challenges. *Cancers (Basel)* **2019**, *11*, 950. [CrossRef] [PubMed]
33. Ihara, T.; Yamamoto, T.; Sugamata, M.; Okumura, H.; Ueno, Y. The process of ultrastructural changes from nuclei to apoptotic body. *Virchows Arch.* **1998**, *433*, 443–447. [CrossRef] [PubMed]
34. Crescitelli, R.; Lässer, C.; Szabó, T.G.; Kittel, A.; Eldh, M.; Dianzani, I.; Buzás, E.I.; Lötvall, J. Distinct RNA profiles in subpopulations of extracellular vesicles: Apoptotic bodies, microvesicles and exosomes. *J. Extracell. Vesicles* **2013**, *2*, 2. [CrossRef]
35. Verweij, F.J.; Bebelman, M.P.; Jimenez, C.R.; Garcia-Vallejo, J.J.; Janssen, H.; Neefjes, J.; Knol, J.C.; Haas, R.D.G.D.; Piersma, S.R.; Baglio, S.R.; et al. Correction: Quantifying exosome secretion from single cells reveals a modulatory role for GPCR signaling. *J. Cell. Biol.* **2018**, *217*, 1157. [CrossRef]
36. Cashikar, A.G.; Hanson, P.I. A cell-based assay for CD63-containing extracellular vesicles. *PLoS ONE* **2019**, *14*, e0220007. [CrossRef]

37. Kalra, H.; Simpson, R.J.; Ji, H.; Aikawa, E.; Altevogt, P.; Askenase, P.W.; Bond, V.C.; Borràs, F.E.; Breakefield, X.O.; Budnik, V.; et al. Vesiclepedia: A compendium for extracellular vesicles with continuous community annotation. *PLoS Biol.* **2012**, *10*, e1001450. [CrossRef]

Publisher's Note: MDPI stays neutral with regard to jurisdictional claims in published maps and institutional affiliations.

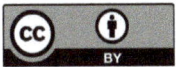 © 2020 by the authors. Licensee MDPI, Basel, Switzerland. This article is an open access article distributed under the terms and conditions of the Creative Commons Attribution (CC BY) license (http://creativecommons.org/licenses/by/4.0/).

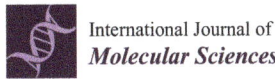

Communication

Three Method-Combination Protocol for Improving Purity of Extracellular Vesicles

Thomas Simon *, Anish Kumaran, Diana-Florentina Veselu and Georgios Giamas *

Department of Biochemistry and Biomedicine, School of Life Sciences, University of Sussex, Brighton BN1 9QG, UK; anish.kumaran26@gmail.com (A.K.); dv80@sussex.ac.uk (D.-F.V.)
* Correspondence: t.simon@sussex.ac.uk (T.S.); g.giamas@sussex.ac.uk (G.G.)

Received: 30 March 2020; Accepted: 24 April 2020; Published: 27 April 2020

Abstract: Extracellular vesicles (EVs) are nanosized structures able to carry proteins, lipids and genetic material from one cell to another with critical implications in intercellular communication mechanisms. Even though the rapidly growing EVs research field has sparked great interest in the last 20 years, many biological and technical aspects still remain challenging. One of the main issues that the field is facing is the absence of consensus regarding methods for EVs concentration from biofluids and tissue culture medium. Yet, not only can classic methods be time consuming, commercialized kits are also often quite expensive, especially when research requires analyzing numerous samples or concentrating EVs from large sample volumes. In addition, EV concentration often results in either low final yield or significant contamination of the vesicle sample with proteins and protein complexes of similar densities and sizes. Eventually, low vesicle yields highly limit any further application and data reproducibility while contamination greatly impacts extensive functional studies. Hence, there is a need for accessible and sustainable methods for improved vesicle concentration as this is a critical step in any EVs-related research study. In this brief report, we describe a novel combination of three well-known methods in order to obtain moderate-to-high yields of EVs with reduced protein contamination. We believe that such methods could be of high benefits for in vitro and in vivo functional studies.

Keywords: extracellular vesicles; size exclusion chromatography; differential ultracentrifugation

---

1. Introduction

Even though extracellular vesicles (EVs) have been described as 'useless cell debris' for decades, they have been recognized lately as key constituents of inter-cellular communication pathways [1,2]. EVs are lipid bilayer membrane-enclosed particles that are naturally released from cells [3]. Such cargo vessels transfer lipids, proteins, various fragments of nucleic acids and metabolic components to adjacent cells or to distant sites in the body, mainly through the circulatory system. For these reasons, EVs have been reported to play central roles in both normal and pathological conditions, such as pregnancy and cancer [1,4,5]. Similarly, EVs also play a unique role in spreading various pathogens like viruses and prions from one cell to another [6].

EVs can be classified into two clearly defined subtypes based on their sizes, namely "small EVs" (sEVs) with a size between 50–200 nm, or "medium/large EVs" (m/l EVs) with a size range between 200 nm–1 µm in diameter. This nomenclature is now preferred to the classic, yet quite vague, terms "exosomes", "microvesicles" or "oncosomes", as high heterogeneity in terms of size, marker expression and origins have been reported for each subpopulation, leading to overlaps between them [2].

Interest in the EVs has significantly grown in the medical research community over the past decade. Indeed, a thorough and comprehensive description of such EVs-dependent pathways may provide new inputs to develop effective treatments [5,7]. Mostly focusing on the sEVs subtype, the field has failed so far to establish essential technical standards, such as an optimal sEVs concentration/isolation method [1,2]. Thus, there is no consensus regarding that important matter whatsoever, raising important concerns regarding data reliance and reproducibility. As a matter of fact, currently available methods for sEVs concentration can hardly provide both high yield and high purity at once [8,9]. Consequently, such lack of effective techniques directly affects biomarker discovery and functional studies for which description of exclusively sEVs-related mechanisms and cargo is needed.

EVs are most commonly separated and concentrated from cell culture conditioned medium or human biofluids by differential ultracentrifugation (UC). This method allows for the separation of small particles, such as m/l and sEVs, from other larger ones, such as cell debris, based on their respective density and size, through successive increases of centrifugation forces and time. Differential UC is easy to perform, moderately time-consuming and does not require much technical expertise. Nonetheless, even when the parameters are optimized, the process results in a mixture of EVs concentrated along with particles of the same buoyant density and size range. In other words, large proteins and protein aggregates contaminate the EVs preparation. The co-isolated non-EVs structures are most often lipoproteins such as APOA1/2 or APOB, and Albumin [10]. Alternatively, researchers use various different methods such as size exclusion chromatography (SEC), filtration, precipitation, density gradients or immuno-isolation [2]. Yet, such protocols are not perfect as the final yield is often low and the purity is not optimal. In addition, these methods are usually commercialized in the form of expensive kits, altogether making them hardly applicable to extensive in vitro functional studies. For all these reasons, combining some of these methods seems to be the only sensitive strategy to substantially improve both the purity and the concentration of the final EVs preparation [2,10]. In theory, SEC makes it possible to separate the EVs from other particles, mainly proteins complexes and lipoproteins based on their size, through running a sample on a column made of resin with a define pore size. Consequently, such methods should help purify EVs samples obtained through UC [11,12].

For all these reasons, the present study has been undertaken in an attempt to improve the purity of sEVs preparation with the extra goal to maintain an important final concentration so that extensive functional studies are feasible. To do so, we have: (1) concentrated putative sEVs through UC, followed by (2) SEC in order to exclude protein contaminants from the assumed sEVs preparation. Finally, (3) an extra step was performed post-SEC using a centrifugal filter device in order to improve the concentration of the final sEVs samples. The final concentrated sEVs are therefore less contaminated as compare to sEVs separated using UC. Moreover, although there was a marginal loss during the process, we observed that the structure and size of sEVs were intact following all these steps.

2. Results and Discussion

Despite a constant and rapid evolution of the techniques and methods in the EVs field, researchers are yet to reach a consensus regarding the particle concentration step that is critical for any EVs-focused study [13]. However, they largely agree on the higher performance of combinational protocols over single-method approaches, even though proper EVs isolation/purification still seems unrealistic. Indeed, obtaining high concentrations of EVs coupled to acceptable sample purity is still hardly feasible [1,2]. Yet, reaching such a goal would be of high value for current functional studies, as it would make it possible to perform reliable and reproducible experiments for deciphering EVs-specific mechanisms. Indeed, as mentioned in the latest update to the MISEV2018, highly purified EVs should be used when one wants to associate a function or marker expression to vesicles as compared with other potentially present particles [2].

In the present study, conditioned medium was collected from confluent glioblastoma (GBM) cells. Differential UC was then performed so that the original putative sEVs samples could be obtained. Following, nanoparticles analysis (NTA) was employed to determine the concentration of particles in the original samples (1.63×10^{11} particles/mL, Figure 1A).

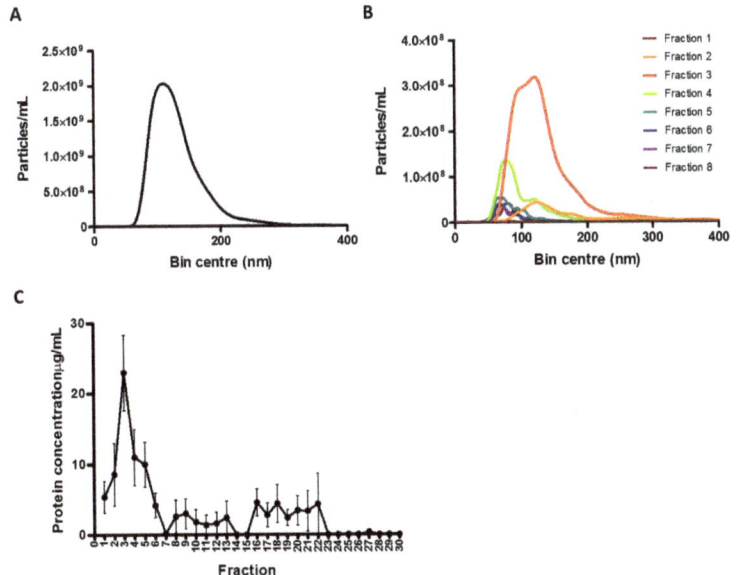

Figure 1. Nanoparticle tracking analysis and protein concentration measurement in initial ultracentrifugation sample and fractions from size exclusion chromatography (Step 1 and 2). Particle samples obtained following step 1 and 2 of the 3 method-combination protocol were processed to nanoparticle analysis (NTA) and protein concentration measurement. (**A**) NTA of the initial ultracentrifugation (UC) sample. Sample was diluted (1/50) in filtered sterile phosphate buffer solution (PBS) and measured using a Nanosight NS300. (**B**) NTA of the fractions from size exclusion chromatography (SEC). The initial UC sample was processed through SEC and fractions were measured by NTA. Fractions were diluted (1/20) in filtered PBS and measured using a Nanosight NS300. (**C**) Protein concentration measurement in the SEC fractions. Protein concentration was measured using a Nanodrop 200. The mean ± SEM of $n = 5$ independent experiments is shown.

SEC was performed following this initial step. As shown in Figure 1B, NTA measurements revealed the presence of particles of the sEVs sizes mainly in SEC fractions 2, 3 and 4 (0.43, 2.70 and 0.74×10^{10} particles/mL, respectively). In addition, further Nanodrop analysis showed that SEC fractions 2, 3 and 4 (8.6, 23 and 11 µg/mL, respectively) showed the highest protein content, confirming the detection of putative EVs in the earliest fractions (detection of sEVs-associated proteins) and suggesting the presence of protein contaminants in the latest (Figure 1C).

Accordingly, fraction 3 was pooled with either fraction 2 or 4 and concentrated in a 100 µL of sterile phosphate buffer solution (PBSs). NTA of this final sample showed a particle concentration of 3.84×10^{10} particles/mL, which was 4.2× lower as compared to the original concentration obtained by UC (Figure 2A,B).

Western blotting for sEVs markers, namely CD9 and HSP70, fibronectin (FN1) and described EVs sample contaminant albumin (BSA), was then performed. Data revealed exclusive expression of CD9 and HSP70 in both the original UC and final putative sEVs samples, validating the EVs concentration by both the UC method and the three method-combination protocol. The expression of EVs markers was lower in the final sEVs as compared to the UC sample (Figure 3A). BSA expression was mostly observed in the initial UC sample, fraction 5, fraction 6 and fraction 10. In addition, as shown in Figure 3A, a decrease of the FN1 expression was observed in the final sEVs sample as compared to the original UC sample. Yet, FN1 expression was also detected in all the SEC fractions with a slight decrease in fractions 7 and 8, and a slight increase in fractions 9 and 10.

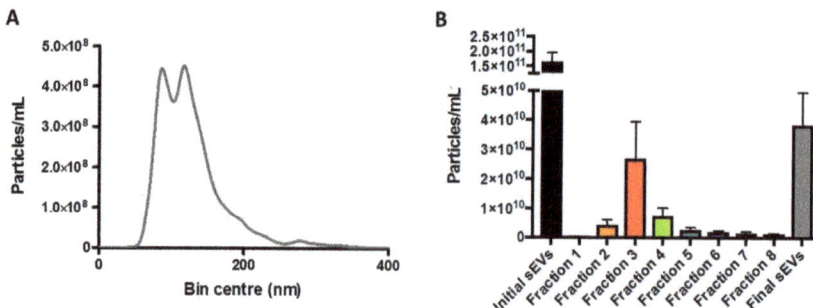

Figure 2. Comparison of particle concentration in final putative sEVs sample versus ultracentrifugation sample and fractions from size exclusion chromatography (Step 3). Final putative sEV sample was obtained following concentration of selected size exclusion chromatography (SEC) fractions using an Amicon Ultra 0.5 device – 30k. (**A**) Nanoparticle tracking analysis (NTA) of the final putative sEV sample. Sample was diluted (1/50) in filtered PBS and analyzed using a Nanosight NS300. (**B**) Particle concentration of the initial UC sample, fractions from SEC and final putative sEVs sample. The mean ± SEM of $n = 5$ independent experiments is shown.

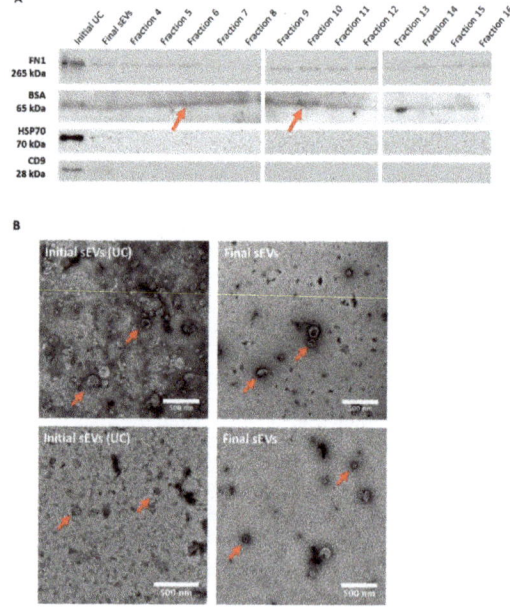

Figure 3. Validation of sEV concentration and decreased protein contamination. (**A**) Western blotting detection of fibronectin (FN1), bovine serum albumin (BSA), HSP70 and CD9 in initial (UC), final sEVs and SEC fractions. (**B**) TEM detection of sEVs (×20k magnification and zoom). Red arrows show sEVs. Representative pictures are shown. Scale bar = 500 µm.

Finally, transmission electron microscopy (TEM) was performed in order to observe the structure/membrane integrity of the final sEVs sample as compare to the original UC one (Figure 3B). As seen in Figure 3B, final particles appear very similar structure wise as compare to original ones from the UC sample, displaying an apparently intact lipid bilayer membrane. Particle concentration appeared much lower in the final sample as compare to the original UC sample, confirming the NTA observations. Moreover, fewer debris and sEVs aggregates could be observed in TEM pictures of the final sEVs sample, as compared to the original UC one.

Using our combination of methods, we observed that our final sEVs samples presented with fewer debris and particle aggregates as compared to our original samples obtained by UC. Altogether, it appears that our three method-combination protocol produced concentrated sEVs samples with enhanced purity as compared to the commonly used UC protocol. We can therefore confirm that combining UC and then SEC, in this order, allows: 1) to use large amounts of cell culture conditioned medium/biofluids for high sEVs concentrations and 2) to separate particles from protein contaminants found in the UC concentrated preparations. Final centrifugal concentration then allows for reducing sample dilution due to SEC.

Our present method might be especially valuable for in vitro functional studies, as one of the strengths here is to make possible using very large volumes (>100 mL) of starting material. The final concentration of sEVs in this way is high enough to perform multiple validation and further functional/phenotypic experiments with the same sample, thus increasing data impact. In addition, even though SEC columns that allow for EVs separation from large volumes are finally emerging, they are still very costly and a few of them would be required in case of repeated usage. Our present UC/SEC combination takes advantage of the SEC impact on sample quality without the requirement of multiple columns in order to process such starting material. Alternatively, here we propose a rather cheap and sustainable method that consecutively has more potential for a wide use and would allow for a better standardization of techniques among teams. As the EVs community is in need of a general improvement of data specificity, we believe our easily accessible alternative could be of great help, especially to small research teams.

For the same reasons, our method combination could also benefit the biomarker discovery in EVs [5]. For instance, better separation of EVs from freely circulating material, such as apolipoproteins, in blood would allow for improved identification of EVs-specific biomarkers. As, for example, cancer-derived EVs are believed to travel very long distances to set up metastatic sites, improved plasma-derived EVs concentration could have highly sensitive clinical applications [5]. Nevertheless, as mentioned in the MISEV2018, definitive association of a biomarker with EVs might not be essential to such application. According to the authors, even if it just co-isolates with EVs, such biomarker is valuable as long as it can be associated to any clinical benefit (for diagnosis or prognosis for example) [2]. Yet, one could argue that better EVs separation leading to higher sample purity might provide more specific and thus more effective and stringent EVs-associated biomarkers.

Despite that such a novel method can represent progress towards standardization, there is still room for improvement. For instance, while the decrease of particle concentration we could observe at the end of the protocol should be mostly due, in theory, to the actual purification process, it could also be due to material loss during the many handling, transfer and filtration steps. Furthermore, as we used only one GBM cell line for the present study, we have to acknowledge that our three method-protocol might present variable efficacy when performed with CM derived from cell lines or primary cells of different origins. Indeed, as we also observed in previous studies, EVs production and cargo are highly affected by their cell origin [5]. Nevertheless, even though an extended work would confirm such assumption, we believe that our present three method-protocol to be applicable to any sorts of biofluids, including CM from immortalized and primary cell lines. Furthermore, extended comparison of our present protocol to other available method combinations will be needed in the near future in order to fully assess its efficacy [14]. Finally, while the present protocol is optimized for the specific recovery of sEVs, which received most of the field attention over the last 10 years, interest in m/lEVs and larger particles is slowly growing [15]. As these EVs sub-populations might also be involved in key mechanisms in both normal and pathological conditions, there is a growing need for innovative methods for precise and reliable separation of these different EVs sub-populations. For instance, an additional SEC step could be added to the present protocol, following the $10,000\times g$

UC step in order to separate m/lEVs from other membrane debris and contaminants. Such work would then be a highly valuable follow-up study to the present report.

3. Materials and Methods

3.1. Cells and Reagents

U118 glioblastoma (GBM) cells (ATCC) were maintained in Dulbecco's Modified Eagle Medium (DMEM, Sigma-Aldrich, Gillingham, UK). Cell line culture medium was supplemented with 100 Units mL^{-1} penicillin, 100 µg mL^{-1} streptomycin, 2 mM L-glutamine (PSG, Sigma-Aldrich, Gillingham, UK) and 10% heat inactivated fetal bovine serum (FBS, Sigma-Aldrich, Gillingham, UK).

3.2. Differential Ultracentrifugation for Extracellular Vesicle Concentration

In order to collect sEVs derived from GBM cells, cells were seeded in 4 to 5×175 cm^2 flasks and grown in 10% FCS medium until they reach confluence. Then, cells were washed with sterile PBS and 15 mL of corresponding serum free medium was added to each flask for 24 h. Following this incubation, conditioned medium (CM) was collected from each flask, pooled together in 2×50 mL falcon tubes and kept at either 4 °C for a very short time (up to 24 h) or at −20 °C for longer periods (up to 6 months) before sEV concentration. In accordance with the latest Minimal Information for Studies of Extracellular Vesicles (MISEV2018), cell count at time of collection was recorded and used to normalize the final sEV concentration (particles mL^{-1} per cell). Cell number and viability were measured using a Countess ™ cell counter (Thermo Fisher Scientific, Life Technologies, Paisley, UK) following mixing of the cell suspension with 0.4% Trypan blue. Only CMs harvested from cell culture with >90% viability were stored.

Concentration of sEVs was performed using an UC-based protocol [13]. Every step of the concentration protocol was performed at 4 °C. In total, 20 mL of stored CM was pipetted into each UC tube. An initial $300\times g$ centrifugation was performed for 10 min to discard any floating cells from the CM, followed by a 10 min centrifugation step at $2000\times g$ to remove any floating cell debris and dead cells (Hettich Universal 320R centrifuge, DJB Labcare Ltd., Newport Pagnell, UK). A $10,000\times g$ UC step (Beckman optima LE 80-k ultracentrifuge, Beckman Type 70 Ti rotor, Beckman polypropylene centrifuge 14×89 mm tubes, full dynamic braking, $k_{adj} = 15,638$, Beckman Coulter Ltd., High Wycombe, UK) was then performed for 30 min to remove any further cell debris and potential large vesicles (m/lEVs) from the CM. Finally, a first $100,000\times g$ UC run was performed for 1 h 30 min to pellet the putative sEVs from the CM (Beckman optima LE 80-k ultracentrifuge, Beckman Type 70 Ti rotor, Beckman polypropylene centrifuge 14×89 mm tubes, full dynamic braking, $k_{adj} = 494$). Supernatant was stored at −20 °C. The UC pellet was then washed in filtered sterile PBS and centrifuged again for 1 h 30 min at $100,000\times g$ in order to discard contaminants. The final pellet was re-suspended in 100 µL filtered sterile PBS and immediately characterized through nanoparticle tracking analysis (NTA). Protein concentration (µg/mL) of the final UC preparation was determined using a Nanodrop 200 spectrophotometer (Thermofisher Scientific, Life Technologies, Paisley, UK) (Figure 4).

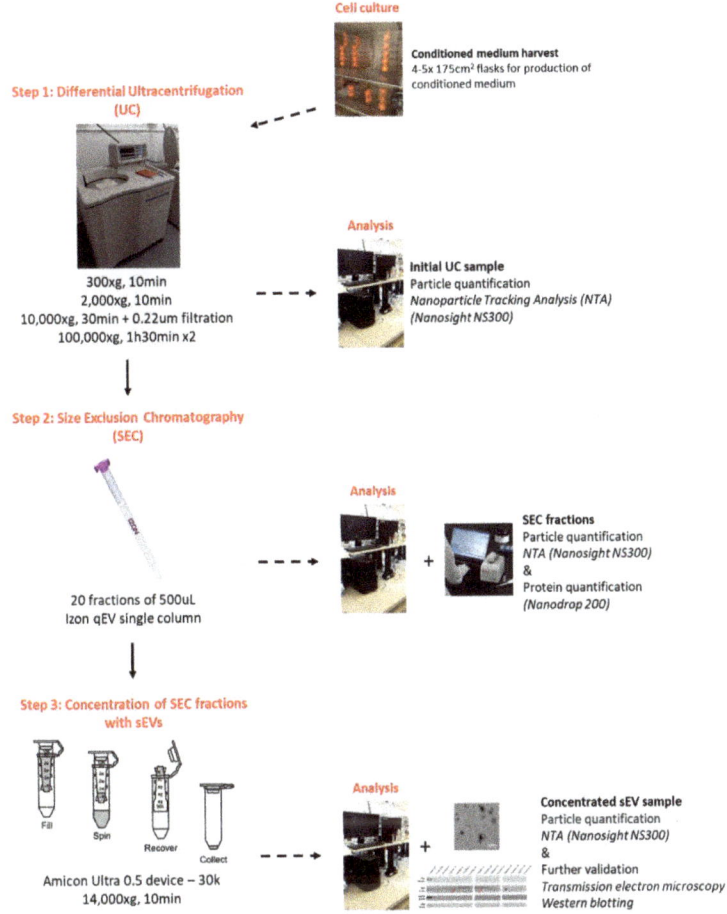

Figure 4. Three method-combination for concentrating EVs derived from cell culture medium. Cells are grown to confluence in 4 × 175 cm² flasks to produce conditioned medium. Conditioned medium is then processed through the differential ultracentrifugation (UC) protocol in order to obtain an initial UC sample (step 1). The initial UC sample is then processed through a size exclusion chromatography column (SEC - Izon qEV single column) in the aim to separate putative EVs from protein contaminants (step 2). Following measurement of the particle and protein concentration, SEC fractions of interest are then pooled together and concentrated using Amicon ultra 0.5 devices (step 3). Final validation experiments confirm the sEVs concentration and the decreased protein contamination of the sample.

3.3. Size Exclusion Chromatography for Extracellular Vesicle Separation from Protein Contaminants

Following the initial UC step, 20 µL of the original preparation (out of 100 µL) was kept at −20 °C for further analysis. The rest of the preparation (~80 µL) was diluted in filtered sterile PBS in order to reach a final volume of 150 µL. SEC was performed using qEV single size exclusion columns (separation size = 70 nm, iZON science, Oxford, UK). According to the manufacturer's recommendations, the SEC column was first equilibrated using sterile PBS before the sample (150 µL) was loaded. As stated by the manufacturer, loading a 150 µL sample at the top of the column results in a 1 mL void volume and fractions of 500 µL. Following loading of the sample at the top of the column, fractions (20 in total) of 500 µL were immediately collected and kept on ice. First 7 fractions were then characterized through NTA. Protein concentration (µg/mL) of all fractions was determined using a Nanodrop 200 spectrophotometer (Thermofisher Scientific, Life Technologies, Paisley, UK). Fractions were then stored at −20 °C (Figure 4).

3.4. Concentration of SEC Fractions

SEC fractions with the highest concentrations of particles (as stated, based on NTA data) were concentrated in an Amicon Ultra 0.5 device – 30k (Merck milipore, Watford, UK). The centrifugal filter device was pre-rinsed with filtered PBS. Samples (500 µL at once) were loaded to the filter device and centrifuged at 14,000× g for 5–10 min at 4 °C. The putative concentrated sEVs preparation was characterized through NTA and was further processed or stored at −20 °C (Figure 4).

3.5. Nanoparticles Tracking Analysis (NTA)

Vesicle concentration and size were determined using a Nanosight© NS300 and the Nanosight© NTA 3.2 software (Malvern Instruments, Malvern, UK). The following conditions were applied for the NTA analysis at the Nanosight instrument: temperature was 20–25 °C; viscosity was ~0.98cP; camera type was sCMOS; laser type was Blue488; camera levels were either 14 or 15; syringe Pump Speed was set to 70 AU; 5 measurements of 60 s each were recorded. Graphs show an average of at least 4 experiments.

3.6. Coomassie Blue Staining

Samples were loaded, as stated, on 10% tris-glycine gels and run at 180 V and 40 mA for 100 min. The gels were then stained with Quick Coomassie Stain (Generon, Slough, UK) at room temperature overnight. Excess stain was removed through deionized water washes. Gels were viewed and captured by Criterion Stain Free Imager (Biorad, Watford, UK).

3.7. Western Blotting

Characterization of the sEVs was performed through western blotting by measuring the expression of the EV membrane associated marker CD9 (mainly associated with light sEVs) and Fibronectin (mainly associated with dense sEVs), and EV cytosolic marker HSP70 [2,15]. Standard western blotting protocol was performed as described before [16]. For the EV marker analysis, comparable amount of sEVs (as stated) was loaded on the SDS gel. Primary antibodies: anti-BSA (Merck Millipore 07–248, 1/500 dilution, Merck-Millipore, Watford, UK), anti-CD-9 (System Biosciences EXOAB-CD9A-1, 1/10000 dilution), anti-Fibronectin (Abcam ab2413, 1/1000 dilution), anti-HSP-70 (System Biosciences EXOAB-HSP70A-1,1/10000 dilution, Cambridge Bioscience, Cambridge, UK). Secondary antibodies used: Polyclonal Goat Anti-Rabbit/Mouse Immunoglobulins/HRP (Dako P0447/8, 1/3000 dilution, Agilent, CA, USA) antibodies and Anti-Rabbit Immunoglobulins/HRP (ExoAb antibody Kit, System Biosciences EXO-AB-HRP, 1/3000 dilution, Cambridge Bioscience, Cambridge, UK). Chemiluminescence was observed using a UVP Chemstudio instrument (Analytik Jena, London, UK) and the Vision Works software. All experiments have been repeated at least 3 times.

3.8. Transmission Electron Microscopy

Transmission electron microscopy (TEM) has been performed on putative sEVs preparation in order to visualize and assess/confirm the size range of the vesicles, as described before [13]. Samples were visualized using a JEOL JEM1400-Plus (120 kV, LaB6) microscope (JEOL Ltd., Welwyn Garden City, UK) equipped with a Gatan OneView 4K camera at × 20 k magnification. In total, 10–15 pictures per grid were taken.

4. Conclusions

Overall, the present study establishes an easy and affordable method for sEVs separation that provides both improved sample purity and particles' concentration. We believe that the present 3 method-combination protocol will have a great potential for future in vitro functional studies.

Author Contributions: T.S. and G.G. conceived the idea. A.K., D.-F.V. and T.S. performed the experiments and the analysis of the data. T.S. and G.G. wrote the manuscript. All authors have read and agreed to the published version of the manuscript.

Funding: This work was supported by Action Against Cancer.

Acknowledgments: We would like to thank Pascale Schellenberger for helping with transmission electron microscopy at the University of Sussex's Electron microscopy imaging center, funded by the School of Life Sciences, the Wellcome Trust (095605/Z/11/A, 208348/Z/17/Z) and the RM Philips Trust.

Conflicts of Interest: The authors declare no conflicts of interest.

References

1. Margolis, L.; Sadovsky, Y. The biology of extracellular vesicles: The known unknowns. *PLoS Boil.* **2019**, *17*, e3000363. [CrossRef] [PubMed]
2. Théry, C.; Witwer, K.W.; Aikawa, E.; Alcaraz, M.J.; Anderson, J.D.; Andriantsitohaina, R.; Antoniou, A.; Arab, T.; Archer, F.; Atkin-Smith, G.K.; et al. Minimal information for studies of extracellular vesicles 2018 (MISEV2018): A position statement of the International Society for Extracellular Vesicles and update of the MISEV2014 guidelines. *J. Extracell. Vesicles* **2018**, *7*, 1535750. [CrossRef] [PubMed]
3. Wendler, F.; Favicchio, R.; Simon, T.; Alifrangis, C.; Stebbing, J.; Giamas, G. Extracellular vesicles swarm the cancer microenvironment: From tumor–stroma communication to drug intervention. *Oncogene* **2016**, *36*, 877–884. [CrossRef] [PubMed]
4. Wendler, F.; Stamp, G.W.; Giamas, G. Tumor–Stromal Cell Communication: Small Vesicles Signal Big Changes. *Trends Cancer* **2016**, *2*, 326–329. [CrossRef] [PubMed]
5. Lane, R.; Simon, T.; Vintu, M.; Solkin, B.; Koch, B.; Stewart, N.; Benstead-Hume, G.; Pearl, F.M.; Critchley, G.; Stebbing, J.; et al. Cell-derived extracellular vesicles can be used as a biomarker reservoir for glioblastoma tumor subtyping. *Commun. Boil.* **2019**, *2*, 1–12. [CrossRef] [PubMed]
6. Qin, J.; Xu, Q. Functions and application of exosomes. *Acta Pol. Pharm. - Drug Res.* **2014**, *71*, 537–543.
7. Simon, T.; Pinioti, S.; Schellenberger, P.; Rajeeve, V.; Wendler, F.; Cutillas, P.R.; King, A.; Stebbing, J.; Giamas, G. Shedding of bevacizumab in tumour cells-derived extracellular vesicles as a new therapeutic escape mechanism in glioblastoma. *Mol. Cancer* **2018**, *17*, 132. [CrossRef] [PubMed]
8. Gardiner, C.; Di Vizio, L.; Sahoo, S.; Théry, C.; Witwer, K.W.; Wauben, M.; Hill, A.F. Techniques used for the isolation and characterization of extracellular vesicles: Results of a worldwide survey. *J. Extracell. Vesicles* **2016**, *5*, 27066. [CrossRef] [PubMed]
9. Helwa, I.; Cai, J.; Drewry, M.D.; Zimmerman, A.; Dinkins, M.B.; Khaled, M.L.; Seremwe, M.; Dismuke, W.M.; Bieberich, E.; Stamer, W.D.; et al. A Comparative Study of Serum Exosome Isolation Using Differential Ultracentrifugation and Three Commercial Reagents. *PLoS ONE* **2017**, *12*, e0170628. [CrossRef] [PubMed]
10. Takov, K.; Yellon, D.M.; Davidson, S.M. Comparison of small extracellular vesicles isolated from plasma by ultracentrifugation or size-exclusion chromatography: Yield, purity and functional potential. *J. Extracell. Vesicles* **2018**, *8*, 1560809. [CrossRef] [PubMed]
11. Lozano-Ramos, I.; Bancu, I.; Oliveira-Tercero, A.; Armengol, M.P.; Menezes-Neto, A.; Del Portillo, H.A.; Lauzurica-Valdemoros, R.; Borràs, F.E. Size-exclusion chromatography-based enrichment of extracellular vesicles from urine samples. *J. Extracell. Vesicles* **2015**, *4*, 27369. [CrossRef] [PubMed]
12. Guerreiro, E.M.; Vestad, B.; Steffensen, L.A.; Aass, H.C.D.; Saeed, M.; Øvstebø, R.; Costea, D.E.; Galtung, H.K.; Søland, T.M. Efficient extracellular vesicle isolation by combining cell media modifications, ultrafiltration, and size-exclusion chromatography. *PLoS ONE* **2018**, *13*, e0204276. [CrossRef] [PubMed]
13. Théry, C.; Amigorena, S.; Raposo, G.; Clayton, A. Isolation and Characterization of Exosomes from Cell Culture Supernatants and Biological Fluids. *Curr. Protoc. Cell Boil.* **2006**, *30*, 3.22.1–3.22.29. [CrossRef] [PubMed]

14. Kowal, J.; Arras, G.; Colombo, M.; Jouve, M.; Morath, J.P.; Primdal-Bengtson, B.; Dingli, F.; Loew, D.; Tkach, M.; Théry, C. Proteomic comparison defines novel markers to characterize heterogeneous populations of extracellular vesicle subtypes. *Proc. Natl. Acad. Sci. USA* **2016**, *113*, E968–E977. [CrossRef] [PubMed]
15. Giamas, G.; Hirner, H.; Shoshiashvili, L.; Grothey, A.; Gessert, S.; Kuhl, M.; Henne-Bruns, D.; Vorgias, C.E.; Knippschild, U. Phosphorylation of CK1δ: Identification of Ser370 as the major phosphorylation site targeted by PKA in vitro and in vivo. *Biochem. J.* **2007**, *406*, 389–398. [CrossRef] [PubMed]
16. Corso, G.; Mäger, I.; Lee, Y.; Görgens, A.; Bultema, J.; Giebel, B.; Wood, M.; Nordin, J.; El Andaloussi, S. Reproducible and scalable purification of extracellular vesicles using combined bind-elute and size exclusion chromatography. *Sci. Rep.* **2017**, *7*, 11561. [CrossRef] [PubMed]

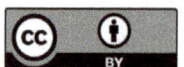 © 2020 by the authors. Licensee MDPI, Basel, Switzerland. This article is an open access article distributed under the terms and conditions of the Creative Commons Attribution (CC BY) license (http://creativecommons.org/licenses/by/4.0/).

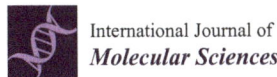

Article

Optimized Protocol for Isolation of Small Extracellular Vesicles from Human and Murine Lymphoid Tissues

Marie Bordas [1,2], Géraldine Genard [3], Sibylle Ohl [1], Michelle Nessling [4], Karsten Richter [4], Tobias Roider [5], Sascha Dietrich [5], Kendra K. Maaß [6,7,†] and Martina Seiffert [1,*,†]

1. Division of Molecular Genetics, German Cancer Research Center (DKFZ), 69120 Heidelberg, Germany; m.bordas@dkfz.de (M.B.); s.ohl@dkfz.de (S.O.)
2. Faculty of Biosciences, University of Heidelberg, 69120 Heidelberg, Germany
3. Division of Biomedical Physics in Radiation Oncology, German Cancer Research Center (DKFZ), 69120 Heidelberg, Germany; g.genard@dkfz-heidelberg.de
4. Central Unit Electron Microscopy, DKFZ, 69120 Heidelberg, Germany; m.nessling@dkfz.de (M.N.); k.richter@dkfz.de (K.R.)
5. Department of Medicine V, Hematology, Oncology and Rheumatology, University of Heidelberg, 69120 Heidelberg, Germany; Tobias.Roider@med.uni-heidelberg.de (T.R.); Sascha.Dietrich@med.uni-heidelberg.de (S.D.)
6. Hopp-Children's Cancer Center Heidelberg (KiTZ), 69120 Heidelberg, Germany; k.maass@kitz-heidelberg.de
7. Division of Pediatric Neurooncology, German Cancer Research Center (DKFZ), 69120 Heidelberg, Germany
* Correspondence: m.seiffert@dkfz.de; Tel.: +49-6221-42-4586
† These authors contributed equally to this work.

Received: 6 July 2020; Accepted: 31 July 2020; Published: 4 August 2020

Abstract: Small extracellular vesicles (sEVs) are nanoparticles responsible for cell-to-cell communication released by healthy and cancer cells. Different roles have been described for sEVs in physiological and pathological contexts, including acceleration of tissue regeneration, modulation of tumor microenvironment, or premetastatic niche formation, and they are discussed as promising biomarkers for diagnosis and prognosis in body fluids. Although efforts have been made to standardize techniques for isolation and characterization of sEVs, current protocols often result in co-isolation of soluble protein or lipid complexes and of other extracellular vesicles. The risk of contaminated preparations is particularly high when isolating sEVs from tissues. As a consequence, the interpretation of data aiming at understanding the functional role of sEVs remains challenging and inconsistent. Here, we report an optimized protocol for isolation of sEVs from human and murine lymphoid tissues. sEVs from freshly resected human lymph nodes and murine spleens were isolated comparing two different approaches (1) ultracentrifugation on a sucrose density cushion and (2) combined ultracentrifugation with size-exclusion chromatography. The purity of sEV preparations was analyzed using state-of-the-art techniques, including immunoblots, nanoparticle tracking analysis, and electron microscopy. Our results clearly demonstrate the superiority of size-exclusion chromatography, which resulted in a higher yield and purity of sEVs, and we show that their functionality alters significantly between the two isolation protocols.

Keywords: extracellular vesicles; exosomes; small extracellular vesicles; isolation; purification; size-exclusion chromatography; ultracentrifugation; sucrose density cushion; lymph node; spleen; solid tissue

1. Introduction

Extracellular vesicles (EVs) are lipid bilayer-enveloped nanovesicles secreted by both eukaryotic and prokaryotic cells and carrying cargos of proteins, lipids, and nucleic acids [1,2]. EVs contain both surface and luminal factors which can be used as markers for specific EV populations representing the different biogenesis pathways [3,4]. Although the definition of EVs is continuously being refined, currently three main subtypes of eukaryotic cell-derived EVs can be distinguished based on their size, composition, and cellular origin—small EVs (sEVs or exosomes, 30–150 nm), microvesicles (MVs, 100 nm^{-1} µm), and apoptotic bodies (1–5 µm) [5,6]. Unlike MVs, which originate from direct budding of the plasma membrane, sEVs stem from the endocytic compartment and are released after fusion of multivesicular bodies with the plasma membrane [5,7]. Due to the secretory release mechanism of MVs, it is well recognized that their cargo mirrors the cytoplasmic and surface composition of the parental cell. In contrast, several studies on sEV loading reported a specific enrichment or depletion of cellular proteins or RNAs in their cargoes, and several sorting mechanisms have been suggested [8–12].

sEVs have been shown to be taken up by various recipient cell types such as myeloid, stromal, and neuronal cells, among many others [13]. The delivery of sEV cargoes into recipient cells can lead to both transcriptional and proteomic changes as a result [1,14,15]. Depending on the origin of the sEVs and the recipient cells, sEV uptake can affect diverse biologic processes, e.g., inflammation, angiogenesis, immune response, or composition of the extracellular matrix [1]. Besides their functional properties, sEVs and their content, in particular microRNAs, are also discussed for their potential as diagnostic and prognostic biomarkers in pathological conditions [1,16]. More recently, researchers explored sEVs as a new therapeutic tool for targeted drug delivery [17,18].

Due to their large spectrum of action, the interest of the scientific community for sEVs has increased exponentially over the last few years. However, many technical limitations are encountered during isolation and purification of sEVs. In particular, the isolation of sEVs from solid tissues remains challenging, limiting studies with primary patient material and causing a biased use of cell line-derived sEVs. To overcome this limitation, we aimed to improve the isolation and purification of sEVs from lymphoid tissues of human and murine specimens by comparing two different isolation protocols. The first protocol is based on differential centrifugation combined with ultracentrifugation on a sucrose density cushion as previously described [19], whereas the second protocol combines differential centrifugation with size-exclusion chromatography (SEC) using the commercially available single qEV 35 nm columns from IZON (Izon, Christchurch, New Zealand) [20]. Previous studies have already compared the efficiency of qEV IZON columns with other accepted sEV isolation techniques and reported higher yields and quality of the final product, in particular for isolation of sEVs from plasma samples [21,22].

As starting material, we used three biopsies of lymph nodes (LNs) collected from patients with B-cell lymphoma and three spleens from a B-cell lymphoma mouse model [23,24]. By directly comparing the amount, purity, and functionality of sEVs obtained for both sample types with the two protocols, we demonstrate the superiority of the SEC-based isolation technique for lymphoid tissues.

2. Results

2.1. Isolation and Purification of sEVs from Human Lymph Nodes

Two protocols for sEV isolation from lymphoid tissues were performed in parallel on the same starting material to compare their efficiency in terms of (1) total amount of recovered sEVs, (2) purity of sEV preparation, and (3) reproducibility. After manual dissociation of LN biopsies of three B-cell lymphoma patients, the supernatants of the cell suspensions were collected and processed by differential centrifugation. The resulting pellets (100 K pellet) containing sEVs and soluble proteins and lipids was resuspended and split into two equal parts each, which were then combined either with SEC on IZON columns or differential centrifugation combined with ultracentrifugation on a 40% sucrose density cushion as illustrated in Figure 1. An identical volume of PBS (250 µL) was used for the final resuspension of sEVs isolated from IZON columns and the sucrose density cushions ("cushion"). Nanoparticle tracking analysis (NTA) revealed that the resuspended pellet from the "cushion" preparation as well as fractions 1 and 2 collected from the IZON column were enriched in the characteristic sEV size profile, with IZON fraction 2 accounting for the peak fraction (Figure 2A, left). SEV size profiles were also detected in the IZON fraction 3, although in lower concentrations. The absolute number of particles yielded from IZON peak fractions as assessed by NTA was 3.9- to 10.3-fold higher than the sEV particle number recovered using the sucrose density cushion (Figure 2A, right). We then performed protein quantification using a bicinchoninic acid (BCA) assay (Figure 2B, left). Due to their smaller size, protein complexes are able to enter the pores of the IZON column, and their elution is delayed, which can be observed as a second protein peak in the fraction F7 collected later [20,25]. The absolute amount of proteins recovered from IZON peak fractions was lower than the one obtained in the respective "cushion" preparation (1.4- to 2.2-fold lower; Figure 2B, right) which was less than the fold change detected by NTA for particle numbers. Calculation of the particle/protein ratios revealed lower values for "cushion" preparations compared to IZON fractions in two of the three samples (Figure 2D). Therefore, we hypothesized that the sucrose density cushion approach led to a larger amount of protein complexes co-isolated with the sEVs. The mean particle size and size distribution of sEVs were similar in IZON fractions 1 and 2 and the "cushion" preparation with 153, 157, and 148 nm for the peak IZON fractions, and 155, 163, and 152 nm for the corresponding "cushion" preparations (Figure 2C,E). In line with our hypothesis, immunoblot analysis revealed a lower signal for exosomal surface markers FLOTILLIN-1, CD81, CD9, and the luminal marker TSG101 in the "cushion" preparations compared to IZON fractions 1 and 2 for the same amount of protein loaded (Figure 2F and Figure S1). As our study is one of the first to focus on solid tissues, we thoroughly validated the presence of contaminant proteins as recommended by the MISEV guidelines [26]. We neither detected the Golgi marker GM130 nor the mitochondrial marker CYTOCHROME C in both preparations. Surprisingly, we detected the endoplasmic reticulum (ER) protein CALNEXIN in sEVs isolated with both protocols. However, the amount of CALNEXIN in the sEV preparations was lower in comparison to the parental cell lysate (Figure 2F and Figure S1). Although partial contamination of the samples with cellular debris cannot be excluded, the presence of CALNEXIN but no markers from other cell organelles might be indicative for a specific sEV biogenesis pathway involving the ER in lymphoma cells. In addition, the IZON fraction F2 and "cushion" samples were analyzed by transmission electron microscopy (TEM). The results illustrate that the SEC isolated samples allow a clear identification of sEVs for all of the three samples. However, we observed a higher heterogeneity in the "cushion" preparations, with sEVs barely detected in two out of three samples (Figure 2G). Employing immuno-electron microscopy, we confirmed the presence of the immune receptor MHC Class II (HLA-DR) on the surface of sEVs isolated by both approaches and thereby validate their immune cell origin (Figure 2H).

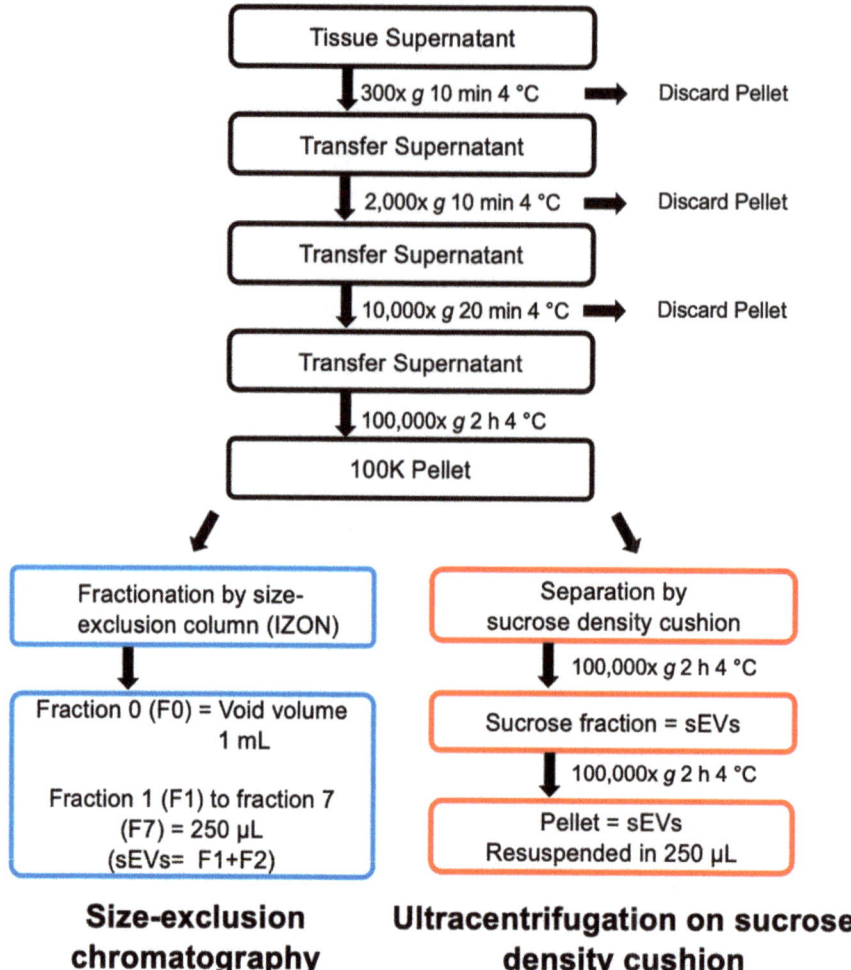

Figure 1. Experimental outline of the comparison of size-exclusion column-based (SEC) versus density-based small extracellular vesicle (sEV) isolations. Supernatant of dissociated lymphatic tissues was separated by differential ultracentrifugation and the resulting 100 K pellet was resuspended and split into two equal parts for direct method comparison. Equal volumes were loaded on either SEC columns or on a sucrose density cushion. Resulting sEV fractions were compared for yield, purity and functionality.

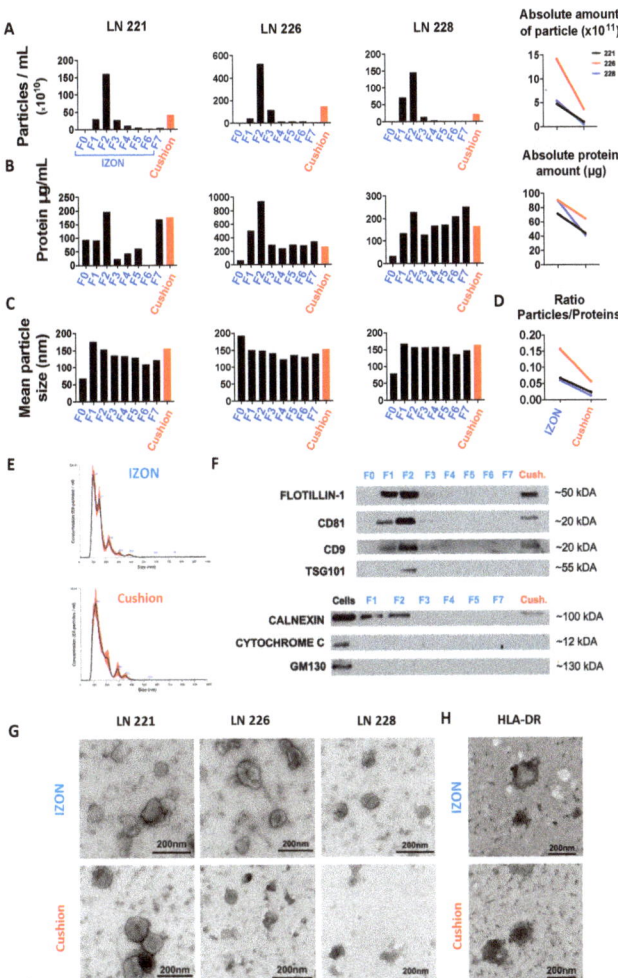

Figure 2. Comparative isolation and characterization of sEVs from human lymph nodes (LN). Size-exclusion column (SEC) fractions (F0 = void volume, 1 mL; F1, F2, F3, F4, F5, F6, F7 = serial fractions, 250 µL) and cushion fraction (pellet resuspended in 250 µL) were analyzed by nanosight tracking analysis (NTA), bicinchoninic acid (BCA) protein quantification, immunoblotting, and transmission electron microscopy (TEM). (**A**) Left: particle concentrations in IZON fractions F0–F7 and "cushion" fraction for three different human LN samples measured by NTA. Right: Absolute number of detected particles as sum of fraction 1 and fraction 2. For each sample, the particle concentration was normalized to the final volume of elution. (**B**) Left: BCA protein quantification for IZON fraction F0–F7 and the "cushion" fraction. Right: Absolute amount of protein in fraction 1 and fraction 2 (the protein concentration was normalized to the final volume of elution). (**C**) Mean particle size for IZON fraction F0–F7 and the "cushion" fraction analyzed by NTA. (**D**) Ratios of particles per protein amount are plotted for IZON and "cushion" fraction. (**E**) Representative particle distribution profile for IZON fraction 2 sample (left) and "cushion" sample analyzed by NTA (Sample LN221). (**F**) Immunoblotting analysis of FLOTILLIN-1, CD81, CD9, TSG101, CALNEXIN, CYTOCHROME C, and GM130 for indicated IZON fractions, the "cushion" fraction and parental cell lysates for one LN sample. (**G**) TEM images of IZON fraction 2 and the "cushion" fraction for the three indicated samples. (**H**) Immunogold electron microscopy for HLA-DR of one human LN sample (sample LN221). Scale bar: 200 µm.

2.2. Isolation and Purification of sEVs from Murine Spleen

Spleens from three mice with B-cell lymphoma were dissociated and processed as outlined in Figure 1. Similar to human LN samples, NTA results revealed an enriched particle concentration in IZON fractions 1 and 2, with fraction 2 being the peak fraction (Figure 3A, left). For one of the samples, sEVs were mainly detected in fractions 2 and 3, a difference we attribute to manual loading and elution of the IZON column. The absolute number of particles isolated was 4.8- to 27.7-fold higher in the IZON peak fractions in comparison to the respective cushion preparations (Figure 3A, right). The protein concentrations measured by BCA were more similar between IZON fractions and "cushion" and might be attributed to protein complexes co-isolated with the sEVs in the "cushion" preparation (Figure 3B, left). The absolute amount of proteins recovered was 1.4- to 2.6-fold higher in the IZON preparations in comparison to the respective cushion preparations (Figure 3B, right). In line with these results, the particle/protein ratios were drastically reduced for "cushion" preparations in comparison to IZON fractions (Figure 3D). The mean particle sizes were 154, 142, and 157 nm in the IZON peak fractions, and 114, 143, and 155 nm for the corresponding "cushion" preparations (Figure 3C). Those results imply that, for one preparation at least, the obtained product was different when using the SEC or the sucrose density cushion approach. Additionally, we observed a difference in the size distribution profile depending on the isolation protocol used, which might be explained by different EV subpopulations isolated by the different approaches (Figure 3E). Immunoblot results confirmed the exosomal identity of the particles in fractions 1, 2, and 3 and the cushion fraction by positive bands for the surface marker FLOTILLIN-1 but also the luminal markers ALIX and TSG101 in the IZON fractions 1–3 and in the "cushion" preparations (Figure 3F and Figure S2). FLOTILLIN-1 was only detected in IZON fractions, and TSG101 showed varying intensities being highly present in the "cushion" fraction while only weakly detected in the IZON fractions. Together with the variance in NTA size profiles, the immunoblotting results further suggested that different sEV subpopulations were isolated. Irrespective, we could exclude mitochondrial contaminations by ATP5A being absent from all sEV fractions (Figure 3F and Figure S2). In concordance with the human LN data, CALNEXIN could again be detected in sEV fractions from both protocols. The quality and purity of the sEV isolations was further assessed by TEM (Figure 3G). We noted a high heterogeneity among the samples for the "cushion" preparations, with one sample highly enriched in lipidic structures (Figure 3G). Interestingly, we noticed the recurrent presence of small dark structures of an approximate size of 10 nm exclusively in "cushion" preparations (Black arrows, Figure 3G). A closer look at the particles revealed a specific geometrical shape, typical for ferritin (Figure 3H) [27,28]. We further observed a red color of the sEV pellets and suspensions which is typical for a contamination with erythrocyte-derived protein, strengthening our hypothesis (Figure 3I).

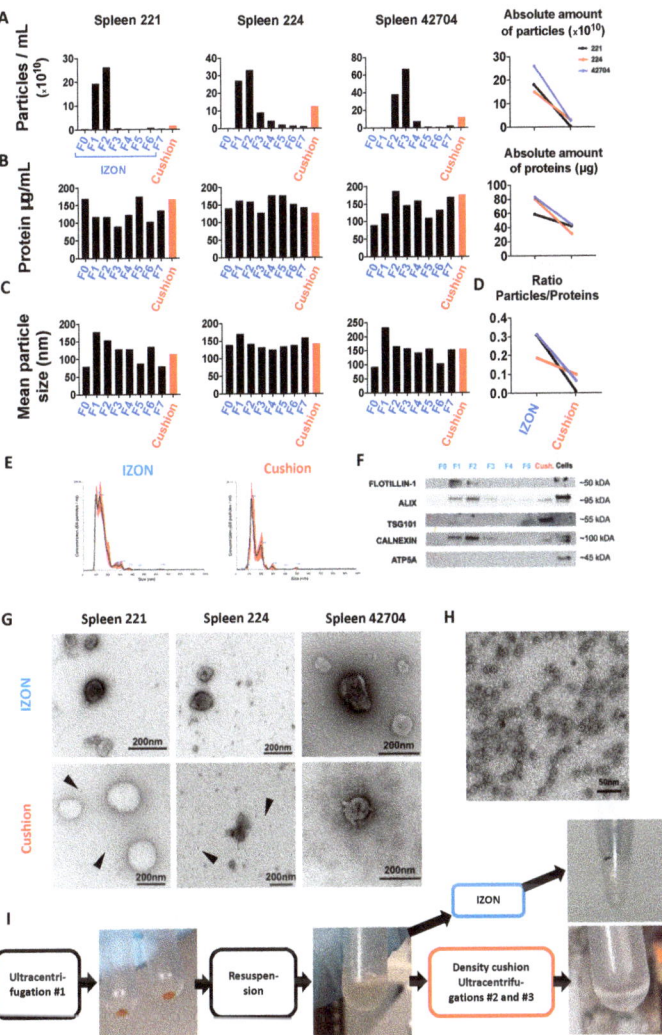

Figure 3. Isolation and characterization of murine spleen sEVs. (**A**) Left: SEV concentration in the different IZON Fractions and "cushion" preparations for three samples analyzed by NTA. Right: Absolute number of particles in indicated preparations. For each sample, the particle concentration in the two peak fractions or in the cushion product was normalized to the final volume of elution. (**B**) Left: protein quantification in the indicated preparations assessed by BCA assay. Right: absolute amount of protein in indicated preparations (the protein concentration was normalized to the final volume of elution). (**C**) Mean particle size of all fractions and the "cushion" preparations analyzed by NTA. (**D**) Ratios of particles per protein amount are plotted for IZON and "cushion" fraction. (**E**) One representative particle distribution profile for an IZON fraction 2 (left) and a "cushion" preparation analyzed by NTA (Spleen 42704). (**F**) Immunoblotting analysis of FLOTILLIN-1, ALIX, TSG101, CALNEXIN, and ATP5A for the different IZON fractions, the "cushion" preparation and parental cells for one spleen sample (spleen 224). (**G**) Transmission electron microscopy (TEM) images of IZON peak fraction and "cushion" preparation for the three indicated samples. (**H**) TEM image of ferritin-like structures found in "cushion" preparations. (**I**) Pictures of the sEV pellet, resuspended sEVs prior to application on the sucrose density cushion, and final pellet in PBS before resuspension.

2.3. Functional Analysis of sEVs Isolated by the Two Different Protocols

We and others have previously reported that tumor-derived sEVs (TEX) are able to induce an immunosuppressive phenotype in monocytes in vitro, with a typical upregulation of surface PD-L1 and HLA-DR [29–31]. We compared the potential of murine TEX isolated from three spleen samples using the two different approaches regarding their ability to induce such a phenotype. Both TEX preparations (IZON and "cushion") induced PD-L1 upregulation in monocytes, although to various degrees (Figure 4A and Figure S3 for gating strategy). However, for two of the three samples, "cushion" preparations did not induce an upregulation of HLA-DR (Figure 4B). These results indicate that both protocols resulted in sEV samples that induce a different immunosuppressive phenotype in monocytes. We also analyzed the expression of the activation marker ICAM-1 (CD54) in monocytes treated with TEX, which showed a much more drastic upregulation with the "cushion" preparations compared to the SEC-isolated TEX in all 3 analyzed samples (Figure 4C).

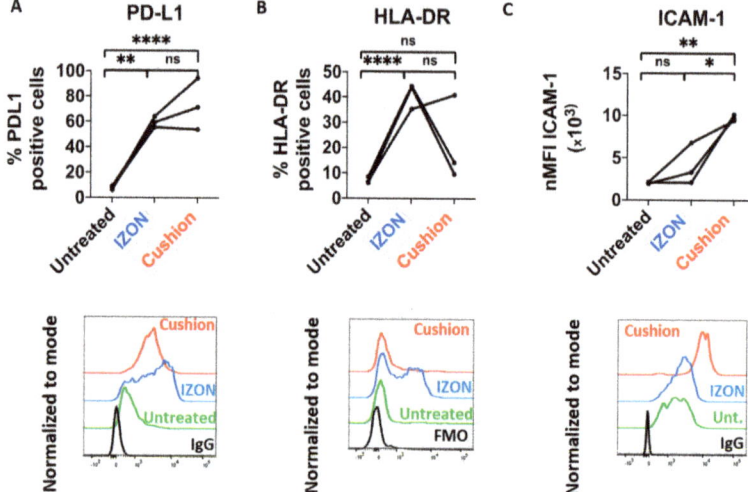

Figure 4. Response of murine monocytes upon tumor-derived sEVs (TEX) treatment. Bone marrow-derived monocytes were treated with 5 µg of the indicated sEV preparations for 8 h and analyzed by flow cytometry gating on CD11b+F4/80+$^+$CX3CR1+Ly6C+ cells (n = 3 mice per sEV preparation). (**A**) Top: percentage of PD-L1 positive cells among CD11b+F4/80+CX3CR1+Ly6C+ monocytes. Bottom: representative histogram including isotype antibody staining as negative control (IgG). (**B**) Percentage of MHC-II/HLA-DR positive cells among CD11b+F4/80+CX3CR1+Ly6C+ monocytes. Bottom: representative histogram including fluorescence-minus-one (FMO) staining as negative control. (**C**) Top: ICAM-1/CD54 expression presented as normalized mean fluorescence intensity (nMFI). Bottom: representative histogram. p-values were determined by one-way ANOVA with Tukey's multiple comparisons test. * $p < 0.05$; ** $p < 0.0021$; *** $p < 0.0002$; **** $p < 0.0001$.

3. Discussion

Multiple isolation approaches have been proposed for sEV preparations, including commercially available kits, ultrafiltration, polymer precipitation, immune-affinity capture, size-exclusion chromatography, ultracentrifugation, and ultracentrifugation combined with density cushion [32,33]. The selection of the isolation technique must consider the subsequent usage of the sEV preparations. Yield is generally prioritized when performing RNA or DNA sequencing. However, contamination with protein or lipid complexes must be avoided for proteomic analysis or functional assays. The sources and risk of protein contamination are even higher when isolation of sEVs is performed from solid tissues that require mechanical or enzymatic dissociation. Here, we compared two different protocols to isolate sEVs from solid lymphoid tissues: differential centrifugation combined to SEC using commercially available IZON columns and differential centrifugation combined to ultracentrifugation on sucrose density cushions. Although a total of three human LN and three mouse spleens are shown in our manuscript, our results are representative of larger cohorts of samples regularly analyzed in our laboratory. Both approaches led to efficient isolation of sEVs as shown by size characterization based on NTA analysis and the presence of exosomal markers by immunoblotting. However, further characterization of the preparations using BCA assay, TEM, and functional assay led us to conclude that the SEC approach is superior in terms of purity, quantity, and reproducibility.

In particular, our results strongly suggest that isolation of sEVs by the sucrose density cushion isolation protocol results in a more severe co-isolation of protein complexes with the sEVs. Using immunoblotting, we excluded contamination by mitochondrial and Golgi-derived proteins. We speculate that the presence of cellular debris in the supernatant of the dissociated tissues, which would lead to the sample contamination, was efficiently avoided by the rapid isolation of sEVs following organs' resection. However, the ER-derived protein CALNEXIN was found in sEV preparations using both isolation approaches. Such contamination likely results from the tissue dissociation. However, further investigations are required to verify that the presence of ER-proteins but not of proteins of other organelles could be the result of a specific packaging mechanism of tumor-derived sEVs. Furthermore, we also observed the presence of ferritin-like proteins in spleen sEVs isolated by the sucrose density cushion but not the SEC approach. The presence of ferritin seems to indicate an erythrocyte contamination. However, addition of erythrocyte lysis buffer to the supernatant would result in an increased release of hemoglobin. As erythrocytes are easier to separate from sEVs than hemoglobin, we do not recommend the usage of such buffer.

Previous studies focusing on plasma-derived sEVs reported lipoproteins as the main contaminants of sEV preparations [34–37]. Unfortunately, lipoproteins cannot be efficiently discriminated from sEVs when performing NTA analysis. However, contamination by lipoproteins of low and high density in sEV preparations seem less important when using the SEC-isolation approach [34–36]. In our study, we noticed the presence of large lipidic structures in one of the three murine samples isolated with the sucrose density cushion but not with SEC. Additional immunoblots are required to conclude on lipoprotein contamination in sEVs isolated with both approaches. A solution to limit lipoprotein contamination would be the combination of both SEC and sucrose density cushion. However, combination of isolation methods often results in a drastic loss of material. Other possible sources of contamination include secreted proteins, and extracellular matrix proteins. Investigations on such contaminants remain challenging, as these proteins could be considered as well as of exosomal origin.

We also would like to emphasize that ultracentrifugation combined with density cushion and differential centrifugation combined with SEC are isolation techniques that are based on the density or the size of EVs, respectively. Thus, it is possible that the use of a unique isolation protocol may impact on the distribution of sEV subpopulations in the preparations. In line with this hypothesis, different sEV marker proteins were enriched in sEVs isolated from spleens by the two different methods: sEV preparations obtained using the SEC approach were enriched in FLOTILIN-1 and ALIX but not TSG101, whereas the "cushion" preparations did show an enrichment in ALIX and TSG101 but not in FLOTILIN-1.

We previously reported that treatment of monocytes with TEX induces the upregulation of surface PD-L1 and major histocompatibility complex (MHC) II/HLA-DR. We compared the capability of TEX preparations of both isolation protocols to induce such a phenotype, using an identical amount of sEVs based on protein quantification. Treatment of monocytes with "cushion" preparations resulted in a more heterogeneous response of those two markers in comparison to SEC preparations, indicating different amounts of contaminant proteins from one "cushion" preparation to another. In particular, MHC II surface expression was increased when monocytes were treated with IZON preparations but not with "cushion" preparations, for two of three preparations. Yet, it is known that sEVs secreted by antigen-presenting cells are enriched in MHC II molecules, and that sEVs can promote the transfer of functional MHC II/antigen complexes to recipient cells [38,39]. On the contrary, we observed a higher upregulation of the monocyte activation marker ICAM-1 upon treatment with "cushion" preparations. These results highlight that contaminant proteins can interfere with biological results and lead to an incorrect conclusion of sEV-induced phenotypes. ICAM-1 expression on monocytes is a general activation marker and its upregulation can be induced by cytokines, lipoproteins, LPS etc. [40,41]. Given these results, we suspect that the PD-L1 upregulation observed in monocytes treated either with the IZON preparations or the "cushion" preparations is the consequence of monocytes' activation mainly by sEVs, whereas induced expression of ICAM-1 results from both sEVs and non-sEV contaminants. These results raise the hypothesis that soluble pro-inflammatory cytokines, secreted in B-cell lymphoma microenvironments, might contribute to the contamination in the "cushion" preparations, although further investigations would be required for firm conclusion.

As a conclusion, we strongly recommend the usage of SEC for sEV isolation from solid tissue represented here by lymphoid tissues. Multiple controls should be performed to validate the purity of the samples. Such controls include extensive immunoblotting of positive and negative exosomal markers. Reaching a complete purity of sEVs from biofluids or solid tissue seems unrealistic. Nevertheless, immunoblotting results in parallel to NTA analysis can provide a reliable estimation of preparations' contamination by protein complexes. TEM remains an indispensable tool to validate the presence and integrity of sEVs and to assess the amount of contamination by lipid complexes.

4. Materials and Methods

4.1. Animals

Eµ-TCL1 mice on C57BL/6 background were kindly provided by Carlo Croce (Ohio State University). C57BL/6 wild-type (WT) mice were purchased from Charles River Laboratories (Sulzfeld, Germany). Adoptive transfer of Eµ-TCL1 tumors was performed as previously described [42,43]. Briefly, $1-2 \times 10^7$ B-cells enriched from Eµ-TCL1 splenocytes were transplanted intraperitoneally (i.p.) into C57BL/6N WT animals. B-cell enrichment was performed using EasySep™ Mouse Pan-B Cell Isolation Kit (Stemcell Technologies, Vancouver, BC, Canada), yielding a purity above 95% of CD5+ CD19+ cells. Tumor load was assessed in the blood every week using flow cytometry as the proportion of CD5+ CD19+ cells among CD45+ cells. Animals with a tumor load >90% in peripheral blood were sacrificed; spleen was isolated and mechanically dissociated in PBS. All animal experiments were carried out according to institutional and governmental guidelines approved by the local authorities (Regierungspräsidium Karlsruhe, permit number G98/16, approved on 13 July 2016).

4.2. SEV-Free RPMI Medium

Fetal calf serum (FCS) (Gibco, Carlsbad, CA, USA) was ultra-centrifuged at 100,000× g for 18 h at 4 °C. FCS supernatant was filtered through a 0.22 µm filter. RPMI 1640 medium (Thermo Fisher Scientific Inc., Waltham, MA, USA) was supplemented with 10% sEV-free FCS and 1% penicillin/streptomycin (Gibco, Carlsbad, CA, USA). The medium was filtered through a 0.22 µm filter prior to use.

4.3. Isolation of Lymph Node Supernatants

Patient lymph node (LN) samples were obtained after the study protocols' approval by local ethics' committees from the Department of Medicine V of the University Clinic Heidelberg according to the declaration of Helsinki, and with patients' informed consent. LN samples were collected directly after biopsies from patients with diverse B-cell lymphomas. LNs were placed in 0.9% NaCl solution and processed immediately. Each LN was cut in small pieces with a maximum size of 2 mm. Cells were released in 50 mL of RPMI medium supplemented with sEV-free FCS (10%), Penicillin-Streptomycin (1%) and L-Glutamine (1%).

4.4. Isolation of Murine Spleen Supernatants

Entire spleens from three adoptively transferred Eµ-TCL1 mice were collected in 7 mL of 0.22 µm-filtered PBS each. Spleens were mechanically dissociated using MACS dissociator (Miltenyi Biotec, Bergisch Gladbach, Germany), using the program "m_spleen_01".

4.5. Differential Centrifugation

Collected supernatants of human LN and mouse spleen were centrifuged at 300× g for 10 min at 4 °C in a swing-out centrifuge to remove cellular debris. Resulting supernatants were transferred into new collection tubes and centrifuged at 2000× g for 20 min at 4 °C to remove larger apoptotic bodies. Resulting 2000× g supernatants were transferred into new collection tubes and centrifuged at 10,000× g for 40 min at 4 °C to remove MVs. Resulting 10,000× g supernatants were transferred into ultracentrifugation tubes (#5031, Seton Sci., Petaluma, CA, USA), and centrifuged at 100,000× g for 2 h at 4 °C on a Beckman Optima L-70 ultracentrifuge (Beckman Coulter GmbH, Krefeld, Germany) using a 40 Ti Swinging-Bucket Rotor. Resulting 100,000× g pellets were resuspended in 400 µL of 0.22-µm-filtered PBS and split in half for direct method comparison described below.

4.6. SEV Isolation on Sucrose Density Cushion

This protocol was adapted from a previous protocol established in our lab [19]. The half volume of the resuspended 100,000× g pellet was filled up with 0.22-µm-filtered PBS to 7 mL. The diluted pellet fraction was carefully applied onto 4 mL of a 40% sucrose cushion with a density of 1.12 g/mL without disturbing the cushion and centrifuged at 100,000× g for 2 h at 4 °C. The most upper PBS phase of around 6.5 mL was discarded. The following 3.5 mL high-density sucrose fraction containing the sEVs was recovered. The pellet was left untouched to avoid contaminating the sEV fraction with high molecular weight protein complexes. The sEVs were recovered by washing in 0.22-µm-filtered PBS by adding 7 mL of 0.22-µm-filtered PBS and centrifugation at 100,000× g for 2 h at 4 °C. The resulting sEV pellet was resuspended in 250 µL of 0.22-µm-filtered PBS.

4.7. SEV Isolation on Single qEV 35nm Columns, IZON

Single qEV 35 nm columns (Izon, Christchurch, New Zealand) were allowed to reach room temperature for 30 min. The resuspended pellet fraction (200 µL) was added onto the column. As soon as the sample volume was taken up by the column, 0.22-µm-filtered PBS was added to the top of the column tube. The following fractions were collected: F0 (1 mL = void volume of the column) and F1 to F7 (250 µL each), according to the manufacturer's instructions.

4.8. Bicinchonic Acid (BCA) Assay and Nanoparticle Tracking Analyzis (NTA)

Protein concentration of sEV samples was assessed employing Pierce™ BCA Protein Assay Kit (Thermo Fisher Scientific Inc., Waltham, MA, USA). 9 µL of each sEV sample was lysed with 1 µL of 10× RIPA buffer (Abcam, Cambridge, UK) and incubated for 30 min on a rotating wheel at 4 °C. Samples were then centrifuged at 17,000× g for 20 min at 4 °C. Resulting supernatants were subjected to the BCA assay according to the manufacturer's instructions. Absorbance was assessed with the use of a MITHRAS LB 940 plate reader (Berthold Technologies, Bad Wildbad, Germany). Particle quantification of sEV samples was performed via NTA using NanoSight LM10 equipped with a 405 nm laser (Malvern Instruments, Malvern, UK). For the NTA analysis, samples were diluted 1:500 to 1:1000 in 0.22-µm-filtered PBS. Camera level and detection threshold were set up at 13 and 5, respectively. The absence of background was verified using 0.2-µm-filtered PBS. For each sample, four videos of 60 s each were recorded and analyzed using the NTA 3.0 software version (Malvern Instruments, Malvern, UK).

4.9. Immunoblotting

SEVs and respective parental cells were lysed in RIPA buffer (Abcam, Cambridge, UK), and whole protein lysates were quantified via BCA™ Protein Assay Kit (Thermo Fisher Scientific Inc., Waltham, MA, USA). Per lane, 2.8 µg (human samples) or 3.4 µg (mouse samples) of protein were loaded onto 10% polyacrylamide gels. Following SDS-PAGE and protein transfer, membranes were blocked in 5% bovine serum albumin in Tris-buffered saline (TBS)-Tween 0.1%, and primary antibodies against FLOTILLIN-1 (1:1,000, Cell Signaling Technology, Danvers, MA, USA, #18634), CD81 (1:400, ProSci Inc., San Diego, CA, USA, #5195), CD9 (1:1000, Cell Signalling Technology, Danvers, MA, USA, #13174), TSG101 (1:1000, BD Bioscience, San Jose, CA, USA, #612697), ALIX (1:1000, Cell Signalling Technology, Danvers, MA, USA, #2171) CALNEXIN (1:500, GeneScript, Piscataway, NJ, USA, #A0124040), CYTOCHROME C (1:750, GeneScript, Piscataway, NJ, USA, #A0150740), GM130 (1:1000, Cell Signaling Technology, Danvers, MA, USA, #12480), ATP5A (1:1,000, Abcam, Cambridge, UK, #ab14748) were used in indicated dilutions in 5% bovine serum albumin in TBS-Tween 0.1%. Signals were visualized after secondary antibody hybridization by chemiluminescence detection reagent (Bio-Rad Lab, Hercules, CA, USA, #1705061) with GE Healthcare Amersham Imager 600 (GE Healthcare, Chicago, IL, USA).

4.10. Electron Microscopy (EM)

SEV fractions were adsorbed onto glow discharged carbon coated grids, washed in aqua bidest and negatively stained with 2% aqueous uranyl acetate. For immuno-EM, carbon-coated formvar grids were used and the immune reaction was performed after buffer wash including incubation with blocking agent (Aurion, Wageningen, The Netherlands), dilution series of primary antibody HLA-DR (Santa Cruz, Dallas, TX, USA #sc-51618) and Protein A-Au reporter (CMC, UMC Utrecht, The Netherlands). Micrographs were taken with a Zeiss EM 910 or EM 912 at 100 kV (Carl Zeiss, Oberkochen, Germany) using a slow scan CCD camera (TRS, Moorenweis, Germany).

4.11. Functional Assay

Murine monocytes were isolated from the bone marrow of C57BL/6 mice by magnetic depletion (EasySep™ Mouse Monocyte Isolation Kit, STEMCELL Technologies Inc., Vancouver, BC, Canada). 5×10^4 cells were cultured in 48-well plates in sEV-free RPMI medium and treated for 8 h with 5 µg of the respective sEV fractions referred above, as determined by BCA assay. Changes in PD-L1, HLA-DR and ICAM-1 expression were evaluated by flow cytometry (BD LSR Fortessa, BD Biosciences, San Jose, CA, USA). The following antibodies were used: PD-L1-PerCP (Biolegend, San Diego, CA, USA, #46-5982-82), HLA-DR-AlexaFluor700 (eBiosciences, San Diego, CA, USA, #56-5321-82), CD54-PE (Biolegend, San Diego, CA, USA, #116108), CX3CR1-BV711 (Biolegend, San Diego, CA, USA, #149031), Ly6C-APC-Cy7 (Biolegend, San Diego, CA, USA, #128015), CD11b-PeCy7 (Biolegend, San Diego, CA, USA, #101216), F4/80-FITC (Biolegend, San Diego, CA, USA, #123107), and the viability dye eFluorTM 506 (eBiosciences, San Diego, CA, USA, #65-0866).

4.12. Statistical Analysis

Results of the functional analysis were analyzed for statistical significance with GraphPad PRISM 8.0 software (GraphPad Software, San Diego, CA, USA), using one-way analysis of variance (ANOVA), followed by Tukey's multiple comparisons. The differences between means were considered significant if $p \leq 0.05$. The results are expressed as the means ± standard deviation.

4.13. EV Track

We have submitted all relevant data of our experiments to the EV-TRACK knowledgebase (EV-TRACK ID: EV200073) (Van Deun J, et al. EV-TRACK: transparent reporting and centralizing knowledge in extracellular vesicle research. Nature methods. 2017;14(3):228–32).

You may access and check the submission of experimental parameters to the EV-TRACK knowledgebase via the following URL: http://evtrack.org/review.php. Please use the EV-TRACK ID (EV200073) and the last name of the first author (Bordas) to access our submission.

Supplementary Materials: Supplementary materials can be found at http://www.mdpi.com/1422-0067/21/15/5586/s1.

Author Contributions: Conceptualization, M.B., G.G., K.K.M., and M.S.; methodology, M.B., G.G., S.O., M.N., K.R. and K.K.M.; resources, T.R. and S.D.; writing—original draft preparation, M.B. and G.G.; writing—review and editing, K.K.M. and M.S.; visualization, M.B., G.G., M.N. and K.R.; supervision, K.K.M. and M.S.; funding acquisition, M.S. All authors have read and agreed to the published version of the manuscript.

Funding: This study was supported by the Deutsche Forschungsgemeinschaft (DFG, project EV-RNA).

Acknowledgments: The authors thank Carolin Kolb, Mareike Knoll, and Angela Lenze for their help in collecting LN supernatants, and Franziska Haderk and Mariana Coelho for their critical review of the paper.

Conflicts of Interest: The authors declare no conflict of interest.

Abbreviations

BCA	Bicinchoninic acid
ER	Endoplasmatic reticulum
EVs	Extracellular vesicles
FCS	Fetal calf serum
i.p.	Intraperitoneal
LN	Lymph node
MHC	Major histocompatibility complex
MVs	Microvesicles
NTA	Nanoparticle Tracking Analysis
SEC	Size-exclusion chromatography
sEVs	Small extracellular vesicles
TEM	Transmission electron microscopy
TEX	Tumor-derived sEVs
WT	Wild-type

References

1. Kalluri, R.; LeBleu, V.S. The biology, function, and biomedical applications of exosomes. *Science* **2020**, *367*, eaau6977. [CrossRef] [PubMed]
2. Samanta, S.; Rajasingh, S.; Drosos, N.; Zhou, Z.; Dawn, B.; Rajasingh, J. Exosomes: New molecular targets of diseases. *Acta Pharmacol. Sin.* **2018**, *39*, 501–513. [CrossRef] [PubMed]
3. Campos-Silva, C.; Suárez, H.; Jara-Acevedo, R.; Linares-Espinós, E.; Martinez-Piñeiro, L.; Yáñez-Mó, M.; Valés-Gómez, M. High sensitivity detection of extracellular vesicles immune-captured from urine by conventional flow cytometry. *Sci. Rep.* **2019**, *9*, 1–12. [CrossRef] [PubMed]
4. Wu, D.; Yan, J.; Shen, X.; Sun, Y.; Thulin, M.; Cai, Y.; Wik, L.; Shen, Q.; Oelrich, J.; Qian, X.; et al. Profiling surface proteins on individual exosomes using a proximity barcoding assay. *Nat. Commun.* **2019**, *10*, 1–10. [CrossRef]
5. Maas, S.L.N.; Breakefield, X.O.; Weaver, A.M. Extracellular Vesicles: Unique Intercellular Delivery Vehicles. *Trends Cell Biol.* **2017**, *27*, 172–188. [CrossRef]
6. Raposo, G.; Stahl, P.D. Extracellular vesicles: A new communication paradigm? *Nat. Rev. Mol. Cell Biol.* **2019**, *20*, 509–510. [CrossRef]
7. Colombo, M.; Moita, C.; Van Niel, G.; Kowal, J.; Vigneron, J.; Benaroch, P.; Manel, N.; Moita, L.F.; Théry, C.; Raposo, G. Analysis of ESCRT functions in exosome biogenesis, composition and secretion highlights the heterogeneity of extracellular vesicles. *J. Cell Sci.* **2013**, *126*, 5553–5565. [CrossRef]
8. Palma, J.; Yaddanapudi, S.C.; Pigati, L.; Havens, M.A.; Jeong, S.; Weiner, G.A.; Weimer, K.M.E.; Stern, B.; Hastings, M.L.; Duelli, D.M. MicroRNAs are exported from malignant cells in customized particles. *Nucleic Acids Res.* **2012**, *40*, 9125–9138. [CrossRef]

9. Villarroya-Beltri, C.; Baixauli, F.; Gutiérrez-Vázquez, C.; Sánchez-Madrid, F.; Mittelbrunn, M. Sorting it out: Regulation of exosome loading. *Semin. Cancer Biol.* **2014**, *28*, 3–13. [CrossRef]
10. Leidal, A.M.; Huang, H.H.; Marsh, T.; Solvik, T.; Zhang, D.; Ye, J.; Kai, F.B.; Goldsmith, J.; Liu, J.Y.; Huang, Y.H.; et al. The LC3-conjugation machinery specifies the loading of RNA-binding proteins into extracellular vesicles. *Nat. Cell Biol.* **2020**, *22*, 187–199. [CrossRef]
11. Koppers-Lalic, D.; Hackenberg, M.; Bijnsdorp, I.V.; van Eijndhoven, M.A.J.; Sadek, P.; Sie, D.; Zini, N.; Middeldorp, J.M.; Ylstra, B.; de Menezes, R.X.; et al. Nontemplated nucleotide additions distinguish the small RNA composition in cells from exosomes. *Cell Rep.* **2014**, *8*, 1649–1658. [CrossRef] [PubMed]
12. Jeppesen, D.K.; Fenix, A.M.; Franklin, J.L.; Higginbotham, J.N.; Zhang, Q.; Zimmerman, L.J.; Liebler, D.C.; Ping, J.; Liu, Q.; Evans, R.; et al. Reassessment of Exosome Composition. *Cell* **2019**, *177*, 428–445.e18. [CrossRef] [PubMed]
13. Mathieu, M.; Martin-Jaular, L.; Lavieu, G.; Théry, C. Specificities of secretion and uptake of exosomes and other extracellular vesicles for cell-to-cell communication. *Nat. Cell Biol.* **2019**, *21*, 9–17. [CrossRef] [PubMed]
14. El Andaloussi, S.; Mäger, I.; Breakefield, X.O.; Wood, M.J.A. Extracellular vesicles: Biology and emerging therapeutic opportunities. *Nat. Rev. Drug Discov.* **2013**, *12*, 347–357. [CrossRef] [PubMed]
15. Zhang, X.; Yuan, X.; Shi, H.; Wu, L.; Qian, H.; Xu, W. Exosomes in cancer: Small particle, big player. *J. Hematol. Oncol.* **2015**, *8*, 83. [CrossRef]
16. Reclusa, P.; Taverna, S.; Pucci, M.; Durendez, E.; Calabuig, S.; Manca, P.; Serrano, M.J.; Sober, L.; Pauwels, P.; Russo, A.; et al. Exosomes as diagnostic and predictive biomarkers in lung cancer. *J. Thorac. Dis.* **2017**, *9*, S1373–S1382. [CrossRef]
17. Liu, Y.; Li, D.; Liu, Z.; Zhou, Y.; Chu, D.; Li, X.; Jiang, X.; Hou, D.; Chen, X.; Chen, Y.; et al. Targeted exosome-mediated delivery of opioid receptor Mu siRNA for the treatment of morphine relapse. *Sci. Rep.* **2015**, *5*, 17543. [CrossRef]
18. Yong, T.; Zhang, X.; Bie, N.; Zhang, H.; Zhang, X.; Li, F.; Hakeem, A.; Hu, J.; Gan, L.; Santos, H.A.; et al. Tumor exosome-based nanoparticles are efficient drug carriers for chemotherapy. *Nat. Commun.* **2019**, *10*, 3838. [CrossRef]
19. Haderk, F.; Hanna, B.; Richter, K.; Schnölzer, M.; Zenz, T.; Stilgenbauer, S.; Lichter, P.; Seiffert, M. Extracellular vesicles in chronic lymphocytic leukemia. *Leuk. Lymphoma* **2013**, *54*, 1826–1830. [CrossRef]
20. Böing, A.N.; van der Pol, E.; Grootemaat, A.E.; Coumans, F.A.W.; Sturk, A.; Nieuwland, R. Single-step isolation of extracellular vesicles by size-exclusion chromatography. *J. Extracell. Vesicles* **2014**, *3*. [CrossRef]
21. Lobb, R.J.; Becker, M.; Wen, S.W.; Wong, C.S.F.; Wiegmans, A.P.; Leimgruber, A.; Möller, A. Optimized exosome isolation protocol for cell culture supernatant and human plasma. *J. Extracell. Vesicles* **2015**, *4*, 27031. [CrossRef] [PubMed]
22. Stranska, R.; Gysbrechts, L.; Wouters, J.; Vermeersch, P.; Bloch, K.; Dierickx, D.; Andrei, G.; Snoeck, R. Comparison of membrane affinity-based method with size-exclusion chromatography for isolation of exosome-like vesicles from human plasma. *J. Transl. Med.* **2018**, *16*, 1–9. [CrossRef] [PubMed]
23. Bichi, R.; Shinton, S.A.; Martin, E.S.; Koval, A.; Calin, G.A.; Cesari, R.; Russo, G.; Hardy, R.R.; Croce, C.M. Human chronic lymphocytic leukemia modeled in mouse by targeted TCL1 expression. *Proc. Natl. Acad. Sci. USA* **2002**, *99*, 6955–6960. [CrossRef] [PubMed]
24. Gorgun, G.; Ramsay, A.G.; Holderried, T.A.W.; Zahrieh, D.; Dieu, R.L.; Liu, F.; Quackenbush, J.; Croce, C.M.; Gribben, J.G. Eμ-TCL1 mice represent a model for immunotherapeutic reversal of chronic lymphocytic leukemia-induced T-cell dysfunction. *Proc. Natl. Acad. Sci. USA* **2009**, *106*, 6250–6255. [CrossRef] [PubMed]
25. Gámez-Valero, A.; Monguió-Tortajada, M.; Carreras-Planella, L.; Franquesa, M.; Beyer, K.; Borràs, F.E. Size-Exclusion Chromatography-based isolation minimally alters Extracellular Vesicles' characteristics compared to precipitating agents. *Sci. Rep.* **2016**, *6*, 33641. [CrossRef] [PubMed]
26. Théry, C.; Witwer, K.W.; Aikawa, E.; Alcaraz, M.J.; Anderson, J.D.; Andriantsitohaina, R.; Antoniou, A.; Arab, T.; Archer, F.; Atkin-Smith, G.K.; et al. Minimal information for studies of extracellular vesicles 2018 (MISEV2018): A position statement of the International Society for Extracellular Vesicles and update of the MISEV2014 guidelines. *J. Extracell. Vesicles* **2018**, *7*, 1535750. [CrossRef]
27. Sana, B.; Johnson, E.; Sheah, K.; Poh, C.L.; Lim, S. Iron-based ferritin nanocore as a contrast agent. *Biointerphases* **2010**, *5*, FA48–FA52. [CrossRef]

28. Falvo, E.; Tremante, E.; Arcovito, A.; Papi, M.; Elad, N.; Boffi, A.; Morea, V.; Conti, G.; Toffoli, G.; Fracasso, G.; et al. Improved Doxorubicin Encapsulation and Pharmacokinetics of Ferritin–Fusion Protein Nanocarriers Bearing Proline, Serine, and Alanine Elements. *Biomacromolecules* **2015**, *17*, 514–522. [CrossRef]
29. Fleming, V.; Hu, X.; Weller, C.; Weber, R.; Groth, C.; Riester, Z.; Hüser, L.; Sun, Q.; Nagibin, V.; Kirschning, C.; et al. Melanoma extracellular vesicles generate immunosuppressive myeloid cells by upregulating PD-L1 via TLR4 signaling. *Cancer Res.* **2019**, *79*, 4715–4728. [CrossRef]
30. Gabrusiewicz, K.; Li, X.; Wei, J.; Hashimoto, Y.; Marisetty, A.L.; Ott, M.; Wang, F.; Hawke, D.; Yu, J.; Healy, L.M.; et al. Glioblastoma stem cell-derived exosomes induce M2 macrophages and PD-L1 expression on human monocytes. *OncoImmunology* **2018**, *7*, e1412909. [CrossRef]
31. Haderk, F.; Schulz, R.; Iskar, M.; Cid, L.L.; Worst, T.; Willmund, K.V.; Schulz, A.; Warnken, U.; Seiler, J.; Benner, A.; et al. Tumor-derived exosomes modulate PD-L1 expression in monocytes. *Sci. Immunol.* **2017**, *2*, 1–12. [CrossRef] [PubMed]
32. Gurunathan, S.; Kang, M.H.; Jeyaraj, M.; Qasim, M.; Kim, J.H. Review of the Isolation, Characterization, Biological Function, and Multifarious Therapeutic Approaches of Exosomes. *Cells* **2019**, *8*, 307. [CrossRef] [PubMed]
33. Gardiner, C.; Di Vizio, D.; Sahoo, S.; Théry, C.; Witwer, K.M.; Wauben, M.; Hill, A.F. Techniques used for the isolation and characterization of extracellular vesicles: Results of a worldwide survey. *J. Extracell. Vesicles* **2016**, *5*, 32945. [CrossRef] [PubMed]
34. Yuana, Y.; Levels, J.; Grootemaat, A.; Sturk, A.; Nieuwland, R. Co-isolation of extracellular vesicles and high-density lipoproteins using density gradient ultracentrifugation. *J. Extracell. Vesicles* **2014**, *3*. [CrossRef] [PubMed]
35. Karimi, N.; Cvjetkovic, A.; Jang, C.J.; Crescitelli, S.; Feizi, M.A.H.; Nieuwland, R.; Lötvall, J.; Lässer, C. Detailed analysis of the plasma extracellular vesicle proteome after separation from lipoproteins. *Cell. Mol. Life Sci.* **2018**, *75*, 2873–2886. [CrossRef]
36. Brennan, K.; Martin, K.; FitzGerald, S.P.; O'Sullivan, J.; Wu, Y.; Blanco, A.; Richardson, C.; Mc Gee, M.M. A comparison of methods for the isolation and separation of extracellular vesicles from protein and lipid particles in human serum. *Sci. Rep.* **2020**, *10*. [CrossRef]
37. Takov, K.; Yellon, D.M.; Davidson, S. Comparison of small extracellular vesicles isolated from plasma by ultracentrifugation or size-exclusion chromatography: Yield, purity and functional potential. *J. Extracell. Vesicles* **2018**, *8*, 1560809. [CrossRef]
38. Raposo, G.; Nijman, H.W.; Stoorvogel, W.; Liejendekker, R.; Harding, C.V.; Melief, C.K.; Geuze, H.J. B Lymphocytes Secrete Antigen-Presenting Vesicles. *J. Exp. Med.* **1996**, *1*, 1161–1172. [CrossRef]
39. André, F.; Chaput, N.; Schartz, N.E.C.; Flament, C.; Aubert, N.; Bernard, J.; Lemonnier, F.; Raposo, G.; Escudier, B.; Hsu, D.-H.; et al. Exosomes as Potent Cell-Free Peptide-Based Vaccine. I. Dendritic Cell-Derived Exosomes Transfer Functional MHC Class I/Peptide Complexes to Dendritic Cells. *J. Immunol.* **2004**, *172*, 2126–2136.
40. Möst, J.; Schwaeble, W.; Drach, J.; Sommerauer, A.; Dierich, M.P. Regulation of the Expression of ICAM-1 on Human Monocytes and Monocytic Tumor Cell Lines. *J. Immunol.* **1992**, *148*, 1635–1642.
41. Fujihara, M.; Ikebuchi, K.; Yamaguchi, M.; Abe, H.; Niwa, K.; Sekiguchi, S. Effects of Liposome-Encapsulated Hemoglobin on Phorbol Ester-Induced Superoxide Production and Expression of Costimulatory Molecules by Monocytes in Vitro. *Artif. Cells Blood Substit. Immobil. Biotechnol.* **1998**, *26*, 487–495. [CrossRef] [PubMed]
42. McClanahan, F.; Riches, J.C.; Miller, S.; Day, W.P.; Kotsiou, E.; Neuberg, D.; Croce, C.M.; Capasso, M.; Gribben, J.G. Mechanisms of PD-L1/PD-1–mediated CD8 T-cell dysfunction in the context of aging-related immune defects in the Eµ-TCL1 CLL mouse model. *Blood* **2015**, *126*, 212–221. [CrossRef] [PubMed]
43. Hanna, B.; McClanahan, F.; Yazdanparast, H.; Zaborsky, N.; Kalter, V.; Rössner, P.M.; Benner, A.; Dürr, C.; Egle, A.; Gribben, J.G.; et al. Depletion of CLL-associated patrolling monocytes and macrophages controls disease development and repairs immune dysfunction in vivo. *Leukemia* **2016**, *30*, 570–579. [CrossRef] [PubMed]

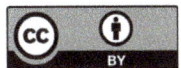

© 2020 by the authors. Licensee MDPI, Basel, Switzerland. This article is an open access article distributed under the terms and conditions of the Creative Commons Attribution (CC BY) license (http://creativecommons.org/licenses/by/4.0/).

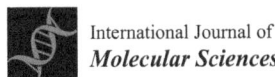

Article

Measuring Extracellular Vesicles by Conventional Flow Cytometry: Dream or Reality?

Donatella Lucchetti [1], Alessandra Battaglia [2], Claudio Ricciardi-Tenore [1], Filomena Colella [1], Luigi Perelli [1], Ruggero De Maria [1], Giovanni Scambia [3], Alessandro Sgambato [4,*] and Andrea Fattorossi [3]

[1] Department of Translational Medicine and Surgery, Università Cattolica del Sacro Cuore, 00168 Rome, Italy; dnlucchetti@gmail.com (D.L.); c.ricciarditenore@hotmail.it (C.R.-T.); colella.filomena@gmail.com (F.C.); luigi.perelli19934@libero.it (L.P.); demariaruggero@gmail.com (R.D.M.)

[2] Department of Life Science and Public Health, Università Cattolica del Sacro Cuore, 00168 Rome, Italy; alessandra.battaglia@unicatt.it

[3] Laboratory of Cytometry and Immunology, Department of Obstetrics and Gynecology, Università Cattolica del Sacro Cuore, Fondazione Policlinico Universitario A. Gemelli IRCCS, 00168 Rome, Italy; giovanni.scambia@policlinicogemelli.it (G.S.); andrea.fattorossi@guest.policlinicogemelli.it (A.F.)

[4] Centro di Riferimento Oncologico della Basilicata (IRCCS-CROB), Rionero in Vulture (PZ), 85028 Potenza, Italy

* Correspondence: alessandro.sgambato@crob.it

Received: 25 June 2020; Accepted: 27 August 2020; Published: 29 August 2020

Abstract: Intense research is being conducted using flow cytometers available in clinically oriented laboratories to assess extracellular vesicles (EVs) surface cargo in a variety of diseases. Using EVs of various sizes purified from the HT29 human colorectal adenocarcinoma cell line, we report on the difficulty to assess small and medium sized EVs by conventional flow cytometer that combines light side scatter off a 405 nm laser with the fluorescent signal from the EVs general labels Calcein-green and Calcein-violet, and surface markers. Small sized EVs (~70 nm) immunophenotyping failed, consistent with the scarcity of monoclonal antibody binding sites, and were therefore excluded from further investigation. Medium sized EVs (~250 nm) immunophenotyping was possible but their detection was plagued by an excess of coincident particles (swarm detection) and by a high abort rate; both factors affected the measured EVs concentration. By running samples containing equal amounts of Calcein-green and Calcein-violet stained medium sized EVs, we found that swarm detection produced false double positive events, a phenomenon that was significantly reduced, but not totally eliminated, by sample dilution. Moreover, running highly diluted samples required long periods of cytometer time. Present findings raise questions about the routine applicability of conventional flow cytometers for EV analysis.

Keywords: extracellular vesicles; exosomes; flow cytometry; immunophenotyping; swarm detection

1. Introduction

Extracellular vesicles (EVs) are membrane-surrounded structures released in the intercellular environment and blood stream by a large variety of cells. EVs shuttle lipids, proteins, RNA, DNA, and other metabolites between cells and tissues. They diverge into two main subgroups according to their biogenesis and release mechanism: microvesicles (150–1000 nm in diameter, MVs) shed from the plasma membrane, and exosomes, which are generally smaller in size (30–150 nm in diameter, EXOs) originating from the endosome as intraluminal vesicles enclosed within multivesicular bodies [1]. EVs are central in regulating multiple physiological processes—e.g., tissue repair, stem cell maintenance and coagulation—and pathophysiological processes—e.g., cancer, neurodegenerative diseases and viral infections [2]—because of their ability to transfer biological content. Since EVs are found in accessible body fluids and express a variety of bioactive molecules of the cells of origin, intense research is being conducted to understand EVs' potential as biomarkers for personalized medicine, and to develop relatively simple and fast methods to assess EVs in translational studies using high-throughput technologies.

Indeed, a number of techniques are potentially suited to assess individual EVs, including electron microscopy, resistive pulse sensing, nanoparticle tracking analysis, dynamic light scatter (DLS), and flow cytometry [3]. However, only the latter technique is able to combine high-throughput and adequate speed allowing EVs evaluation in translational studies and in a routine clinical setting. Several custom-constructed flow cytometers or last generation modified cell sorter, with optimized fluidics and flow cell design, have been developed to detect extremely small particles [4,5]. However, these instruments are not optimally suited for other more common applications in clinical settings, mostly cell immunophenotyping. Paradoxically, it is in the clinical setting that EVs are currently most extensively investigated by flow cytometry in a variety of pathological processes.

The current generation of commercial flow cytometers include highly complex and sensitive instruments, which are optimized to assess lymphocytes and other similar sized cells. Commercially available flow cytometers routinely measure light scatter in the forward scatter (FSC) and right angle, or side scatter (SSC), directions, and the two parameters combined provide a good foundation to begin cell population analysis. To identify a particle, the scattered light must exceed the triggering threshold, which must be set to exclude the optical and electronic noise. This is easily accomplished when analyzing micrometer-sized particles, such as cells and the largest EVs, e.g., apoptotic bodies. Conversely, smaller EVs generate scatter signals that may be extremely low and fall within the range of the optical and electronic noise; because the intensity of the scattered light attenuates exponentially with size (the sixth power of particle size) [6], these EVs remain hidden in the background.

In the cytometry of EVs with conventional flow cytometers, FSC is generally less used than SSC, as only particles with a diameter larger than the typical 488 nm wavelength excitation provided by the standard blue laser preferentially scatter (in fact diffract) light in the "forward" direction. SSC is better suited to identify particles with diameters smaller than the wavelength of the incident laser light, because SSC is a measure of mostly refracted and reflected light. However, SSC signal intensity also depends on the ratio between the particle size and the wavelength of the incident laser light. To improve resolution, conventional flow cytometers have been developed to measure the SSC off the violet laser (hereafter referred to as VSSC) instead of blue laser SSC (hereafter referred to as BSSC), as the 405 nm wavelength of the violet laser compared with the 488 nm wavelength of the blue laser is closer to EVs size [7].

In the present study, we explored the feasibility to identify small/medium sized EVs (size range 70 to 300 nm) by a conventional flow cytometer, equipped with blue and violet laser excitation sources, designed to be used in clinical setting for a wide range of applications (CytoFLEX S, Beckman Coulter, Milano, Italy) [8].

We demonstrate that immunophenotyping of small sized EVs (in the 100 nm size range) is in fact not feasible, not even when the staining involves very abundant surface molecules, showing that conventional flow cytometry is inadequate for these EVs assessment. Additionally, we show that the flow cytometry analysis of medium sized EVs (around 250 nm) is plagued by an excess of coincident particles (swarm detection)—a limitation that must be considered when formulating schemes for EVs studies using conventional flow cytometers.

2. Results

2.1. EVs Generation and Flow Cytometer Set Up

EVs were obtained from the HT29 (human colorectal adenocarcinoma) cell line. EVs isolation and characterization are detailed in [9] and Supplementary Information) and shown in Figure S1.

The window of analysis was determined by VSSC and fluorescence parameters using fluorescent Megamix-Plus FSC polystyrene microbeads (Figure S2). The superiority of VSSC over BSSC in terms of resolution is shown in Figure S2. During apoptotic cell death, apoptotic exosome-like vesicles similar in size and in certain surface marker expression—e.g., CD63—are released in culture supernatant [10], so we collected supernatant for EVs purification only when cell culture viability exceeded 90% by trypan blue exclusion.

2.2. Identification of Small and Medium Sized EVs by VSSC and Calceins

In the cytometry of EVs, fluorescence is less affected by background noise than light scatter. Thus, the poor resolution of dim light scatter signals generated by EVs can be improved by adding a fluorescent label as parameter. Among several available fluorescent labels potentially useful for EVs staining [11], we chose Calceins (Calcein-green and Calcein-violet) [12]. Calcein probes are best suited to avoid possible interferences related to staining of cell membrane fragments and non-intact EVs following ultracentrifugation procedures [13], because they require hydrolysis by intracellular esterases to become fluorescent, and, therefore, identify only metabolically active, intact vesicles, which can transform the non-fluorescent dye into the fluorescent form [12]. Moreover, these probes have little to no spectral overlap with each other and with the other fluorochromes we used, minimizing compensation and spreading error [14].

Unless otherwise stated, we adopted 1.5 µg/mL of EVs (by Bradford assay) in a solution with either Calcein-green or Calcein-violet at final concentration of 1 µM in filtered PBS. Most experiments were performed using Calcein-green; thus, Calcein will refer to Calcein-green, unless otherwise stated (Figure 1).

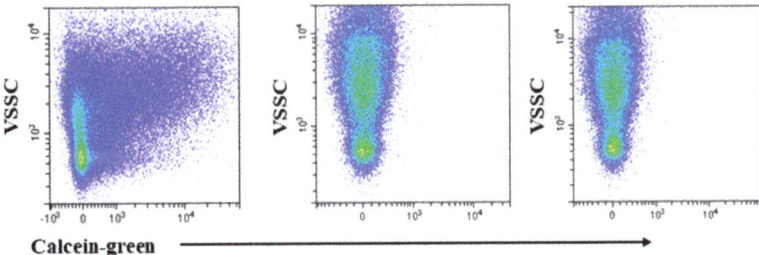

Figure 1. Calcein stains intact extracellular vesicles (EVs). Violet side scatter (VSSC)/Calcein-green fluorescence profile of EVs incubated with Calcein-green at 37 °C (left and right panels) and 4 °C (middle panel). The low temperature prevented the non-fluorescent Calcein from being converted into the green fluorescent form inside EVs, indicating that free dye does not contribute to the observed fluorescence pattern. Triton-X-100 treatment abrogates Calcein fluorescence at 37 °C (right panel). Using Calcein-violet produced identical results.

To confirm previous observation [12] that Calceins only stain intact EVs, an EVs sample was incubated with the dyes at 4 °C, as this temperature inhibits internal esterase activity and, therefore, prevents the non-fluorescent Calcein form conversion to the fluorescent form. Data in the left and middle panel of Figure 1 were generated by staining samples with Calcein at 37 °C and 4 °C, respectively. EVs remained non-fluorescent when incubated at low temperature. Subsequently, as any disruption of plasma membrane, obtained with detergents, leads to leakage of the dye from particle, we treated Calcein-stained EVs with Triton-X-100. In accordance with a previous report [12], positive events disappeared following Triton-X-100 treatment, thus excluding the contribution of free esterases to Calcein signal (Figure 1, right panel).

Calcein staining was dim to moderate, yet the distinction between positive and negative events, remained discernible by visual inspection (Figure 1, left panel). These findings seem at odds with those of De Rond et al. [15] that deemed Calcein as scarcely sensitive. We can only conjecture as to why our findings differ from previous results because the lack of a detailed description of the gating strategy and particle size in the De Rond study [15] make a comparison difficult.

After demonstrating that the inclusion of Calcein as a second parameter was viable to identify EVs, we applied this procedure to purified medium and small sized EVs

The left panel of Figure 2a shows that, in purified medium sized EVs preparations, most Calcein positive events generated a VSSC signal that roughly corresponded to that of the 100 nm microbeads (Figure S2a, left panel). Thus, owing to the medium sized EVs distribution of 210 ± 49 nm (Figure S1), it can be inferred that these EVs generated a scatter signal with intensity comparable to that of the 100 nm polystyrene beads. This is well in line with the notion that the inner refractive index of EVs is less than 1.4, which is considerably lower than that of polymer beads (generally ~1.6) [16].

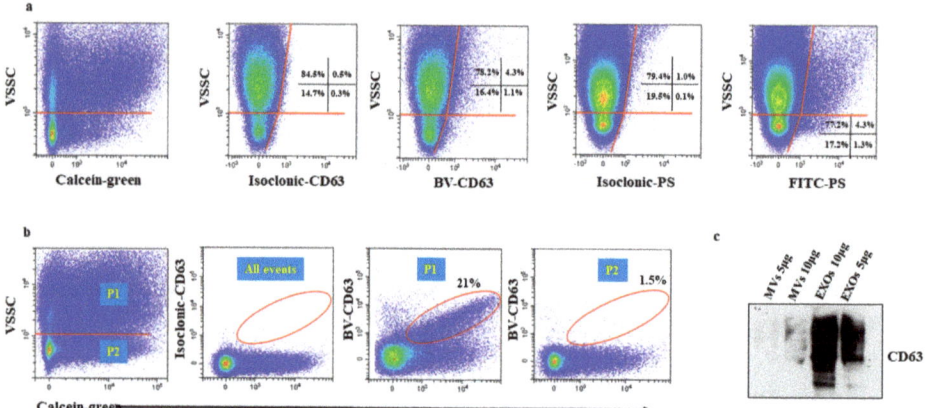

Figure 2. Immunostaining of purified medium and small sized EVs, (**a**) and (**b**), respectively. Both in (**a**) and (**b**), two populations can be visually discerned based on the intensity of the VSSC signal (horizontal red line). (**a**) Left panel, in this representative experiment the percentage of events with high VSSC signal intensity was 84%. Second panel from left, to demonstrate specificity of staining and set the quad markers, the binding of brilliant violet-conjugated CD63 (BV-CD63) moAb was blocked by pre-incubation with unlabelled CD63 moAb prior to staining with the BV-CD63 moAb (isoclonic control). Third panel from left, only a marginal amount of events reacted with the BV-CD63 moAb, consistent with the non-exosomes (EXOs) nature of these particles. Fourth panel from left, to demonstrate specificity of staining and set the quad markers, the binding of FITC (Fluorescein isothiocyanate)-conjugated anti- Phosphatidylserine (PS) moAb was blocked by pre-incubation with unlabelled anti-PS moAb prior to staining with the anti-PS moAb (isoclonic control). Right panel, a detectable proportion of medium sized EVs expressed PS demonstrating that immunophenotyping EVs of that size is feasible. (**b**) Left panel, in this representative experiment, the percentage of events with high VSSC (P1) and low (P2) signal intensity was 43% and 57%, respectively. Middle panel, isoclonic control. Right and far right panels, BV-CD63 staining in P1 and P2 populations, respectively. BV-CD63 moAb reacted only with events in the P1 region, consistent with the EXOs nature of these particles. Values in regions show percentages of positive events. We addressed the issue of possible BV-CD63 fluorescence quenching by Calcein because of the spectral characteristics of BV fluorochrome and run side by side small sized EVs stained with only BV-CD63 or double stained with BV-CD63 and Calcein. (**c**) Representative western bot assay showing the preferential expression of CD63 by small sized EVs. Red lines = analysis gates; red circles = EVs population analyzed.

A Calcein positive particle population (~15% in six independent experiments) with a clearly lower VSSC signal intensity was also visible (Figure 2a left panel). We hypothesized that these events reflected contaminating small sized EVs deriving from imperfect ultracentrifugation procedures, which remained undetected by the DLS analysis because of their low frequency. EVs are defined according to their modality of generation, rather than size. However, microvesicles (MVs) are generally larger than exosomes (EXOs), thus, we inferred that small sized EVs samples were mostly EXOs and medium sized EVs samples were mostly MVs. It is known that CD63 and CD9, two tetraspanins, are specially enriched in EXOs membranes and scarcely expressed by MVs [17,18], and Western blot analysis of small and medium sized EVs samples showed that only the former exhibited a strong reactivity for CD63 (Figure 2c). Thus, Calcein-stained medium sized EVs samples were incubated with monoclonal antibodies (moAbs) to CD63 and CD9, to determine the origin of particles with lower VSSC signal intensity in medium sized EVs samples. Virtually no particle stained positive for CD63 (Figure 2a, second panel from left). Although these findings suggests a non-EXOs nature of these particles, this issue will be discussed again below. The moAb to CD63 marginally stained particles in the high VSSC region—a finding consistent with the low CD63 expression by MVs [17,18].

MVs stained positive for anti-Phosphatidylserine (PS) antibody, demonstrating that the immunophenotyping of medium sized EVs is possible [19] (right panel, Figure 2).

Running purified small sized EVs, we observed that a large proportion of Calcein positive particles was located in the high VSSC region (Figure 2b, left panel), which is a region that corresponds to that of the ~250 nm sized particles (Figure 2a, left panel) and therefore, visibly exceeds the size of these EVs (68 ± 7 nm by DLS, Figure S1). We reasoned that these particles could be aggregates, possibly generated by high-speed centrifugation [20]. In the cytometry of cells, the aggregate issue is usually addressed by checking the height, area, and width of the FSC and/or SSC pulse. In the cytometry of EVs, the exceedingly small pulse makes this conventional doublet discrimination impossible, because the magnitude of difference in any pulse parameter between an aggregate and a single event is small, and requires the resolution of a linear scale, which is unfeasible, as scatter parameters require a logarithmic scale. To determine the origin of larger particles in small sized EVs samples, we incubated small sized EVs samples with the moAb to CD63 and CD9, and analyszd the staining in relationship with VSSC signal intensity. Figure 2b, third panel from left, shows that CD63 staining was detectable only in particles with high VSSC signal intensity (Figure 2b, right panel), particles with low VSSC signal intensity remained non-fluorescent. These data supports our hypothesis that particles with high VSSC signal intensity were aggregates. However, it remains unclear why such a large proportion of aggregates remained undetected by DLS analysis. Although it is held that DLS fails to detect small proportions of aggregates in otherwise homogeneous EVs preparations [21], the proportion of aggregates we observed in our experiments is too large to remain undetected. We hypothesize that the cytometer preferentially detected aggregates due to their larger size, while most non-aggregated particles are below the VSSC threshold, and are simply not "seen" by the instrument. An alternative, not mutually exclusive explanation, is that the larger particles are coincident events (swarm detection), an issue that is addressed below.

2.3. Particles in the Low VSSC Signal Region Do Not Stain for Tetraspanins Because of an Insufficient Number of Binding Sites

As outlined above, findings in Figure 2 indicated that the nature of the events in the low VSSC region in both the small and medium sized EVs samples could not be assessed by staining for the typical small sized EVs (mostly EXOs) markers. The analyses of medium sized EVs indicated that ~250 nm EVs were positioned in the high VSSC region (Figure 2a), and the intensity of the scattered light attenuates exponentially with size [21], so we infer that the EVs size in the low VSSC region should be considerably lower, possibly around 70 nm, in line with DLS data. Studies showed that the number of antigenic sites, which can react with a fluorochrome-labelled moAb on the surface of an EV in this size range, is around 10/15 epitopes, which is too scarce to generate a fluorescence signal detectable by a commercial flow cytometer [22–24]. Thus, we hypothesized that the absence of EVs immunolabeling in the low VSSC region reflected insufficient target epitopes. To verify this hypothesis, we mimicked fluorescence generated by the anti-tetraspanins fluorochrome-conjugated moAbs using FITC-conjugated mouse IgG (Immunoglobulin G) bound to 50 nm–sized anti-mouse IgG microbeads. The experiments were performed at various microbeads/FITC-conjugated mouse IgG ratios. No fluorescence signal was ever detected in the low VSSC region (Figure 3 left and middle panel). To insure that the amount of FITC-conjugated mouse IgG was enough to produce a detectable fluorescence signal in the presence of particles carrying a suitable number of binding sites, the lowest amount of FITC-conjugated mouse IgG, which was incubated with the 50 nm microbeads, was incubated with larger (3μm) microbeads coated with anti-mouse IgG. In this condition, FITC-conjugated mouse IgG generated a brilliant fluorescence signal (Figure 3 right panel). We also ascertained by fluorescence microscopy that FITC-conjugated mouse IgG made the 50 nm–sized anti-mouse IgG microbeads fluorescent (Figure 3, lower panels).

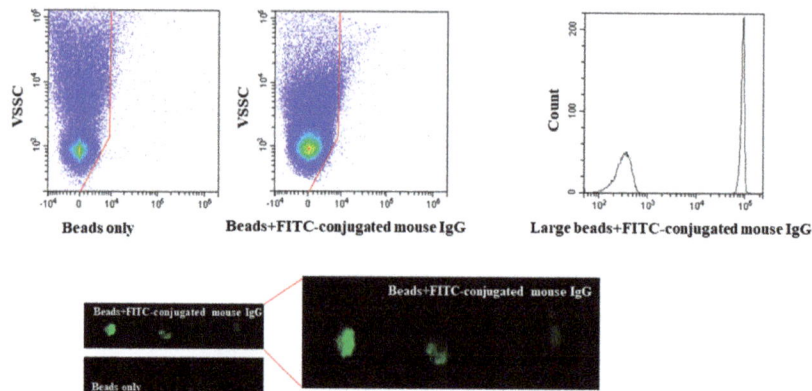

Figure 3. Fifty nm-sized anti-mouse IgG microbeads do not bind enough FITC-conjugated mouse IgG to generate a measurable fluorescence signal. Anti-mouse IgG microbeads background fluorescence (**top left panel**) and anti-mouse IgG microbeads coated with FITC-conjugated mouse IgG fluorescence (**top middle panel**). The same amount of FITC-conjugated mouse IgG generates a brilliant fluorescence signal when incubated with larger-sized (3 μm) microbeads coated with anti-mouse IgG (**top right panel**). Fluorescence microscopy analysis of anti-mouse IgG microbeads carrying FITC-conjugated mouse IgG (**lower panel**). Red lines in top panel = analysis gates.

Thus, assessing the surface cargo of small sized EVs is a difficult task using conventional flow cytometers, because the fluorescence signal may remain hidden in the background.

2.4. Swarming and Abort Rate Affect EVs Detection

Unlike cells, EVs are not prone to align and traverse the laser path in a single row and separated from each other because of their small size. Therefore, swarm detection is the most common cause for spurious or artifactual results in the cytometry of EVs. As outlined above, we found that immunophenotyping of small sized EVs (in the size range of most EXOs) was essentially impossible. In a clinical setting, immunophenotyping is the most common approach to identify the EVs populations of interest in bodily fluids. Therefore, small sized EVs were excluded from further investigation, and we focused on medium sized EVs to investigate how swarm detection affected their analysis.

Studies suggested that the occurrence of swarming detection can be verified by serial sample dilution experiments [24–26]; upon dilution, the number of particles simultaneously traversing the laser beam should progressively reduce to a single particle, and the number of counted events should then decrease linearly in response to further dilution. Concomitantly, the intensity of fluorescence signal generated by the many particles coincidentally traversing the laser beam should progressively decline upon dilution and finally remain stable, which is consistent with analysis of single particles.

Thus, we quantitated changes in measured medium sized EVs concentrations and fluorescence intensity at various sample dilutions. Concentration (events/l) was calculated using the volumetric measurement featured in the CytoFLEX S cytometer (CytoFLEX S, Beckman Coulter, Milano, Italy).

A relation between particle concentrations measured by the cytometer and sample dilutions was noted, which was more evident at higher dilutions, leading to hypothesize the occurrence of detection as single event (Figure 4, left panel). However, the fluorescence signal intensity never levelled completely (Figure 4 center panel). Collectively, these findings suggest that dilution reduces but does not fully prevent swarm detection.

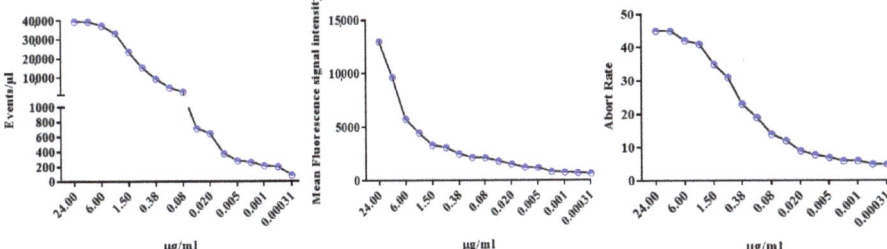

Figure 4. Four-fold dilutions experiments comparing changes in estimated Calcein-stained MVs concentration, fluorescence intensity and abort rate yielded not univocal results. **Left panel**, the measured MVs concentration decreased in proportion to the dilution suggesting single particle detection. **Middle** and **right panel**, fluorescence intensities and the abort rate, respectively, almost levelled only at the last four dilutions as it is the case for single particle detection. Data are from one experiment representative for the other four experiments conducted.

As a result of swarming, the flow cytometry of EVs is plagued by a high abort rate; the electronics is still processing the previous pulse and aborts the new event that, consequently, is lost to analysis. Thus, we hypothesized that if EVs were detected as single events as a consequence of dilution, the abort rate would be concomitantly reduced. Figure 4, right panel, shows that the abort rate declined upon dilution, a finding that concurs with data shown in the left and center panels, supporting the progressive decrease of swarm detection. Of note, minimizing swarm detection required a progressive increase of flow cytometry time; at the highest dilution a single run required ~40 min (including washing to prevent carry-over) to collect at least 5000 Calcein positive events.

Subsequently, we approached the issue of swarm detection using a model that included Calcein-green MVs mixed with Calcein-violet medium sized EVs (final concentration in the tube 0.325 µg/mL each) at a 1:1 ratio just before the flow cytometry run. Under these experimental conditions, any double-stained event undoubtedly denotes more than one EVs coincidentally traversing the laser beam. Data in Figure 5a demonstrate the presence of a sizeable number of double positive events in samples containing Calcein-green and Calcein-violet medium sized EVs, consistent with swarm detection. Consistent with the concomitant presence of several particles in the flow chamber, the VSCC signal of Calcein-green/Calcein-violet double positive EVs was higher than that of either Calcein-green or Calcein-violet single positive EVs.

To provide further experimental evidence of swarm detection and its impact, medium sized EVs samples, containing Calcein-green medium sized EVs mixed with Calcein-violet medium sized EVs, were run at higher flow rates to increase the sample fluid stream size and to boost coincidences. Thus, the samples were run at 10 µL/min—the lowest flow rate allowed by the instrument—30 µL/min and 60 µL/min. Consistent with a progressive increase of particles, simultaneously illuminated by the laser beam, the percentage of the double stained population increased in step with the flow rate (Figure 5b left panel) [23–25]. Additionally, the abort rate was enhanced, which further indicated the concomitant presence of several particles simultaneously traversing the laser beam, which were too close together to be processed as single events (Figure 5b right panel). Interestingly, swarm detection and the concomitant high abort rate reduced the number of particles detected. In the experiment depicted in Figure 5, the number of particles/µL was 25.2×10^3, 17.3×10^3 and 10.6×10^3 at 10 µL/min, 30 µL/min and 60 µL/min, respectively.

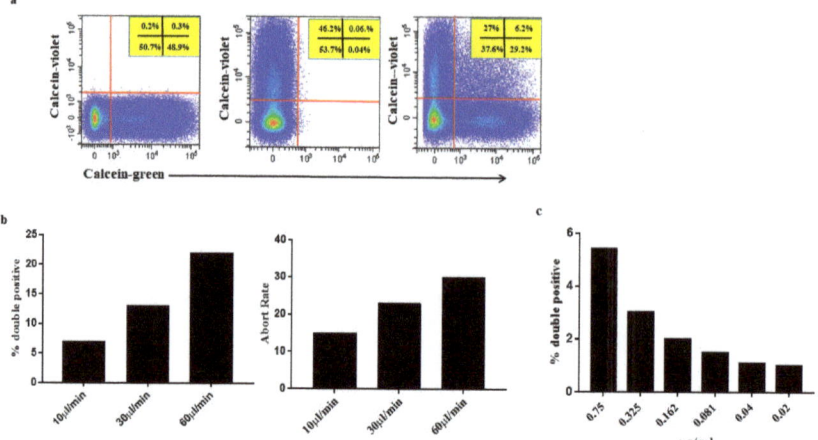

Figure 5. Two aliquots of the same medium sized EVs preparation were separately labelled, one with Calcein-green and the other with Calcein-violet, kept refrigerated and mixed at 1:1 ratio just before analysis. (**a**) Flow cytometry profile (green and violet fluorescence) of medium sized EVs marked individually with Calcein-green (left plot) and Calcein-violet (middle plot). The two Calceins stained medium sized EVs with comparable efficiency and the fluorescence signal of each dye did not interfere with the other. In the mixture (right plot), the two dyes identified single stained particles (either Calcein-green or Calcein-violet) and double-stained particles. Double-stained particles are visible in the upper right quadstat gate. These particles are indicative of coincident events, as there should not be double positive events when the two markers in comparison (Calcein-green and Calcein-violet) are not present on the same event. Samples were run at 10 µL/min. Values in panels show percentages of positive events. (**b**) Same sample as in (**a**), but run at the different flow rates featured in the cytometer. The frequency of double stained events (left panel) increased in step with the flow rate indicating that several particles were simultaneously traversing the laser beam as a consequence of the enlarged size of sample fluid stream. Consistent with the presence of several particles in the laser beam illuminated simultaneously, the abort ratio also increased (right panel) in step with the flow rate. Data are from one experiment representative for the other three experiments conducted. (**c**) The mixture of Calcein-green and Calcein-violet medium sized EVs were diluted to further explore the effect of high dilution on swarm recognition. Samples were run at 10 µL/min. The percentage of double positive events declined with dilution and close to zero at the lowest concentrations. Red lines = analysis gates.

After demonstrating swarm detection impact on EVs analysis, we used the Calcein-green/Calcein-violet model, to test again how dilution may reduce coincidences contributing to overcome the problem. To this end, the Calcein-green/Calcein-violet medium sized EVs mixture was progressively diluted yielding a final concentration of 0.04 µg/tube, and the samples were run at the lowest flow rate allowed by the instrument. The proportion of double positive events declined with dilution and approximated to zero (Figure 5c), comforting data obtained in the dilution experiments carried out using Calcein-green stained medium sized EVs (Figure 4). Confirming the preceding experiments (Figure 4), minimizing double positive events entailed a long flow cytometer time ($\geq$ 40 min).

3. Discussion

In the era of precision medicine, considerable interest using flow cytometry exists to assess both quantitative and phenotypic EVs characteristics in patients suffering from a variety of diseases in the hope to reveal clinically relevant EVs subpopulations. Moreover, the presence of EVs in readily accessible sources e.g., blood, urine, and cerebrospinal fluid, makes EV flow cytometric characterization particularly appealing to monitor diseases in longitudinal studies. Unfortunately, EVs size, which is well below that of whole cells, pushes flow cytometry to the edge of its lower reliability limits.

Within recent years, several dedicated flow cytometric approaches have been developed and refined for single EVs counting and for studying EVs heterogeneity in terms of surface markers [4]. Such methods generally demand extensive operator expertise for sample preparation and, most importantly, require dedicated instrumentation for sample acquisition and data analysis, which is unfeasible for most clinically oriented flow cytometry facilities using standard nonspecialized instruments.

In the present study, we investigated in depth whether small/medium-sized EVs (50 to 250 nm size range) can be detected by a conventional flow cytometer (CytoFLEX S, Beckman Coulter) designed primarily for common applications, mostly cell immunophenotyping. Using calibrated microbeads, we were able to show that the VSSC, i.e., the SSC signal off the 405 nm laser, is much more effective than the BSSC signal, i.e., the SSC signal off the 488 nm laser in detecting EVs, as already reported [7]. However, even the VSSC signal fells short to discriminate EVs over the background generated by particulate, which survived extensive buffer filtering, and by electronic noise of the system. In fact, EVs recognition was only possible by the concomitant assessment of VSSC and the fluorescence signal produced by the general fluorescent Calcein dyes.

Perhaps the most important application of flow cytometry in the EVs study is the purported ability to evaluate their surface cargo by staining with fluorochrome-conjugated monoclonal antibodies. We found that immunophenotyping of small sized EVs, i.e., below the 100 nm range, in our experience, was impossible. Our data show that the immunofluorescent signal generated by EVs of that size becomes measurable only when generated by multiple particles that traverse the laser beam at the same time and emit enough fluorescence to be detected, whereas single particles remain underneath the fluorescence sensitivity. Notably, these conclusions were drawn by staining for markers expressed at the highest possible level on the surface of the particle, emphasizing that they will extend to all the less expressed surface markers. While we cannot exclude that effective staining may depend on type/source of EVs and the markers being evaluated, the present findings cast doubts on the view that conventional flow cytometer is a convenient tool to explore such small sized EVs. This view is in line with the early literature indicating that a single EV of that size carries around 10 epitopes; one would not expect this particle to bind enough fluorescent moAb molecules to be detected by conventional flow cytometers [22,23]. Thus, great caution must be exerted when interpreting immunophenotyping data on small sized EVs. Additional uncertainties exist performing small EVs immunophenotyping; early work showed that the attachment of large labels to antibody molecules resulted in reduced antibody binding even to surface antigens of whole cells [27]. Notably, some of the commonly used fluorophores (PE—240 kDa, PE-Cy7—255 kDa) exceed the antibody size itself and attenuation by bulky fluorophores in multicolor flow cytometry has been reported [28].

The conclusion that assessing surface cargo of EVs in the EXOs size range (50–70 nm) by conventional flow cytometry is questionable seems to be in contrast with some earlier data, in which anti-CD63 moAb reportedly stained EXOs [29]. Comparisons are difficult because of several factors that might have affected the results, such as the modality to set the boundary between negative and positive events, the use of an isotype rather than of a more reliable isoclonic control, and the type of instrument. However, differences in the capabilities of the Apogee A 50 dedicated cytometer used in that study [24], and the CytoFLEX S conventional cytometer in our study, to resolve artificial particles of ~100 nm size, do not seem to be relevant; the Apogee A 50 depicts large angle light scatter (LALS) compared with fluorescence profiles of FITC-labelled latex beads included in our study, which closely resemble plots depicting VSSC/FITC-labelled beads. Moreover, a comparison of our results with those by Van der Pol et al. [24], suggests that the sensitivity of the scatter signals of the Apogee A 50 dedicated cytometer and the CytoFLEX S conventional cytometer is similar, as the Apogee A 50 dedicated cytometer was able to detect single 102 nm polystyrene beads [30], as we did with the CytoFLEX S. However, it should be emphasized that our conclusions, which are based on 50 nm beads as a model for small particles immunophenotyping, cannot be generalized, as different fluorescent dyes and/or different excitation sources and/or different detection devices might provide different results. This issue, as well as other related questions, will be addressed in future studies. In this scenario, in a recent paper, the CytoFLEX was reported to detect EVs as small as 60 nm, triggering with VSSC and immunophenotyping [8]. While it is possible that the surface antigen density on the EVs used in that study was much higher than that of the EVs we tested here, it should be noted that the swarming issue was not addressed, so that it cannot be excluded that multiple small sized EVs coincidentally traversing the laser spot may have contributed to the detected fluorescence signal.

Immunophenotyping was possible in larger EVs, in the 250 nm size range. However, their assessment was plagued by swarming—a finding in line with several earlier publications [24–26]. We also confirmed that swarming could be minimized by extensive sample dilution [24–26]. Unfortunately, in translational studies, particle concentration in a given sample is most often unknown, and quite hard to predict. Thus, one should measure each given sample at various dilutions, which is unfeasible in clinically oriented laboratories. Moreover, minimizing coincidences by running high diluted samples comes at the cost of very long cytometry times (up to more than half an hour in our experience) to collect enough events of interest—a constraint hardly compatible with applications in clinical research. Notably, a (unknown) portion of double stained EVs reported in immunophenotyping studies may in fact represent coincident events, because overlooked swarm detection injects 'polluted' events into the cytometry data [22].

In conclusion, our study emphasizes the inherent difficulties in investigating the surface cargo of small sized EVs (in the EXOs size range ~50–70 nm). Conventional flow cytometry does detect surface cargo of relatively large sized EVs (in the MVs size range ~200–300 nm). However, we must be aware of the intrinsic limitations due to swarm detection.

A limitation of the present study is that data were generated using CytoFLEX S as example of a commercially available last generation flow cytometer designed for a wide spectrum of applications, which does not necessitate labor intensive manual hardware adjustments and calibrations. We do not have direct knowledge of the performance of other commercial instruments offering the same features to assess EVs, and we are not aware of side-by-side comparative tests performed using the same EVs preparation. This latter point is quite an important one, as knowing what size and level of fluorescence a given platform is able to detect will allow for comparisons amongst different instruments, and even of the same producer, which is an important issue for standardization, and, therefore, reproducibility. We are now designing studies to allow the conversion of scattering intensity in arbitrary units to diameter distribution and of fluorescence intensity to MESF (Molecules of Equivalent Soluble Fluorochrome) to better define the detection limits of each instrument [31].

4. Methods

4.1. Reagents

Calcein-AM green (referred to as Calcein-green) and Calcein-AM violet (referred to as Calcein-violet) were purchased from Life Technologies. Both dyes were solubilized in DMSO to produce a 100x stock solution (1 mM). The nonionic detergent Triton X-100 was purchased from Thermofisher. Mouse anti-human brilliant violet-conjugated CD63 (BV-CD63, clone H5C6) and mouse anti-human R-phycoerythrin (PE)-conjugated CD9 (PE-CD9, clone HI9a) monoclonal antibodies (moAbs), as well as unconjugated identical (isoclonic control) CD63 and CD9 moAbs were purchased from BioLegend, Inc. Fluorochrome-conjugated moAbs were centrifuged before using to minimize the antibody aggregates commonly found in commercial preparations. Fifty nm sized microbeads carrying goat anti-mouse IgG (H+L) F (ab')2 fragments were purchased from Miltenyi Biotec (referred to as anti-mouse IgG microbeads). These beads are made of very dense material to be paramagnetic, a feature that implies a refraction index at least comparable to that of polystyrene beads. The VSSC threshold we used in all experiments included events producing a signal one and half decade lower than that generated by the smallest polystyrene beads (100 nm) included in the Megamix-Plus FSC mix (Supplementary Figure S2a and Supplementary Information), so we speculated that the Miltenyi 50 nm beads might become visible if made fluorescent. FITC Mouse IgG1, κ Isotype Control (clone MOPC-21) was purchased from BD Biosciences. Megamix-Plus FSC consisting in 100 nm, 300 nm, 500 nm, and 900 nm microbeads were purchased from BioCytex. Rainbow Calibration Particles consisting in a series of beads with eight different predefined levels of fluorescence intensity, including nonfluorescent beads, were purchased from BD Biosciences. VersaComp 3μm beads were purchased from Beckman Coulter.

4.2. EVs Staining by Calcein-Green and Calcein-Violet, and Anti-Tetraspanins moAbs

Calcein-green and Calcein-violet are essentially colorless and non-fluorescent until hydrolyzed. Once inside the EVs, the lipophilic blocking groups are cleaved by nonspecific esterases. As a result, Calceins are trapped inside the EV and emit a green or a violet fluorescence signal (emission max 516 nm and 450 nm, respectively) following excitation with a blue (488 nm) or violet (405 nm) laser. After some preliminary experiments, the incubation time was set at 20 min at 37 °C, final concentration 1 μM All staining steps were carried out in filtered PBS.

In immunophenotyping experiments, EVs, which had been previously loaded with Calcein, were incubated with moAbs to CD63, CD9, Anti-Phosphatidylserine for 30 min at room temperature (RT). All moAbs were used at concentration of 1.25 μg/mL^{-1}. All moAbs were used at 1:20 final dilution. To assess moAb non-specific binding, Calcein-loaded MVs and EXOs were incubated with a five-fold excess of identical unlabelled moAb (isoclonic control) before being reacted with the fluorochrome-conjugated moAb. Under these conditions, all specific binding sites of the fluorochrome-conjugated moAb are blocked by the large excess of unconjugated antibody and non-specific staining can be measured. Summary of reagents used for flow cytometry experiment are shown in Table 1.

To avoid false positive events, moAbs were centrifuged using 0.22 μm centrifugal filter tubes and a fixed angle single speed centrifuge (~750× g) at RT for 2 min. The flow through was collected and used for immunophenotyping experiments. In each staining session, the moAbs were run in filtered PBS alone to check signal from antibody aggregates that survived centrifugation.

4.3. Microbead Experiments

The 50 nm anti-mouse IgG microbeads served to mimic the low amount of binding sites available on an EXO-sized particle. These microbeads are designed to bind the largest possible number of moAb molecules per surface unit. The microbeads (5 to 10 μL directly from original bottle) were incubated with FITC-conjugated mouse IgG (final dilution 1:20 in filtered PBS) for 30' at 4 °C in rotation. For comparison, the same amount of FITC-conjugated mouse IgG was incubated with 5 μL of larger sized beads (VersaComp 3 μm beads, Beckman Coulter, CytoFLEX S, Beckman Coulter, Milano, Italy), coated with anti-mouse IgG.

Table 1. Summary of reagents.

Characteristic[s] Measured	Analyte	Analyte Detector	Reporter	Isotype	Clone	Final Concentration	Manufacturer	Catalogue. Number	Lot Number
Intracellular Esterase activity	Vesicles esterases	Calcein-green	Green-fluorescent calcein	NA	NA	1 µM	Life Technologies	C3100MP	1837717
		Calcein-violet	Violet-fluorescent calcein	NA	NA	1 µM	Life Technologies	C34858	2018203
Cell surface protein	Human CD63	Anti-human CD63 antibody	Brilliant Violet 421™	Mouse IgG1k	H5C6	1.25 µg/mL^{-1}	BioLegend	353030	B275650
	Human CD63	Anti-human CD63 antibody	NA	Mouse IgG1k	H5C6	5 µg/mL^{-1}	BD Pharmingen	556019	VP036
Membrane Phospholipids	Phosphatidylserine	Anti-Phosphatidylserine Antibody	Alexa Fluor 488	Mouse IgG1	1H6	1.25 µg/mL^{-1}	Millipore	16-256	2926493
		Anti-Phosphatidylserine Antibody	NA	Mouse IgG1	1H6	5 µg/mL^{-1}	Millipore	05-719	2867579
Mouse IgG1 Fluorescein-conjug. Antibody	Miltenyi Microbeads	50 nm-microbeads	Fluorescein	Mouse IgG1k	N/A	Dilution 1/20	R&D system	IC002F	1171
Anti-mouse IgG MicroBeads, human	NA	NA	NA	Mouse IgG1	NA	5 µl from the bottle	Miltenyi Biotec	130-057-501	5171201227

NA= not applicable.

4.4. Flow Cytometry

EVs were analysed using a CytoFLEX S instrument equipped with blue (488 nm) and violet laser (405 nm) excitation sources. The instrument is able to collect SSC off the blue laser (BSSC) and the violet laser (VSSC). The set-up of the instrument is a critical point for EVs analysis, so the flow cytometer was first calibrated using the 8-Peak Rainbow Beads. The linear regression equation between the predefined fluorescence intensity values of the fluorescent microbeads and the instrument's response in histogram channel values was then computed at several photodiode gains. The best gain was then determined for each fluorescent channel and used throughout all experiments. The Megamix-Plus FSC beads emitting a FITC-like fluorescent light of different sizes (100, 300, 500, and 900 nm), used throughout all experiments, served to establish the best photodiode gains for BSSC and VSSC, which produced the smallest coefficient of variation. Megamix-Plus FSC beads were also used for daily standardization. All signals were collected in log area mode, except the VSSC, which was also collected in log height mode and served as threshold parameter. Time delays between lasers were optimized and controlled by the standard daily QC start-up procedure.

To ensure system and reagent cleanliness, the sample line was washed with sterile distilled water filtered through 100 nm filter before each flow cytometry run, and the same fluid was used as sheath fluid. The sheath fluid tank was thoroughly rinsed with the filtered water. In between samples, the sample line was flushed by boosting filtered PBS and Coulter Clenz® Cleaning Agent (Beckman Coulter, CytoFLEX S, Beckman Coulter, Milano, Italy) and clean distilled water to minimize carry-over.

Unless otherwise stated, EVs samples were run at the lowest rate allowed by the instrument (10 µL/min) to maintain the diameter of the sample stream as small as possible. Data were acquired and analysed by the CytExpert 2.2™ software (version 2.2, CytoFLEX S, Beckman Coulter, Milano, Italy). EVs number was measured using the cell-counting feature of the instrument that relies on a calibrated peristaltic pump for sample delivery.

To tighten the pulse window and thus reducing the background for small-particle analyses, the event rate setting feature implemented in the CytoFLEX S instrument was set to "high", according to manufacturer's instructions.

4.5. Western Blot Analysis

The EVs (microvesicles or exosomes) were lysed using lysis buffer (50 mmol/L Tris-HCl pH 7.2, 5 mmol/L MgCl2, 50 mmol/L NaCl, 0.25%, 0.1% SDS, and 1% Triton X-100) containing protease inhibitors (2 mmol/L phenyl methyl sulfonyl fluoride, 10 mg/mL aprotinin, and 2 mmol/L Na3VO4, 100 mmol/L NaF). Protein concentration was assessed using the Bradford method (Bradford protein assay kit II, Bio-Rad, Hercules, CA, USA), with BSA used as a standard. EVs extracted proteins (5–10 µg) were resolved by SDS PAGE (Sodium Dodecyl Sulfate PolyAcrylamide Gel Electrophoresis) 10% under reducing or non-reducing conditions, and were transferred to PVDF blotting membranes (GE Healthcare, Solingen, Germany) and analyzed using the enhanced chemiluminescence kit for Western blotting detection (Advansta, WesternBright TM ECL, Bering Drive San Jose, CA, USA). CD63 primary monoclonal antibody was used following suppliers' (dilution, 1:500; sc-5275; Santa Cruz Biotechnology, Inc., Dallas, TX, USA). This antibody recognizes the glycosylated forms of CD63 (30–60 kDa).

4.6. Fluorescence Microscopy

The 50 nm anti-mouse IgG microbeads (5 µL directly from original bottle) were incubated with FITC-conjugated mouse IgG (final dilution 1:20 in filtered PBS) for 30' at 4 °C in rotation. All images were collected with a Nikon ECLIPSE TE2000-S (Chiyoda, Tokyo, Japan) inverted microscope equipped with: 20× objective (Numerical aperture 0.4), filters TRITC, FITC, and UV, and a Nikon Digital Camera DXM1200F (Chiyoda, Tokyo, Japan). The images were analyzed with NIS Elements BR 2.10 software.

Supplementary Materials: The following are available online at http://www.mdpi.com/1422-0067/21/17/6257/s1, Figure S1: Size and morphology of isolated MVs and EXOs from HT29 cell line supernatant following differential centrifugation. Figure S2: VSSC is superior to BSSC to detect nanosized particles.

Author Contributions: Authors' individual contributions: Conceptualization, D.L. and A.F.; Methodology, C.R.-T. and F.C.; Formal Analysis, L.P.; Resources, R.D.M. and G.S.; Writing–Original Draft Preparation, A.F. and D.L.; Writing–Review A.B. and A.S. All authors have read and agreed to the published version of the manuscript.

Funding: This study was supported by funding from Università Cattolica del Sacro Cuore (Linea D1) and PRIN 2017AHTCK7 (LS7) to A.S.

Conflicts of Interest: The authors declare no conflict of interest.

References

1. Lane, R.E.; Korbie, D.; Hill, M.M.; Trau, M. Extracellular vesicles as circulating cancer biomarkers: Opportunities and challenges. *Clin. Transl. Med.* **2019**, *7*, 14. [CrossRef] [PubMed]
2. Meldolesi, J. Extracellular vesicles, news about their role in immune cells: Physiology, pathology and diseases. *Clin. Exp. Immunol.* **2019**, *196*, 318–327. [CrossRef]
3. Lucchetti, D.; Fattorossi, A.; Sgambato, A. Extracellular Vesicles in Oncology: Progress and Pitfalls in the Methods of Isolation and Analysis. *Biotechnol. J.* **2019**, *14*, e1700716. [CrossRef] [PubMed]
4. Zhu, S.; Ma, L.; Wang, S.; Chen, C.; Zhang, W.; Yang, L.; Hang, W.; Nolan, J.P.; Wu, L.; Yan, X. Light-scattering detection below the level of single fluorescent molecules for high-resolution characterization of functional nanoparticles. *ACS Nano* **2014**, *8*, 10998–11006. [CrossRef]
5. Morales-Kastresana, A.; Musich, T.A.; Welsh, J.A.; Telford, W.; Demberg, T.; Wood, J.; Bigos, M.; Ross, C.D.; Kachynski, A.; Dean, A.; et al. High-fidelity detection and sorting of nanoscale vesicles in viral disease and cancer. *J. Extracell. Vesicles* **2019**, *8*, 1597603. [CrossRef] [PubMed]
6. Chýlek, P. Absorption and scattering of light by small particles. By C. F. Bohren and d. R. Huffman. *Appl. Opt.* **1986**, *25*, 3166. [PubMed]
7. McVey, M.J.; Spring, C.M.; Kuebler, W.M. Improved resolution in extracellular vesicle populations using 405 instead of 488 nm side scatter. *J. Extracell. Vesicles* **2018**, *7*. [CrossRef]
8. Brittain, G.C.; Chen, Y.Q.; Martinez, E.; Tang, V.A.; Renner, T.M.; Langlois, M.A.; Gulnik, S. A Novel Semiconductor-Based Flow Cytometer with Enhanced Light-Scatter Sensitivity for the Analysis of Biological Nanoparticles. *Sci. Rep.* **2019**, *9*, 1–13. [CrossRef]
9. Lucchetti, D.; Calapà, F.; Palmieri, V.; Fanali, C.; Carbone, F.; Papa, A.; De Maria, R.; De Spirito, M.; Sgambato, A. Differentiation Affects the Release of Exosomes from Colon Cancer Cells and Their Ability to Modulate the Behavior of Recipient Cells. *Am. J. Pathol.* **2017**, *187*, 1633–1647. [CrossRef]
10. Park, S.J.; Kim, J.M.; Kim, J.; Hur, J.; Park, S.; Kim, K.; Shin, H.-J.; Chwae, Y.J. Molecular mechanisms of biogenesis of apoptotic exosome-like vesicles and their roles as damage-associated molecular patterns. *Proc. Natl. Acad. Sci. USA* **2018**, *11*, E11721–E11730. [CrossRef]
11. Tsien, R.Y. Fluorescent probes of cell signaling. *Annu. Rev. Neurosci.* **1989**, *12*, 227–253. [CrossRef] [PubMed]
12. Gray, W.D.; Mitchell, A.J.; Searles, C.D. An accurate, precise method for general labeling of extracellular vesicles. *MethodsX* **2015**, *2*, 360–367. [CrossRef] [PubMed]
13. Nordin, J.Z.; Lee, Y.; Vader, P.; Mäger, I.; Johansson, H.J.; Heusermann, W.; Wiklander, O.P.; Hällbrink, M.; Seow, Y.; Bultema, J.; et al. Ultrafiltration with size-exclusion liquid chromatography for high yieldisolation of extracellular vesicles preserving intact biophysical and functional properties. *Nanomedicine* **2015**, *11*, 879–883. [CrossRef] [PubMed]
14. Roederer, M. Spectral compensation for flow cytometry: Visualization artifacts, limitations, and caveats. *Cytometry* **2001**, *45*, 194–205. [CrossRef]
15. de Rond, L.; Libregts, S.; Rikkert, L.G.; Hau, C.M.; van der Pol, E.; Nieuwland, R.; van Leeuwen, T.G.; Coumans, F. Refractive index to evaluate staining specificity of extracellular vesicles by flow cytometry. *J. Extracell. Vesicles* **2019**, *8*, 1643671. [CrossRef]
16. Coumans, F.; Brisson, A.R.; Buzas, E.I.; Dignat-George, F.; Drees, E.; El-Andaloussi, S.; Emanueli, C.; Gasecka, A.; Hendrix, A.; Hill, A.; et al. Methodological Guidelines to Study Extracellular Vesicles. *Circ. Res.* **2017**, *120*, 1632–1648. [CrossRef]

17. Escola, J.-M.; Kleijmeer, M.J.; Stoorvogel, W.; Griffith, J.; Yoshie, O.; Geuze, H.J. Selective enrichment of tetraspan proteins on the internal vesiclesof multivesicular endosomes and exosomes secreted by humanB-lymphocytes. *J. Biol. Chem.* **1998**, *273*, 20121–20127. [CrossRef]
18. Chutipongtanate, S.; Greis, K.D. Multiplex Biomarker Screening Assay for Urinary Extracellular Vesicles Study: A Targeted Label-Free Proteomic Approach. *Sci. Rep.* **2018**, *9*, 15039. [CrossRef]
19. Arraud, N.; Linares, R.; Tan, S.; Gounou, C.; Pasquet, J.M.; Mornet, S.; Brisson, A.R. Extracellular vesicles from blood plasma: Determination of their morphology, size, phenotype and concentration. *J. Thromb. Haemost.* **2014**, *12*, 614–627. [CrossRef]
20. Linares, R.; Tan, S.; Gounou, C.; Arraud, N.; Brisson, A.R. High-speed centrifugation induces aggregation of extracellular vesicles. *J. Extracell. Vesicles* **2015**, *4*, 29509. [CrossRef]
21. Maas, S.L.; de Vrij, J.; van der Vlist, E.J.; Geragousian, B.; van Bloois, L.; Mastrobattista, E.; Schiffelers, R.M.; Wauben, M.H.; Broekman, M.L.; Nolte-'t Hoen, E.N. Possibilities and limitations of current technologies for quantification of biological extracellular vesicles and synthetic mimics. *J. Control. Release* **2015**, *200*, 87–96. [CrossRef] [PubMed]
22. Nolan, J.P.; Jones, J.C. Detection of platelet vesicles by flow cytometry. *Platelets* **2017**, *28*, 256–262. [CrossRef] [PubMed]
23. Welsh, J.A.; Holloway, J.A.; Wilkinson, J.S.; Englyst, N.A. Extracellular Vesicle Flow Cytometry Analysis and Standardization. *Front. Cell Dev. Biol.* **2017**, *5*, 78. [CrossRef] [PubMed]
24. Van der Pol, E.; van Gemert, M.J.; Sturk, A.; Nieuwland, R.; van Leeuwen, T.G. Single vs swarm detection of microparticles and exosomes by flow cytometry. *J. Thromb. Haemost.* **2012**, *10*, 919–930. [CrossRef] [PubMed]
25. Kormelink, T.G.; Arkesteijn, G.J.; Nauwelaers, F.A.; van den Engh, G.; Nolte-'t Hoen, E.N.; Wauben, M.H. Prerequisites for the analysis and sorting of extracellular vesicle subpopulations by high-resolution flow cytometry. *Cytom. Part A* **2016**, *89*, 135–147. [CrossRef] [PubMed]
26. Libregts, S.F.W.M.; Arkesteijn, G.J.A.; Németh, A.; Nolte-'t Hoen, E.N.M.; Wauben, M.H.M. Flow cytometric analysis of extracellular vesicle subsets in plasma: Impact of swarm by particles of non-interest. *J. Thromb. Haemost.* **2018**, *16*, 1423–1436. [CrossRef] [PubMed]
27. Kent, S.P.; Ryan, K.H.; Siegel, A.L. Steric hindrance as a factor in the reaction of labeled antibody with cell surface antigenic determinants. *J. Histochem. Cytochem.* **1978**, *26*, 618–621. [CrossRef] [PubMed]
28. De Vita, M.; Catzola, V.; Buzzonetti, A.; Fossati, M.; Battaglia, A.; Zamai, L.; Fattorossi, A. Unexpected interference in cell surface staining by monoclonal antibodies to unrelated antigens. *Cytom. Part B Clin. Cytom.* **2015**, *88*, 352–354. [CrossRef]
29. Kibria, G.; Ramos, E.K.; Lee, K.E.; Bedoyan, S.; Huang, S.; Samaeekia, R.; Athman, J.J.; Harding, C.V.; Lötvall, J.; Harris, L.; et al. A rapid, automated surface protein profiling of single circulating exosomes in human blood. *Sci. Rep.* **2016**, *6*, 36502. [CrossRef]
30. Van der Pol, E.; Coumans, F.A.; Grootemaat, A.E.; Gardiner, C.; Sargent, I.L.; Harrison, P.; Sturk, A.; van Leeuwen, T.G.; Nieuwland, R. Particle size distribution of exosomes and microvesicles determined by transmission electron microscopy, flow cytometry, nanoparticle tracking analysis, and resistive pulse sensing. *J. Thromb. Haemost.* **2014**, *12*, 1182–1192. [CrossRef]
31. Welsh, J.A.; Horak, P.; Wilkinson, J.S.; Ford, V.J.; Jones, J.C.; Smith, D. FCMPASS Software Aids Extracellular Vesicle Light Scatter Standardization. *Cytom. Part A* **2000**, *97*, 569–581. [CrossRef] [PubMed]

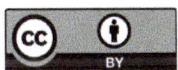

© 2020 by the authors. Licensee MDPI, Basel, Switzerland. This article is an open access article distributed under the terms and conditions of the Creative Commons Attribution (CC BY) license (http://creativecommons.org/licenses/by/4.0/).

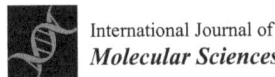

Review

Tiny Actors in the Big Cellular World: Extracellular Vesicles Playing Critical Roles in Cancer

Ancuta Jurj [1,†], Cecilia Pop-Bica [1,†], Ondrej Slaby [2,3], Cristina D. Ștefan [4], William C. Cho [5], Schuyler S. Korban [6] and Ioana Berindan-Neagoe [1,7,*]

1. Research Center for Functional Genomics, Biomedicine and Translational Medicine, "Iuliu Hațieganu" University of Medicine and Pharmacy, 400337 Cluj-Napoca, Romania; ancajurj15@gmail.com (A.J.); cecilia.bica8@gmail.com (C.P.-B.)
2. Central European Institute of Technology, Masaryk University, 625 00 Brno, Czech Republic; on.slaby@gmail.com
3. Department of Pathology, Faculty Hospital Brno and Faculty of Medicine, Masaryk University, 625 00 Brno, Czech Republic
4. SingHealth Duke-NUS Global Health Institute, Singapore 169857, Singapore; cristinastefan10@gmail.com
5. Department of Clinical Oncology, Queen Elizabeth Hospital, Hong Kong, China; chocs@ha.org.hk
6. Department of Natural Resources and Environmental Sciences, University of Illinois at Urbana-Champaign, Urbana, IL 61801, USA; korban@illinois.edu
7. Department of Functional Genomics and Experimental Pathology, "Prof. Dr. Ion Chiricuta" Oncology Institute, 400015 Cluj-Napoca, Romania
* Correspondence: ioananeagoe29@gmail.com
† These authors contribution equally.

Received: 26 August 2020; Accepted: 15 October 2020; Published: 17 October 2020

Abstract: Communications among cells can be achieved either via direct interactions or via secretion of soluble factors. The emergence of extracellular vesicles (EVs) as entities that play key roles in cell-to-cell communication offer opportunities in exploring their features for use in therapeutics; i.e., management and treatment of various pathologies, such as those used for cancer. The potential use of EVs as therapeutic agents is attributed not only for their cell membrane-bound components, but also for their cargos, mostly bioactive molecules, wherein the former regulate interactions with a recipient cell while the latter trigger cellular functions/molecular mechanisms of a recipient cell. In this article, we highlight the involvement of EVs in hallmarks of a cancer cell, particularly focusing on those molecular processes that are influenced by EV cargos. Moreover, we explored the roles of RNA species and proteins carried by EVs in eliciting drug resistance phenotypes. Interestingly, engineered EVs have been investigated and proposed as therapeutic agents in various in vivo and in vitro studies, as well as in several clinical trials.

Keywords: extracellular vesicles; cancer; therapeutic agents; cell-to-cell communication

1. Introduction

Both solid and hematological malignant tumors are not isolated entities. In fact, they involve complex systemic networks involving cell-to-cell communications between tumor cells and accompanying modified cells. Moreover, both tumor progression and invasion are sustained by a complex microenvironment. This is comprised of networks of components, including cancer-associated fibroblasts, endothelial cells, lymphocytes, and macrophages, as well as secreted factors and elements of the extracellular matrix. Interactions among neighboring cells through a direct cell–cell contact is essential for tumor growth and development, while intercellular communication provides a complex system of secreted factors [1].

To manage all components present in multicellular organisms, cellular communication is critical. McCrea et al. wrote an inspirational quote on the intercellular communication "the music that the nucleus hears" [2]. Communication involves sharing of information through several signaling mechanisms that are either direct (intracrine/autocrine and juxtacrine) and/or indirect (endocrine, paracrine, and synaptic) communications [3]. In this regard, all types of cells have been shown to release and receive both soluble factors and membrane-derived vesicles, the latter receiving increasing attention in the past decades [4]. The first instance of the presence of membrane-derived vesicles is observed in reticulocytes, wherein released vesicles would remove transferrin receptors from the cell, an important step in their maturation to erythrocytes [5]. Early on, these membrane-derived vesicles have been initially deemed as cellular "garbage bags". Subsequently, numerous studies have been undertaken to investigate membrane-derived vesicles detected on primary cells [6]; i.e., primary cells of the immune and nervous systems, and cancer cell lines [7]. It has been reported that extracellular vesicles (EVs) can be isolated from various bodily fluids, as they play important roles in the management of various normal physiological processes, including stem cell maintenance [8], immune surveillance [9], tissue repair [10], and blood coagulation [4].

It is reported that physical and molecular characteristics of EVs have impacts on various biological processes, including cancer development, progression, and metastasis [11]. Moreover, small sizes of EVs offer critical properties, including immune system escape, biocompatibility, and biodegradability, as well as transfer of their contents into both neighboring and distant cells. During biogenesis, EVs acquire important bioactive molecules that regulate several biological processes. Thus, cancer-derived EVs have been largely described as possessing both pro- and antitumor functions. For example, tumor-derived EVs interact with immune cells by delivering negative signals and interfering with their antitumor functions. By suppressing immune cell functions, EVs promote cancer progression and facilitate tumor escape. Moreover, EVs carry important molecules and factors that either directly or indirectly influence several processes, including development and maturation, as well as antitumor activities in immune cells [11]. Conversely, antitumor effects of EVs have been observed in dendritic cell-derived EVs, and these are capable of being used in immunotherapy [12].

It has been observed that EVs are tightly linked to tumorigenesis [13], spread of pathogenic agents and viruses (e.g., the Human Immunodeficiency Virus-1 [HIV-1]), amyloid-β-derived peptides [14], and α-synuclein [15] (linked to Alzheimer's and Parkinson's diseases). Due to varied compositions of EVs, they have been deemed useful in the fields of both diagnostics and therapeutics [16]. Moreover, EVs can be potentially useful in serving as drug delivery vehicles by transporting several molecular species as part of normal cell-to-cell communication.

In this review, we will discuss the potential and role(s) of EVs in modulating both physiological and pathological processes, as well as how these entities can be used as therapeutic agents [17].

2. The War Waged Inside the Cell

EVs are described based on their size, cellular origin (endosome- or plasma membrane-derived), biological function, and biogenesis process. Moreover, when described based on their biogenesis, EVs are cataloged into apoptotic bodies, microvesicles, and exosomes [18]. These major classes are cell-based vesicles having diameters ranging between 30 and 2000 nm (Table 1). Furthermore, these entities exhibit different properties that help distinguish them among all main classes of EVs. Differences among different EV classes are based on the content, size, route of biogenesis, and surface markers [19].

One of the largest cell-based vesicles is those of apoptotic bodies that are released by any type of cell once apoptotic processes are activated. Specifically, apoptotic EVs are generated during plasma membrane blebbing during apoptosis, as these are phagocytosed by macrophages and then fused with lysosomes [20]. Generally, these EVs are known to carry nuclear fragments and cellular organelles as a result of cell fragmentation [20]. Furthermore, these EVs are characterized by a flip of phosphatidylserine along an external layer, a permeable membrane, and expression of phagocytosis-promoting signals (calreticulin [21] and calnexin [22]), as well as chemokines and adhesion molecules, including ICAM3 and CX3CL1/fractalkine, and MHC class II molecules [23]. These are all important for direct antigen presentation CD4+ T cells and immunological memory activation [23].

Microvesicles, also known as ectosomes, are usually larger than 0.2 µm in size, and they are released outward from the plasma membrane via budding or shedding into the extracellular matrix. The process of microvesicle formation is mediated through a complex process involving cytoskeletal protein contraction and phospholipid redistribution [24]. During biogenesis, microvesicles are mainly composed of a plasma membrane and of cytosolic-associated proteins [19]. Microvesicles are involved in several key functions, including intercellular communication, signal transduction, and immune regulation. In particular, these entities mediate tumor invasion, inflammation, metastases, stem-cell renewal, and expansion [25]. During biogenesis, microvesicles receive important structural components, including Flotillin-2, Annexin V, integrins, selectin, CD40, and metalloproteinase [26].

In contrast, exosomes are between 30–100 nm in size, and are generated using the endosomal pathway [25]. Exosome biogenesis begins with the formation of early endosomes that undergo inward (or reverse) budding and then subsequent formation of intraluminal vesicles (ILVs), and referred to as multivesicular bodies (MVBs) or late endosomes. As a final step, late endosomes may either directly fuse with lysosomes, wherein the endocytosed cargo is degraded, or they may fuse with the plasmalemma releasing its ILVs (exosomes) to the extracellular space [25,27]. ESCRT (endosomal sorting complexes required for transport) is a molecular complex that plays an important role in MVB formation and regulation (Figure 1). Specifically, ESCRT is formed from the other four molecular complexes, including ESCRT-0, -I, -II, and -III. These multi-protein complexes are responsible for different functions, depending on their components. ESCRT-0 is dependent on ubiquitin and determines clustering of the cargo, ESCRT-I and ESCRT-II play important roles in bud formation, and ESCRT-III determines scission of vesicles. In addition, accessory proteins (VPS4 ATPase) are implicated in the final steps of ESCRT functions, namely of dissociation and recycling. In many studies, other ESCRT-independent pathways of MVB formation have been observed [28]. Some classes of molecules implicated in ESCRT-independent mechanisms of exosome biogenesis are represented by proteolipid proteins, tetraspanins, and heat shock proteins [29].

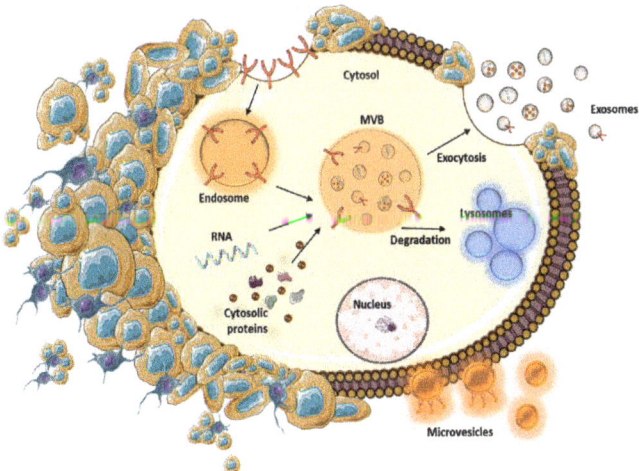

Figure 1. Biogenesis mechanisms of EVs, exosomes, and microvesicles. Endocytosis, an active process, begins with the generation of endosomes after cells are internalized within the extracellular fluid material to form internal vesicles and early and late endosomes. Furthermore, multivesicular bodies (MVBs) are formed via inward budding of a late endosomal membrane. Moreover, MVBs can fuse with either the plasmalemma, releasing their cargo into extracellular space, or with lysosomes, wherein their contents are degraded.

In general, following MVB fusion with the plasmalemma, exosomes are secreted from cells. This mechanism is regulated via two mechanisms, constitutive and inducible. The constitutive mechanism is managed by a plethora of molecules, including heterotrimeric G-proteins, flotillins, and glycosphingolipids [30], while inducible secretion is determined by stress stimuli, including thrombin, DNA damage, hypoxia, heat shock, and lipopolysaccharide (LPS) stimulation [27].

Table 1. Major characteristics of EVs.

Characteristics	Exosome	Multivesicular Body	Apoptotic Body	References
Size	Homologous 30–100 nm	Heterogenous 100–1000 nm	Heterogenous 1–5 µm	[31–33]
Origin	Multivesicular bodies fusion with cellular membrane	Direct outward budding or blebbing from the cellular membrane	Cellular membrane blebbing during cell death, cellular debris	[33,34]
Density	1.13–1.19 g/mL	1.25–1.30 g/mL	1.16–1.28 g/mL	[35]
Contents	Nucleic acids (DNA, mRNAs, miRs), lipids, specific proteins	Nucleic acids (DNA, mRNAs, miRs), lipids, specific proteins	Cellular organelles, cytosolic content (RNAs, fragmented DNA, proteins)	[33]
Protein components	Multivesicular body biogenesis (ALIX, TSG101), tetraspanins (CD9, CD63, CD81, CD82)	Death receptors (CD40 ligands), Cell adhesion (selectins, integrins)	Transcription and protein synthesis (histones)	[25,36]
Lipids	Lipidic molecules from the donor cells (include BMP)	Lipids from plasma membrane and resemble the donor cells (without BMP)	Characterized by phosphatidylserine externalization	[36,37]
Mechanism of release	Constitutive and/or cellular activation, depends on the cell type of origin	Cytoskeleton rearrangements, generation of membrane curvature, vesicle release, relocation of phospholipids to the outer membrane	Rho-associated kinase I and myosin ATPase activity	[37–39]
Determinant of controlled contents	The cellular origin and physiological state of the cell	No direct correlation	The cellular origin and stimuli	[35]
Markers	Membrane impermeable (PI negative), CD63, TSG101, Alix, flotillin, tetraspanins, HSP70, HSP90	Membrane impermeable (PI negative), selectin, integrin, flotillin-2, Annexin A1	Membrane permeable (PI positive), histone, DNA, Annexin V	[25,32]

MV, microvesicle; BMP, bone morphogenetic protein; PI, propidium iodide.

During biogenesis, exosomes receive critical bioactive molecules from donor cells, including nucleic acids, lipids, and proteins, that are specific for each cell type [40]. For composition of both exosomes and microvesicles, the following components are important: mRNAs, microRNAs (miR), non-coding RNAs, DNAs (mtDNA, ssDNA, and dsDNA), mRNA cytoplasmic proteins, and lipid raft-interacting proteins (Figure 2) [41]. Recent attention has focused on understanding how DNAs are packaged within EVs. In this regard, several research groups have reported on the presence of DNAs (mtDNA, ssDNA, and dsDNA) in EVs secreted from various types of malignancies, including melanoma, breast, lung, pancreas, and prostate cancer [42]. However, there is little knowledge of the origin, biological significance, and mechanism of DNA packaging in EVs. Conversely, few studies have reported that DNA is located along the outer surface and not within EVs [43,44]. Thus, it is proposed that outer surfaces of EVs are capable of interacting with proteins, nucleic acids, and other molecules regulating motility, aggregation, and various other important processes for EVs [45]. Furthermore, cargos within these vesicles can influence recipient cells [46], thus suggesting that exchanges of EV cargos between either normal or cancer cells may represent an effective and efficient intercellular communication when cells have particular physiological behaviors, but these are dramatically altered in cancer cells. Alongside nucleic acids, exosomal proteins are specific, and they are present in endocytic compartments of donor cell membranes, as well as in cellular membranes, the nucleus, the cytosol, and the Golgi apparatus, as well as in the endoplasmic reticulum and mitochondria, but at lower frequencies for these latter two organelles [47]. Tetraspanins (CD9, CD63, CD81, and CD82) are among some of the most typical proteins present in exosomes, alongside GPI-anchored proteins and receptors. Moreover, within interiors of exosomes, several molecular species of a parent cell are encased, and these are represented by structural components, heat shock proteins, chaperones, and enzymes involved in metabolic processes, among many others (Figure 2) [17,27].

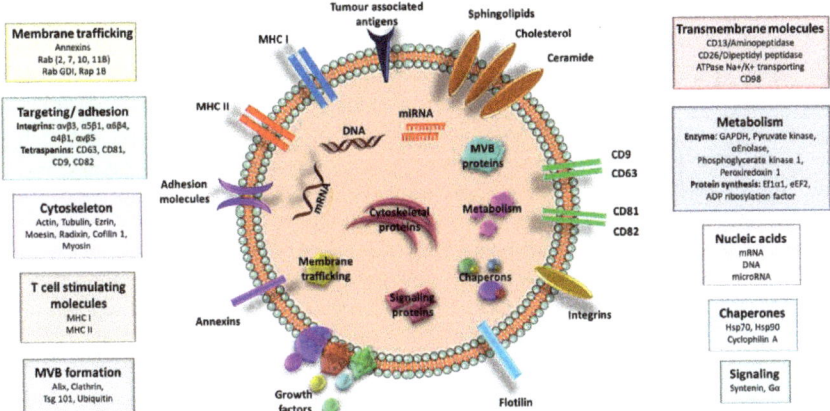

Figure 2. EVs' cargo profile. EVs are secreted by a wide range of cells, normal and tumor, having the capacity to deliver various bioactive molecules including nucleic acids, specific proteins, and lipids from the donor cells to recipient cells

Interestingly, EVs are carriers of essential soluble immune mediators, including cytokines and chemokines. Several cytokines, such as IL-1α, IL-1β, IL-6, IL18, and IL-32, are engulfed within EVs. In endothelial cell-derived apoptotic bodies, IL-1α is present; whereas, IL-18 is associated with EVs shed from surfaces of macrophages. Additionally, IL-6 and IL-32 are secreted by mast cells upon IL-1 stimulation [48]. Moreover, heat-stressed tumor cells have been shown to release EVs with different CCL compositions compared to their nonstressed counterpart [49].

3. EVs Isolation and Characterization

EVs can be isolated from different biological fluids (plasma, serum, saliva, milk, and urine, among others), as well as from cell culture supernatants. There are several available methodologies to remove undesirable particles from samples of interest. In cell cultures, EVs are separated from other components of cell media using differential centrifugation. This technique utilizes centrifugal force to separate contaminants from EVs, along with several necessary steps to remove cells, cell debris, and large microvesicles in order to obtain purified EVs [50]. Another isolation technique, density gradient centrifugation, separates EVs into specific layers in different solutions (sucrose, iohexol, and iodixanol) depending on their buoyant densities [51]. In this method, subcellular components, including mitochondria, endosomes, and peroxisomes, are successfully separated into distinct layers within the density gradient solution [52]. In yet another method, size-exclusion chromatography utilizes porous beads to separate biomolecules based on their hydrodynamic radii [53]; thus, biological samples are filtered through a column of porous beads of radii smaller than those of EVs [54]. Similarly, filter-based enrichment methods also depend on the sizes of EVs for separation, but instead of porous beads, sieves are used. Further, antibody enrichment methods are based on selecting for markers specific for EVs, such as CD9, CD63, and CD81, thus serving as complementary to size-based methods, thereby capable of specific selection of EVs [55]. Recently, acoustics and/or microfluidics methods have been developed that will isolate EVs in label-free and contact-free manners [56,57]. In addition, EVs can be separated from biological samples via precipitation using different chemicals, such as polyethylene glycol (PEG), sodium acetate, or protamine. It has been reported that using PEG, both EVs and proteins are precipitated into a pellet that can be further analyzed [58]. Similarly, magnetic beads coated with antibodies for common EV surface proteins (CD9, CD63, and CD81) are used [59]; whereas, a fluidic technique, ExoTIC (exosome total isolation kit), utilizes step-wise nanoporous membranes to trap molecules or particles of specific sizes, thereby allowing for smaller molecules and particles to flow through a membrane filter [60]. This latter method may be deemed as the most accurate size-based method used to isolate EVs from biological samples with a high yield of intact EV structures.

As EVs, of nano-sizes, must be quantified and evaluated for purity, there are several methods that can determine the numbers of vesicles released and cell type (detection of surface antigens), as well as EV morphological traits [61]. Dynamic light scattering (DLS) is based on a particle's Brownian motion in solution, used to measure the size distribution of particles, as well as their zeta potentials, measuring diameters of particles ranging between 1 nm and 6 μm [62]. However, this technique does not provide any biochemical data of purified EVs [62]. In another technique similar to DLS, nanoparticle tracking analysis (NTA) is used to measure concentration, count, and size distribution of EVs based on their Brownian motion; moreover, this technique can measure smaller-sized EVs, ranging from 1 to 1000 nm [63]. In yet another technique, flow cytometry is used to indirectly quantify EVs as it is based on using specific antibodies that accurately recognize EV markers from a liquid medium. However, flow cytometry cannot evaluate the complex profiles of subsets of EVs. Similar to DLS and NTA, flow cytometry is capable of providing data on EV size, count, and distribution [64]. Finally, both EV purity and quality can be determined using transmission electron microscopy (TEM) wherein standard traits, such as cup-like structures and lipid bilayers, can be determined [65]; whereas, EV purity can be assessed based on presence or absence of protein markers [50].

4. Biological Roles of EVs

EVs, particularly exosomes, play important roles in cells by influencing several biological processes. Their effects on receptor cells can be exerted via various mechanisms, such as phagocytosis, direct receptor binding, and receptor-dependent internalization. Thus, EVs can deliver information through a wide range of mechanisms, thereby playing important roles in tissue repair [10], stem cell maintenance [8], and immune surveillance [9]. Due to their pleiotropic actions, EVs have been, time and time again, deemed as signalomes.

It has been reported that EVs can influence activities of immune cells present both in the tumor microenvironment and in the circulatory system [66]. Once EVs are internalized into targeted cells, they release their cargo and exert their role by activating different biological mechanisms. EVs can mediate the activation of immune cells by promoting proliferation and survival of hematopoietic stem cells, as well as activation of monocytes [67], B lymphocytes [66], and NK cells [68]. EVs can also inhibit immune responses via regulation of NK and CD8$^+$ cell activities [69] and activation of Treg cells, as well as inhibition of dendritic cell (DC) maturation [70] and formation [71]. For those EVs derived from stem cells, they have been demonstrated to regulate stem cell maintenance with implications in tissue regeneration [72]. In addition, it has also been shown that EVs can modify stem cells to develop into either a liver cell phenotype [73] or a lung phenotype [74].

5. Pathological Roles of EVs

It is important to point out that EVs can be secreted by malignant or deregulated cells. During biogenesis processes, EVs are loaded with important bioactive molecules from malignant cells that influence the phenotype(s) of target cells. It has been reported that EVs are implicated in the formation of a premetastatic milieu throughout the body [75]. Moreover, EVs are also involved in other critical biological processes and have the capability of stimulating tumor progression [13]. This process is sustained by EVs via delivery and release of their targets into a target cell(s). Alongside tumor progression, EVs have the capability of carrying out other critical processes, including cell proliferation, tumor growth [76], angiogenesis [77–85], matrix remodeling, metastasis [75,86–96], immune escape [69,97–109], resistance to apoptosis [110–113], deregulation of energetic metabolism [114–117], sustaining proliferative signaling [94,118–120], evading growth suppression [121–123], deregulating and tumor-promoting inflammation [100,124,125] (Figure 3).

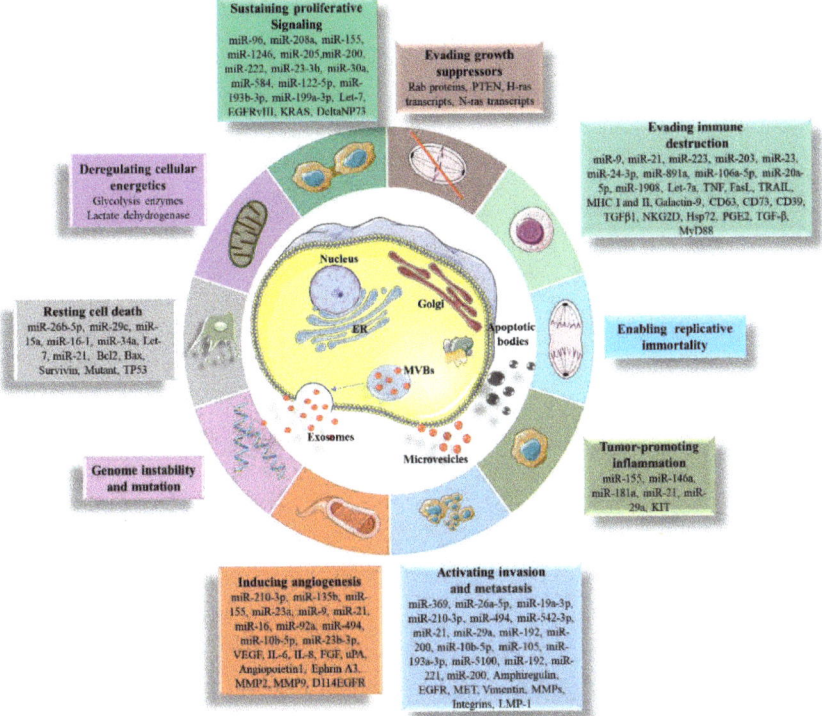

Figure 3. A schematic representation of the impact of tumor-derived EVs on the hallmarks of cancer. Pro-oncogenic molecules can be transported through the cellular membrane by EVs and microvesicles. Molecules transported via EVs have been reported to contribute to each of the hallmarks of cancer. Abbreviations: ER, endoplasmic reticulum; MVBs, multivesicular bodies

5.1. Promoting Cell Proliferation and Resistance to Apoptosis

EV transfer can modify particular signaling pathways in the target cell, modifying proliferation and resistance to apoptosis, among other processes. For example, it has been reported that in gastric cancer, cell proliferation can be enhanced through exosomal transfer of CD97 that activates the Mitogen-Activated Protein Kinase (MAPK) pathway [126]. In chronic myeloid leukemia, it has been observed that cellular proliferation is promoted via induction of phosphatidylinositol 3-kinase (PI3K)/protein kinase B (AKT) and MAPK pathways [127]. For instance, melanoma-derived EVs transfer PDGFR-8, which in turn activates the PI3K/AKT pathway in target cells [128]. Moreover, PI3K/AKT and MAPK pathways are reported to be activated in both gastric and bladder carcinomas by EVs [129]. In addition, EVs derived from glioblastoma are reported to promote cell proliferation in a CLIC1-dependent manner [130]. Soekmadji et al. have demonstrated that EVs derived from prostate cancer cells cultured in the presence of androgens are enriched in CD9, which promotes proliferation of androgen-deprived cells [131]; whereas, Matsumoto et al. have reported that mice injected with melanoma-derived EVs result in accelerated in vivo growth of murine melanomas [132].

EVs can also alter target cell(s) via their miR content as it has been shown that miR-93-5 from esophageal cancer-derived EVs inhibits phosphatase and tensin protein (PTEN) expression stimulating cell proliferation [133]. Other important examples of EVs' role in stimulating cell proliferation has been reported in colon cancer wherein EVs carry higher levels of miR-200b and miR-193a [134] and of pancreatic cancer-derived EVs loaded with miR-23b-3p and of papillary thyroid cancer-derived EVs loaded with miR-222 [135]. Furthermore, it has been observed that tumor-derived EVs actively transfer miR-106a-5p, miR-891a, miR-24-3p, and miR-20a-5p that promote cell proliferation via alteration of Microtubule Affinity-Regulating Kinase1 (MARK1) signaling in human nasopharynx cancer [136]. Moreover, EV miR-302b is delivered from lung carcinoma cell lines to target cells, leading to cell growth inhibition via the TGFβRII/ERK signaling pathway [137], while EV miR-584 accelerates cell proliferation in hepatocellular cancer cells [138].

5.2. Promoting Cell Migration

In addition to their effects on cell proliferation, EVs secreted by tumor cells can also alter the migratory status of malignant cells. EVs derived from nasopharyngeal carcinoma carrying epithelial-mesenchymal transition (EMT)-inducing signals, including HIF1α, TGFβ [98], and matrix metalloproteinases (MMPs), were reported to improve the migratory capacity of tumor cells [139]. Interestingly, EVs from a hypoxic prostate cell line have been shown to lead to increased mobility and invasiveness in a naïve human prostate cancer cells [140]. Moreover, EVs secreted from muscle-invasive bladder cancer contributed to decreased levels of E-cadherin as well as to enhanced migration and invasion in uroepithelial cells [141,142]. In another study, EV miR-105 was reported to stimulate invasion in both the respiratory and central nervous systems by inhibiting ZO-1 in endothelial cells, leading to enhanced cell migration [143]. Furthermore, it has been observed that EV miR-21 stimulates invasion of esophageal tumor cells by activating the programmed cell death 4 (PDCD4)/c-Jun NH_2-terminal kinase (JNK) axis [90].

5.3. Sustaining Angiogenesis

It has been reported that induction of a mutated epidermal growth factor receptor variant III (EGFRvIII) in glioma cells would lead to increased vesiculation and transfer of the mutated EGFRvIII to other cells and to increased vascular endothelial growth factor (VEGF) production [94]. In addition, it has been observed that EVs from primary glioblastoma cells are loaded with miRs that influence angiogenesis [76]. Recently, it has been demonstrated that EGFR can be transferred to endothelial cells wherein expression of VEGF is induced along with subsequent autocrine activation of VEGF-R2 [77]. Thus, these findings suggest that EVs can result in tumor growth by stimulating cancer cell proliferation and activating angiogenesis in adjacent endothelial cells [77]. Kim et al. have reported that sphingomyelin expressed on tumor cells-derived EVs stimulate processes, such as migration and angiogenesis, in endothelial cells [144]. It has been observed that such EVs secreted by tumor cells are enriched in MMPs as well as in CD147. These components have been proposed to play roles in both hydrolysis of the extracellular matrix and initiation of angiogenesis [145]. Interestingly, it has also been observed that pSTAT5 can be transferred to endothelial cells via EVs, and that it is capable of activating ERK1/2 along with subsequent angiogenesis stimulation [146]. Moreover, miR-214 is also responsible for promoting angiogenesis by suppressing Ataxia Telangiectasia Mutated (ATM) expression and preventing senescence [147]. In fact, mesenchymal stem cells-derived EVs have also been shown to stimulate the angiogenesis process, as demonstrated in vivo in an ischemic heart model [148].

Colon cancer cells have been shown to transfer miR-25-3p to endothelial cells not only by stimulating angiogenesis but also by increasing vascular permeability [149]. EVs secreted by hepatocellular carcinoma cells have been shown to transfer miR-103 to endothelial cells, leading to a reduction in the integrity of endothelial junctions, and thereby increasing vascular permeability [150]. The angiogenesis process has also been shown to be stimulated by miR-145-5p and miR-14-3p from lung cancer-derived EVs [151]. Moreover, in lung cancer cells, release of EV miR-21 stimulates angiogenesis in nontumor lung cells [90]. In another study, miR-9 exhibits proangiogenic activity by reducing expression levels of the *SOCS5* gene and by promoting Janus kinase/signal transducers and activators of transcription (JAK-STAT) signaling, thereby supporting migration of endothelial cells and tumor angiogenesis [152]. Furthermore, increased expression levels of EV miR-9 can differentiate an osteoblast precursor cell line into osteoblast cells and upregulate angiogenesis via an AMPK-dependent pathway [153].

From a therapeutic perspective, it has been observed that EVs can be used to shed bevacizumab, an anti-VEGF antibody, thus leading to decreased efficacy in glioblastoma [154]. Additionally, some cancers are capable of secreting VEGF isoforms with reduced affinities for bevacizumab, leading to another therapy escape mechanism [155]. Another antiangiogenic agent commonly used throughout the field of oncology is sorafenib. Hepatocellular carcinoma-derived EVs have been shown to activate the HGF/MET/AKT pathway in sensitive hepatocellular carcinoma cells, thereby inducing sorafenib resistance. Moreover, it has been observed that more invasive cell lines are capable of better inducing sorafenib resistance compared to less invasive cell lines, thus demonstrating that different malignant subclones are capable of sharing their acquired resistance [156].

It has been reported that sorafenib induces increased expression of linc-ROR in EVs secreted by hepatocellular carcinoma cells [157]. EVs have also been shown to transfer resistance to sunitinib, a similar compound to sorafenib, to hepatocellular carcinoma subclones [157], as well as to different subclones of renal cell carcinoma [158].

5.4. Immune System Evasion

One of the important functions of the immune system is to recognize and to destroy particular cells that present alterations when compared to self-antigens of unaltered (normal) cells. However, this function can be evaded by malignant cells either by changing surface antigens of malignant cells or by influencing the immune system. The role(s) of EVs in this process has been reported in various studies [80]. It has been demonstrated that EVs secreted from tumor-derived macrophages are enriched with particular miRs that enhance the local invasion of breast cancer cells [103]. In fact, the effects induced by EVs are related to modulation of the immune response. Furthermore, it has been demonstrated that EVs of tumor cells are capable of promoting immune escape by determining regulatory T cell expansion [159] and by shedding FAS ligand (FASL), as well as by inducing $CD8^+T$ cell apoptosis and increasing expression of the *MMP9* gene in melanoma cells [79,160].

Recently, it has been reported that EVs can express PD-L1, thus suppressing activities of antitumor T-cells [161]. Moreover, it has been observed that EV PD-L1 expression is inversely correlated with nivolumab and pembrolizumab response [162]. These findings are of particular importance in checkpoint blockade therapy as this reveals that EVs can act as decoys for therapeutic agents. As checkpoint blockers, this would allow for adjustment of the dosage of therapy by taking into consideration EV expression of particular markers, such as PD-L1. In other cancers, such as head and neck squamous cell carcinoma, it has been observed that there are differences between EV cargos in patients experiencing relapse compared to those who remain in remission at two years following ipilimumab therapy [163]. More specifically, it has been observed that for patients in remission, at two years, have lower numbers of EVs positive for both CD3 and CTLA4. Conversely, it has been shown that patients who relapsed after two years have increased numbers of EVs derived from Treg cells, thus demonstrating the importance of EVs in mirroring the T-cell response to tumor cells [163].

Immunomodulatory effects of EVs have also been reported in gastric cancer [164]. It has been observed that EVs isolated from gastroepiploic veins have shown increased levels of TGF-β1 expression for patients presenting either lymph nodes or distant metastasis. This finding has demonstrated the role of EVs in preparing an immunosuppressive premetastatic niche for engraftment of circulating tumor cells [164]. Although not explored in the abovementioned study, it is likely that checkpoint inhibitors could reverse these observed generated immunosuppressive premetastatic niches along with reduced probability of gastric cancer reaching advanced stages.

In other studies, it has been observed that EV miR-212-3p from pancreatic cancer cells have degraded RFXAP mRNAs in dendritic cells (DCs), leading to immune tolerance by minimizing expression of MHC II [165]. Furthermore, hypoxic tumor cells-derived EVs influence functions of natural killer (NK) cells by delivering miR-23a and TGFβ [166], while miR-214 secreted from human embryonic kidney cells induces immunological tolerance responses in CD4+ T-cells [167].

5.5. Transferring Mutations

Tumor-derived EVs have DNA fragments that can be transferred to recipient cells [45]. It has been reported that resistant melanoma cells can activate the MAPK pathway in sensitive melanoma cells through an EV-mediated truncated ALK transfer [168]. Moreover, EVs positive for EGFRvIII have been shown to activate both MAPK and PI3K/AKT pathways [94]; whereas, β-catenin-mutated colon cancer cells are reported to transfer their mutation to β-catenin wild-type cells along with subsequent activation of the β-catenin/WNT pathway [169]. In addition, a mutated SMAD4 is observed to be transferred from resistant to sensitive ovarian cancer cells, leading to an increased platinum resistance [80].

6. EVs in Cancer Stem Cells

As EVs play important roles in cancer cells, it is known that particular subpopulation(s) within a malignant mass, cancer stem cells (CSCs), present significant chemoresistance and are generally deemed as seeds for relapse [170]. EVs derived from CSCs are reported to transfer particular information to other cells. For example, EVs derived from renal cell carcinoma stem cells have been shown to carry a specific miR signature that influences levels of PTEN in target cells. This change is functionally translated into increased EMT followed by a subsequent increase in frequency of metastasis [88,171].

EVs derived from glioblastoma stem cells contain miR-21, which can be transferred to endothelial cells, leading to upregulation of angiogenesis via the miR-21/VEGF pathway [172]. In another study, macrophages treated with glioblastoma cancer stem cell-derived EVs can skew macrophages to an anti-inflammatory phenotype (M2), associated with increased expression of PD-L1 on surfaces of these cells, thus demonstrating immunosuppressive roles of these EVs [173]. On the other hand, EVs from thyroid CSC spheroids can induce a stem cell-like phenotype in recipient cells by increasing levels of SOX2. Moreover, it has been shown that EVs derived from these cells also increase the EMT through SLUG upregulation [174].

EVs from CSCs have also been shown to influence the immune system, as EVs derived from colorectal CSC are reported to increase IL-1β in neutrophils, thereby inducing a pro-inflammatory environment [175].

7. EVs in Drug Resistance

One of the most heavily investigated characteristics of EVs is their ability to transfer resistance to particular therapeutic compounds. This is due to their capability of transferring specific molecular traits, such as efflux pumps or pathway regulation, thus rendering a phenotype better adapted to a particular selected therapeutic strategy [80]. Often, efflux pumps are transferred from resistant to sensitive cells [176–180]. These efflux pumps induce tumor resistance, corresponding to the transfer of ATP-binding cassette (ABC) family members, of which the multidrug resistance 1 (MDR1) and multidrug resistance-associated protein 1 (MRP1) have attracted attention in oncology [176–180]. More specifically, MRP1 can be transferred from resistant acute promyelocytic leukemia to sensitive cells [176]. Additionally, in breast cancer, MDR1 can be induced by EVs through the activation of NFATc3 [181]. On the other hand, it has been demonstrated that p-STAT3 can be transferred to 5-fluorouracil-sensitive colorectal cancer cells to increase their resistance to 5-fluorouracil [182]. Furthermore, it has been observed that CLIC1 can be transferred to gastric cancer cells, thereby increasing levels of MDR1 and BCL2 and leading both to increased drug efflux and decreased apoptosis [183].

It is important to point out that other important molecular species, including both coding and non-coding RNAs, can also be transferred in EVs, which can also contribute enhanced cell resistance to various drug/compound treatments.

As platinum compounds are important components of the oncology arsenal, studies have been undertaken to assess transfer of resistance to these compounds. Often, it has been demonstrated that miRs influence resistance to platinum. For example, miR-19b influences resistance to platinum in colon cancer [184], while both miR-425-3p and miR-96 influence resistance to platinum in lung cancer cells [185,186]. Moreover, transfer of lncRNA HOTTIP increases resistance to platinum in gastric cancer cells, while increased serum HOTTIP lncRNA is associated with poor response to platinum [187]. Furthermore, coding RNAs are reported to influence sensitivity to platinum. For example, transfer of DNMT1 mRNA increases the resistance of ovarian cancer to platinum compounds [188].

Several other compounds are reported to be transferred through EVs as well For example, resistance to 5-fluorouracil in colon cancer cells is induced by both miR-145 and miR-34a [189], while the resistance of breast cancer cells to both adriamycin and tamoxifen are mediated by miR-222 transfer [190,191], and resistance of pancreatic cancer cells to gemcitabine is mediated by miR-155 transfer, leading to TP53INP1 modulation [192].

Interestingly, some pathways are more frequently targeted by some of the miRs, it has been reported that the PI3K/AKT pathway can be targeted by miR-21 in breast cancer cells [193] and by miR-1238 in glioblastoma cells [194].

8. EVs Used as Diagnostic Markers

EVs have been deemed as useful diagnostic markers in detecting the presence of a disease once the characteristics of malignancy are known. However, current methodologies for isolation and characterization of EVs are costly and not sufficiently standardized for de novo diagnostic protocols.

Nevertheless, one set of markers useful for diagnostics consists of fusion genes present in an assessed disease. These fusions occur more or less frequently depending on various malignancies, with hematologic malignancies, sarcomas, and prostate cancer presenting the most frequent fusion events [195]. For example, presence of *BCR-ABL* fusion genes in EVs, secreted by chronic myelogenous leukemia (CML) [18], in a patient's plasma correlate with remission status in CML patients [196]. Although this approach cannot be directly transferred to a clinical diagnosis, as CML can be easily assessed in a patient's blood, this can serve as an example for use in solid tumors, such as prostate cancer. The prostate cancer malignancy presents gene fusions in ~50% of cases, particularly of the *TMPRSS2–ERG* fusion gene as it is highly frequent [197]. Such an approach requires use of urine samples as isolated EVs present alterations in RNA signature(s) compared to those of control samples, including presence of the *TMPRSS2–ERG* fusion gene [198].

However, several common cancers do not present high frequencies of fusion genes. As a result, alternative strategies must be explored. For example, HER2-HER3 dimers from EVs have been assessed in HER2-positive breast cancer patients participating in a clinical trial (NCT04288141). Although the primary objective of this study was to identify a marker for resistance to anti-HER2 therapy, assessment of HER2-HER3 dimers from EVs may aid in identifying the tumor load in HER2-positive breast cancer patients (NCT04288141).

One of the most common alternative approaches under consideration for use of EVs as biomarkers is that of the dosage of the RNA species, particularly of miRs, determined by qRT-PCR followed by protein assessment, using either ELISA or mass spectrometry [199]. However, a major problem that may arise, particularly in assessing RNAs content in EVs, is that of sensitivity of RNA species to particular transport and storage conditions. Moreover, it has been observed that RNA assessment has rarely made it to a clinical setting, as these assessments have been generally constrained to viral loads, particularly of RNA viruses.

Thus, future studies should focus on either genetic or proteomic markers present in EVs, as these are more likely to be amenable for clinical implementation.

9. EVs Used in Anti-Cancer Therapy

In recent years, accumulated knowledge of characteristics and cargos of EVs has suggested that these structures could serve as valuable biomarkers for diagnostic/prognosis, as well as therapeutic agents for treatment of various pathologies [200]. The emergence of EVs in cancer therapy serves as a valuable nanotechnology to overcome major worldwide cancer management problems [201]. Currently, there are many studies recommending use of EVs as delivery vectors for treatment of various cancer, following manipulation and engineering of these EVs to carry various molecules useful as therapeutic agents (Figure 4) [61,202,203].

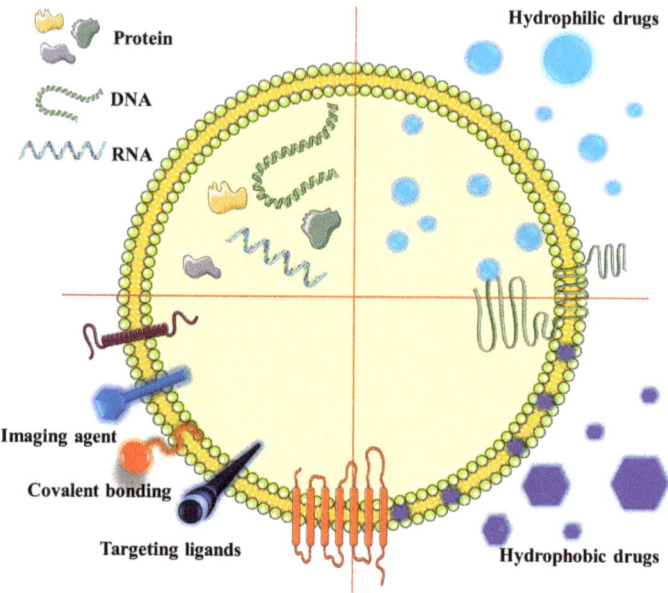

Figure 4. Properties of EVs useful in serving as drug delivery systems. These EVs consist of a lipid bilayer and an aqueous core, as they can incorporate hydrophilic drugs, hydrophobic drugs, nucleic acids (DNA, RNA), and proteins, as well as compounds (targeting ligands, covalent bonding, and imaging agents) that can be specifically attached to surfaces of EVs.

Overall, use of EVs as delivery agents will aid in the transport of internal cargo via enhanced endocytosis, thus protecting the contents from degradation. In contrast to liposomes or other nanoparticles used as carriers, EVs can serve as ideal bioparticles for targeted therapies [204,205]. Interestingly, it is suggested that biodistribution of EVs is influenced by cell origin and characteristics, with cell-specific tropism, thereby highlighting their potential use in the field of precision medicine [206]. In this arena, studies have reported on the efficiency of EVs as biocompatible drug vectors, as well as exhibiting low cytotoxicity and immunogenicity, and demonstrating their internalizing capabilities within a cell, as well as crossing the blood–brain barrier [207,208]. These EVs are capable of encapsulating various molecules, such as siRNA, miR, and various chemotherapeutics [207]. For example, Ma et al. have demonstrated that EVs carrying anti-cancer compounds can be absorbed by regenerated tumor cells, thus offering opportunities for their use in overcoming acquired drug resistance during cancer therapy [208]. Furthermore, it is reported that EVs are more likely to be internalized under acidic conditions; therefore, tumor cells are preferentially targeted by EVs rather than cells from surrounding healthy tissues [209]. Moreover, paclitaxel-loaded EVs have been used to improve the efficiency of treatment in multidrug-resistant tumor cells [210]. Recently, it has been demonstrated that tumor-derived EVs exhibit tropism toward their parental tumor cells [211], wherein engineered EVs, derived from fibrosarcoma and cervical cancer cell lines encapsulating the drug Doxil, are monitored both in vivo and in vitro using either HT1080 or HeLa tumors/cell lines. As expected, mice treated with Doxil-encapsulated EVs have higher levels of Doxil at the tumor site than those treated with Doxil alone, thereby reducing nonspecific cytotoxic effects of this drug [211].

In another study on small cell lung cancer (SCLC), sFlt-1-enriched EVs (soluble fms-like tyrosine kinase-1) are reported to act as tumor suppressors in mice via suppression of angiogenesis and induction of apoptosis in SCLC tumor cells [212].

Furthermore, in vitro and in vivo experiments of colorectal cancer cells revealed that EVs carrying miR-128-3p enhanced sensitivities to oxaliplatin by targeting *Bmi1* and *MRP5* genes [213]. In another study, the inhibitory effects on cell proliferation and EMT of miR-34c were evaluated using EVs derived from mesenchymal stem cells for delivery of miR-34c into nasopharyngeal carcinoma cell lines, and increased sensitivity to radiotherapy was observed [214]. Moreover, EVs delivering miR-199a-3p successfully suppressed both invasion and proliferation of ovarian cancer cell lines [215].

Currently, numerous clinical trials are investigating potential uses of EVs for either diagnostic/prognostic purposes or for therapeutic treatments of cancer (Table 2). These clinical trials assessing the use of microvesicles underlines their critical roles in malignancies. For example, some of these ongoing studies are evaluating engineered EVs for use as therapeutics for the treatment of pancreatic cancer. While in a completed phase II clinical trial, a vaccine developed with tumor antigen-loaded dendritic cell-derived EVs for NSCLC patients responsive to induction chemotherapy have yielded promising results [216]. It is reported dendritic cell-derived EVs manufactured with IFN-γ serve as a viable immunotherapeutic for NSCLC patients [216]. Moreover, this construct boosts NKp30-dependent NK cell functions, but without adverse consequences on antigen-specific T cell responses when used as maintenance immunotherapy for these NSCLC patients [216].

Table 2. Clinical studies exploring the use of EVs in cancer research studies.

Clinical Trial Identifier/Phase Status	Malignancy Investigated	EVs Use
NCT03236675/active, not recruiting	NSCLC	Detection of *EML4-ALK* fusion transcripts and T790M EGFR mutation
NCT03108677/recruiting	Osteosarcoma	Biomarkers for lung metastases, based on the RNS profile
NCT03985696/recruiting	Non-Hodgkin B-cell Lymphomas	Investigate EVs roles in immunotherapy, as carriers of therapeutic targets (CD20, PDL-1)
NCT03217266/recruiting	Soft tissue sarcoma	Detection of cell-free circulating tumor DNA mutations.
NCT02310451/unknown	Melanoma	Investigation of the effect of EVs produced by senescent melanoma cells
NCT03800121/recruiting	Sarcoma	Biomarkers for recurrence.
NCT03102268/unknown	Cholangiocarcinoma	Characterization of the ncRNAs in tumor derived EVs
NCT03911999/recruiting	Prostate cancer	Investigation of the relationship of urinary EVs and the aggressiveness of prostate cancer
NCT03711890/recruiting	Pancreatic cancer	Diagnostic biomarkers
NCT02869685/unknown	NSCLC	Detection of PD-L1 mRNA in plasma EVs
NCT03488134/active, not recruiting	Thyroid cancer	Urine exosomal proteins as biomarkers
NCT04258735/recruiting	Breast cancer	Diagnostic makers in a genomic panel
NCT02862470/active, not recruiting	Thyroid cancer	Urine EVs for the use as prognostic biomarkers
NCT01159288/completed	NSCLC	Treatment as tumor antigen-loaded dendritic cell-derived EVs
NCT04227886/recruiting	Rectal cancer	Biomarkers for toxicities and response to neoadjuvant therapy
NCT03608631/not yet recruiting	Pancreatic cancer	Treatment - mesenchymal stromal cells-derived EVs with KRAS G12D siRNA
NCT01779583/unknown	Gastric cancer	Prognostic and predictive biomarkers
NCT03874559/recruiting	Rectal cancer	Diagnostic biomarkers

Abbreviations: EVs- Extracellular vesicles; ncRNA–non-coding RNA; NSCLC–non-small cell lung cancer; PDL-1- programmed cell death ligand 1; siRNA–silence interfering RNA.

All the abovementioned features of EVs render them as suitable candidates for targeted therapies, especially for cancer. However, there are some challenges in attempts for use in broad applications for cancer therapy, such as lack of standardized methods of isolation and purification of EVs, and challenges in identifying optimized methods for loading EVs with therapeutic compounds [217–219]. As of now, there are several studies on the use of engineered EVs loaded with different molecules/drugs for in vitro and/or in vivo experiments in cancer research, and these are summarized in Table 3.

Table 3. Studies focused on investigating the effect of EVs-based therapy in in vivo and in vitro.

Pathology	EVs/Extracellular Vesicles Derived From	Cargo	Method of Engineering	In Vitro/In Vivo	Effect	Reference
Ovarian cancer	Fibroblasts from normal omentum	miR-199a-3p	Electroporation	SKOV3ip1, OVCAR3, CaOV3 and SKOV3-13	Inhibition of ovarian cancer cell proliferation, invasiveness, and c-Met expression.	[215]
Cancer	M1 macrophages	aCD47 and SIRPα	Polarization and conjugation	4T1 tumor-bearing BALB/c mice	Inhibition of ovarian cancer peritoneal dissemination. enhanced the phagocytosis of macrophages	[220]
Cancer	Bel7402 cell line	Doxorubicin-loaded PSiNPs (porous silicone nanoparticles)	Incubation	BALB/c mice and C57BL/6 mice bearing H22 tumors	Enhanced tumor accumulation of doxorubicin	[221]
Small cell lung cancer	BEAS-2B and NCI-H69 cell lines	sFlt-1	Cloning sFlt-1 into a lentivirus and obtaining engineered cell lines overexpressing sFlt-1	Nude mice with NCI-H69 xenografts	Induction of tumor apoptosis and inhibition tumor cell proliferation.	[212]
Glioma	RAW 264.7 cells	Doxorubicin	Incubation	GL261 cells and RAW264.7 cells	Uptake of loaded EVs is higher in cancer cells than in normal cells	[222]
				C57BL/6 mice	Increased blood circulation time Inhibition of cellular growth	
Breast cancer	Artificial chimeric EVs (ACEs)	Doxorubicin	Integration of RBCs and MCF-7 cell membrane proteins into synthetic phospholipid bilayers.	MCF-7 cells BALB/c nude mice and ICR mice	Doxorubicin accumulation in tumor improving anti-tumor efficacy	[223]
Hepatocellular carcinoma	Plasma of healthy blood donors	miR-31 and miR-451	Electroporation	HepG2 cells	Increased cancer cell apoptosis.	[224]
Breast cancer	MSC	Doxorubicin	Electroporation	BT-474 and MDA-MB231 cells	Reduced cell viability, but with no significant differences between free DOX and EVs encapsulate DOX	[225]
Her2+ Breast Cancer	HEK 293T cells	siRNA	pLEX-LAMP-DARPin lentiviral transduction in HEK 293T cells	SKBR3 cells	Increased suppression of target gene (TPD52) compared to untreated cells and negative control (unloaded EVs)	[226]
Breast cancer	MSC	miR-379	lentiviral transduction of MSCs	BALB/c nude mice	Reduction in tumor size compared to the negative control (NTC extracellular vesicles)	[227]
NSCLC	RAW 264.7 cells	Paclitaxel	Sonication and incubation (including vectorization of EVs-AA-PEG-exoPTX)	C57BL/6 mice with established mCherry-3LL-M27 metastases	Stronger suppression of metastases growth and greater survival time as compared to Taxol, or non-vectorized exoPTX formulation	[228]
Pancreatic cancer	Normal fibroblast-like mesenchymal cells	siRNA or shRNA targeting Kras^G12D	Electroporation	Panc-1 cells	Enhanced apoptosis and decreased proliferation	[229]
				Nu/nu mice with orthotopic Panc-1 tumors	Controlled growth of tumors	
Chronic myeloid leukemia	HEK293T cells	Imatinib (IL3 EVs)	Incubation	LAMA84 and K562R cells	Reduction in cell viability compared to empty imatinib loaded EVs	[230]
				NOD/SCID mice	Reduction in tumor size	
Melanoma	B16BL6 cells	CpG-DNA (SAV-LA EVs)	Incubation	C57BL/6J mice and BALB/c nu/nu mice	Inhibition of tumor growth.	[231]
Breast cancer	immature mouse dendritic cell line (imDC)	Doxorubicin (iRGD-positive EVs)	Electroporation	MDA-MB-231	Inhibition of cell proliferation	[232]
				MDA-MB-231 tumor-bearing BALB/c nude mice	Inhibition of tumor growth due to effective accumulation of Dox at tumor sites	
Breast cancer	HEK293	let-7 (GE11-positive EVs)	lipofection	RAG2−/− mice	Suppression of tumor growth	[233]

Abbreviations: EVs, extracellular vesicles; MSC, mesenchymal stem cells; NSCLC, non-small cell lung cancer; siRNA, small interfering RNA; shRNA, short hairpin RNA; DC, dendritic cells.

10. Conclusions

EVs represent particles released from both normal and malignant cells that have important biological roles in ensuring cell-to-cell communication, not only for neighboring cells but also for distant cells. EVs are classified as EVs, multivesicular bodies and apoptotic bodies, of different sizes, origin, and protein and lipid compositions. These EVs play critical roles in pathological states of cells, regulating all hallmarks of cancer cells and resistance to drug treatments, thus highlighting the potential of these entities in the management of cancer. EV capabilities in carrying different active biomolecules, such as different RNA species, DNA, and proteins for targeting recipient cells without triggering immune responses, have rendered them as valuable biological entities for use as therapeutic agents that can overcome the shortcomings of complex diseases, such as cancer.

Author Contributions: Conceptualization, A.J. and C.P.-B.; methodology, W.C.C.; validation, O.S. and C.D.Ș.; formal analysis, C.D.Ș.; investigation, A.J., C.P.-B., W.C.C., and I.B.-N.; writing—original draft preparation, A.J., C.P.-B., O.S., C.D.Ș., W.C.C., and I.B.-N.; writing—review and editing, W.C.C., S.S.K., and I.B.-N.; visualization, A.J., C.P.-B., O.S., C.D.Ș., W.C.C., and I.B.-N.; supervision, I.B.-N.; project administration, I.B.-N.; funding acquisition, I.B.-N. All authors have read and agreed to the published version of the manuscript.

Funding: This research was funded by H2020-MSCA-RISE-2018 No. 824036/2019'Excellence in research and development of non-coding RNA DIAGnostics in Oncology' (RNADIAGON), project PNCDI III 2015–2020 titled "Increasing the performance of scientific research and technology transfer in translational medicine through the formation of a new generation of young researchers"–ECHITAS, No. 29PFE/18.10.2018 and Competitiveness Operational Program, 2014–2020, titled "Clinical and economic impact of personalized targeted anti-microRNA therapies in reconverting lung cancer chemoresistance"—CANTEMIR, No. 35/01.09.2016, MySMIS 103375.

Conflicts of Interest: The authors declare no conflict of interest.

References

1. Maia, J.; Caja, S.; Strano Moraes, M.C.; Couto, N.; Costa-Silva, B. Exosome-Based Cell-Cell Communication in the Tumor Microenvironment. *Front. Cell Dev. Biol.* **2018**, *6*, 18. [CrossRef] [PubMed]
2. McCrea, P.D.; Gu, D.; Balda, M.S. Junctional Music that the Nucleus Hears: Cell-Cell Contact Signaling and the Modulation of Gene Activity. *Cold Spring Harb. Perspect. Biol.* **2009**, *1*, a002923. [CrossRef] [PubMed]
3. Brücher, B.L.D.M.; Jamall, I.S. Cell-Cell Communication in the Tumor Microenvironment, Carcinogenesis, and Anticancer Treatment. *Cell Physiol. Biochem.* **2014**, *34*, 213–243. [CrossRef] [PubMed]
4. Lee, Y.; EL Andaloussi, S.; Wood, M.J.A. Exosomes and microvesicles: Extracellular vesicles for genetic information transfer and gene therapy. *Hum. Mol. Genet.* **2012**, *21*, R125–R134. [CrossRef] [PubMed]
5. Harding, C.; Heuser, J.; Stahl, P. Endocytosis and intracellular processing of transferrin and colloidal gold-transferrin in rat reticulocytes: Demonstration of a pathway for receptor shedding. *Eur. J. Cell Biol.* **1984**, *35*, 256–263.
6. Lai, R.C.; Chen, T.S.; Lim, S.K. Mesenchymal stem cell exosome: A novel stem cell-based therapy for cardiovascular disease. *Regen. Med.* **2011**, *6*, 481–492. [CrossRef]
7. Guescini, M.; Genedani, S.; Stocchi, V.; Agnati, L.F. Astrocytes and Glioblastoma cells release exosomes carrying mtDNA. *J. Neural Transm.* **2010**, *117*, 1–4. [CrossRef]
8. Ratajczak, J.; Miekus, K.; Kucia, M.; Zhang, J.; Reca, R.; Dvorak, P.; Ratajczak, M.Z. Embryonic stem cell-derived microvesicles reprogram hematopoietic progenitors: Evidence for horizontal transfer of mRNA and protein delivery. *Leukemia* **2006**, *20*, 847–856. [CrossRef]
9. Raposo, G.; Nijman, H.W.; Stoorvogel, W.; Liejendekker, R.; Harding, C.V.; Melief, C.J.; Geuze, H.J. B lymphocytes secrete antigen-presenting vesicles. *J. Exp. Med.* **1996**, *183*, 1161–1172. [CrossRef]
10. Gatti, S.; Bruno, S.; Deregibus, M.C.; Sordi, A.; Cantaluppi, V.; Tetta, C.; Camussi, G. Microvesicles derived from human adult mesenchymal stem cells protect against ischaemia-reperfusion-induced acute and chronic kidney injury. *Nephrol. Dial. Transplant.* **2011**, *26*, 1474–1483. [CrossRef]
11. Olejarz, W.; Dominiak, A.; Żołnierzak, A.; Kubiak-Tomaszewska, G.; Lorenc, T. Tumor-Derived Exosomes in Immunosuppression and Immunotherapy. *J. Immunol. Res.* **2020**, *2020*, 6272498. [CrossRef] [PubMed]
12. Besse, B.; Charrier, M.; Lapierre, V.; Dansin, E.; Lantz, O.; Planchard, D.; Le Chevalier, T.; Livartoski, A.; Barlesi, F.; Laplanche, A.; et al. Dendritic cell-derived exosomes as maintenance immunotherapy after first line chemotherapy in NSCLC. *OncoImmunology* **2016**, *5*, e1071008. [CrossRef] [PubMed]

13. Rak, J.; Guha, A. Extracellular vesicles—Vehicles that spread cancer genes. *Bioessays* **2012**, *34*, 489–497. [CrossRef] [PubMed]
14. Bellingham, S.A.; Guo, B.B.; Coleman, B.M.; Hill, A.F. Exosomes: Vehicles for the Transfer of Toxic Proteins Associated with Neurodegenerative Diseases? *Front. Physiol.* **2012**, *3*, 124. [CrossRef] [PubMed]
15. Emmanouilidou, E.; Melachroinou, K.; Roumeliotis, T.; Garbis, S.D.; Ntzouni, M.; Margaritis, L.H.; Stefanis, L.; Vekrellis, K. Cell-Produced -Synuclein Is Secreted in a Calcium-Dependent Manner by Exosomes and Impacts Neuronal Survival. *J. Neurosci.* **2010**, *30*, 6838–6851. [CrossRef] [PubMed]
16. Tai, Y.-L.; Chu, P.-Y.; Lee, B.-H.; Chen, K.-C.; Yang, C.-Y.; Kuo, W.-H.; Shen, T.-L. Basics and applications of tumor-derived extracellular vesicles. *J. Biomed. Sci.* **2019**, *26*, 35. [CrossRef]
17. EL Andaloussi, S.; Mäger, I.; Breakefield, X.O.; Wood, M.J.A. Extracellular vesicles: Biology and emerging therapeutic opportunities. *Nat. Rev. Drug Discov.* **2013**, *12*, 347–357. [CrossRef]
18. Jurj, A.; Pasca, S.; Teodorescu, P.; Tomuleasa, C.; Berindan-Neagoe, I. Basic knowledge on BCR-ABL1-positive extracellular vesicles. *Biomark. Med.* **2020**, *14*, 451–458. [CrossRef]
19. Gebara, N.; Rossi, A.; Skovronova, R.; Aziz, J.M.; Asthana, A.; Bussolati, B. Extracellular Vesicles, Apoptotic Bodies and Mitochondria: Stem Cell Bioproducts for Organ Regeneration. *Curr. Transpl. Rep.* **2020**, *7*, 105–113. [CrossRef]
20. Kakarla, R.; Hur, J.; Kim, Y.J.; Kim, J.; Chwae, Y.-J. Apoptotic cell-derived exosomes: Messages from dying cells. *Exp. Mol. Med.* **2020**, *52*, 1–6. [CrossRef]
21. Gardai, S.J.; McPhillips, K.A.; Frasch, S.C.; Janssen, W.J.; Starefeldt, A.; Murphy-Ullrich, J.E.; Bratton, D.L.; Oldenborg, P.-A.; Michalak, M.; Henson, P.M. Cell-Surface Calreticulin Initiates Clearance of Viable or Apoptotic Cells through trans-Activation of LRP on the Phagocyte. *Cell* **2005**, *123*, 321–334. [CrossRef] [PubMed]
22. Lunavat, T.R.; Cheng, L.; Kim, D.-K.; Bhadury, J.; Jang, S.C.; Lässer, C.; Sharples, R.A.; López, M.D.; Nilsson, J.; Gho, Y.S.; et al. Small RNA deep sequencing discriminates subsets of extracellular vesicles released by melanoma cells—Evidence of unique microRNA cargos. *RNA Biol.* **2015**, *12*, 810–823. [CrossRef] [PubMed]
23. Caruso, S.; Poon, I.K.H. Apoptotic Cell-Derived Extracellular Vesicles: More Than Just Debris. *Front. Immunol.* **2018**, *9*, 1486. [CrossRef]
24. Akers, J.C.; Gonda, D.; Kim, R.; Carter, B.S.; Chen, C.C. Biogenesis of extracellular vesicles (EV): Exosomes, microvesicles, retrovirus-like vesicles, and apoptotic bodies. *J. Neurooncol.* **2013**, *113*, 1–11. [CrossRef]
25. Jurj, A.; Zanoaga, O.; Braicu, C.; Lazar, V.; Tomuleasa, C.; Irimie, A.; Berindan-Neagoe, I. A Comprehensive Picture of Extracellular Vesicles and Their Contents. Molecular Transfer to Cancer Cells. *Cancers* **2020**, *12*, 298. [CrossRef] [PubMed]
26. Borges, F.T.; Reis, L.A.; Schor, N. Extracellular vesicles: Structure, function, and potential clinical uses in renal diseases. *Braz. J. Med. Biol. Res.* **2013**, *46*, 824–830. [CrossRef]
27. Ailawadi, S.; Wang, X.; Gu, H.; Fan, G.-C. Pathologic function and therapeutic potential of exosomes in cardiovascular disease. *Biochim. Biophys. Acta (BBA) Mol. Basis Dis.* **2015**, *1852*, 1–11. [CrossRef]
28. Kajimoto, T.; Okada, T.; Miya, S.; Zhang, L.; Nakamura, S. Ongoing activation of sphingosine 1-phosphate receptors mediates maturation of exosomal multivesicular endosomes. *Nat. Commun.* **2013**, *4*, 2712. [CrossRef]
29. Kowal, J.; Tkach, M.; Théry, C. Biogenesis and secretion of exosomes. *Curr. Opin. Cell Biol.* **2014**, *29*, 116–125. [CrossRef]
30. Ekström, E.J.; Bergenfelz, C.; von Bülow, V.; Serifler, F.; Carlemalm, E.; Jönsson, G.; Andersson, T.; Leandersson, K. WNT5A induces release of exosomes containing pro-angiogenic and immunosuppressive factors from malignant melanoma cells. *Mol. Cancer* **2014**, *13*, 88. [CrossRef]
31. Chuo, S.T.-Y.; Chien, J.C.-Y.; Lai, C.P.-K. Imaging extracellular vesicles: Current and emerging methods. *J. Biomed. Sci.* **2018**, *25*, 91. [CrossRef] [PubMed]
32. Willms, E.; Cabañas, C.; Mäger, I.; Wood, M.J.A.; Vader, P. Extracellular Vesicle Heterogeneity: Subpopulations, Isolation Techniques, and Diverse Functions in Cancer Progression. *Front. Immunol.* **2018**, *9*, 738. [CrossRef]
33. Doyle, L.; Wang, M. Overview of Extracellular Vesicles, Their Origin, Composition, Purpose, and Methods for Exosome Isolation and Analysis. *Cells* **2019**, *8*, 727. [CrossRef] [PubMed]
34. Xie, C.; Ji, N.; Tang, Z.; Li, J.; Chen, Q. The role of extracellular vesicles from different origin in the microenvironment of head and neck cancers. *Mol. Cancer* **2019**, *18*, 83. [CrossRef] [PubMed]

35. Zhang, Y.; Liu, Y.; Liu, H.; Tang, W.H. Exosomes: Biogenesis, biologic function and clinical potential. *Cell Biosci.* **2019**, *9*, 19. [CrossRef] [PubMed]
36. Zaborowski, M.P.; Balaj, L.; Breakefield, X.O.; Lai, C.P. Extracellular Vesicles: Composition, Biological Relevance, and Methods of Study. *BioScience* **2015**, *65*, 783–797. [CrossRef]
37. Simeone, P.; Bologna, G.; Lanuti, P.; Pierdomenico, L.; Guagnano, M.T.; Pieragostino, D.; Del Boccio, P.; Vergara, D.; Marchisio, M.; Miscia, S.; et al. Extracellular Vesicles as Signaling Mediators and Disease Biomarkers across Biological Barriers. *Int. J. Mol. Sci.* **2020**, *21*, 2514. [CrossRef]
38. Catalano, M.; O'Driscoll, L. Inhibiting extracellular vesicles formation and release: A review of EV inhibitors. *J. Extracell. Vesicles* **2020**, *9*, 1703244. [CrossRef]
39. Joshi, B.S.; de Beer, M.A.; Giepmans, B.N.G.; Zuhorn, I.S. Endocytosis of Extracellular Vesicles and Release of Their Cargo from Endosomes. *ACS Nano* **2020**, *14*, 4444–4455. [CrossRef]
40. Théry, C.; Ostrowski, M.; Segura, E. Membrane vesicles as conveyors of immune responses. *Nat. Rev. Immunol.* **2009**, *9*, 581–593. [CrossRef]
41. Villarroya-Beltri, C.; Baixauli, F.; Gutiérrez-Vázquez, C.; Sánchez-Madrid, F.; Mittelbrunn, M. Sorting it out: Regulation of exosome loading. *Semin. Cancer Biol.* **2014**, *28*, 3–13. [CrossRef]
42. Thakur, B.K.; Zhang, H.; Becker, A.; Matei, I.; Huang, Y.; Costa-Silva, B.; Zheng, Y.; Hoshino, A.; Brazier, H.; Xiang, J.; et al. Double-stranded DNA in exosomes: A novel biomarker in cancer detection. *Cell Res.* **2014**, *24*, 766–769. [CrossRef] [PubMed]
43. Fischer, S.; Cornils, K.; Speiseder, T.; Badbaran, A.; Reimer, R.; Indenbirken, D.; Grundhoff, A.; Brunswig-Spickenheier, B.; Alawi, M.; Lange, C. Indication of Horizontal DNA Gene Transfer by Extracellular Vesicles. *PLoS ONE* **2016**, *11*, e0163665. [CrossRef] [PubMed]
44. Shelke, G.; Jang, S.C.; Yin, Y.; Lässer, C.; Lötvall, J. Human mast cells release extracellular vesicle-associated DNA. *Matters* **2016**, *2*, e201602000034. [CrossRef]
45. Kawamura, Y.; Yamamoto, Y.; Sato, T.-A.; Ochiya, T. Extracellular vesicles as trans-genomic agents: Emerging roles in disease and evolution. *Cancer Sci.* **2017**, *108*, 824–830. [CrossRef]
46. Record, M.; Subra, C.; Silvente-Poirot, S.; Poirot, M. Exosomes as intercellular signalosomes and pharmacological effectors. *Biochem. Pharmacol.* **2011**, *81*, 1171–1182. [CrossRef] [PubMed]
47. Choi, D.-S.; Kim, D.-K.; Kim, Y.-K.; Gho, Y.S. Proteomics, transcriptomics and lipidomics of exosomes and ectosomes. *Proteomics* **2013**, *13*, 1554–1571. [CrossRef]
48. Yáñez-Mó, M.; Siljander, P.R.-M.; Andreu, Z.; Bedina Zavec, A.; Borràs, F.E.; Buzas, E.I.; Buzas, K.; Casal, E.; Cappello, F.; Carvalho, J.; et al. Biological properties of extracellular vesicles and their physiological functions. *J. Extracell. Vesicles* **2015**, *4*, 27066. [CrossRef] [PubMed]
49. Chen, T.; Guo, J.; Yang, M.; Zhu, X.; Cao, X. Chemokine-Containing Exosomes Are Released from Heat-Stressed Tumor Cells via Lipid Raft-Dependent Pathway and Act as Efficient Tumor Vaccine. *J. Immunol.* **2011**, *186*, 2219–2228. [CrossRef]
50. Li, I.; Nabet, B.Y. Exosomes in the tumor microenvironment as mediators of cancer therapy resistance. *Mol. Cancer* **2019**, *18*, 32. [CrossRef]
51. Cvjetkovic, A.; Lötvall, J.; Lässer, C. The influence of rotor type and centrifugation time on the yield and purity of extracellular vesicles. *J. Extracell. Vesicles* **2014**, *3*, 23111. [CrossRef] [PubMed]
52. Konoshenko, M.Y.; Lekchnov, E.A.; Vlassov, A.V.; Laktionov, P.P. Isolation of Extracellular Vesicles: General Methodologies and Latest Trends. *Biomed. Res. Int.* **2018**, *2018*, 8545347. [CrossRef] [PubMed]
53. Böing, A.N.; van der Pol, E.; Grootemaat, A.E.; Coumans, F.A.W.; Sturk, A.; Nieuwland, R. Single-step isolation of extracellular vesicles by size-exclusion chromatography. *J. Extracell. Vesicles* **2014**, *3*, 23430. [CrossRef] [PubMed]
54. Yamamoto, K.R.; Alberts, B.M.; Benzinger, R.; Lawhorne, L.; Treiber, G. Rapid bacteriophage sedimentation in the presence of polyethylene glycol and its application to large-scale virus purification. *Virology* **1970**, *40*, 734–744. [CrossRef]
55. Li, P.; Kaslan, M.; Lee, S.H.; Yao, J.; Gao, Z. Progress in Exosome Isolation Techniques. *Theranostics* **2017**, *7*, 789–804. [CrossRef]
56. Liu, F.; Vermesh, O.; Mani, V.; Ge, T.J.; Madsen, S.J.; Sabour, A.; Hsu, E.-C.; Gowrishankar, G.; Kanada, M.; Jokerst, J.V.; et al. The Exosome Total Isolation Chip. *ACS Nano* **2017**, *11*, 10712–10723. [CrossRef]

57. Wu, M.; Ouyang, Y.; Wang, Z.; Zhang, R.; Huang, P.-H.; Chen, C.; Li, H.; Li, P.; Quinn, D.; Dao, M.; et al. Isolation of exosomes from whole blood by integrating acoustics and microfluidics. *Proc. Natl. Acad. Sci. USA* **2017**, *114*, 10584–10589. [CrossRef]
58. Gallart-Palau, X.; Serra, A.; Wong, A.S.W.; Sandin, S.; Lai, M.K.P.; Chen, C.P.; Kon, O.L.; Sze, S.K. Extracellular vesicles are rapidly purified from human plasma by PRotein Organic Solvent PRecipitation (PROSPR). *Sci. Rep.* **2015**, *5*, 14664. [CrossRef]
59. Heath, N.; Grant, L.; De Oliveira, T.M.; Rowlinson, R.; Osteikoetxea, X.; Dekker, N.; Overman, R. Rapid isolation and enrichment of extracellular vesicle preparations using anion exchange chromatography. *Sci. Rep.* **2018**, *8*, 5730. [CrossRef]
60. Merchant, M.L.; Powell, D.W.; Wilkey, D.W.; Cummins, T.D.; Deegens, J.K.; Rood, I.M.; McAfee, K.J.; Fleischer, C.; Klein, E.; Klein, J.B. Microfiltration isolation of human urinary exosomes for characterization by MS. *Proteom. Clin. Appl.* **2010**, *4*, 84–96. [CrossRef]
61. Usman, W.M.; Pham, T.C.; Kwok, Y.Y.; Vu, L.T.; Ma, V.; Peng, B.; Chan, Y.S.; Wei, L.; Chin, S.M.; Azad, A.; et al. Efficient RNA drug delivery using red blood cell extracellular vesicles. *Nat. Commun.* **2018**, *9*, 2359. [CrossRef]
62. Gercel-Taylor, C.; Atay, S.; Tullis, R.H.; Kesimer, M.; Taylor, D.D. Nanoparticle analysis of circulating cell-derived vesicles in ovarian cancer patients. *Anal. Biochem.* **2012**, *428*, 44–53. [CrossRef] [PubMed]
63. Vestad, B.; Llorente, A.; Neurauter, A.; Phuyal, S.; Kierulf, B.; Kierulf, P.; Skotland, T.; Sandvig, K.; Haug, K.B.F.; Øvstebø, R. Size and concentration analyses of extracellular vesicles by nanoparticle tracking analysis: A variation study. *J. Extracell. Vesicles* **2017**, *6*, 1344087. [CrossRef] [PubMed]
64. Headland, S.E.; Jones, H.R.; D'Sa, A.S.V.; Perretti, M.; Norling, L.V. Cutting-edge analysis of extracellular microparticles using ImageStream(X) imaging flow cytometry. *Sci. Rep.* **2014**, *4*, 5237. [CrossRef] [PubMed]
65. Linares, R.; Tan, S.; Gounou, C.; Brisson, A.R. Imaging and Quantification of Extracellular Vesicles by Transmission Electron Microscopy. *Methods Mol. Biol.* **2017**, *1545*, 43–54. [CrossRef]
66. Sprague, D.L.; Elzey, B.D.; Crist, S.A.; Waldschmidt, T.J.; Jensen, R.J.; Ratliff, T.L. Platelet-mediated modulation of adaptive immunity: Unique delivery of CD154 signal by platelet-derived membrane vesicles. *Blood* **2008**, *111*, 5028–5036. [CrossRef]
67. Baj-Krzyworzeka, M.; Mytar, B.; Szatanek, R.; Surmiak, M.; Węglarczyk, K.; Baran, J.; Siedlar, M. Colorectal cancer-derived microvesicles modulate differentiation of human monocytes to macrophages. *J. Transl. Med.* **2016**, *14*, 36. [CrossRef]
68. Simhadri, V.R.; Reiners, K.S.; Hansen, H.P.; Topolar, D.; Simhadri, V.L.; Nohroudi, K.; Kufer, T.A.; Engert, A.; Pogge von Strandmann, E. Dendritic Cells Release HLA-B-Associated Transcript-3 Positive Exosomes to Regulate Natural Killer Function. *PLoS ONE* **2008**, *3*, e3377. [CrossRef]
69. Clayton, A.; Mitchell, J.P.; Court, J.; Linnane, S.; Mason, M.D.; Tabi, Z. Human Tumor-Derived Exosomes Down-Modulate NKG2D Expression. *J. Immunol.* **2008**, *180*, 7249–7258. [CrossRef]
70. Eken, C.; Gasser, O.; Zenhaeusern, G.; Oehri, I.; Hess, C.; Schifferli, J.A. Polymorphonuclear Neutrophil-Derived Ectosomes Interfere with the Maturation of Monocyte-Derived Dendritic Cells. *J. Immunol.* **2008**, *180*, 817–824. [CrossRef]
71. Yu, S.; Liu, C.; Su, K.; Wang, J.; Liu, Y.; Zhang, L.; Li, C.; Cong, Y.; Kimberly, R.; Grizzle, W.E.; et al. Tumor Exosomes Inhibit Differentiation of Bone Marrow Dendritic Cells. *J. Immunol.* **2007**, *178*, 6867–6875. [CrossRef] [PubMed]
72. Camussi, G.; Deregibus, M.-C.; Bruno, S.; Grange, C.; Fonsato, V.; Tetta, C. Exosome/microvesicle-mediated epigenetic reprogramming of cells. *Am. J. Cancer Res.* **2011**, *1*, 98–110.
73. Jang, Y.-Y.; Collector, M.I.; Baylin, S.B.; Diehl, A.M.; Sharkis, S.J. Hematopoietic stem cells convert into liver cells within days without fusion. *Nat. Cell Biol.* **2004**, *6*, 532–539. [CrossRef]
74. Quesenberry, P.J.; Aliotta, J.M. Cellular phenotype switching and microvesicles. *Adv. Drug Deliv. Rev.* **2010**, *62*, 1141–1148. [CrossRef] [PubMed]
75. Peinado, H.; Alečković, M.; Lavotshkin, S.; Matei, I.; Costa-Silva, B.; Moreno-Bueno, G.; Hergueta-Redondo, M.; Williams, C.; García-Santos, G.; Ghajar, C.; et al. Melanoma exosomes educate bone marrow progenitor cells toward a pro-metastatic phenotype through MET. *Nat. Med.* **2012**, *18*, 883–891. [CrossRef] [PubMed]

76. Skog, J.; Würdinger, T.; van Rijn, S.; Meijer, D.H.; Gainche, L.; Curry, W.T.; Carter, B.S.; Krichevsky, A.M.; Breakefield, X.O. Glioblastoma microvesicles transport RNA and proteins that promote tumour growth and provide diagnostic biomarkers. *Nat. Cell Biol.* **2008**, *10*, 1470–1476. [CrossRef]
77. Al-Nedawi, K.; Meehan, B.; Kerbel, R.S.; Allison, A.C.; Rak, J. Endothelial expression of autocrine VEGF upon the uptake of tumor-derived microvesicles containing oncogenic EGFR. *Proc. Natl. Acad. Sci. USA* **2009**, *106*, 3794–3799. [CrossRef]
78. Hu, C.; Meiners, S.; Lukas, C.; Stathopoulos, G.T.; Chen, J. Role of exosomal microRNAs in lung cancer biology and clinical applications. *Cell Prolif.* **2020**, *53*. [CrossRef]
79. Kumar, A.; Deep, G. Exosomes in hypoxia-induced remodeling of the tumor microenvironment. *Cancer Lett.* **2020**, *488*, 1–8. [CrossRef]
80. Lee, J.-K.; Park, S.-R.; Jung, B.-K.; Jeon, Y.-K.; Lee, Y.-S.; Kim, M.-K.; Kim, Y.-G.; Jang, J.-Y.; Kim, C.-W. Exosomes Derived from Mesenchymal Stem Cells Suppress Angiogenesis by Down-Regulating VEGF Expression in Breast Cancer Cells. *PLoS ONE* **2013**, *8*, e84256. [CrossRef]
81. Umezu, T.; Ohyashiki, K.; Kuroda, M.; Ohyashiki, J.H. Leukemia cell to endothelial cell communication via exosomal miRNAs. *Oncogene* **2013**, *32*, 2747–2755. [CrossRef] [PubMed]
82. Kalinina, N.; Klink, G.; Glukhanyuk, E.; Lopatina, T.; Efimenko, A.; Akopyan, Z.; Tkachuk, V. miR-92a regulates angiogenic activity of adipose-derived mesenchymal stromal cells. *Exp. Cell Res.* **2015**, *339*, 61–66. [CrossRef]
83. Liu, Y.; Luo, F.; Wang, B.; Li, H.; Xu, Y.; Liu, X.; Shi, L.; Lu, X.; Xu, W.; Lu, L.; et al. STAT3-regulated exosomal miR-21 promotes angiogenesis and is involved in neoplastic processes of transformed human bronchial epithelial cells. *Cancer Lett.* **2016**, *370*, 125–135. [CrossRef] [PubMed]
84. Mao, G.; Liu, Y.; Fang, X.; Liu, Y.; Fang, L.; Lin, L.; Liu, X.; Wang, N. Tumor-derived microRNA-494 promotes angiogenesis in non-small cell lung cancer. *Angiogenesis* **2015**, *18*, 373–382. [CrossRef]
85. Grange, C.; Tapparo, M.; Collino, F.; Vitillo, L.; Damasco, C.; Deregibus, M.C.; Tetta, C.; Bussolati, B.; Camussi, G. Microvesicles Released from Human Renal Cancer Stem Cells Stimulate Angiogenesis and Formation of Lung Premetastatic Niche. *Cancer Res.* **2011**, *71*, 5346–5356. [CrossRef] [PubMed]
86. Sidhu, S.S.; Mengistab, A.T.; Tauscher, A.N.; LaVail, J.; Basbaum, C. The microvesicle as a vehicle for EMMPRIN in tumor–stromal interactions. *Oncogene* **2004**, *23*, 956–963. [CrossRef] [PubMed]
87. Le, M.T.N.; Hamar, P.; Guo, C.; Basar, E.; Perdigão-Henriques, R.; Balaj, L.; Lieberman, J. miR-200–containing extracellular vesicles promote breast cancer cell metastasis. *J. Clin. Invest.* **2014**, *124*, 5109–5128. [CrossRef] [PubMed]
88. Liao, J.; Liu, R.; Shi, Y.-J.; Yin, L.-H.; Pu, Y.-P. Exosome-shuttling microRNA-21 promotes cell migration and invasion-targeting PDCD4 in esophageal cancer. *Int. J. Oncol.* **2016**, *48*, 2567–2579. [CrossRef]
89. Zhou, W.; Fong, M.Y.; Min, Y.; Somlo, G.; Liu, L.; Palomares, M.R.; Yu, Y.; Chow, A.; O'Connor, S.T.F.; Chin, A.R.; et al. Cancer-secreted miR-105 destroys vascular endothelial barriers to promote metastasis. *Cancer Cell* **2014**, *25*, 501–515. [CrossRef]
90. Wang, L.; He, J.; Hu, H.; Tu, L.; Sun, Z.; Liu, Y.; Luo, F. Lung CSC-derived exosomal miR-210-3p contributes to a pro-metastatic phenotype in lung cancer by targeting FGFRL1. *J. Cell Mol. Med.* **2020**, *24*, 6324–6339. [CrossRef]
91. Higginbotham, J.N.; Demory Beckler, M.; Gephart, J.D.; Franklin, J.L.; Bogatcheva, G.; Kremers, G.-J.; Piston, D.W.; Ayers, G.D.; McConnell, R.E.; Tyska, M.J.; et al. Amphiregulin Exosomes Increase Cancer Cell Invasion. *Curr. Biol.* **2011**, *21*, 779–786. [CrossRef]
92. Al-Nedawi, K.; Meehan, B.; Micallef, J.; Lhotak, V.; May, L.; Guha, A.; Rak, J. Intercellular transfer of the oncogenic receptor EGFRvIII by microvesicles derived from tumour cells. *Nat. Cell Biol.* **2008**, *10*, 619–624. [CrossRef]
93. Fong, M.Y.; Zhou, W.; Liu, L.; Alontaga, A.Y.; Chandra, M.; Ashby, J.; Chow, A.; O'Connor, S.T.F.; Li, S.; Chin, A.R.; et al. Breast-cancer-secreted miR-122 reprograms glucose metabolism in premetastatic niche to promote metastasis. *Nat. Cell Biol.* **2015**, *17*, 183–194. [CrossRef] [PubMed]
94. Garnier, D.; Magnus, N.; Meehan, B.; Kislinger, T.; Rak, J. Qualitative changes in the proteome of extracellular vesicles accompanying cancer cell transition to mesenchymal state. *Exp. Cell Res.* **2013**, *319*, 2747–2757. [CrossRef] [PubMed]

95. Tauro, B.J.; Mathias, R.A.; Greening, D.W.; Gopal, S.K.; Ji, H.; Kapp, E.A.; Coleman, B.M.; Hill, A.F.; Kusebauch, U.; Hallows, J.L.; et al. Oncogenic H-Ras Reprograms Madin-Darby Canine Kidney (MDCK) Cell-derived Exosomal Proteins Following Epithelial-Mesenchymal Transition. *Mol. Cell Proteom.* **2013**, *12*, 2148–2159. [CrossRef]
96. Aga, M.; Bentz, G.L.; Raffa, S.; Torrisi, M.R.; Kondo, S.; Wakisaka, N.; Yoshizaki, T.; Pagano, J.S.; Shackelford, J. Exosomal HIF1α supports invasive potential of nasopharyngeal carcinoma-associated LMP1-positive exosomes. *Oncogene* **2014**, *33*, 4613–4622. [CrossRef] [PubMed]
97. Cai, Z.; Yang, F.; Yu, L.; Yu, Z.; Jiang, L.; Wang, Q.; Yang, Y.; Wang, L.; Cao, X.; Wang, J. Activated T Cell Exosomes Promote Tumor Invasion via Fas Signaling Pathway. *J. Immunol.* **2012**, *188*, 5954–5961. [CrossRef]
98. Gao, F.; Zhao, Z.-L.; Zhao, W.-T.; Fan, Q.-R.; Wang, S.-C.; Li, J.; Zhang, Y.-Q.; Shi, J.-W.; Lin, X.-L.; Yang, S.; et al. miR-9 modulates the expression of interferon-regulated genes and MHC class I molecules in human nasopharyngeal carcinoma cells. *Biochem. Biophys. Res. Commun.* **2013**, *431*, 610–616. [CrossRef]
99. Fabbri, M.; Paone, A.; Calore, F.; Galli, R.; Gaudio, E.; Santhanam, R.; Lovat, F.; Fadda, P.; Mao, C.; Nuovo, G.J.; et al. MicroRNAs bind to Toll-like receptors to induce prometastatic inflammatory response. *Proc. Natl. Acad. Sci. USA* **2012**, *109*, E2110–E2116. [CrossRef]
100. Ma, X.; Chen, Z.; Hua, D.; He, D.; Wang, L.; Zhang, P.; Wang, J.; Cai, Y.; Gao, C.; Zhang, X.; et al. Essential role for TrpC5-containing extracellular vesicles in breast cancer with chemotherapeutic resistance. *Proc. Natl. Acad. Sci. USA* **2014**, *111*, 6389–6394. [CrossRef]
101. Klibi, J.; Niki, T.; Riedel, A.; Pioche-Durieu, C.; Souquere, S.; Rubinstein, E.; Le Moulec, S.; Guigay, J.; Hirashima, M.; Guemira, F.; et al. Blood diffusion and Th1-suppressive effects of galectin-9–containing exosomes released by Epstein-Barr virus–infected nasopharyngeal carcinoma cells. *Blood* **2009**, *113*, 1957–1966. [CrossRef]
102. Yang, M.; Chen, J.; Su, F.; Yu, B.; Su, F.; Lin, L.; Liu, Y.; Huang, J.-D.; Song, E. Microvesicles secreted by macrophages shuttle invasion-potentiating microRNAs into breast cancer cells. *Mol. Cancer* **2011**, *10*, 117. [CrossRef] [PubMed]
103. Zhou, M.; Chen, J.; Zhou, L.; Chen, W.; Ding, G.; Cao, L. Pancreatic cancer derived exosomes regulate the expression of TLR4 in dendritic cells via miR-203. *Cell. Immunol.* **2014**, *292*, 65–69. [CrossRef] [PubMed]
104. Berchem, G.; Noman, M.Z.; Bosseler, M.; Paggetti, J.; Baconnais, S.; Le cam, E.; Nanbakhsh, A.; Moussay, E.; Mami-Chouaib, F.; Janji, B.; et al. Hypoxic tumor-derived microvesicles negatively regulate NK cell function by a mechanism involving TGF-β and miR23a transfer. *OncoImmunology* **2016**, *5*, e1062968. [CrossRef]
105. Huber, V.; Fais, S.; Iero, M.; Lugini, L.; Canese, P.; Squarcina, P.; Zaccheddu, A.; Colone, M.; Arancia, G.; Gentile, M.; et al. Human Colorectal Cancer Cells Induce T-Cell Death Through Release of Proapoptotic Microvesicles: Role in Immune Escape. *Gastroenterology* **2005**, *128*, 1796–1804. [CrossRef] [PubMed]
106. Clayton, A.; Mitchell, J.P.; Court, J.; Mason, M.D.; Tabi, Z. Human Tumor-Derived Exosomes Selectively Impair Lymphocyte Responses to Interleukin-2. *Cancer Res.* **2007**, *67*, 7458–7466. [CrossRef] [PubMed]
107. Ashiru, O.; Boutet, P.; Fernandez-Messina, L.; Aguera-Gonzalez, S.; Skepper, J.N.; Vales-Gomez, M.; Reyburn, H.T. Natural Killer Cell Cytotoxicity Is Suppressed by Exposure to the Human NKG2D Ligand MICA*008 That Is Shed by Tumor Cells in Exosomes. *Cancer Res.* **2010**, *70*, 481–489. [CrossRef]
108. Condamine, T.; Ramachandran, I.; Youn, J.-I.; Gabrilovich, D.I. Regulation of Tumor Metastasis by Myeloid-Derived Suppressor Cells. *Annu. Rev. Med.* **2015**, *66*, 97–110. [CrossRef] [PubMed]
109. Xiang, X.; Poliakov, A.; Liu, C.; Liu, Y.; Deng, Z.; Wang, J.; Cheng, Z.; Shah, S.V.; Wang, G.-J.; Zhang, L.; et al. Induction of myeloid-derived suppressor cells by tumor exosomes. *Int. J. Cancer* **2009**, *124*, 2621–2633. [CrossRef]
110. Khan, S.; Jutzy, J.M.S.; Aspe, J.R.; McGregor, D.W.; Neidigh, J.W.; Wall, N.R. Survivin is released from cancer cells via exosomes. *Apoptosis* **2011**, *16*, 1–12. [CrossRef]
111. Cappellesso, R.; Tinazzi, A.; Giurici, T.; Simonato, F.; Guzzardo, V.; Ventura, L.; Crescenzi, M.; Chiarelli, S.; Fassina, A. Programmed cell death 4 and microRNA 21 inverse expression is maintained in cells and exosomes from ovarian serous carcinoma effusions: PDCD4 and miR-21 Expression in OSC and Exosomes. *Cancer Cytopathol.* **2014**, *122*, 685–693. [CrossRef] [PubMed]
112. Taylor, D.D.; Gercel-Taylor, C. MicroRNA signatures of tumor-derived exosomes as diagnostic biomarkers of ovarian cancer. *Gynecol. Oncol.* **2008**, *110*, 13–21. [CrossRef]
113. Yu, X.; Harris, S.L.; Levine, A.J. The Regulation of Exosome Secretion: A Novel Function of the p53 Protein. *Cancer Res.* **2006**, *66*, 4795–4801. [CrossRef] [PubMed]

114. Xavier, C.P.R.; Caires, H.R.; Barbosa, M.A.G.; Bergantim, R.; Guimarães, J.E.; Vasconcelos, M.H. The Role of Extracellular Vesicles in the Hallmarks of Cancer and Drug Resistance. *Cells* **2020**, *9*, 1141. [CrossRef]
115. Graner, M.W.; Alzate, O.; Dechkovskaia, A.M.; Keene, J.D.; Sampson, J.H.; Mitchell, D.A.; Bigner, D.D. Proteomic and immunologic analyses of brain tumor exosomes. *FASEB J.* **2009**, *23*, 1541–1557. [CrossRef] [PubMed]
116. Webber, J.; Stone, T.C.; Katilius, E.; Smith, B.C.; Gordon, B.; Mason, M.D.; Tabi, Z.; Brewis, I.A.; Clayton, A. Proteomics Analysis of Cancer Exosomes Using a Novel Modified Aptamer-based Array (SOMAscan™) Platform. *Mol. Cell Proteom.* **2014**, *13*, 1050–1064. [CrossRef] [PubMed]
117. Welton, J.L.; Khanna, S.; Giles, P.J.; Brennan, P.; Brewis, I.A.; Staffurth, J.; Mason, M.D.; Clayton, A. Proteomics Analysis of Bladder Cancer Exosomes. *Mol. Cell Proteom.* **2010**, *9*, 1324–1338. [CrossRef] [PubMed]
118. Demory Beckler, M.; Higginbotham, J.N.; Franklin, J.L.; Ham, A.-J.; Halvey, P.J.; Imasuen, I.E.; Whitwell, C.; Li, M.; Liebler, D.C.; Coffey, R.J. Proteomic Analysis of Exosomes from Mutant KRAS Colon Cancer Cells Identifies Intercellular Transfer of Mutant KRAS. *Mol. Cell Proteom.* **2013**, *12*, 343–355. [CrossRef]
119. Soldevilla, B.; Rodríguez, M.; San Millán, C.; García, V.; Fernández-Periañez, R.; Gil-Calderón, B.; Martín, P.; García-Grande, A.; Silva, J.; Bonilla, F.; et al. Tumor-derived exosomes are enriched in ΔNp73, which promotes oncogenic potential in acceptor cells and correlates with patient survival. *Hum. Mol. Genet.* **2014**, *23*, 467–478. [CrossRef]
120. Ohshima, K.; Inoue, K.; Fujiwara, A.; Hatakeyama, K.; Kanto, K.; Watanabe, Y.; Muramatsu, K.; Fukuda, Y.; Ogura, S.; Yamaguchi, K.; et al. Let-7 MicroRNA Family Is Selectively Secreted into the Extracellular Environment via Exosomes in a Metastatic Gastric Cancer Cell Line. *PLoS ONE* **2010**, *5*, e13247. [CrossRef]
121. Abd Elmageed, Z.Y.; Yang, Y.; Thomas, R.; Ranjan, M.; Mondal, D.; Moroz, K.; Fang, Z.; Rezk, B.M.; Moparty, K.; Sikka, S.C.; et al. Neoplastic Reprogramming of Patient-Derived Adipose Stem Cells by Prostate Cancer Cell-Associated Exosomes: Tumor Exosomes Trigger Stem Cell Transformation. *Stem Cells* **2014**, *32*, 983–997. [CrossRef]
122. Ostenfeld, M.S.; Jeppesen, D.K.; Laurberg, J.R.; Boysen, A.T.; Bramsen, J.B.; Primdal-Bengtson, B.; Hendrix, A.; Lamy, P.; Dagnaes-Hansen, F.; Rasmussen, M.H.; et al. Cellular Disposal of miR23b by RAB27-Dependent Exosome Release Is Linked to Acquisition of Metastatic Properties. *Cancer Res.* **2014**, *74*, 5758–5771. [CrossRef] [PubMed]
123. Putz, U.; Howitt, J.; Doan, A.; Goh, C.-P.; Low, L.-H.; Silke, J.; Tan, S.-S. The Tumor Suppressor PTEN Is Exported in Exosomes and Has Phosphatase Activity in Recipient Cells. *Sci. Signal.* **2012**, *5*, ra70. [CrossRef]
124. Meehan, K.; Vella, L.J. The contribution of tumour-derived exosomes to the hallmarks of cancer. *Crit. Rev. Clin. Lab. Sci.* **2016**, *53*, 121–131. [CrossRef]
125. Xiao, H.; Lässer, C.; Shelke, G.V.; Wang, J.; Rådinger, M.; Lunavat, T.R.; Malmhäll, C.; Lin, L.H.; Li, J.; Li, L.; et al. Mast cell exosomes promote lung adenocarcinoma cell proliferation—Role of KIT-stem cell factor signaling. *Cell Commun. Signal.* **2014**, *12*, 64. [CrossRef]
126. Li, C. CD97 promotes gastric cancer cell proliferation and invasion through exosome-mediated MAPK signaling pathway. *World J. Gastroenterol. WJG* **2015**, *21*, 6215. [CrossRef] [PubMed]
127. Qu, J.-L.; Qu, X.-J.; Zhao, M.-F.; Teng, Y.-E.; Zhang, Y.; Hou, K.-Z.; Jiang, Y.-H.; Yang, X.-H.; Liu, Y.-P. Gastric cancer exosomes promote tumour cell proliferation through PI3K/Akt and MAPK/ERK activation. *Dig. Liver Dis.* **2009**, *41*, 875–880. [CrossRef] [PubMed]
128. Vella, L.J.; Behren, A.; Coleman, B.; Greening, D.W.; Hill, A.F.; Cebon, J. Intercellular Resistance to BRAF Inhibition Can Be Mediated by Extracellular Vesicle–Associated PDGFRβ. *Neoplasia* **2017**, *19*, 932–940. [CrossRef]
129. Yang, L.; Wu, X.-H.; Wang, D.; Luo, C.-L.; Chen, L.-X. Bladder cancer cell-derived exosomes inhibit tumor cell apoptosis and induce cell proliferation in vitro. *Mol. Med. Rep.* **2013**, *8*, 1272–1278. [CrossRef] [PubMed]
130. Setti, M.; Osti, D.; Richichi, C.; Ortensi, B.; Del Bene, M.; Fornasari, L.; Beznoussenko, G.; Mironov, A.; Rappa, G.; Cuomo, A.; et al. Extracellular vesicle-mediated transfer of CLIC1 protein is a novel mechanism for the regulation of glioblastoma growth. *Oncotarget* **2015**, *6*, 31413–31427. [CrossRef]
131. The Australian Prostate Cancer Collaboration BioResource; Soekmadji, C.; Riches, J.D.; Russell, P.J.; Ruelcke, J.E.; McPherson, S.; Wang, C.; Hovens, C.M.; Corcoran, N.M.; Hill, M.M.; et al. Modulation of paracrine signaling by CD9 positive small extracellular vesicles mediates cellular growth of androgen deprived prostate cancer. *Oncotarget* **2017**, *8*, 52237–52255. [CrossRef] [PubMed]

132. Matsumoto, A.; Takahashi, Y.; Nishikawa, M.; Sano, K.; Morishita, M.; Charoenviriyakul, C.; Saji, H.; Takakura, Y. Accelerated growth of B16 BL 6 tumor in mice through efficient uptake of their own exosomes by B16 BL 6 cells. *Cancer Sci.* **2017**, *108*, 1803–1810. [CrossRef]
133. Liu, M.X.; Liao, J.; Xie, M.; Gao, Z.K.; Wang, X.H.; Zhang, Y.; Shang, M.H.; Yin, L.H.; Pu, Y.P.; Liu, R. miR-93-5p Transferred by Exosomes Promotes the Proliferation of Esophageal Cancer Cells via Intercellular Communication by Targeting PTEN. *Biomed. Environ. Sci.* **2018**, *31*, 171–185. [CrossRef]
134. Teng, Y.; Ren, Y.; Hu, X.; Mu, J.; Samykutty, A.; Zhuang, X.; Deng, Z.; Kumar, A.; Zhang, L.; Merchant, M.L.; et al. MVP-mediated exosomal sorting of miR-193a promotes colon cancer progression. *Nat. Commun.* **2017**, *8*, 14448. [CrossRef]
135. Lee, J.C.; Zhao, J.-T.; Gundara, J.; Serpell, J.; Bach, L.A.; Sidhu, S. Papillary thyroid cancer–derived exosomes contain miRNA-146b and miRNA-222. *J. Surg. Res.* **2015**, *196*, 39–48. [CrossRef] [PubMed]
136. Graner, M.W.; Schnell, S.; Olin, M.R. Tumor-derived exosomes, microRNAs, and cancer immune suppression. *Semin. Immunopathol.* **2018**, *40*, 505–515. [CrossRef] [PubMed]
137. Lässer, C.; Théry, C.; Buzás, E.I.; Mathivanan, S.; Zhao, W.; Gho, Y.S.; Lötvall, J. The International Society for Extracellular Vesicles launches the first massive open online course on extracellular vesicles. *J. Extracell. Vesicles* **2016**, *5*, 34299. [CrossRef] [PubMed]
138. Kogure, T.; Lin, W.-L.; Yan, I.K.; Braconi, C.; Patel, T. Intercellular nanovesicle-mediated microRNA transfer: A mechanism of environmental modulation of hepatocellular cancer cell growth. *Hepatology* **2011**, *54*, 1237–1248. [CrossRef]
139. You, Y.; Shan, Y.; Chen, J.; Yue, H.; You, B.; Shi, S.; Li, X.; Cao, X. Matrix metalloproteinase 13-containing exosomes promote nasopharyngeal carcinoma metastasis. *Cancer Sci.* **2015**, *106*, 1669–1677. [CrossRef]
140. Ramteke, A.; Ting, H.; Agarwal, C.; Mateen, S.; Somasagara, R.; Hussain, A.; Graner, M.; Frederick, B.; Agarwal, R.; Deep, G. Exosomes secreted under hypoxia enhance invasiveness and stemness of prostate cancer cells by targeting adherens junction molecules: Hypoxic-exosomes role in pca aggressiveness. *Mol. Carcinog.* **2015**, *54*, 554–565. [CrossRef] [PubMed]
141. Franzen, C.A.; Blackwell, R.H.; Todorovic, V.; Greco, K.A.; Foreman, K.E.; Flanigan, R.C.; Kuo, P.C.; Gupta, G.N. Urothelial cells undergo epithelial-to-mesenchymal transition after exposure to muscle invasive bladder cancer exosomes. *Oncogenesis* **2015**, *4*, e163. [CrossRef] [PubMed]
142. Rahman, M.A.; Barger, J.F.; Lovat, F.; Gao, M.; Otterson, G.A.; Nana-Sinkam, P. Lung cancer exosomes as drivers of epithelial mesenchymal transition. *Oncotarget* **2016**, *7*, 54852–54866. [CrossRef] [PubMed]
143. Fabbri, M.; Paone, A.; Calore, F.; Galli, R.; Croce, C.M. A new role for microRNAs, as ligands of Toll-like receptors. *RNA Biol.* **2013**, *10*, 169–174. [CrossRef]
144. Kim, C.W.; Lee, H.M.; Lee, T.H.; Kang, C.; Kleinman, H.K.; Gho, Y.S. Extracellular membrane vesicles from tumor cells promote angiogenesis via sphingomyelin. *Cancer Res.* **2002**, *62*, 6312–6317. [PubMed]
145. Kholia, S.; Ranghino, A.; Garnieri, P.; Lopatina, T.; Deregibus, M.C.; Rispoli, P.; Brizzi, M.F.; Camussi, G. Extracellular vesicles as new players in angiogenesis. *Vasc. Pharmacol.* **2016**, *86*, 64–70. [CrossRef] [PubMed]
146. Lombardo, G.; Dentelli, P.; Togliatto, G.; Rosso, A.; Gili, M.; Gallo, S.; Deregibus, M.C.; Camussi, G.; Brizzi, M.F. Activated Stat5 trafficking Via Endothelial Cell-derived Extracellular Vesicles Controls IL-3 Pro-angiogenic Paracrine Action. *Sci. Rep.* **2016**, *6*, 25689. [CrossRef] [PubMed]
147. van Balkom, B.W.M.; de Jong, O.G.; Smits, M.; Brummelman, J.; den Ouden, K.; de Bree, P.M.; van Eijndhoven, M.A.J.; Pegtel, D.M.; Stoorvogel, W.; Würdinger, T.; et al. Endothelial cells require miR-214 to secrete exosomes that suppress senescence and induce angiogenesis in human and mouse endothelial cells. *Blood* **2013**, *121*, 3997–4006. [CrossRef] [PubMed]
148. Teng, X.; Chen, L.; Chen, W.; Yang, J.; Yang, Z.; Shen, Z. Mesenchymal Stem Cell-Derived Exosomes Improve the Microenvironment of Infarcted Myocardium Contributing to Angiogenesis and Anti-Inflammation. *Cell Physiol. Biochem.* **2015**, *37*, 2415–2424. [CrossRef]
149. Zeng, Z.; Li, Y.; Pan, Y.; Lan, X.; Song, F.; Sun, J.; Zhou, K.; Liu, X.; Ren, X.; Wang, F.; et al. Cancer-derived exosomal miR-25-3p promotes pre-metastatic niche formation by inducing vascular permeability and angiogenesis. *Nat. Commun.* **2018**, *9*, 5395. [CrossRef]
150. Fang, J.; Zhang, Z.; Shang, L.; Luo, Y.; Lin, Y.; Yuan, Y.; Zhuang, S. Hepatoma cell-secreted exosomal microRNA-103 increases vascular permeability and promotes metastasis by targeting junction proteins. *Hepatology* **2018**, *68*, 1459–1475. [CrossRef]

151. Lawson, J.; Dickman, C.; MacLellan, S.; Towle, R.; Jabalee, J.; Lam, S.; Garnis, C. Selective secretion of microRNAs from lung cancer cells via extracellular vesicles promotes CAMK1D-mediated tube formation in endothelial cells. *Oncotarget* **2017**, *8*, 83913–83924. [CrossRef] [PubMed]
152. Zhuang, G.; Wu, X.; Jiang, Z.; Kasman, I.; Yao, J.; Guan, Y.; Oeh, J.; Modrusan, Z.; Bais, C.; Sampath, D.; et al. Tumour-secreted miR-9 promotes endothelial cell migration and angiogenesis by activating the JAK-STAT pathway. *EMBO J.* **2012**, *31*, 3513–3523. [CrossRef]
153. Qu, J.; Lu, D.; Guo, H.; Miao, W.; Wu, G.; Zhou, M. MicroRNA-9 regulates osteoblast differentiation and angiogenesis via the AMPK signaling pathway. *Mol. Cell. Biochem.* **2016**, *411*, 23–33. [CrossRef] [PubMed]
154. Simon, T.; Pinioti, S.; Schellenberger, P.; Rajeeve, V.; Wendler, F.; Cutillas, P.R.; King, A.; Stebbing, J.; Giamas, G. Shedding of bevacizumab in tumour cells-derived extracellular vesicles as a new therapeutic escape mechanism in glioblastoma. *Mol. Cancer* **2018**, *17*, 132. [CrossRef] [PubMed]
155. Feng, Q.; Zhang, C.; Lum, D.; Druso, J.E.; Blank, B.; Wilson, K.F.; Welm, A.; Antonyak, M.A.; Cerione, R.A. A class of extracellular vesicles from breast cancer cells activates VEGF receptors and tumour angiogenesis. *Nat. Commun.* **2017**, *8*, 14450. [CrossRef]
156. Qu, Z.; Wu, J.; Wu, J.; Luo, D.; Jiang, C.; Ding, Y. Exosomes derived from HCC cells induce sorafenib resistance in hepatocellular carcinoma both in vivo and in vitro. *J. Exp. Clin. Cancer Res.* **2016**, *35*, 159. [CrossRef]
157. Takahashi, K.; Yan, I.K.; Kogure, T.; Haga, H.; Patel, T. Extracellular vesicle-mediated transfer of long non-coding RNA ROR modulates chemosensitivity in human hepatocellular cancer. *FEBS Open Bio* **2014**, *4*, 458–467. [CrossRef]
158. Stone, L. Exosome transmission of sunitinib resistance. *Nat. Rev. Urol.* **2016**, *13*, 297. [CrossRef]
159. Wieckowski, E.U.; Visus, C.; Szajnik, M.; Szczepanski, M.J.; Storkus, W.J.; Whiteside, T.L. Tumor-Derived Microvesicles Promote Regulatory T Cell Expansion and Induce Apoptosis in Tumor-Reactive Activated CD8 + T Lymphocytes. *J. Immunol.* **2009**, *183*, 3720–3730. [CrossRef]
160. Vu, L.T.; Peng, B.; Zhang, D.X.; Ma, V.; Mathey-Andrews, C.A.; Lam, C.K.; Kiomourtzis, T.; Jin, J.; McReynolds, L.; Huang, L.; et al. Tumor-secreted extracellular vesicles promote the activation of cancer-associated fibroblasts via the transfer of microRNA-125b. *J. Extracell. Vesicles* **2019**, *8*, 1599680. [CrossRef]
161. Poggio, M.; Hu, T.; Pai, C.-C.; Chu, B.; Belair, C.D.; Chang, A.; Montabana, E.; Lang, U.E.; Fu, Q.; Fong, L.; et al. Suppression of Exosomal PD-L1 Induces Systemic Anti-tumor Immunity and Memory. *Cell* **2019**, *177*, 414–427.e13. [CrossRef] [PubMed]
162. Del Re, M.; Marconcini, R.; Pasquini, G.; Rofi, E.; Vivaldi, C.; Bloise, F.; Restante, G.; Arrigoni, E.; Caparello, C.; Bianco, M.G.; et al. PD-L1 mRNA expression in plasma-derived exosomes is associated with response to anti-PD-1 antibodies in melanoma and NSCLC. *Br. J. Cancer* **2018**, *118*, 820–824. [CrossRef] [PubMed]
163. Theodoraki, M.-N.; Yerneni, S.; Gooding, W.E.; Ohr, J.; Clump, D.A.; Bauman, J.E.; Ferris, R.L.; Whiteside, T.L. Circulating exosomes measure responses to therapy in head and neck cancer patients treated with cetuximab, ipilimumab, and IMRT. *OncoImmunology* **2019**, *8*, e1593805. [CrossRef] [PubMed]
164. Yen, E.-Y.; Miaw, S.-C.; Yu, J.-S.; Lai, I.-R. Exosomal TGF-β1 is correlated with lymphatic metastasis of gastric cancers. *Am. J. Cancer Res.* **2017**, *7*, 2199–2208.
165. Que, R.; Lin, C.; Ding, G.; Wu, Z.; Cao, L. Increasing the immune activity of exosomes: The effect of miRNA-depleted exosome proteins on activating dendritic cell/cytokine-induced killer cells against pancreatic cancer. *J. Zhejiang Univ. Sci. B* **2016**, *17*, 352–360. [CrossRef]
166. Feitelson, M.A.; Arzumanyan, A.; Kulathinal, R.J.; Blain, S.W.; Holcombe, R.F.; Mahajna, J.; Marino, M.; Martinez-Chantar, M.L.; Nawroth, R.; Sanchez-Garcia, I.; et al. Sustained proliferation in cancer: Mechanisms and novel therapeutic targets. *Semin. Cancer Biol.* **2015**, *35*, S25–S54. [CrossRef]
167. Yin, Y.; Cai, X.; Chen, X.; Liang, H.; Zhang, Y.; Li, J.; Wang, Z.; Chen, X.; Zhang, W.; Yokoyama, S.; et al. Tumor-secreted miR-214 induces regulatory T cells: A major link between immune evasion and tumor growth. *Cell Res.* **2014**, *24*, 1164–1180. [CrossRef]
168. Cesi, G.; Philippidou, D.; Kozar, I.; Kim, Y.J.; Bernardin, F.; Van Niel, G.; Wienecke-Baldacchino, A.; Felten, P.; Letellier, E.; Dengler, S.; et al. A new ALK isoform transported by extracellular vesicles confers drug resistance to melanoma cells. *Mol. Cancer* **2018**, *17*, 145. [CrossRef]
169. Kalra, H.; Gangoda, L.; Fonseka, P.; Chitti, S.V.; Liem, M.; Keerthikumar, S.; Samuel, M.; Boukouris, S.; Al Saffar, H.; Collins, C.; et al. Extracellular vesicles containing oncogenic mutant β-catenin activate Wnt signalling pathway in the recipient cells. *J. Extracell. Vesicles* **2019**, *8*, 1690217. [CrossRef]

170. Yadav, A.K.; Desai, N.S. Cancer Stem Cells: Acquisition, Characteristics, Therapeutic Implications, Targeting Strategies and Future Prospects. *Stem Cell Rev. Rep.* **2019**, *15*, 331–355. [CrossRef]
171. Wang, L.; Yang, G.; Zhao, D.; Wang, J.; Bai, Y.; Peng, Q.; Wang, H.; Fang, R.; Chen, G.; Wang, Z.; et al. CD103-positive CSC exosome promotes EMT of clear cell renal cell carcinoma: Role of remote MiR-19b-3p. *Mol. Cancer* **2019**, *18*, 86. [CrossRef] [PubMed]
172. Sun, Z.; Wang, L.; Dong, L.; Wang, X. Emerging role of exosome signalling in maintaining cancer stem cell dynamic equilibrium. *J. Cell Mol. Med.* **2018**, *22*, 3719–3728. [CrossRef] [PubMed]
173. Gabrusiewicz, K.; Li, X.; Wei, J.; Hashimoto, Y.; Marisetty, A.L.; Ott, M.; Wang, F.; Hawke, D.; Yu, J.; Healy, L.M.; et al. Glioblastoma stem cell-derived exosomes induce M2 macrophages and PD-L1 expression on human monocytes. *OncoImmunology* **2018**, *7*, e1412909. [CrossRef]
174. Hardin, H.; Helein, H.; Meyer, K.; Robertson, S.; Zhang, R.; Zhong, W.; Lloyd, R.V. Thyroid cancer stem-like cell exosomes: Regulation of EMT via transfer of lncRNAs. *Lab. Invest.* **2018**, *98*, 1133–1142. [CrossRef] [PubMed]
175. Hwang, W.-L.; Lan, H.-Y.; Cheng, W.-C.; Huang, S.-C.; Yang, M.-H. Tumor stem-like cell-derived exosomal RNAs prime neutrophils for facilitating tumorigenesis of colon cancer. *J. Hematol. Oncol.* **2019**, *12*, 10. [CrossRef]
176. Bouvy, C.; Wannez, A.; Laloy, J.; Chatelain, C.; Dogné, J.-M. Transfer of multidrug resistance among acute myeloid leukemia cells via extracellular vesicles and their microRNA cargo. *Leuk. Res.* **2017**, *62*, 70–76. [CrossRef] [PubMed]
177. Aung, T.; Chapuy, B.; Vogel, D.; Wenzel, D.; Oppermann, M.; Lahmann, M.; Weinhage, T.; Menck, K.; Hupfeld, T.; Koch, R.; et al. Exosomal evasion of humoral immunotherapy in aggressive B-cell lymphoma modulated by ATP-binding cassette transporter A3. *Proc. Natl. Acad. Sci. USA* **2011**, *108*, 15336–15341. [CrossRef]
178. Bebawy, M.; Combes, V.; Lee, E.; Jaiswal, R.; Gong, J.; Bonhoure, A.; Grau, G.E.R. Membrane microparticles mediate transfer of P-glycoprotein to drug sensitive cancer cells. *Leukemia* **2009**, *23*, 1643–1649. [CrossRef]
179. Lu, J.F.; Luk, F.; Gong, J.; Jaiswal, R.; Grau, G.E.R.; Bebawy, M. Microparticles mediate MRP1 intercellular transfer and the re-templating of intrinsic resistance pathways. *Pharmacol. Res.* **2013**, *76*, 77–83. [CrossRef] [PubMed]
180. Lu, J.F.; Pokharel, D.; Bebawy, M. A novel mechanism governing the transcriptional regulation of ABC transporters in MDR cancer cells. *Drug Deliv. Transl. Res.* **2017**, *7*, 276–285. [CrossRef]
181. Dong, Y.; Pan, Q.; Jiang, L.; Chen, Z.; Zhang, F.; Liu, Y.; Xing, H.; Shi, M.; Li, J.; Li, X.; et al. Tumor endothelial expression of P-glycoprotein upon microvesicular transfer of TrpC5 derived from adriamycin-resistant breast cancer cells. *Biochem. Biophys. Res. Commun.* **2014**, *446*, 85–90. [CrossRef]
182. Zhang, Q.; Liu, R.-X.; Chan, K.-W.; Hu, J.; Zhang, J.; Wei, L.; Tan, H.; Yang, X.; Liu, H. Exosomal transfer of p-STAT3 promotes acquired 5-FU resistance in colorectal cancer cells. *J. Exp. Clin. Cancer Res.* **2019**, *38*, 320. [CrossRef] [PubMed]
183. Zhao, K.; Wang, Z.; Li, X.; Liu, J.; Tian, L.; Chen, J. Exosome-mediated transfer of CLIC1 contributes to the vincristine-resistance in gastric cancer. *Mol. Cell Biochem.* **2019**, *462*, 97–105. [CrossRef]
184. Gu, Y.Y.; Yu, J.; Zhang, J.F.; Wang, C. Suppressing the secretion of exosomal miR-19b by gw4869 could regulate oxaliplatin sensitivity in colorectal cancer. *Neoplasma* **2019**, *66*, 39–45. [CrossRef]
185. Ma, Y.; Yuwen, D.; Chen, J.; Zheng, B.; Gao, J.; Fan, M.; Xue, W.; Wang, Y.; Li, W.; Shu, Y.; et al. Exosomal Transfer Of Cisplatin-Induced miR-425-3p Confers Cisplatin Resistance In NSCLC Through Activating Autophagy. *Int. J. Nanomed.* **2019**, *14*, 8121–8132. [CrossRef]
186. Wu, H.; Zhou, J.; Mei, S.; Wu, D.; Mu, Z.; Chen, B.; Xie, Y.; Ye, Y.; Liu, J. Circulating exosomal microRNA-96 promotes cell proliferation, migration and drug resistance by targeting LMO7. *J. Cell. Mol. Med.* **2017**, *21*, 1228–1236. [CrossRef] [PubMed]
187. Wang, J.; Lv, B.; Su, Y.; Wang, X.; Bu, J.; Yao, L. Exosome-Mediated Transfer of lncRNA HOTTIP Promotes Cisplatin Resistance in Gastric Cancer Cells by Regulating HMGA1/miR-218 Axis. *OncoTargets Therapy* **2019**, *12*, 11325–11338. [CrossRef]
188. Cao, Y.-L.; Zhuang, T.; Xing, B.-H.; Li, N.; Li, Q. Exosomal DNMT1 mediates cisplatin resistance in ovarian cancer. *Cell Biochem. Funct.* **2017**, *35*, 296–303. [CrossRef]

189. Akao, Y.; Khoo, F.; Kumazaki, M.; Shinohara, H.; Miki, K.; Yamada, N. Extracellular Disposal of Tumor-Suppressor miRs-145 and -34a via Microvesicles and 5-FU Resistance of Human Colon Cancer Cells. *Int. J. Mol. Sci.* **2014**, *15*, 1392–1401. [CrossRef]
190. Yu, D.; Wu, Y.; Zhang, X.; Lv, M.; Chen, W.; Chen, X.; Yang, S.; Shen, H.; Zhong, S.; Tang, J.; et al. Exosomes from adriamycin-resistant breast cancer cells transmit drug resistance partly by delivering miR-222. *Tumor Biol.* **2016**, *37*, 3227–3235. [CrossRef]
191. Wei, Y.; Lai, X.; Yu, S.; Chen, S.; Ma, Y.; Zhang, Y.; Li, H.; Zhu, X.; Yao, L.; Zhang, J. Exosomal miR-221/222 enhances tamoxifen resistance in recipient ER-positive breast cancer cells. *Breast Cancer Res. Treat.* **2014**, *147*, 423–431. [CrossRef] [PubMed]
192. Mikamori, M.; Yamada, D.; Eguchi, H.; Hasegawa, S.; Kishimoto, T.; Tomimaru, Y.; Asaoka, T.; Noda, T.; Wada, H.; Kawamoto, K.; et al. MicroRNA-155 Controls Exosome Synthesis and Promotes Gemcitabine Resistance in Pancreatic Ductal Adenocarcinoma. *Sci. Rep.* **2017**, *7*, 42339. [CrossRef]
193. de Souza, P.S.; Cruz, A.L.S.; Viola, J.P.B.; Maia, R.C. Microparticles induce multifactorial resistance through oncogenic pathways independently of cancer cell type. *Cancer Sci.* **2015**, *106*, 60–68. [CrossRef] [PubMed]
194. Yin, J.; Zeng, A.; Zhang, Z.; Shi, Z.; Yan, W.; You, Y. Exosomal transfer of miR-1238 contributes to temozolomide-resistance in glioblastoma. *EBioMedicine* **2019**, *42*, 238–251. [CrossRef] [PubMed]
195. Powers, M.P. The ever-changing world of gene fusions in cancer: A secondary gene fusion and progression. *Oncogene* **2019**, *38*, 7197–7199. [CrossRef]
196. Li, Q.; Zhong, Z.; Zeng, C.; Meng, L.; Li, C.; Luo, Y.; Wang, H.; Li, W.; Wang, J.; Cheng, F.; et al. A clinical observation of Chinese chronic myelogenous leukemia patients after discontinuation of tyrosine kinase inhibitors. *Oncotarget* **2016**, *7*. [CrossRef]
197. Kumar-Sinha, C.; Tomlins, S.A.; Chinnaiyan, A.M. Recurrent gene fusions in prostate cancer. *Nat. Rev. Cancer* **2008**, *8*, 497–511. [CrossRef]
198. Fujita, K.; Nonomura, N. Urinary biomarkers of prostate cancer. *Int. J. Urol.* **2018**, *25*, 770–779. [CrossRef]
199. Wong, C.-H.; Chen, Y.-C. Clinical significance of exosomes as potential biomarkers in cancer. *World J. Clin. Cases* **2019**, *7*, 171–190. [CrossRef]
200. Schey, K.L.; Luther, J.M.; Rose, K.L. Proteomics characterization of exosome cargo. *Methods* **2015**, *87*, 75–82. [CrossRef]
201. Mohammadi, S.; Yousefi, F.; Shabaninejad, Z.; Movahedpour, A.; Mahjoubin Tehran, M.; Shafiee, A.; Moradizarmehri, S.; Hajighadimi, S.; Savardashtaki, A.; Mirzaei, H. Exosomes and cancer: From oncogenic roles to therapeutic applications. *IUBMB Life* **2020**, *72*, 724–748. [CrossRef] [PubMed]
202. Luan, X.; Sansanaphongpricha, K.; Myers, I.; Chen, H.; Yuan, H.; Sun, D. Engineering exosomes as refined biological nanoplatforms for drug delivery. *Acta Pharm. Sin.* **2017**, *38*, 754–763. [CrossRef] [PubMed]
203. Liang, G.; Kan, S.; Zhu, Y.; Feng, S.; Feng, W.; Gao, S. Engineered exosome-mediated delivery of functionally active miR-26a and its enhanced suppression effect in HepG2 cells. *Int. J. Nanomed.* **2018**, *13*, 585–599. [CrossRef]
204. Vader, P.; Mol, E.A.; Pasterkamp, G.; Schiffelers, R.M. Extracellular vesicles for drug delivery. *Adv. Drug Deliv. Rev.* **2016**, *106*, 148–156. [CrossRef]
205. Li, Y.; Zheng, Q.; Bao, C.; Li, S.; Guo, W.; Zhao, J.; Chen, D.; Gu, J.; He, X.; Huang, S. Circular RNA is enriched and stable in exosomes: A promising biomarker for cancer diagnosis. *Cell Res.* **2015**, *25*, 981–984. [CrossRef]
206. Wiklander, O.P.B.; Nordin, J.Z.; O'Loughlin, A.; Gustafsson, Y.; Corso, G.; Mäger, I.; Vader, P.; Lee, Y.; Sork, H.; Seow, Y.; et al. Extracellular vesicle in vivo biodistribution is determined by cell source, route of administration and targeting. *J. Extracell. Vesicles* **2015**, *4*, 26316. [CrossRef] [PubMed]
207. Johnsen, K.B.; Gudbergsson, J.M.; Skov, M.N.; Pilgaard, L.; Moos, T.; Duroux, M. A comprehensive overview of exosomes as drug delivery vehicles—Endogenous nanocarriers for targeted cancer therapy. *Biochim. Biophys. Acta (BBA) Rev. Cancer* **2014**, *1846*, 75–87. [CrossRef]
208. Ma, J.; Zhang, Y.; Tang, K.; Zhang, H.; Yin, X.; Li, Y.; Xu, P.; Sun, Y.; Ma, R.; Ji, T.; et al. Reversing drug resistance of soft tumor-repopulating cells by tumor cell-derived chemotherapeutic microparticles. *Cell Res.* **2016**, *26*, 713–727. [CrossRef]
209. Parolini, I.; Federici, C.; Raggi, C.; Lugini, L.; Palleschi, S.; De Milito, A.; Coscia, C.; Iessi, E.; Logozzi, M.; Molinari, A.; et al. Microenvironmental pH Is a Key Factor for Exosome Traffic in Tumor Cells. *J. Biol. Chem.* **2009**, *284*, 34211–34222. [CrossRef]

210. Kim, M.S.; Haney, M.J.; Zhao, Y.; Mahajan, V.; Deygen, I.; Klyachko, N.L.; Inskoe, E.; Piroyan, A.; Sokolsky, M.; Okolie, O.; et al. Development of exosome-encapsulated paclitaxel to overcome MDR in cancer cells. *Nanomed. Nanotechnol. Biol. Med.* **2016**, *12*, 655–664. [CrossRef]
211. Qiao, L.; Hu, S.; Huang, K.; Su, T.; Li, Z.; Vandergriff, A.; Cores, J.; Dinh, P.-U.; Allen, T.; Shen, D.; et al. Tumor cell-derived exosomes home to their cells of origin and can be used as Trojan horses to deliver cancer drugs. *Theranostics* **2020**, *10*, 3474–3487. [CrossRef] [PubMed]
212. Hao, D.; Li, Y.; Zhao, G.; Zhang, M. Soluble fms-like tyrosine kinase-1-enriched exosomes suppress the growth of small cell lung cancer by inhibiting endothelial cell migration. *Thorac. Cancer* **2019**, *10*, 1962–1972. [CrossRef] [PubMed]
213. Liu, T.; Zhang, X.; Du, L.; Wang, Y.; Liu, X.; Tian, H.; Wang, L.; Li, P.; Zhao, Y.; Duan, W.; et al. Exosome-transmitted miR-128-3p increase chemosensitivity of oxaliplatin-resistant colorectal cancer. *Mol. Cancer* **2019**, *18*, 43. [CrossRef] [PubMed]
214. Wan, F.-Z.; Chen, K.-H.; Sun, Y.-C.; Chen, X.-C.; Liang, R.-B.; Chen, L.; Zhu, X.-D. Exosomes overexpressing miR-34c inhibit malignant behavior and reverse the radioresistance of nasopharyngeal carcinoma. *J. Transl. Med.* **2020**, *18*, 12. [CrossRef]
215. Kobayashi, M.; Sawada, K.; Miyamoto, M.; Shimizu, A.; Yamamoto, M.; Kinose, Y.; Nakamura, K.; Kawano, M.; Kodama, M.; Hashimoto, K.; et al. Exploring the potential of engineered exosomes as delivery systems for tumor-suppressor microRNA replacement therapy in ovarian cancer. *Biochem. Biophys. Res. Commun.* **2020**, *527*, 153–161. [CrossRef]
216. Tian, H.; Li, W. Dendritic cell-derived exosomes for cancer immunotherapy: Hope and challenges. *Ann. Transl. Med.* **2017**, *5*, 221. [CrossRef]
217. Liu, C.; Guo, J.; Tian, F.; Yang, N.; Yan, F.; Ding, Y.; Wei, J.; Hu, G.; Nie, G.; Sun, J. Field-Free Isolation of Exosomes from Extracellular Vesicles by Microfluidic Viscoelastic Flows. *ACS Nano* **2017**, *11*, 6968–6976. [CrossRef]
218. Chen, T.; Arslan, F.; Yin, Y.; Tan, S.; Lai, R.; Choo, A.; Padmanabhan, J.; Lee, C.; de Kleijn, D.P.; Lim, S. Enabling a robust scalable manufacturing process for therapeutic exosomes through oncogenic immortalization of human ESC-derived MSCs. *J. Transl. Med.* **2011**, *9*, 47. [CrossRef]
219. Lener, T.; Gimona, M.; Aigner, L.; Börger, V.; Buzas, E.; Camussi, G.; Chaput, N.; Chatterjee, D.; Court, F.A.; del Portillo, H.A.; et al. Applying extracellular vesicles based therapeutics in clinical trials—An ISEV position paper. *J. Extracell. Vesicles* **2015**, *4*, 30087. [CrossRef]
220. Nie, W.; Wu, G.; Zhang, J.; Huang, L.; Ding, J.; Jiang, A.; Zhang, Y.; Liu, Y.; Li, J.; Pu, K.; et al. Responsive Exosome Nano-bioconjugates for Synergistic Cancer Therapy. *Angew. Chem. Int. Ed.* **2020**, *59*, 2018–2022. [CrossRef]
221. Yong, T.; Zhang, X.; Bie, N.; Zhang, H.; Zhang, X.; Li, F.; Hakeem, A.; Hu, J.; Gan, L.; Santos, H.A.; et al. Tumor exosome-based nanoparticles are efficient drug carriers for chemotherapy. *Nat. Commun.* **2019**, *10*, 3838. [CrossRef] [PubMed]
222. Bai, L.; Liu, Y.; Guo, K.; Zhang, K.; Liu, Q.; Wang, P.; Wang, X. Ultrasound Facilitates Naturally Equipped Exosomes Derived from Macrophages and Blood Serum for Orthotopic Glioma Treatment. *ACS Appl. Mater. Interfaces* **2019**, *11*, 14576–14587. [CrossRef]
223. Zhang, K.-L.; Wang, Y.-J.; Sun, J.; Zhou, J.; Xing, C.; Huang, G.; Li, J.; Yang, H. Artificial chimeric exosomes for anti-phagocytosis and targeted cancer therapy. *Chem. Sci.* **2019**, *10*, 1555–1561. [CrossRef]
224. Pomatto, M.A.C.; Bussolati, B.; D'Antico, S.; Ghiotto, S.; Tetta, C.; Brizzi, M.F.; Camussi, G. Improved Loading of Plasma-Derived Extracellular Vesicles to Encapsulate Antitumor miRNAs. *Mol. Ther. Methods Clin. Dev.* **2019**, *13*, 133–144. [CrossRef] [PubMed]
225. Gomari, H.; Forouzandeh Moghadam, M.; Soleimani, M. Targeted cancer therapy using engineered exosome as a natural drug delivery vehicle. *OncoTargets Therapy* **2018**, *11*, 5753–5762. [CrossRef] [PubMed]
226. Limoni, S.K.; Moghadam, M.F.; Moazzeni, S.M.; Gomari, H.; Salimi, F. Engineered Exosomes for Targeted Transfer of siRNA to HER2 Positive Breast Cancer Cells. *Appl. Biochem. Biotechnol.* **2019**, *187*, 352–364. [CrossRef]
227. O'Brien, K.P.; Khan, S.; Gilligan, K.E.; Zafar, H.; Lalor, P.; Glynn, C.; O'Flatharta, C.; Ingoldsby, H.; Dockery, P.; De Bhulbh, A.; et al. Employing mesenchymal stem cells to support tumor-targeted delivery of extracellular vesicle (EV)-encapsulated microRNA-379. *Oncogene* **2018**, *37*, 2137–2149. [CrossRef]

228. Kim, M.S.; Haney, M.J.; Zhao, Y.; Yuan, D.; Deygen, I.; Klyachko, N.L.; Kabanov, A.V.; Batrakova, E.V. Engineering macrophage-derived exosomes for targeted paclitaxel delivery to pulmonary metastases: In vitro and in vivo evaluations. *Nanomed. Nanotechnol. Biol. Med.* **2018**, *14*, 195–204. [CrossRef]
229. Kamerkar, S.; LeBleu, V.S.; Sugimoto, H.; Yang, S.; Ruivo, C.F.; Melo, S.A.; Lee, J.J.; Kalluri, R. Exosomes facilitate therapeutic targeting of oncogenic KRAS in pancreatic cancer. *Nature* **2017**, *546*, 498–503. [CrossRef]
230. Bellavia, D.; Raimondo, S.; Calabrese, G.; Forte, S.; Cristaldi, M.; Patinella, A.; Memeo, L.; Manno, M.; Raccosta, S.; Diana, P.; et al. Interleukin 3-receptor targeted exosomes inhibit in vitro and in vivo Chronic Myelogenous Leukemia cell growth. *Theranostics* **2017**, *7*, 1333–1345. [CrossRef]
231. Morishita, M.; Takahashi, Y.; Matsumoto, A.; Nishikawa, M.; Takakura, Y. Exosome-based tumor antigens–adjuvant co-delivery utilizing genetically engineered tumor cell-derived exosomes with immunostimulatory CpG DNA. *Biomaterials* **2016**, *111*, 55–65. [CrossRef] [PubMed]
232. Tian, Y.; Li, S.; Song, J.; Ji, T.; Zhu, M.; Anderson, G.J.; Wei, J.; Nie, G. A doxorubicin delivery platform using engineered natural membrane vesicle exosomes for targeted tumor therapy. *Biomaterials* **2014**, *35*, 2383–2390. [CrossRef] [PubMed]
233. Ohno, S.; Takanashi, M.; Sudo, K.; Ueda, S.; Ishikawa, A.; Matsuyama, N.; Fujita, K.; Mizutani, T.; Ohgi, T.; Ochiya, T.; et al. Systemically Injected Exosomes Targeted to EGFR Deliver Antitumor MicroRNA to Breast Cancer Cells. *Mol. Ther.* **2013**, *21*, 185–191. [CrossRef] [PubMed]

Publisher's Note: MDPI stays neutral with regard to jurisdictional claims in published maps and institutional affiliations.

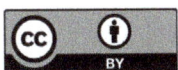

© 2020 by the authors. Licensee MDPI, Basel, Switzerland. This article is an open access article distributed under the terms and conditions of the Creative Commons Attribution (CC BY) license (http://creativecommons.org/licenses/by/4.0/).

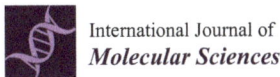

Review

Exosomes in Prostate Cancer Diagnosis, Prognosis and Therapy

Tomasz Lorenc [1,*], Katarzyna Klimczyk [2,3], Izabela Michalczewska [2,3], Monika Słomka [2,3], Grażyna Kubiak-Tomaszewska [2,3] and Wioletta Olejarz [2,3]

1. 1st Department of Clinical Radiology, Medical University of Warsaw, 02-004 Warsaw, Poland
2. Department of Biochemistry and Pharmacogenomics, Faculty of Pharmacy, Medical University of Warsaw, 02-097 Warsaw, Poland; kasiaklimczyk6@gmail.com (K.K.); izabela1356@gmail.com (I.M.); slomka.monika.94@gmail.com (M.S.); grazyna.kubiak-tomaszewska@wum.edu.pl (G.K.-T.); wolejarz@wum.edu.pl (W.O.)
3. Centre for Preclinical Research, Medical University of Warsaw, 02-097 Warsaw, Poland
* Correspondence: tomasz.lorenc@wum.edu.pl

Received: 28 February 2020; Accepted: 17 March 2020; Published: 19 March 2020

Abstract: Prostate cancer (PCa) is the second most common cause of cancer-related mortality among men in the developed world. Conventional anti-PCa therapies are not effective for patients with advanced and/or metastatic disease. In most cases, cancer therapies fail due to an incomplete depletion of tumor cells, resulting in tumor relapse. Exosomes are involved in tumor progression, promoting the angiogenesis and migration of tumor cells during metastasis. These structures contribute to the dissemination of pathogenic agents through interaction with recipient cells. Exosomes may deliver molecules that are able to induce the transdifferentiation process, known as "epithelial to mesenchymal transition". The composition of exosomes and the associated possibilities of interacting with cells make exosomes multifaceted regulators of cancer development. Extracellular vesicles have biophysical properties, such as stability, biocompatibility, permeability, low toxicity and low immunogenicity, which are key for the successful development of an innovative drug delivery system. They have an enhanced circulation stability and bio-barrier permeation ability, and they can therefore be used as effective chemotherapeutic carriers to improve the regulation of target tissues and organs. Exosomes have the capacity to deliver different types of cargo and to target specific cells. Chemotherapeutics, natural products and RNA have been encapsulated for the treatment of prostate cancers.

Keywords: extracellular vesicle; precision oncology; cancer biomarker; prostate cancer

---

1. Introduction

Prostate cancer (PCa) is the most common solid malignancy, with a high mortality in men [1]. In many cases, successful treatment of prostate cancer is difficult due to the late detection and rate of metastasis [2]. Importantly, the tumors of many patients with prostate cancer become refractory to androgen therapy and progress to metastatic castration-resistant disease [3]. An effective treatment course of prostate cancer patients requires predictive biomarkers in metastatic castration-resistant prostate cancer that support individual therapy [4]. Liquid biopsies, circulating tumor cells, exosomes and circulating nucleic acids have been developed as minimally invasive assays to monitor PCa patients [5]. Exosomes are extracellular vesicles (EVs), which may serve as novel tools for various therapeutic approaches, including drug delivery [6], anti-tumor therapy, pathogen vaccination, immune-modulatory and regenerative therapies. They are secreted by cells and detected in various biological fluids, and they can serve as biomarkers for cancer diagnosis, prognosis and therapy [7]. The presence of EVs in urine was discovered in 2004 [8]. It is believed that urinary EVs originate from epithelial cells of the urogenital system, which includes the organs involved in reproduction and urine excretion. Urine has additional advantages relating to cancers of the urogenital system, since the composition of urine directly reflects changes in the function of associated organs. Blood-specific prostate antigen (PSA) remains the most widely used biomarker in the detection of early prostate cancer, but new biomarkers, like exosomal miRNAs, have been proposed to increase specificity and distinguish aggressive from non-aggressive PCas [9]. It has been shown that urinary markers can aid in the decision-making process regarding whether to carry out a prostate biopsy and in the design of a therapeutic strategy [10]. Urinary exosomes and their cargo, especially miR-21 and miR-375, have become an emerging source of biomarkers in the detection and prognosis of PCa [11]. Moreover, the expression of serum exosomal miRNAs induced by radiotherapy may have potential value as prognostic and predictive biomarkers PCa [12]. Exosomes are also promising carriers of drugs and other therapeutic molecules targeting prostate cancer, but there are still several challenges relating to their use as drug carriers [13].

2. Structure and Function of Exosomes

Exosomes are small (from 30 to 120 nm in diameter) extracellular vesicles (EVs) (Figure 1). Their lipid bilayer membrane, with a width of 5 nm, protects them from the negative action of RNases and proteases. Exosomes have a longer retention in circulation in comparison to polymersomes or liposomes [14]. This characteristic originates from transmembrane protein (CD47-SIRPα), which prevents exosomes from being phagocytosed [15]. Moreover, the double membrane structures contain various cargo, such as miRNAs, proteins (e.g., tetraspanin CD63, CD81, CD82, CD53 and CD37, as well as cystolic proteins), lipids (e.g., sphingomyelin, cholesterol and generally saturated fats) and viral particles [16], and their presence depends on the origin cells and organism's health conditions. The proteins in exosomes include endosomal, plasma and nuclear proteins [17]. Therefore, in comparison to cellular proteins in prostate cancer, those in exosomes have a higher level of glycosylation [18]. Moreover, proteins enriched in exosomes include those relevant for individual exosomal biogenesis pathways and for exosome secretion. The Minimal Information for Studies of Extracellular Vesicles 2018 highlights three categories of markers that must be found in isolated extracellular exosomes. They include at least one transmembrane/lipidbound protein or cytosolic protein and one negative protein marker [19]. The cargo present in extracellular vesicles can be transferred and alter signaling pathways in recipient cells [13]. For example, exosomes from metastatic prostate cancer cells showed high contents of miR-21 and miR-141, which are responsible for the regulation of osteoclastogenesis and osteoblastogenesis. Cancer-derived exosomes can promote epithelial–mesenchymal transition (EMT) via miRNAs. They play an important role in the conversion from benign to malignant cancers [13] and in the regulation of the response to docetaxel, such as miR-34 in prostate cancer cells and cell-derived exosomes targeting Bcl-2. This shows the great influence of extracellular vesicles on the drug resistance of prostate cancer cells.

Exosomes are released by the exocytosis of multivesicular bodies (MVBs), developed from early and then late endosomes [20]. Those naturally occurring membrane particles mediate intercellular communication by delivering molecular information between cancer and stromal cells, especially cancer-associated fibroblast (CAFs) [14]. Cancer cell-derived EVs cause very diverse effects and may depend on their target cells, which appear to take them up in several ways, such as receptor/lipid raft endocytosis, phagocytosis, micropinocytosis or fusion with the plasma membrane [17]. Some exosomes can reduce the anti-cancer immune response, interact with specific membrane receptors [9] and promote a suitable microenvironment, while others may cause drug resistance and the failure of antibody therapy involving RNA species and protein delivery [21]. Recent studies point out that exosomes released from the tumor microenvironment can regulate (also by tethering TGFβ) a proliferation, a reduction of apoptosis, a promotion of angiogenesis and, finally, an evasion of immune surveillance (Figure 2). Moreover, exosomes can provide candidate biomarkers for prostate cancer, contribute to tumor progression and, after a loss of environment homeostasis, promote tumor metastasis [18].

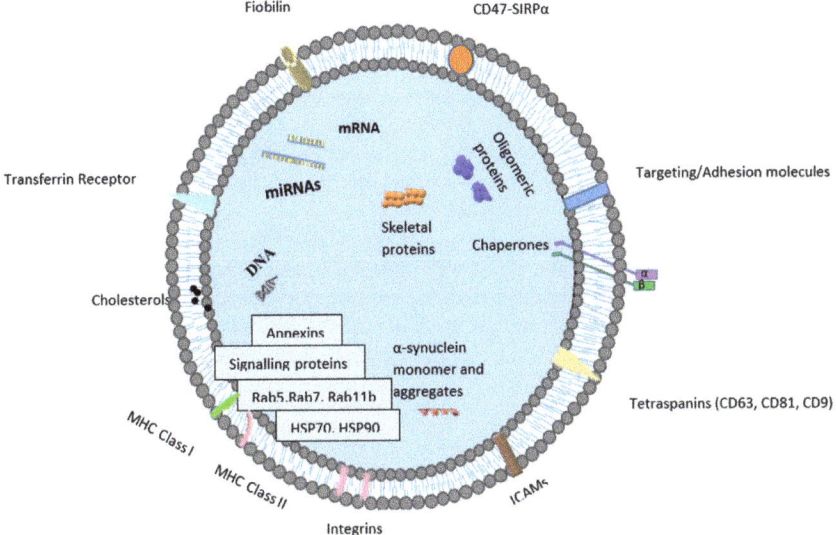

Figure 1. Schematic diagram of an exosome.

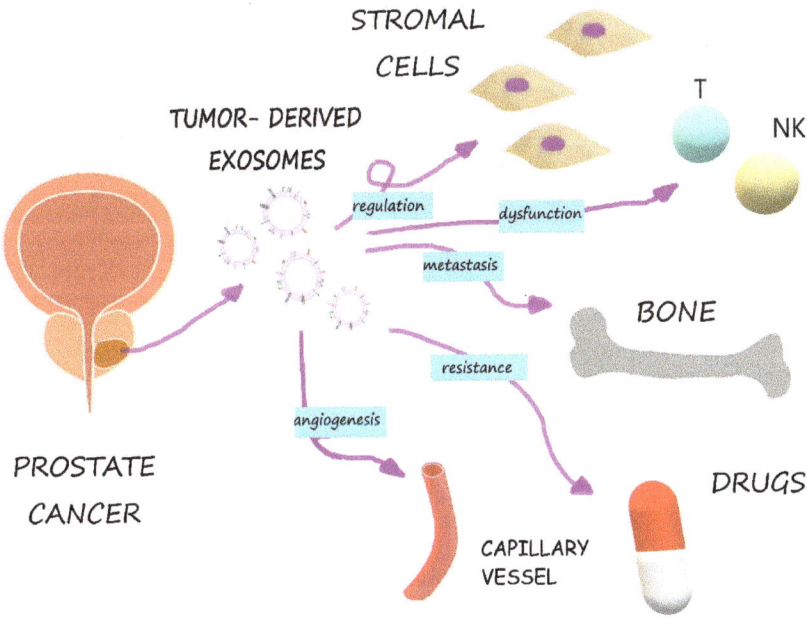

Figure 2. Role of prostate cell-derived exosomes in cancer progression. Exosomes regulate stromal cells, impair immune cells and alter the microenvironment, which could lead to tumor growth and metastasis. Exosomes are also responsible for drug resistance.

3. Tumor-Derived Exosomes in Cancer Progression

3.1. Tumorigenesis

Tumorigenesis or carcinogenesis is the process of an uncontrolled multiplication of cells or deregulated apoptotic cell death, which leads to the formation of cancer. Exosomes derived from prostate cancer cells, which have become the common object of scientists' interest, are implicated in creating a premetastatic niche [13]. It is a microenvironment that is especially favorable to cancer cells composed of different cell types, like fibroblasts, lymphocytes, epithelial cells, matrix molecules, factors, such as growth factors, and cytokines [22]. Exosomes influence the immune system in a premetastatic niche through various mechanisms. Prostate cells are involved in producing tumor-derived secreted factors (TDSFs), including VEGF, TNF-α and interleukins in response to the local inflammatory niche. First, TDSFs stimulate the recruitment of myeloid cells and immune cells to the pre-metastatic niche. Furthermore, the expression of inflammatory factors is upregulated by stromal cells under the influence of TDSFs. Moreover, tumor-derived exosome content enhances the pre-metastatic niche [23]. Tumor exosomes possess the capacity to support the migration of immune cells, like neutrophils, macrophages and regulatory T to secondary sites, thereby reducing immune response against tumors and inhibiting antigen-presenting cells, such as dendritic cells. These nanoparticles could impair the function of T-cells and NK-cells via the blocking, proliferation, activation and provision of apoptosis [23,24].

3.2. Tumor Progression

Recent research suggests that exosomes isolated from the prostate cancer microenvironment are an important factor in the progression of this type of cancer. The increase in the mass of prostate tumors may be the result of tumor stem cell proliferation, which possess a self-renewing ability [13,25]. Prostate cancer exosomes, as the carriers of many lipids, proteins and RNAs, can affect the proliferation, angiogenesis and survival of cancer cells, as well as their ability to avoid immune surveillance [26]. Exosomes, which form in the tumor microenvironment, transport, among other things, miRNAs (miRs, short noncoding RNAs that are responsible for the regulation of gene expression). miR-20a, miR-21 and miR-125b cause the inhibition of apoptosis and survival, promoting the effects of cancer cells. miRNA-221 and miR-222 are responsible for cancer growth. miR-92a and miR-17-92 are involved in the promotion of angiogenesis, as a result of an increased proliferation and migration of endothelial cells. It has been shown that miR-210 is responsible for the induction of metastasis by EMT promotion. miR-21, miR-100 and miR-139 induce fibroblast migration by increasing the expression of MMP-2, MMP-9, MMP-13 and RANKL. miR-21, miR375 and miR-141 overcome low androgen conditions during distant metastasis. miR-1290 and miR-375 are connected with a poor patient prognosis. miR-409 downregulates tumor suppressors, like RSU1 and STAG2, and promotes cancer cell tumorigenesis. The ANXA6/LRP1/TSP1 complex causes tumor growth induction. miR-126 and miR-146a are involved in tumor suppression [27–30]. Moreover, exosomes, with a structure rich in lipids, especially cholesterol and sphingomyelin, can modulate the lipid composition of the target cells, disturbing their homeostasis. A study on prostate cancer has shown that the accumulation of cholesterol esters in prostate cancer cells is associated with tumor progression and metastasis. This was confirmed by studies, using synthetic exosomes carried out by the Lombardo Group, which showed that exosomal lipids can increase the tumor aggressiveness, metastatic progression and drug resistance of pancreatic cancer cells [31].

It is well known that exosomes secreted by prostate cancer cells under hypoxic conditions increase the invasiveness, mobility and EMT in native PC cells and promote the transformation of fibroblasts into myofibroblasts. Moreover, under these conditions, lipid accumulation (triglycerides, bis-monoacylglycerolphosphate, ceramides, cholesterol, etc.) increase in PCs, which leads to increased exosome secretion by hypoxic tumor cells [32].

Exosomes also participate in the regulation of the progression of prostatic tumors, as the carriers of numerous proteins. These vesicular structures, as carriers of TGF-β, can induce the above-mentioned transformation of fibroblasts into myofibroblasts (CAFs) by the activation of TGF-β/Smad3 signaling or independent SMAD signaling pathways and promote neoangiogenesis. Webber found that exosomal TGFβ1 induces a highly aggressive myofibroblast phenotype, with a high proangiogenic activity [13,33]. ITGA3, ITGB1, ITGB4 and ITGB3 are exosomal proteins involved in the progression of prostate cancers. These integrins are responsible for the promotion of the migration and invasion of epithelial cells by the activation of Src phosphorylation in recipient cells. The matrix metalloproteinases MMP-9 and MMP-14 promote cancer cell protection from apoptosis and intensify their mobility through the stimulation of ERK1/2 phosphorylation. Subsequently, they prepare the metastatic site [26,27]. The next group, ligands for the NKG2D and Fas receptors, causes tumor immune evasion by receptor downregulation and silences the cytotoxic activity of NK cells and CD8+ cells. Caveolin-1 increases the survival of cancer cells and their independence from androgens, and they also promote distant metastasis by the positive regulation of fatty acid synthase activity. Hypoxia-inducible factor 1α (HIF-1α) promotes the initiation and progression of metastasis by promoting the loss of E-cadherin. The tetraspanin–integrin complex increases the adhesion of exosomes to the right cells. The epidermal growth factor receptor (EGFR) induces tumor angiogenesis by the activation of the autocrine VEGF/VEGFR-2 pathway in endothelial cells. Tyrosine-protein kinase Met induces metastasis and promotes a phenotype resistant to castration therapy. Other exosomal proteins, c-Src tyrosine kinase, IGF-1R and FAK, induce angiogenesis by the stimulation of the VEGF transcription within the tumor microenvironment [34–39].

It has also been shown that tumor-derived exosomes enhance interleukin-6 production in myeloid-derived suppressor cells through the activation of Toll-like receptor 2 via the membrane-linked heat shock protein, which promotes the autocrine phosphorylation of Stat3 and enhances the effect of the immunosuppression of the immune system and the promotion of prostate cancer [40].

Exosomes secreted by prostate cancer cells are also involved in tumor metastasis in bone, which is common in patients with this type of cancer. Recent studies have shown that prostate cancer cell-derived exosomes mediate cell–cell communication in osteoblastic metastasis. On the other hand, osteoblast-derived exosomes may regulate prostate cancer cell proliferation at the original site of tumor development [41].

Exosomes secreted by tumor cells affect the stromal cells by stimulating the formation of pro-proliferative and proangiogenic phenotypes in these cells. It has been shown that exosomes secreted by cancer-associated fibroblasts increase the ability of prostate cancer cells to proliferate and survive in low-oxygen and low-nutrient environments by inhibiting mitochondrial oxidative phosphorylation and increasing anaerobic glycolysis [33,42].

3.3. Angiogenesis

Exosomes obtained from prostate cancer stem cells support tumorigenesis by promoting angiogenesis, which, as a process of developing a new vasculature, is crucial for tumor growth and migrations and is the main cause of metastasis and malignancy. A recent report has shown that some conditions, like hypoxia or acidosis, enhance secreting exosomes in bodily fluids, and these exosomes cause angiogenesis more frequently [30]. Studies have also reported that the expression of E-cadherin and carbonic anhydrase 9 in exosomes could contribute to the angiogenesis process [43]. In the case of prostate cancer, the process of vascularization is supported by the transfer of sphingomyelin and CD147 via exosomes into endothelial cells [44]. Newly formed blood vessels are created to facilitate tumor growth by transporting TDSFs and circulating tumor cells (CTCs) into secondary tissues, thereby beginning vascular leakage [23]. Prostate cancer cell-derived exosomes, via the activation of TGF-β\SMAD3 signaling, lead to the transformation of fibroblasts into myofibroblasts, referred to as CAFs. The exosomes derived from these special kinds of cells are able to cause an explosive growth of prostate cancer cells by transferring the miRNAs (miR-21 and miR-409) into neighboring epithelia. miR-21 suppresses the expression of APAF1 (apoptotic peptidase activating factor 1) and PDCD4 (programmed cell death 4) to inhibit apoptosis and make cancer cells resistant to chemotherapeutics [13]. Increased angiogenesis and vascular permeability promote metastasis.

3.4. Metastasis

Tumor metastasis is a complicated process, including vascular leakiness and an alteration of the microenvironment, in which exosomes are also involved. Initially, exosomes begin an epithelial–mesenchymal transition (EMT) via miRNAs by losing their junction and adhesion ability. Thus, epithelial tumor cells obtain mesenchymal cell properties and are responsive to malignancy [45].

Exosomes support the formation of a pre-metastatic niche, and cells could then be found at the vascularized organs, but metastasis cannot be developed randomly, but rather only in preferential sites under the direction of exosomes. In the process of this expansion, the special kind of CTCs (metastases-initiating cells (MICs)) are involved [46]. MICs can act on other cells by secreting exosomes that reprogram adjacent stromal cells to create a more favorable tumor microenvironment in order to support cancer growth and progression. As mentioned above, cancer-derived exosomes determine organotropism. Prostate cancer possesses an affinity with bone. Exosomes obtained from prostate cancer cells by osteoclast fusion and differentiation support transmission to this destination [47]. Furthermore, exosomes derived therefrom, through the activation of RANKL, FOXM1 and c-Myc, support EMT [46]. As described previously, cancer cell-derived exosomes transfer various substances, including integrins, which are responsible for organotropism. Integrin σ3 and β1 lead to the migration and dissemination of epithelial cells. In addition, integrin avb6, expressed on the surface, is responsible for the metastatic phenotype [48]. The tumor microenvironment contributes to the regulation of prostate cancer progression through proliferation, angiogenesis and metastasis, and it also regulates immunity.

3.5. Tumor Immune Escape

The immune system is able to recognize transformed cells and eliminate them. Thus, tumors use diverse mechanisms to escape from immune-mediated surveillance. Exosomes derived from prostate cancer cells impair the cytotoxic function of lymphocytes and induce the apoptosis of CD8+ T cells [23]. In the first step, exosomes activate the T cell receptor, and the expression of Fas on the T cell is then upregulated. Subsequently, FasL induces apoptosis directly via receptor CD 95/APO1 or indirectly using dendritic cells [49]. Fas-mediated apoptosis, as an immune-evasive mechanism, may lead to tumorigenesis, but it may also be responsible for drug resistance [49]. Some other mechanisms and molecules may also contribute to T cell apoptosis. Among the substances carried by exosomes is the programmed death ligand 1 (PDL-1). Exosomal PDL-1 plays the same role as tumor PDL-1. PDL-1 binds to its receptor, PD-1, expressed on the surface of activated T and B cells or macrophages, and enables T cell apoptosis [50]. On the other hand, cancer-derived exosomes can not only cause the dysfunction of T and NK cells by blocking the activation and proliferation or induction of apoptosis, but also inhibit antigen-presenting cells and antitumor immune response [23]. While exosomes are characterized by heterogeneity and a risk of developing metastasis, those nanoparticles could be used as diagnostic and prognostic biomarkers for various cancers and as promising drug carriers.

4. The Potential of Exosomes in Prostate Cancer Diagnosis and Monitoring

EVs may be key biomarkers in the early diagnosis of prostate cancer and in a personalized approach to treatment and to future patients' prognosis [26]. EVs in the blood and urine of prostate cancer patients contain unique prostate-cancer-specific contents, which are biomarkers of prostate cancer and cancer metastasis [51,52]. Exosomes present many different proteins on their surface. These proteins can act as epitopes, which are recognized using different mono- or polyclonal antibodies. A dedicated assay has been established to determine if the exosomes in blood plasma can serve as markers for prostate cancer [51]. Additionally, several EV-derived proteins have been investigated as potential cancer biomarkers in clinical settings [53]. Several urinary exosome proteins showed a high sensitivity and specificity for prostate cancer as individual biomarkers, and combining them in a multi-panel test has the potential for a full differentiation of prostate cancer from non-disease controls [52]. Liu et al. showed that exosomes from prostate cancer are highly enriched with PSA, representing characteristics of the original PCa cells [54]. Current evidence indicates that the strongest candidates for intercellular communications in PCa are exosomal RNAs [55]. The EV-derived RNAs have also been assessed in terms of their potential as cancer biomarkers in clinical samples. Yang et al. confirmed, through meta-analysis, that plasma exosomal miRNAs have a high diagnostic value for prostate cancer patients [56]. Hessvik et al. identified 36 exosomal miRNAs as biomarker candidates for PCa in clinical studies [57]. In prostate cancer, plasma vesicles, isolated using the precipitation-based ExoQuick method, identified miR-1290 and miR-375 as potential prognostic biomarkers in castration-resistant prostate cancer (CRPC), since their level correlates with a poorer overall survival ($p < 0.004$) [58,59]. Joncas et al. demonstrated that the exosomal androgen receptor splice variant (AR-V7) is correlated with lower sex steroid levels and with a poor prognosis in CRPC patients [60]. For prostate cancer, the expression of the AR-V7 RNA in CTCs was identified as a predictive marker for response to enzalutamide (anti-androgen) and abiraterone (anti-androgen and CYP17 inhibitor) [61]. Whether the AR-V7 transcript can also be measured in plasma EVs and serve as a biomarker was investigated by Del Re et al. [62]. Using the exoRNeasy purification method, EV-RNA was extracted, and the AR-V7 transcript was detected, preferentially in patients resistant to enzalutamide or abiraterone treatment. This study, as well as other studies, shows the biomarker potential of plasma-derived EV-RNA and the advantages with respect to the cost, ease of workflow and likelihood that all (heterogeneous) tumors are represented by a specific EV population. Communication between a tumor and its environment in PCa via extracellular vesicle (EV) RNAs is a potential mechanism of bone metastasis [63]. It has been shown that exosomal miR-375 significantly promoted osteoblast activity [64]. Krishn et al. proved that prostate cancer sheds the $\alpha v \beta 3$ integrin in vivo through exosomes. The exosomal $\alpha v \beta 3$ integrin has been shown to promote aggressive phenotypes in many types of cancers and may be clinically useful as a non-invasive biomarker to follow prostate cancer progression [65]. Another paper has reported survivin as a plasma-derived EV biomarker through the isolation of total EVs by the ultracentrifugation-based method for prostate cancer [66]. It has been shown that exosomes released by irradiated prostate cancer cells are enriched in B7-H3 protein (CD276), which has been identified as a diagnostic marker [67]. Furthermore, the serum exosomes of prostate cancer patients undergoing radiotherapy had increased levels of HSP72, which plays a key role in the stimulation of pro-inflammatory immune responses [68]. Additionally, urinary exosomes are a promising non-invasive biomarker, with a potential use in the diagnosis, prognosis and monitoring of prostate cancer [69].

5. The Potential of Exosomes in Prostate Cancer Therapy

5.1. Exosomes as Drug Carriers for Prostate Cancer Therapy

Extracellular vesicles have biophysical properties, such as stability, biocompatibility, permeability, low toxicity and low immunogenicity, which are key to successful drug delivery systems [70]. They have an enhanced circulation stability and bio-barrier permeation ability, and they can therefore be used as effective chemotherapeutics carriers to improve the regulation of target tissues and organs [71]. Chemotherapeutics, natural products and RNA were combined for the treatment of prostate, breast, pancreatic, and lung cancers, as well as glioblastoma [14]. Exosomes have the capacity to deliver different types of cargo and to target specific cells (Figure 3). They have been tested for the delivery of different therapeutic agents in in vitro and in vivo experiments [72]. EVs can be used as carriers to deliver therapeutic agents to tumor cells, leading to an effective tumor cell killing, while minimizing the side effects of the drugs [73]. It has been shown that mesenchymal stromal cells are able to package and deliver active drugs through their membrane microvesicles (MVs) [74]. Additionally, Tian et al. demonstrated that exosomes modified by targeting ligands can be used therapeutically for the delivery of doxorubicin to tumors [75]. Additionally, Qi et al. confirmed that drug-loaded exosomes enhanced cancer cell targeting under an external magnetic field and suppressed tumor growth [76]. Saari et al. confirmed that cancer cell-derived EVs can be used as effective carriers of Paclitaxel to autologous prostate cancer cells by increasing its cytotoxicity [21]. The simultaneous application of either radiation technology or nuclear medicine with exosomes are promising tools for the realization of the enhancement of targeting strategies using radiation technology [77].

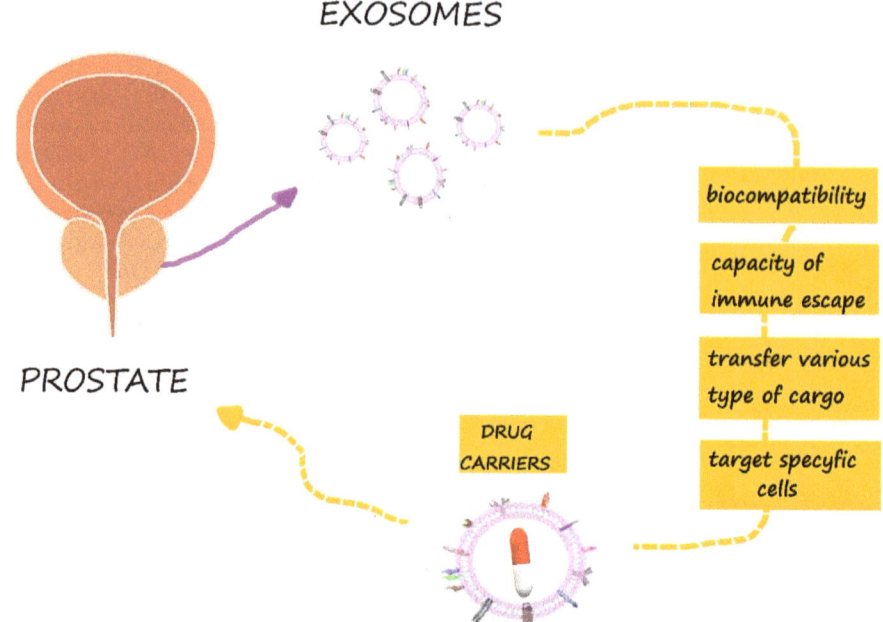

Figure 3. Exosomes are promising drug carriers in prostate cancer therapy.

5.2. Precision Therapy

Exosomes have been shown to be crucial for the development of drug resistance in patients with prostate tumor. In 2017, Del Re et al. assessed AR-V7 as a predictor of resistance to hormonal therapy by highly sensitive digital droplet polymerase chain reaction in plasma-derived exosomal RNA. They found that both the median progression-free survival (20 vs. 3 months; $p < 0.001$) and overall survival (8 months vs. not reached; $p < 0.001$) were significantly longer in AR-V7-negative vs. AR-V7-positive patients [62]. Exosome-derived microRNAs also contribute to PCa chemoresistance [78] and can act as surrogate biomarkers of tumor response to taxanes [79]. It has been observed that the transfer of exosomes (in particular, MDR-1/P-gp) from docetaxel-resistant cell lines to the DU145, 22Rv1, and LNCap PCa cell lines induces an acquired resistance to this drug [80]. In the same view, Kawakami et al. reported that β4 (ITGB4) and VCL in exosomes could be useful markers of PCa progression, which is correlated with taxane resistance [81]. Interestingly, high serum exosomal P-glycoprotein levels are associated with resistance to docetaxel, but not to cabazitaxel, thus representing a potential biomarker for guiding the decision-making process of PCa patients [82].

There is currently also a list of challenges that remain in the era of individualized or person-specific targeting of cancer. EVs are being pursued as intercellular vectors for RNA-based therapy (both miRNAs and siRNAs), with a documented efficacy in animal models of disease. For example, the in vivo suppression of prostate cancer has been achieved through the exosome delivery of the tumor suppressor miRNA, miR-143, in mice [83].

6. Concluding Remarks and Future Directions

Increasingly, studies confirm the potential of exosomes as therapeutic vehicles for cancer treatment. Exosomes can transfer cargos with both an immunoregulatory potential and genetic information. They can decrease tumor cell invasion, migration and proliferation by enhancing immune response, cell death and sensitivity to chemotherapy. Exosomes have a high potential for both as diagnostic and therapeutic agents in immune therapy, vaccination trials and regenerative medicine. The native structure and unique cellular functions of exosomes give them a great potential as natural drug/gene delivery vehicles, but developing efficient and reliable isolation methods is necessary to fully utilize their potential [84]. The use of exosomes in clinical applications must be further investigated in order to establish standards for exosome characterization and manipulation [85]. The most important thing is to choose optimal methods for engineering exosomes and ensuring the safety of engineered exosomes in clinical trials [86]. Furthermore, the translation of EVs into clinical therapies requires their categorization as active drug components or drug delivery vehicles [6]. It is also necessary to clarify the composition and action mechanism of the various substances in exosomes and determine how to obtain highly purified exosomes and the right dosage for their clinical use [15]. Another important therapeutic use of EVs could be cancer vaccination [87]. In brief, exosomes are very promising tools for the future theranostics of prostate cancer, but their use first requires solutions for the many challenging issues remaining.

Funding: This research received no external funding.

Conflicts of Interest: The authors declare no conflicts of interest.

Abbreviations

APAF1	apoptotic peptidase-activating factor 1
AR-V7	androgen receptor variant 7
CAFs	cancer-associated fibroblast
CRPC	castrate-resistant prostate cancer
CTCs	circulating tumor cells
EGFR	epidermal growth factor receptor
EMT	epithelial–mesenchymal transition
EV	extracellular vesicles
FASL	ligand Fas
HIF-1α	hypoxia-inducible factor 1α
HSP	heat shock proteins
ITGB4	integrin β4
MICs	metastases-initiating cells
miR	micro RNA
MMP	matrix metalloproteinase
MVBs	multivesicular bodies
PCa	prostate cancer
PDCD4	programmed cell death 4
PDL-1	programmed death ligand 1
PSA	prostate specific antigen
RANKL	receptor activator for nuclear factor κB ligand
RSU1	Ras suppressor protein 1
siRNA	small interfering RNA
STAG2	cohesin subunit SA-2
TDSFs	tumor-derived secreted factors
TGFβ	transforming growth factor β
VCL	vinculin

References

1. Siegel, R.L.; Miller, K.D.; Jemal, A. Cancer statistics, 2019. *CA Cancer J. Clin.* **2019**, *69*, 7–34. [CrossRef]
2. Kim, S.J.; Kim, S.I. Current treatment strategies for castration-resistant prostate cancer. *Korean J. Urol.* **2011**, *52*, 157–165. [CrossRef] [PubMed]
3. Ingrosso, G.; Detti, B.; Scartoni, D.; Lancia, A.; Giacomelli, I.; Baki, M.; Carta, G.; Livi, L.; Santoni, R. Current therapeutic options in metastatic castration-resistant prostate cancer. *Semin. Oncol.* **2018**, *45*, 303–315. [PubMed]

4. Kretschmer, A.; Tilki, D. Biomarkers in prostate cancer—Current clinical utility and future perspectives. *Crit. Rev. Oncol. Hematol.* **2017**, *120*, 180–193. [CrossRef] [PubMed]
5. Lu, Y.T.; Delijani, K.; Mecum, A.; Goldkorn, A. Current status of liquid biopsies for the detection and management of prostate cancer. *Cancer Manag. Res.* **2019**, *11*, 5271–5291. [CrossRef]
6. Lener, T.; Gimona, M.; Aigner, L.; Borger, V.; Buzas, E.; Camussi, G.; Chaput, N.; Chatterjee, D.; Court, F.A.; Del Portillo, H.A.; et al. Applying extracellular vesicles based therapeutics in clinical trials—An ISEV position paper. *J. Extracell. Vesicles* **2015**, *4*, 30087. [CrossRef]
7. Jiang, L.; Gu, Y.; Du, Y.; Liu, J. Exosomes: Diagnostic Biomarkers and Therapeutic Delivery Vehicles for Cancer. *Mol. Pharm.* **2019**, *16*, 3333–3349. [CrossRef] [PubMed]
8. Pisitkun, T.; Shen, R.F.; Knepper, M.A. Identification and proteomic profiling of exosomes in human urine. *Proc. Natl. Acad. Sci. USA* **2004**, *101*, 13368–13373. [CrossRef] [PubMed]
9. Filella, X.; Foj, L. Prostate Cancer Detection and Prognosis: From Prostate Specific Antigen (PSA) to Exosomal Biomarkers. *Int. J. Mol. Sci.* **2016**, *17*, 1784. [CrossRef]
10. Fujita, K.; Nonomura, N. Urinary biomarkers of prostate cancer. *Int. J. Urol.* **2018**, *25*, 770–779. [CrossRef]
11. Foj, L.; Ferrer, F.; Serra, M.; Arevalo, A.; Gavagnach, M.; Gimenez, N.; Filella, X. Exosomal and Non-Exosomal Urinary miRNAs in Prostate Cancer Detection and Prognosis. *Prostate* **2017**, *77*, 573–583. [CrossRef] [PubMed]
12. Malla, B.; Aebersold, D.M.; Pra, A.D. Protocol for serum exosomal miRNAs analysis in prostate cancer patients treated with radiotherapy. *J. Transl. Med.* **2018**, *16*, 223. [CrossRef] [PubMed]
13. Pan, J.; Ding, M.; Xu, K.; Yang, C.; Mao, L.J. Exosomes in diagnosis and therapy of prostate cancer. *Oncotarget* **2017**, *8*, 97693–97700. [CrossRef] [PubMed]
14. Pullan, J.E.; Confeld, M.I.; Osborn, J.K.; Kim, J.; Sarkar, K.; Mallik, S. Exosomes as Drug Carriers for Cancer Therapy. *Mol. Pharm.* **2019**, *16*, 1789–1798. [CrossRef] [PubMed]
15. Di, C.; Zhang, Q.; Wang, Y.; Wang, F.; Chen, Y.; Gan, L.; Zhou, R.; Sun, C.; Li, H.; Zhang, X.; et al. Exosomes as drug carriers for clinical application. *Artif. Cells Nanomed. Biotechnol.* **2018**, *46*, S564–S570. [CrossRef]
16. Qin, J.; Xu, A.Q. Functions and application of exosomes. *Acta Pol. Pharm.* **2014**, *71*, 537–543.
17. Guo, W.; Gao, Y.; Li, N.; Shao, F.; Wang, C.; Wang, P.; Yang, Z.; Li, R.; He, J. Exosomes: New players in cancer (Review). *Oncol. Rep.* **2017**, *38*, 665–675. [CrossRef]
18. Liu, C.M.; Hsieh, C.L.; Shen, C.N.; Lin, C.C.; Shigemura, K.; Sung, S.Y. Exosomes from the tumor microenvironment as reciprocal regulators that enhance prostate cancer progression. *Int. J. Urol.* **2016**, *23*, 734–744. [CrossRef]
19. Thery, C.; Witwer, K.W.; Aikawa, E.; Alcaraz, M.J.; Anderson, J.D.; Andriantsitohaina, R.; Antoniou, A.; Arab, T.; Archer, F.; Atkin-Smith, G.K.; et al. Minimal information for studies of extracellular vesicles 2018 (MISEV2018): A position statement of the International Society for Extracellular Vesicles and update of the MISEV2014 guidelines. *J. Extracell. Vesicles* **2018**, *7*, 1535750. [CrossRef]
20. Panigrahi, G.K.; Deep, G. Exosomes-based biomarker discovery for diagnosis and prognosis of prostate cancer. *Front. Biosci.* **2017**, *22*, 1682–1696.
21. Saari, H.; Lazaro-Ibanez, E.; Viitala, T.; Vuorimaa-Laukkanen, E.; Siljander, P.; Yliperttula, M. Microvesicle- and exosome-mediated drug delivery enhances the cytotoxicity of Paclitaxel in autologous prostate cancer cells. *J. Control. Release* **2015**, *220*, 727–737. [CrossRef] [PubMed]
22. Egeblad, M.; Nakasone, E.S.; Werb, Z. Tumors as organs: Complex tissues that interface with the entire organism. *Dev. Cell* **2010**, *18*, 884–901. [CrossRef] [PubMed]
23. Guo, Y.; Ji, X.; Liu, J.; Fan, D.; Zhou, Q.; Chen, C.; Wang, W.; Wang, G.; Wang, H.; Yuan, W.; et al. Effects of exosomes on pre-metastatic niche formation in tumors. *Mol. Cancer* **2019**, *18*, 39. [CrossRef] [PubMed]
24. Liu, Y.; Xiang, X.; Zhuang, X.; Zhang, S.; Liu, C.; Cheng, Z.; Michalek, S.; Grizzle, W.; Zhang, H.G. Contribution of MyD88 to the tumor exosome-mediated induction of myeloid derived suppressor cells. *Am. J. Pathol.* **2010**, *176*, 2490–2499. [CrossRef] [PubMed]
25. Alzahrani, F.A.; El-Magd, M.A.; Abdelfattah-Hassan, A.; Saleh, A.A.; Saadeldin, I.M.; El-Shetry, E.S.; Badawy, A.A.; Alkarim, S. Potential Effect of Exosomes Derived from Cancer Stem Cells and MSCs on Progression of DEN-Induced HCC in Rats. *Stem Cells Int.* **2018**, *2018*, 8058763. [CrossRef] [PubMed]
26. Vlaeminck-Guillem, V. Extracellular Vesicles in Prostate Cancer Carcinogenesis, Diagnosis, and Management. *Front. Oncol.* **2018**, *8*, 222. [CrossRef]

27. Giusti, I.; Dolo, V. Extracellular vesicles in prostate cancer: New future clinical strategies? *Biomed. Res. Int.* **2014**, *2014*, 561571. [CrossRef]
28. Umezu, T.; Ohyashiki, K.; Kuroda, M.; Ohyashiki, J.H. Leukemia cell to endothelial cell communication via exosomal miRNAs. *Oncogene* **2013**, *32*, 2747–2755. [CrossRef]
29. Wang, Z.; Tan, Y.; Yu, W.; Zheng, S.; Zhang, S.; Sun, L.; Ding, K. Small role with big impact: miRNAs as communicators in the cross-talk between cancer-associated fibroblasts and cancer cells. *Int. J. Biol. Sci.* **2017**, *13*, 339–348. [CrossRef]
30. Mashouri, L.; Yousefi, H.; Aref, A.R.; Ahadi, A.M.; Molaei, F.; Alahari, S.K. Exosomes: Composition, biogenesis, and mechanisms in cancer metastasis and drug resistance. *Mol. Cancer* **2019**, *18*, 75. [CrossRef] [PubMed]
31. Brzozowski, J.S.; Jankowski, H.; Bond, D.R.; McCague, S.B.; Munro, B.R.; Predebon, M.J.; Scarlett, C.J.; Skelding, K.A. Lipidomic profiling of extracellular vesicles derived from prostate and prostate cancer cell lines. *Lipids Health Dis.* **2018**, *17*, 211. [CrossRef] [PubMed]
32. Deep, G.; Schlaepfer, I.R. Aberrant Lipid Metabolism Promotes Prostate Cancer: Role in Cell Survival under Hypoxia and Extracellular Vesicles Biogenesis. *Int. J. Mol. Sci.* **2016**, *17*, 1061. [CrossRef] [PubMed]
33. Webber, J.P.; Spary, L.K.; Sanders, A.J.; Chowdhury, R.; Jiang, W.G.; Steadman, R.; Wymant, J.; Jones, A.T.; Kynaston, H.; Mason, M.D.; et al. Differentiation of tumour-promoting stromal myofibroblasts by cancer exosomes. *Oncogene* **2015**, *34*, 290–302. [CrossRef] [PubMed]
34. Bellezza, I.; Aisa, M.C.; Palazzo, R.; Costanzi, E.; Mearini, E.; Minelli, A. Extracellular matrix degrading enzymes at the prostasome surface. *Prostate Cancer Prostatic Dis.* **2005**, *8*, 344–348. [CrossRef] [PubMed]
35. Di Vizio, D.; Sotgia, F.; Williams, T.M.; Hassan, G.S.; Capozza, F.; Frank, P.G.; Pestell, R.G.; Loda, M.; Freeman, M.R.; Lisanti, M.P. Caveolin-1 is required for the upregulation of fatty acid synthase (FASN), a tumor promoter, during prostate cancer progression. *Cancer Biol. Ther.* **2007**, *6*, 1263–1268. [CrossRef]
36. Wu, M.; Wang, G.; Hu, W.; Yao, Y.; Yu, X.F. Emerging roles and therapeutic value of exosomes in cancer metastasis. *Mol. Cancer* **2019**, *18*, 53. [CrossRef]
37. Conigliaro, A.; Cicchini, C. Exosome-Mediated Signaling in Epithelial to Mesenchymal Transition and Tumor Progression. *J. Clin. Med.* **2018**, *8*, 26. [CrossRef]
38. Tian, W.; Liu, S.; Li, B. Potential Role of Exosomes in Cancer Metastasis. *Biomed. Res. Int.* **2019**, *2019*, 4649705. [CrossRef]
39. Lopez, T.; Hanahan, D. Elevated levels of IGF-1 receptor convey invasive and metastatic capability in a mouse model of pancreatic islet tumorigenesis. *Cancer Cell* **2002**, *1*, 339–353. [CrossRef]
40. Chalmin, F.; Ladoire, S.; Mignot, G.; Vincent, J.; Bruchard, M.; Remy-Martin, J.P.; Boireau, W.; Rouleau, A.; Simon, B.; Lanneau, D.; et al. Membrane-associated Hsp72 from tumor-derived exosomes mediates STAT3-dependent immunosuppressive function of mouse and human myeloid-derived suppressor cells. *J. Clin. Invest.* **2010**, *120*, 457–471. [CrossRef]
41. Li, F.X.; Liu, J.J.; Xu, F.; Lin, X.; Zhong, J.Y.; Wu, F.; Yuan, L.Q. Role of tumor-derived exosomes in bone metastasis. *Oncol. Lett.* **2019**, *18*, 3935–3945. [CrossRef] [PubMed]
42. Vander Heiden, M.G.; Cantley, L.C.; Thompson, C.B. Understanding the Warburg effect: The metabolic requirements of cell proliferation. *Science* **2009**, *324*, 1029–1033. [CrossRef] [PubMed]
43. Tang, M.K.S.; Yue, P.Y.K.; Ip, P.P.; Huang, R.L.; Lai, H.C.; Cheung, A.N.Y.; Tse, K.Y.; Ngan, H.Y.S.; Wong, A.S.T. Soluble E-cadherin promotes tumor angiogenesis and localizes to exosome surface. *Nat. Commun.* **2018**, *9*, 2270. [CrossRef] [PubMed]
44. Naito, Y.; Yoshioka, Y.; Yamamoto, Y.; Ochiya, T. How cancer cells dictate their microenvironment: Present roles of extracellular vesicles. *Cell Mol. Life Sci.* **2017**, *74*, 697–713. [CrossRef]
45. Roma-Rodrigues, C.; Mendes, R.; Baptista, P.; Fernandes, A. Targeting Tumor Microenvironment for Cancer Therapy. *Int. J. Mol. Sci.* **2019**, *20*, 840. [CrossRef]
46. Shiao, S.L.; Chu, G.C.; Chung, L.W. Regulation of prostate cancer progression by the tumor microenvironment. *Cancer Lett.* **2016**, *380*, 340–348. [CrossRef]
47. Karlsson, T.; Lundholm, M.; Widmark, A.; Persson, E. Tumor Cell-Derived Exosomes from the Prostate Cancer Cell Line TRAMP-C1 Impair Osteoclast Formation and Differentiation. *PLoS ONE* **2016**, *11*, e0166284. [CrossRef]

48. Bijnsdorp, I.V.; Geldof, A.A.; Lavaei, M.; Piersma, S.R.; van Moorselaar, R.J.; Jimenez, C.R. Exosomal ITGA3 interferes with non-cancerous prostate cell functions and is increased in urine exosomes of metastatic prostate cancer patients. *J. Extracell. Vesicles* **2013**, *2*. [CrossRef]
49. Ichim, T.E.; Zhong, Z.; Kaushal, S.; Zheng, X.; Ren, X.; Hao, X.; Joyce, J.A.; Hanley, H.H.; Riordan, N.H.; Koropatnick, J.; et al. Exosomes as a tumor immune escape mechanism: Possible therapeutic implications. *J. Transl. Med.* **2008**, *6*, 37. [CrossRef]
50. Chen, G.; Huang, A.C.; Zhang, W.; Zhang, G.; Wu, M.; Xu, W.; Yu, Z.; Yang, J.; Wang, B.; Sun, H.; et al. Exosomal PD-L1 contributes to immunosuppression and is associated with anti-PD-1 response. *Nature* **2018**, *560*, 382–386. [CrossRef]
51. Tavoosidana, G.; Ronquist, G.; Darmanis, S.; Yan, J.; Carlsson, L.; Wu, D.; Conze, T.; Ek, P.; Semjonow, A.; Eltze, E.; et al. Multiple recognition assay reveals prostasomes as promising plasma biomarkers for prostate cancer. *Proc. Natl. Acad. Sci. USA* **2011**, *108*, 8809–8814. [CrossRef] [PubMed]
52. Overbye, A.; Skotland, T.; Koehler, C.J.; Thiede, B.; Seierstad, T.; Berge, V.; Sandvig, K.; Llorente, A. Identification of prostate cancer biomarkers in urinary exosomes. *Oncotarget* **2015**, *6*, 30357–30376. [CrossRef] [PubMed]
53. Soekmadji, C.; Corcoran, N.M.; Oleinikova, I.; Jovanovic, L. Extracellular vesicles for personalized therapy decision support in advanced metastatic cancers and its potential impact for prostate cancer. *Prostate* **2017**, *77*, 1416–1423. [CrossRef] [PubMed]
54. Liu, T.; Mendes, D.E.; Berkman, C.E. Functional prostate-specific membrane antigen is enriched in exosomes from prostate cancer cells. *Int. J. Oncol.* **2014**, *44*, 918–922. [CrossRef] [PubMed]
55. Soekmadji, C.; Russell, P.J.; Nelson, C.C. Exosomes in prostate cancer: Putting together the pieces of a puzzle. *Cancers* **2013**, *5*, 1522–1544. [CrossRef]
56. Yang, B.; Xiong, W.Y.; Hou, H.J.; Xu, Q.; Cai, X.L.; Zeng, T.X.; Ha, X.Q. Exosomal miRNAs as Biomarkers of Cancer: A Meta-Analysis. *Clin. Lab.* **2019**. [CrossRef]
57. Hessvik, N.P.; Sandvig, K.; Llorente, A. Exosomal miRNAs as Biomarkers for Prostate Cancer. *Front. Genet.* **2013**, *4*, 36. [CrossRef]
58. Huang, X.; Yuan, T.; Tschannen, M.; Sun, Z.; Jacob, H.; Du, M.; Liang, M.; Dittmar, R.L.; Liu, Y.; Liang, M.; et al. Characterization of human plasma-derived exosomal RNAs by deep sequencing. *BMC Genomics* **2013**, *14*, 319. [CrossRef]
59. Huang, X.; Yuan, T.; Liang, M.; Du, M.; Xia, S.; Dittmar, R.; Wang, D.; See, W.; Costello, B.A.; Quevedo, F.; et al. Exosomal miR-1290 and miR-375 as prognostic markers in castration-resistant prostate cancer. *Eur. Urol.* **2015**, *67*, 33–41. [CrossRef]
60. Joncas, F.H.; Lucien, F.; Rouleau, M.; Morin, F.; Leong, H.S.; Pouliot, F.; Fradet, Y.; Gilbert, C.; Toren, P. Plasma extracellular vesicles as phenotypic biomarkers in prostate cancer patients. *Prostate* **2019**, *79*, 1767–1776. [CrossRef]
61. Antonarakis, E.S.; Lu, C.; Wang, H.; Luber, B.; Nakazawa, M.; Roeser, J.C.; Chen, Y.; Mohammad, T.A.; Chen, Y.; Fedor, H.L.; et al. AR-V7 and resistance to enzalutamide and abiraterone in prostate cancer. *N. Engl. J. Med.* **2014**, *371*, 1028–1038. [CrossRef] [PubMed]
62. Del Re, M.; Biasco, E.; Crucitta, S.; Derosa, L.; Rofi, E.; Orlandini, C.; Miccoli, M.; Galli, L.; Falcone, A.; Jenster, G.W.; et al. The Detection of Androgen Receptor Splice Variant 7 in Plasma-derived Exosomal RNA Strongly Predicts Resistance to Hormonal Therapy in Metastatic Prostate Cancer Patients. *Eur. Urol.* **2017**, *71*, 680–687. [CrossRef] [PubMed]
63. Probert, C.; Dottorini, T.; Speakman, A.; Hunt, S.; Nafee, T.; Fazeli, A.; Wood, S.; Brown, J.E.; James, V. Communication of prostate cancer cells with bone cells via extracellular vesicle RNA; a potential mechanism of metastasis. *Oncogene* **2019**, *38*, 1751–1763. [CrossRef] [PubMed]
64. Li, S.L.; An, N.; Liu, B.; Wang, S.Y.; Wang, J.J.; Ye, Y. Exosomes from LNCaP cells promote osteoblast activity through miR-375 transfer. *Oncol. Lett.* **2019**, *17*, 4463–4473. [CrossRef]
65. Krishn, S.R.; Singh, A.; Bowler, N.; Duffy, A.N.; Friedman, A.; Fedele, C.; Kurtoglu, S.; Tripathi, S.K.; Wang, K.; Hawkins, A.; et al. Prostate cancer sheds the alphavbeta3 integrin in vivo through exosomes. *Matrix Biol.* **2019**, *77*, 41–57. [CrossRef]
66. Khan, S.; Jutzy, J.M.; Valenzuela, M.M.; Turay, D.; Aspe, J.R.; Ashok, A.; Mirshahidi, S.; Mercola, D.; Lilly, M.B.; Wall, N.R. Plasma-derived exosomal survivin, a plausible biomarker for early detection of prostate cancer. *PLoS ONE* **2012**, *7*, e46737. [CrossRef]

67. Lehmann, B.D.; Paine, M.S.; Brooks, A.M.; McCubrey, J.A.; Renegar, R.H.; Wang, R.; Terrian, D.M. Senescence-associated exosome release from human prostate cancer cells. *Cancer Res.* **2008**, *68*, 7864–7871. [CrossRef]
68. Hurwitz, M.D.; Kaur, P.; Nagaraja, G.M.; Bausero, M.A.; Manola, J.; Asea, A. Radiation therapy induces circulating serum Hsp72 in patients with prostate cancer. *Radiother Oncol.* **2010**, *95*, 350–358. [CrossRef]
69. Erozenci, L.A.; Bottger, F.; Bijnsdorp, I.V.; Jimenez, C.R. Urinary exosomal proteins as (pan-)cancer biomarkers: Insights from the proteome. *FEBS Lett.* **2019**, *593*, 1580–1597. [CrossRef]
70. Kim, S.M.; Kim, H.S. Engineering of extracellular vesicles as drug delivery vehicles. *Stem Cell Investig.* **2017**, *4*, 74. [CrossRef]
71. Lin, Y.; Lu, Y.; Li, X. Biological characteristics of exosomes and genetically engineered exosomes for the targeted delivery of therapeutic agents. *J. Drug Target.* **2019**, *28*, 129–141. [CrossRef] [PubMed]
72. Johnsen, K.B.; Gudbergsson, J.M.; Skov, M.N.; Pilgaard, L.; Moos, T.; Duroux, M. A comprehensive overview of exosomes as drug delivery vehicles—Endogenous nanocarriers for targeted cancer therapy. *Biochim. Biophys. Acta* **2014**, *1846*, 75–87. [CrossRef] [PubMed]
73. Tang, K.; Zhang, Y.; Zhang, H.; Xu, P.; Liu, J.; Ma, J.; Lv, M.; Li, D.; Katirai, F.; Shen, G.X.; et al. Delivery of chemotherapeutic drugs in tumour cell-derived microparticles. *Nat. Commun.* **2012**, *3*, 1282. [CrossRef]
74. Pascucci, L.; Cocce, V.; Bonomi, A.; Ami, D.; Ceccarelli, P.; Ciusani, E.; Vigano, L.; Locatelli, A.; Sisto, F.; Doglia, S.M.; et al. Paclitaxel is incorporated by mesenchymal stromal cells and released in exosomes that inhibit in vitro tumor growth: A new approach for drug delivery. *J. Control. Release* **2014**, *192*, 262–270. [CrossRef] [PubMed]
75. Tian, Y.; Li, S.; Song, J.; Ji, T.; Zhu, M.; Anderson, G.J.; Wei, J.; Nie, G. A doxorubicin delivery platform using engineered natural membrane vesicle exosomes for targeted tumor therapy. *Biomaterials* **2014**, *35*, 2383–2390. [CrossRef] [PubMed]
76. Qi, H.; Liu, C.; Long, L.; Ren, Y.; Zhang, S.; Chang, X.; Qian, X.; Jia, H.; Zhao, J.; Sun, J.; et al. Blood Exosomes Endowed with Magnetic and Targeting Properties for Cancer Therapy. *ACS Nano* **2016**, *10*, 3323–3333. [CrossRef]
77. Bakht, M.K.; Oh, S.W.; Hwang, D.W.; Lee, Y.S.; Youn, H.; Porter, L.A.; Cheon, G.J.; Kwak, C.; Lee, D.S.; Kang, K.W. The Potential Roles of Radionanomedicine and Radioexosomics in Prostate Cancer Research and Treatment. *Curr. Pharm. Des.* **2017**, *23*, 2976–2990. [CrossRef]
78. Li, J.; Yang, X.; Guan, H.; Mizokami, A.; Keller, E.T.; Xu, X.; Liu, X.; Tan, J.; Hu, L.; Lu, Y.; et al. Exosome-derived microRNAs contribute to prostate cancer chemoresistance. *Int. J. Oncol.* **2016**, *49*, 838–846. [CrossRef]
79. Kharaziha, P.; Chioureas, D.; Rutishauser, D.; Baltatzis, G.; Lennartsson, L.; Fonseca, P.; Azimi, A.; Hultenby, K.; Zubarev, R.; Ullen, A.; et al. Molecular profiling of prostate cancer derived exosomes may reveal a predictive signature for response to docetaxel. *Oncotarget* **2015**, *6*, 21740–21754. [CrossRef]
80. Corcoran, C.; Rani, S.; O'Brien, K.; O'Neill, A.; Prencipe, M.; Sheikh, R.; Webb, G.; McDermott, R.; Watson, W.; Crown, J.; et al. Docetaxel-resistance in prostate cancer: Evaluating associated phenotypic changes and potential for resistance transfer via exosomes. *PLoS ONE* **2012**, *7*, e50999. [CrossRef]
81. Kawakami, K.; Fujita, Y.; Kato, T.; Mizutani, K.; Kameyama, K.; Tsumoto, H.; Miura, Y.; Deguchi, T.; Ito, M. Integrin beta4 and vinculin contained in exosomes are potential markers for progression of prostate cancer associated with taxane-resistance. *Int. J. Oncol.* **2015**, *47*, 384–390. [CrossRef] [PubMed]
82. Kato, T.; Mizutani, K.; Kameyama, K.; Kawakami, K.; Fujita, Y.; Nakane, K.; Kanimoto, Y.; Ehara, H.; Ito, H.; Seishima, M.; et al. Serum exosomal P-glycoprotein is a potential marker to diagnose docetaxel resistance and select a taxoid for patients with prostate cancer. *Urol. Oncol.* **2015**, *33*, 385.e15–385.e20. [CrossRef] [PubMed]
83. Kosaka, N.; Iguchi, H.; Yoshioka, Y.; Hagiwara, K.; Takeshita, F.; Ochiya, T. Competitive interactions of cancer cells and normal cells via secretory microRNAs. *J. Biol. Chem.* **2012**, *287*, 1397–1405. [CrossRef] [PubMed]
84. Li, X.; Corbett, A.L.; Taatizadeh, E.; Tasnim, N.; Little, J.P.; Garnis, C.; Daugaard, M.; Guns, E.; Hoorfar, M.; Li, I.T.S. Challenges and opportunities in exosome research-Perspectives from biology, engineering, and cancer therapy. *APL Bioeng.* **2019**, *3*, 011503. [CrossRef]
85. Gilligan, K.E.; Dwyer, R.M. Engineering Exosomes for Cancer Therapy. *Int. J. Mol. Sci.* **2017**, *18*, 1122. [CrossRef]

86. Rahbarghazi, R.; Jabbari, N.; Sani, N.A.; Asghari, R.; Salimi, L.; Kalashani, S.A.; Feghhi, M.; Etemadi, T.; Akbariazar, E.; Mahmoudi, M.; et al. Tumor-derived extracellular vesicles: Reliable tools for Cancer diagnosis and clinical applications. *Cell Commun. Signal.* **2019**, *17*, 73. [CrossRef] [PubMed]
87. Giulietti, M.; Santoni, M.; Cimadamore, A.; Carrozza, F.; Piva, F.; Cheng, L.; Lopez-Beltran, A.; Scarpelli, M.; Battelli, N.; Montironi, R. Exploring Small Extracellular Vesicles for Precision Medicine in Prostate Cancer. *Front. Oncol.* **2018**, *8*, 221. [CrossRef] [PubMed]

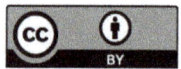

© 2020 by the authors. Licensee MDPI, Basel, Switzerland. This article is an open access article distributed under the terms and conditions of the Creative Commons Attribution (CC BY) license (http://creativecommons.org/licenses/by/4.0/).

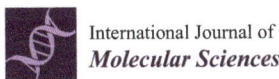

Article

Potential Use of Extracellular Vesicles Generated by Microbubble-Assisted Ultrasound as Drug Nanocarriers for Cancer Treatment

Yuana Yuana [1,2,*], Banuja Balachandran [1], Kim M. G. van der Wurff-Jacobs [3], Raymond M. Schiffelers [4] and Chrit T. Moonen [1]

1. Imaging Division, University Medical Center Utrecht, 3584 CX Utrecht, The Netherlands
2. Department of Biomedical Engineering, TU Eindhoven, 5600 MB Eindhoven, The Netherlands
3. Department of Pharmaceutical Sciences, University of Utrecht, 3584 CG Utrecht, The Netherlands
4. Laboratory of Clinical Chemistry and Haematology, University Medical Center Utrecht, 3584 CX Utrecht, The Netherlands
* Correspondence: Y.yuana@tue.nl; Tel.: +31-0-402-473-075

Received: 1 April 2020; Accepted: 22 April 2020; Published: 24 April 2020

Abstract: Extracellular vesicles (EVs)-carrying biomolecules derived from parental cells have achieved substantial scientific interest for their potential use as drug nanocarriers. Ultrasound (US) in combination with microbubbles (MB) have been shown to trigger the release of EVs from cancer cells. In the current study, the use of microbubbles-assisted ultrasound (USMB) to generate EVs containing drug cargo was investigated. The model drug, CellTracker™ green fluorescent dye (CTG) or bovine serum albumin conjugated with fluorescein isothiocyanate (BSA FITC) was loaded into primary human endothelial cells in vitro using USMB. We found that USMB loaded CTG and BSA FITC into human endothelial cells (HUVECs) and triggered the release of EVs containing these compounds in the cell supernatant within 2 h after treatment. The amount of EV released seemed to be correlated with the increase of US acoustic pressure. Co-culturing these EVs resulted in uptake by the recipient tumour cells within 4 h. In conclusion, USMB was able to load the model drugs into endothelial cells and simultaneously trigger the release of EVs-carrying model drugs, highlighting the potential of EVs as drug nanocarriers for future drug delivery in cancer.

Keywords: drug delivery; extracellular vesicles; lysosome; nanocarriers; ultrasound

1. Introduction

A major problem of drug delivery in cancer is that drugs cannot always efficiently bypass the multiple biological barriers. In most of the tissues, the endothelial lining is dense and does not permit the rapid exchange of materials such as drugs between the blood and the interstitial tumour space. Improvements in the drug delivery system to treat cancer including the delivery vehicles may improve the efficacy and safety of drugs [1,2].

Nanosized-lipid bilayer vesicles, known as extracellular vesicles (EVs), carry biomolecules such as proteins, lipids and genetic information that originated from the host cells [3]. The nanometre size and targeting modalities enable EVs to penetrate the interstitial tumour space. When EVs are loaded with a drug, this drug cargo can be delivered and transferred to dedicated cancer cells [1,4]. In general, drugs can be loaded into host cells allowing their natural mechanism to package drugs into EVs, also known as endogenous loading [5]. Drugs also can be exogenously loaded into EVs after isolation/purification steps using physical or chemical methods [6]. The feasibility and safety of EVs also have been shown in human clinical trials [7]. Thus, EVs hold potentials as drug nanocarriers.

Ultrasound (US) in combination with gaseous microbubbles (MB), beyond their common use for diagnosis, represents an emerging approach for localized drug delivery [8,9]. Under the action of US waves, MBs transiently affect the permeability of biological barriers (e.g., cell membrane, endothelial lining), thus leading to the uptake and enhanced accumulation of drugs in the region where the US-induced pressure surpasses a certain threshold [10,11]. Despite the potential benefits of USMB-guided drug delivery, the micron size of MB used in this system limits their action exclusively to the vascular bed [12,13]. Thus, future refinements in USMB-guided drug delivery to enhance drug uptake to the targeted tumour cells are warranted.

Recently, we showed that EVs with a diameter of less than 200 nm were released from head-and-neck cancer cells (FaDu) in vitro for up to 4-fold at 2–4 h after USMB [14]. The fact that USMB triggered a rapid release of EVs shows the significance of this technology to generate EVs and opens opportunities for us to study whether the drug-loaded EVs can be generated following the loading of the drug into the host cells using USMB.

In this study, we used human endothelial cells (HUVECs) as an in vitro model. CellTracker™ green fluorescent dye (CTG) and bovine serum albumin (BSA) with fluorescein isothiocyanate (FITC) conjugate were used as model drugs. These compounds have distinct characteristics: CTG could freely pass through cell membranes and be transformed into a cell-impermeant fluorescent product in the cytosol, whereas BSA FITC conjugate could pass through cell membranes via endocytosis. Different US acoustic pressures (0.6, 0.7 and 0.8 MPa) were applied to load CTG and BSA FITC into HUVECs. Cells and cell supernatants were harvested and measured to investigate if model drugs were present in the cells and EVs. Subsequently, we highlighted the potential use of EVs as drug nanocarriers by demonstrating the uptake of drug-loaded EVs generated by USMB after 4 h being co-cultured with the recipient cancer cells, FaDu and MDA-MB-231 human breast carcinoma cells. Finally, we utilized the Cre-LoxP system to confirm these findings [15].

2. Results

2.1. Loading Model Drugs into Cells

Using the bright-field microscopy, we observed that directly after US application at 0.6, 0.7 and 0.8 MPa, most cells remained attached to the culture chamber (Figure 1A). Increasing the pressure to 1 MPa detached almost 50% of the cells from the surface of the culture chamber, and therefore this condition was not used further in this study (Figure 1A). Untreated and USMB-treated HUVECs (0.6, 0.7 and 0.8 MPa) were harvested and stained using propidium iodide (PI) to determine the percentage of live and dead cells using flow cytometry. The percentages of live and dead cells in treated samples were comparable with the untreated samples (Figure 1B). These results indicated that the US acoustic pressures 0.6, 0.7 and 0.8 MPa could be used safely for loading the model drug into cells in vitro. We observed that HUVECs could be loaded directly with CTG by incubating CTG for 30 min (Figure 1C). However, USMB did not enhance the loading of CTG in HUVECs (Figure 1C).

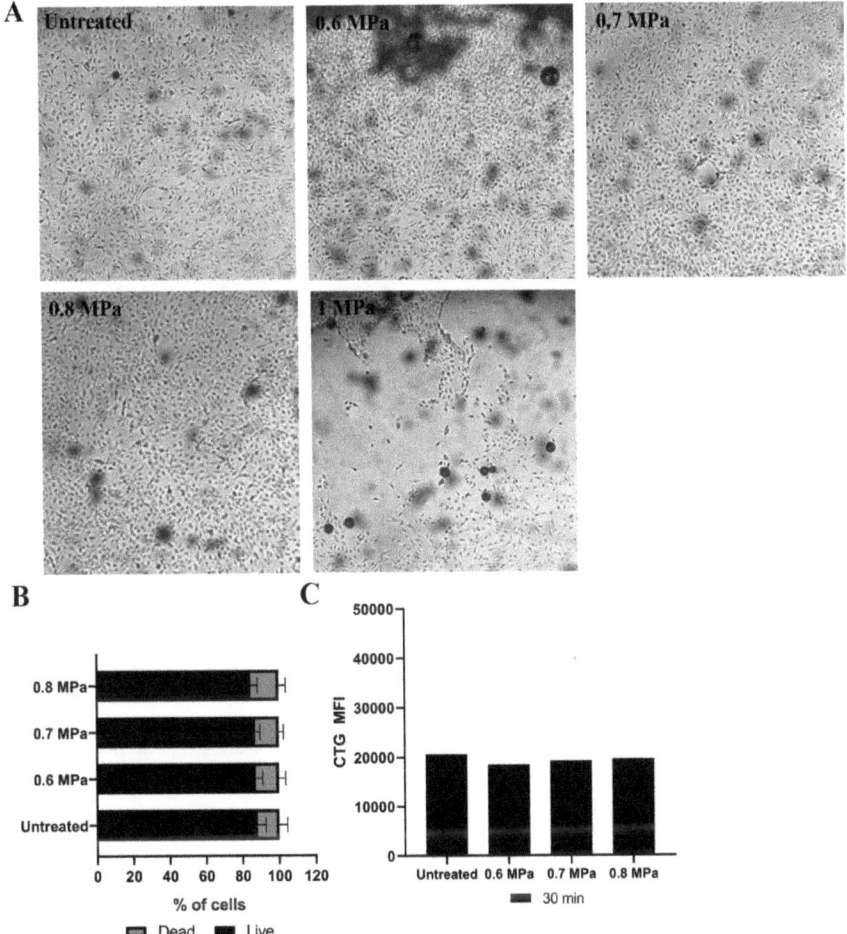

Figure 1. Human endothelial cells (HUVECs) stained with CellTracker™ green fluorescent dye (CTG) and treated at different ultrasound (US) acoustic pressures. Microscopy pictures of HUVECs captured before (untreated) and directly after US treatment (0.6, 0.7, 0.8 and 1 MPa) are presented at 10× magnification (**A**). Afterwards, cells were harvested and stained with PI to determine live and dead cells. The mean percentages of live and dead cells are presented (**B**). US acoustic pressures of 0.6, 0.7 and 0.8 MPa were tested to increase CTG signal intensities in HUVECs after incubation of CTG for 30 min (**C**). Untreated condition was HUVEs after incubation of CTG for 30 min. After 2 h of post-USMB, HUVECs were harvested and measured using flow cytometry (**C**). The mean fluorescent intensities (MFI) of CTG were presented (**C**). As a control, HUVECs without CTG staining were used. MFI results presented are the mean of two independent experiments.

By using USMB, our objective was to increase the delivery of BSA FITC into the cells. We found that loading BSA FITC using different US acoustic pressures was not correlated with the increase of BSA FITC signal in the cells. At 0.6 MPa, BSA FITC signal intensities in HUVECs measured by flow cytometry were the highest compared to untreated and treated HUVECs at 0.7 and 0.8 MPa (Figure 2A). Using a fluorescence microscope, we observed that BSA FITC was present in the HUVECs after treatment with different US acoustic pressures (0.6, 0.7 and 0.8 MPa) and also in the untreated HUVECs (Figure 2B).

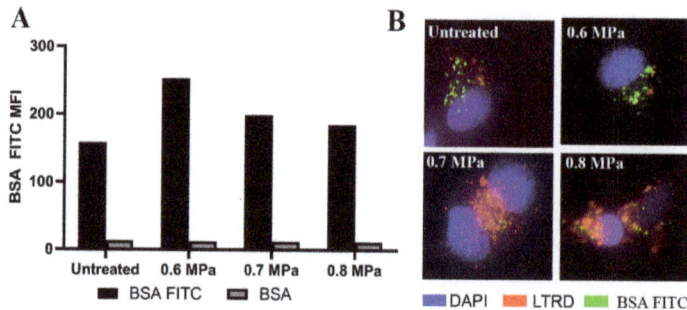

Figure 2. HUVECs loaded with bovine serum albumin conjugated with fluorescein isothiocyanate (BSA FITC) before and after USMB application at different acoustic pressures. After administering BSA FITC with USMB, HUVECs were incubated for 1 h and then, the medium was refreshed. After 2 h, HUVECs were harvested and measured with flow cytometry to quantify the BSA FITC signal, depicted as MFI (**A**). The results presented were the mean of two independent experiments. These cells were also stained with a nuclear stain, DAPI (blue) and a lysosomal marker, LTRD (**B**). Co-localisation of red and green colours indicate the presence of BSA FITC in the lysosomal compartment (**B**). These images were representative images taken at 60× magnification using a fluorescence microscope (Keyence BZ9000, Mechelen, Belgium).

This BSA FITC signal was co-localised with LysoTraker™ Red DND-99 (LTRD) staining in HUVECs, especially after US treatments (Figure 2B). The presence of this molecule in the lysosomal compartment of these cells possibly indicates the degradation of BSA in this compartment. We also co-administered HUVECs with DQ-Red BSA and MB before application of US at 0.6, 0.7 and 0.8 MPa to check if lysosomes were involved in the degradation of BSA. The bright red spots which were indicative for de-quenched fluorescence molecules of DQ-Red BSA when reaching the degradative endo-lysosomes, were detected in HUVECs after US treatment (Figure S1). These red spots were absent in untreated HUVECs (Figure S1). Thus, these results confirmed the presence of BSA in lysosomal compartments after US treatment.

2.2. Triggering EV Release Containing Model Drug Cargo

Using anti-CD9 and anti-CD63-coated magnetic beads, we captured EVs from the cell supernatants of HUVECs which have been incubated with CTG for 30 min and treated with USMB. USMB triggered an increased release of EVs from HUVEC shown by an increased level of mean fluorescent intensity (MFI) of EVs positive for CD9 and CD63 after USMB treatment especially at 0.8 MPa compared to the untreated, 0.6 and 0.7 MPa conditions (Figure 3A,B). EVs captured by anti-CD9 and anti-CD63 beads carried CTG and the MFI levels of CTG seemed to increase when US acoustic pressures were increased (Figure 3A,B). The measurement of the same cell supernatants using a micro flow cytometer showed that the concentrations of EVs exposing CD9 and CD63 increased 2- and 3-fold subsequently after USMB compared to untreated counterparts, especially at 0.7 and 0.8 MPa (Figure 3C). These EVs also carried CTG and their concentration was significantly higher at 0.8 MPa ($p < 0.05$, Figure 3C). The percentages of EVs positive for CD9 or CD63 which carried CTG generated by USMB at 0.8 MPa are about 20% and 37% respectively.

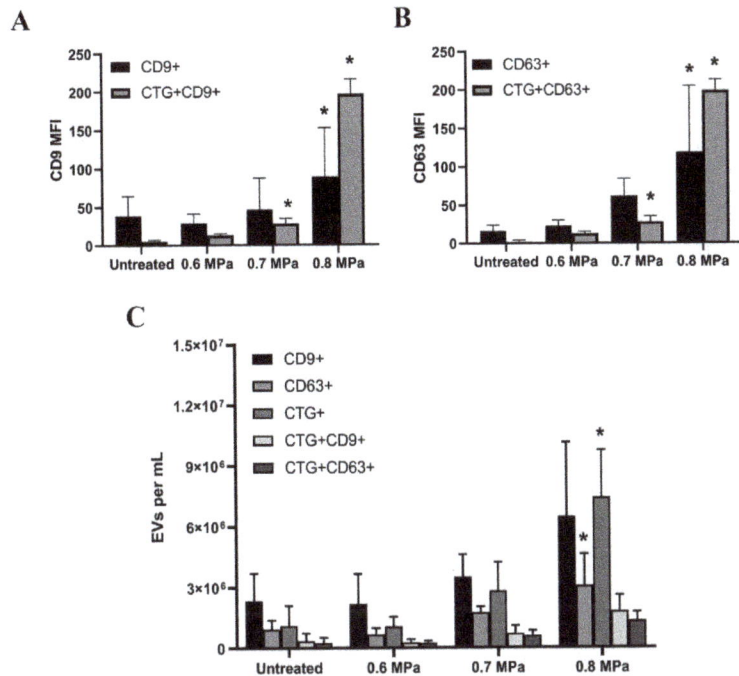

Figure 3. Extracellular vesicles (EVs)-containing supernatants of HUVECs after CTG and USMB treatments measured using flow cytometry. EVs were captured by anti-CD9 and anti-CD63 beads in the supernatants of CTG-stained HUVEC followed by USMB treatment. These EVs were stained with anti-CD9 and anti-CD63 detection antibodies. The MFI of CD9 and CD63 levels in untreated and USMB treated samples (0.6, 0.7 and 0.8 MPa) were quantified using flow cytometry (**A**,**B**). These captured CD9 EVs and CD63 EVs carried CTG (**A**,**B**). Samples were measured in triplicate and these were data from two independent experiments. The same samples were measured using a micro flow cytometer. Anti-CD9 and -CD63 were used to detect EVs bearing CD9 and CD63 antigens present in the cell supernatants (**C**). Total EVs carrying CTG and EVs exposing CD9 or CD63 which carried CTG were also quantified in the same samples (**C**). Results are reported in EVs per mL sample. These were data from two independent experiments. As controls, EVs without CTG were used and all results presented have been corrected from these controls (**A**–**C**). Statistical analysis was performed using one-way ANOVA followed by Tukey's test. The p value < 0.05 was considered significant (*).

HUVECs loaded with BSA FITC also released EVs containing BSA FITC (Figures 4 and 5). These EVs from the cell supernatants were captured by anti-CD9 and anti-CD63 beads (Figure 4A,B). As controls, BSA was used and EVs present in the supernatant of HUVECs were measured. EVs exposing CD9 and CD63 generated by USMB showed higher BSA FITC fluorescent signal (BSA FITC MFI) than the BSA FITC signal detected from EVs generated by untreated counterparts (Figure 4A,B). However, the increased MFI levels of BSA FITC were not correlated with increasing US pressures. Using the micro flow cytometer, we could detect the concentration of EVs carrying BSA FITC increased significantly at the conditions of 0.7 and 0.8 MPa (2.4×10^6/mL and 2.2×10^6/mL; Figure 4C) compared to the untreated conditions. The percentages of EVs positive for CD9 or CD63 which carried BSA FITC generated by USMB at 0.7 MPA are about 12% and 25% respectively, whereas these generated by USMB at 0.8 MPA are about 10% and 18% respectively. Because of the sensitivity of the micro flow cytometer in measuring single EVs, differences in EV concentrations in condition media of HUVEC treated using different US pressures were detectable.

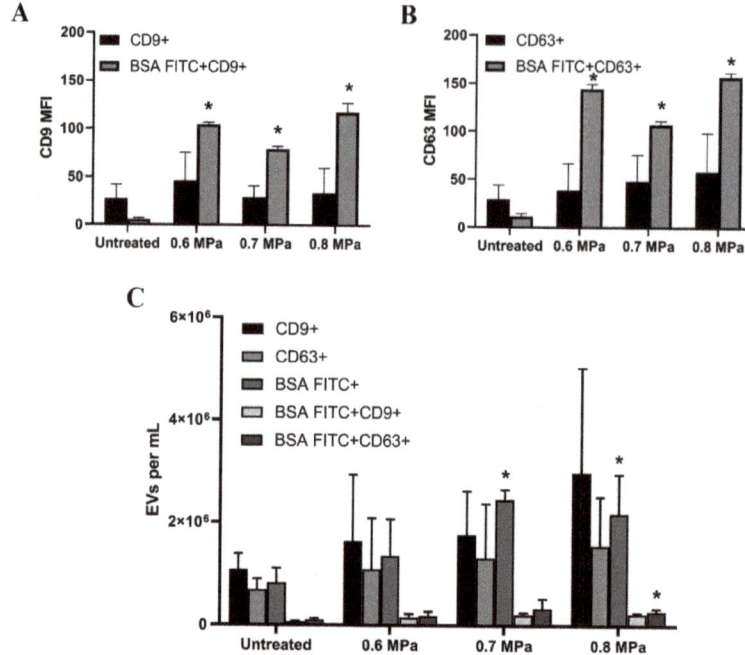

Figure 4. EVs-containing supernatants of HUVECs after co-administration of BSA FITC and MB followed by US treatments measured using flow cytometry. Anti-CD9 and anti-CD63 capture assays coupled to flow cytometry measurement were used to detect CD9 and CD63 EVs present in the conditioned media of HUVEC co-administered with BSA FITC together with MB. Anti-CD9 captured EVs with CD9 on the surface, whereas anti-CD63 captured EVs with CD63 on the surface. Anti-CD9 and anti-CD63 were used as the detection antibodies (**A,B**). The MFI of CD9 and CD63 levels in untreated and USMB treated samples (0.6, 0.7 and 0.8 MPa) and also the BSA FITC signals in these captured CD9 EVs and CD63 were quantified (**A,B**). Samples were measured in triplicate and these were data from two independent experiments. The same samples were measured by the micro flow cytometer. Anti-CD9 and -CD63 were used to detect EVs bearing CD9 and CD63 antigens present in the conditioned media (**C**). Total EVs carrying BSA-FITC, indicated by EVs exposing CD9 and CD63, which carried BSA-FITC were quantified in the same samples (**C**). Results are reported in EVs per mL sample. These were data from two independent experiments. EVs with BSA were used as controls and all results presented have been corrected from these controls (**A–C**). Statistical analysis was performed using one-way ANOVA followed by Tukey's test. The p value < 0.05 was considered significant (*).

To visualise EVs carrying BSA FITC, we also performed immunogold electron microscopy. We used anti-CD9 and anti-CD63 to detect EVs exposing CD9 and CD63 on their surface. Anti-mouse IgG secondary antibody labelled with 6-nm gold particles was used to trace EVs exposing CD9 or CD63. To investigate whether these EVs were carrying BSA FITC, we stained the samples with anti FITC secondary antibody labelled with 10-nm gold particles. We found that CD9-exposing EV carried BSA FITC (Figure 5A). Some CD63-exposing EVs carried BSA FITC (Figure 5B). In Figure 5C, EV carrying BSA FITC was clearly detected. Negative controls were samples containing EVs with BSA (Figure 5D–F). EVs imaged by electron microscopy mostly have a diameter of around 100 nm. This is also confirmed by NTA measurements (Figure S2). These results show that HUVECs which were loaded with BSA FITC released EVs carrying BSA FITC after USMB treatment.

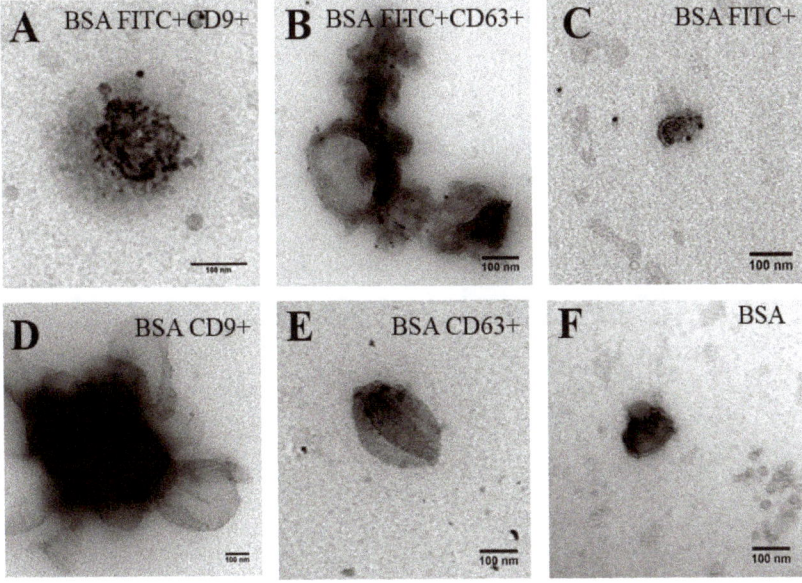

Figure 5. Immunogold electron microscopy of cell supernatant containing EVs derived from HUVEC treated with USMB (0.7 MPa) in the presence of BSA FITC as a model drug. EVs were stained with anti-CD9 or anti-CD63 and the detection antibody was anti mouse IgG secondary antibody labelled with 6-nm gold particles (**A,B**). IgG1 isotype control was used as a control for anti-CD9 and anti-CD63 staining (**C**). Anti FITC secondary antibody labelled with 10-nm gold particles stained BSA FITC present on EVS (**A–C**). As controls, cell supernatant containing EVs with non-conjugated BSA processed and stained in the same manner (**D–F**).

2.3. Uptake of EVs Carrying CTG and BSA FITC

We performed flow cytometry measurement to quantify the EV uptake by FaDu and MDA-MB-231 after 4 h of co-culturing. The uptake of EV carrying CTG or BSA FITC is shown by the percentages of positive cells for CTG or BSA FITC (Figure 6A,B). After co-culturing with undiluted EVs carrying CTG, there were 0.3% FaDU cells and 0.5% MDA-MB-231 cells positive for CTG (Figure 6A). We also monitored the uptake of EVs containing CTG by MDA-MB-231 cells at 0, 2 and 4 h using a fluorescent microscope (Figure S3). After co-culturing for 4 h, only 2–3 cells per 1.7 cm^2 were positive for CTG. Thus, the overall results show that the uptake of EVs containing CTG by these cancer cells was low. The same cancer cells took up more EVs carrying BSA FITC (Figure 6B). Particularly, 9.7% of the FaDu cells and 30.5% of the MDA-MB-231 cells were positive after co-culturing with undiluted EVs carrying BSA FITC as detected by flow cytometry (Figure 6B).

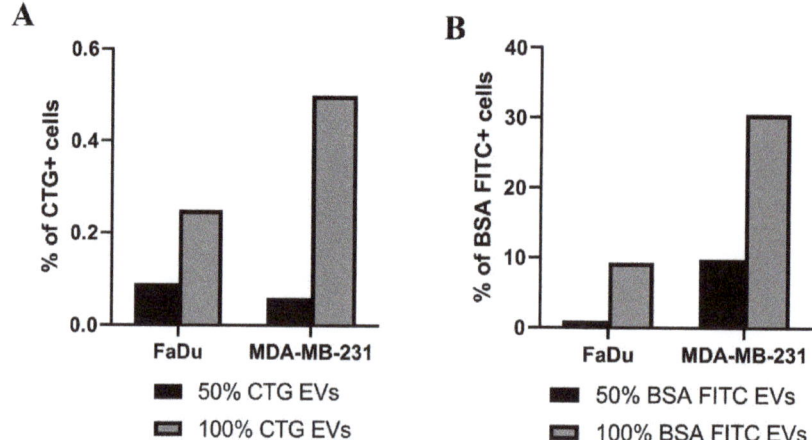

Figure 6. Uptake of EVs containing CTG or BSA-FITC by FaDu and MDA-MB-231 cells. EVs containing CTG (**A**) or BSA-FITC (**B**) at a concentration of 50% and 100% were co-cultured with FaDu or MDA-MB-231 cells for 4 h. The uptake of these EVs was measured by using flow cytometry. Percentages of FaDu and MDA-MB-231 cells exposing CTG or BSA FITC after EV uptake at 4 h-time point are presented (**A**,**B** accordingly). Control conditions were cells co-cultured with EVs which contained no CTG or BSA FITC. Percentages of the positive cells have been corrected for their controls and the uptake of EVs was normalized to 1×10^9 particles/mL.

We also stained the cells with the lysosomal tracker, LTRD, and nucleic acid stain DAPI, to localize the presence of EVs containing BSA FITC in the cells. Using fluorescent and confocal microscopes, we observed that EVs containing BSA FITC were taken up by cells and they were not present in the lysosomal compartment of these cells (Figure 7A,B). The FITC fluorescent signal was observed in the cell cytoplasm or in the vicinity of the cell nucleus (Figure 7A,B accordingly, and Supplementary Video S1).

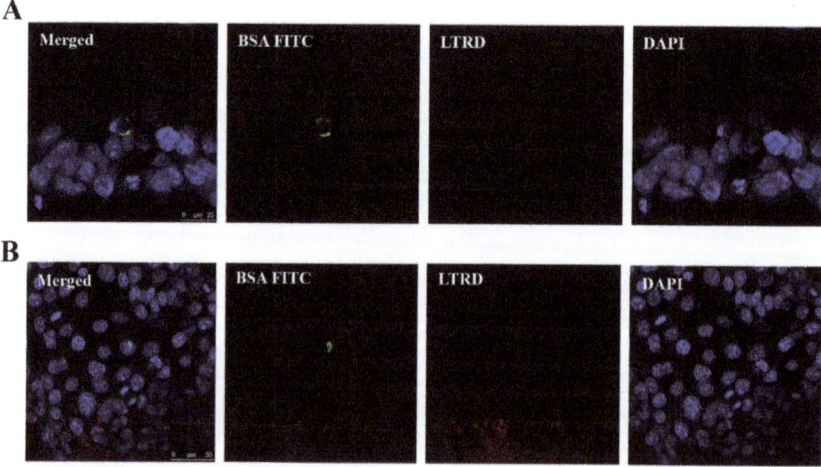

Figure 7. Uptake of EVs containing BSA FITC by FaDu cells. FaDu cells were co-cultured with EVs containing BSA FITC (undiluted). After 4 h, cells were washed with acid wash buffer followed by PBS and fixed prior to staining. LTRD probe (red) was used to stain lysosome and DAPI (blue) to stain the nucleus. Merged images show the uptake of BSA FITC by FaDu cells. BSA FITC signal (green) seems to be present in the cell cytoplasm (**A, merged**) or in the vicinity of the cell nucleus (**B, merged**).

To confirm the uptake of EVs by recipient tumour cells and the release of their cargo in these cells, we co-cultured EVs containing Cre recombinase with T47D receptor cells. The expression of Cre recombinase in EVs has been confirmed by PCR (Figure S4). The colour switch from red to green when receptor cells took up EVs containing Cre recombinase was monitored using a fluorescence microscope and flow cytometer (Figure 8A,B). Using a fluorescent microscope, we monitored the uptake of EVs containing Cre recombinase (100% concentration) at 0, 2 and 4 h (Figure 8A). At 2 h, we could not detect the green Cre-LoxP cells. At 4 h, we located green Cre-LoxP cells (2 cells/0.7 cm^2 chamber slide, Figure 8A white arrow). Flow cytometry analysis also shows that Cre-LoxP cells were present after co-culturing T47D recipient cells with EVs containing Cre recombinase at a concentration of 50% and 100% (Figure 8Bi,ii). Cells co-cultured with EVs without Cre recombinase served as control (Figure 8Biii). The percentage of green Cre-LoxP cells increased with increasing concentration of EV containing Cre recombinase (7.33% to 10.5%; Figure 8Bi–ii). A red-to-green colour switch observed in reporter-expressing T47D human mammary cells after co-culturing USMB-generated EV carrying active cre recombines confirms the uptake of EVs and transfer of their active cargo into the recipient cells.

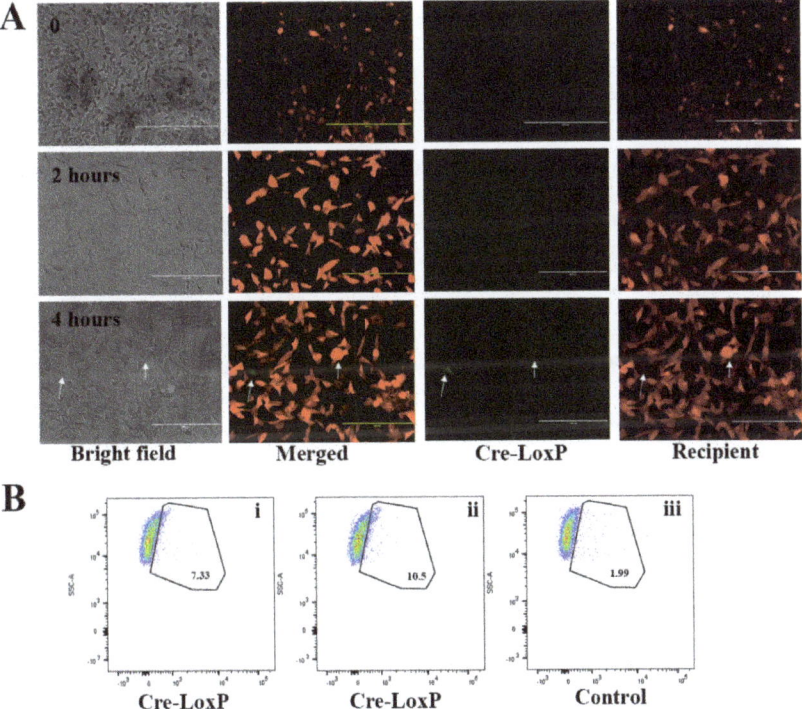

Figure 8. Uptake of EVs carrying Cre recombinase by T47D recipient tumour cells. Undiluted (100%) EVs carrying Cre-recombinase were added to T47D recipient cells (red). At 0, 2 and 4 h, bright field and fluorescent images were taken (**A**). Images were taken at 10× magnification at time point 0. Other images were taken at 20× magnification. Cre-LoxP cells which have a green fluorescent colour were located and shown with a white arrow, both in the bright field and fluorescent images. This uptake was also monitored using flow cytometry. Flow cytometry measurements were performed to assess the presence of Cre-LoxP cells which exposed green fluorescent signal after the co-culturing of EVs carrying Cre recombinase at a concentration of 50% and 100% for 4 h (**Bi–ii**). Controls were cells that were co-cultured with EVs without Cre recombinase (**Biii**).

3. Discussion

In the current study, we observed that increased US acoustic pressure is not always favourable for drug loading. By increasing US acoustic pressure to 1 MPa, cells were already detached from the culture chamber. Lammertink et al. [16] reported that HUVEC detachment was already observed after the application of 0.5 MPa. However, in that study HUVEC was grown on collagen-coated OptiCells™ which may explain this discrepancy. We also noticed that as CTG could freely pass through cell membranes, incubation for 30 min was already sufficient to stain/load HUVECs with CTG and therefore, applying USMB had no additional effect. In the case of BSA FITC loading, applying USMB at 0.6 MPa enhanced the loading. However, increasing US acoustic pressure to 0.7 or 0.8 MPa did not further enhance the loading of this molecule into cells. Based on the degradation of DQ-Red BSA and the de-quenching of the fluorescence after USMB loading, it was likely that our model drug was trapped and degraded in the lysosomal compartment. In conclusion, the type of the model drug is one of parameters which may influence the loading using USMB. It is also clear that this loading would not be optimal if the model drug would be trapped in the lysosomal compartment.

Our previous findings indicated that levels of EVs exposing CD9 or CD63 significantly increased at 2 and 4 h after USMB [14]. Therefore, we measured EVs containing CTG or BSA FITC in the cell supernatant 2 h after USMB treatment. The concentration of EVs containing CTG was 3-fold higher than the concentration of EVs containing BSA FITC, especially when the highest US acoustic pressure was applied (0.8 MPa). This difference may be caused by the mechanism through which these compounds are taken up and sorted by the cells [17]. As CTG could freely enter cell membranes and reside in the cytosol, this compound may avoid endosomal entrapment and perhaps easily be packed into EVs. In contrast, BSA FITC which was internalised by cells via endocytosis may lead to the delivery of endocytosed cargo into the endosomal-lysosomal degradative pathway, influencing the packing of this cargo into EVs [18,19]. It may be necessary to reduce the lysosomal function to prevent the drug compound degradation after internalization and eventually increase the release of EV containing drug [19,20].

Multiple different cellular entry routes are available for EVs and other nanoparticles to cross a cell's plasma membrane during in vitro and in vivo cell exposure. This cell uptake likely depends on the type of recipient cells and the EV cargo [17,21,22]. In our study, EVs prepared in a similar manner were internalised 2–3-fold more by MDA-MB-231 than FaDu cells. We observed that EVs containing CTG were taken up less than EVs containing BSA FITC. As EVs containing BSA FITC were not observed in the lysosomal compartment indicating that multiple or perhaps independently contributing pathways are involved in EV internalisation processes.

In conclusion, we have demonstrated the feasibility of USMB to load model drugs into endothelial cells allowing the cell's natural mechanism to generate EVs and package this compound into EVs. Co-culturing these EVs with FaDu and MDA-MB-231 cells resulted in the uptake of EVs and the release of model drug cargo in these cells. These results highlight the potential of EVs as drug nanocarriers for drug delivery.

4. Materials and Methods

4.1. Cell Culture

HUVECs (pooled donors, Lonza, Verviers, Belgium) were cultured in endothelial cell growth medium 2 with supplement mix (PromoCell GmbH, Heidelberg, Germany). MDA-MB-231 (ATCC® HTB-26™, LGC Standards GmbH, Wesel, Germany) and FaDu (ATCC® HTB-43™) cells were cultured in high glucose Dulbecco's modified Eagle medium (DMEM) (Sigma-Aldrich, Zwijndrecht, The Netherlands) and 10% foetal bovine serum (FBS) (Sigma-Aldrich). For FaDu cells, this medium was also supplemented with 1% non-essential amino acid (Sigma-Aldrich, Zwijndrecht, The Netherlands). MDA-MB-231 expressing Cre recombinase and T47D receptor cells were a kind gift from Prof. Raymond Schiffelers and these stable cell lines have been generated as described by Zomer et al. [15]. MDA-MB231 cells expressing Cre recombinase were cultured in high glucose DMEM, whereas T47D receptor cells were cultured in DMEM: F12 medium (Lonza, Breda, The Netherlands). In these culture media, 10% FBS, 1% penicillin-streptomycin (Fisher Scientific, Landsmeer, The Netherlands) and 5 μg/mL puromycin (Fisher scientific) were added. All cells were maintained in standard cell culture flasks in a humidified incubator at 37 °C and 5% CO_2 and passaged twice a week to maintain 80% confluency.

4.2. Cell Preparation for USMB

For USMB experiments, cells were prepared according to our previously reported method [14]. Briefly, cells were seeded in cell culture chambers (treated CLINIcell® 175 μm thick polycarbonate walls, 25 cm^2) (Mabio, Tourcoing, France) 1 day prior to USMB. Media used for maintaining cells in the culture chambers are the same media for maintaining cells in the culture flasks. Except for HUVECs, medium M199 containing L-glutamine (Sigma-Aldrich) and 20% FBS was used. Prior to USMB treatment, these culture media were filtered using 100 KDa centrifugal filter units (Amicon ultra-15, Merck Millipore, Amsterdam, The Netherlands) to deplete EVs related to bovine serum.

4.3. Loading Model Drug Using USMB

SonoVue™ (Bracco, Milan, Italy) lipid shelled MB, encapsulating sulphur hexafluoride gas (SF6) were used in the USMB experiments [23]. Microbubbles (MB) were prepared according to the manufacturer's guidelines.

For co-administrating CTG, cells were first washed with phosphate-buffered saline (PBS) and incubated with 10 nM CTG in serum-free medium for 30 min. As a negative control, cells without CTG were used. Prior to USMB, MB (700 μL) were mixed with 9.5 mL EV-depleted serum-containing medium. This MB-containing medium (final concentration of $0.7–3.5 \times 10^8$ MB) was then injected and the cell culture chamber was placed upside down, allowing the MB to rise by floatation towards the cells, ensuring close contact between cells and MB. For co-administrating BSA FITC, cells were first starved for 4 h in serum-free medium before BSA FITC (50 μg/mL) and MB were administered. As a negative control, non-conjugated BSA was administered at the same concentration. We also used DQ-Red BSA (Fisher scientific) to observe the loading of BSA by USMB. Once DQ-Red BSA has reached the degradative endo-lysosomes, it is broken down into smaller fragments which lead to fluorescence de-quenching shown as bright red spots in endo-lysosomes [24], and therefore tracking the location of this molecule in the cell.

Cells and MB were exposed to pulsed ultrasound (10% duty cycle, 1 kHz pulse repetition frequency and 100 μs pulse duration) with varying acoustic pressures at 0.6, 0.7 and 0.8 MPa peak negative pressure (PNP) as was calibrated using a 125 μm glass fibre hydrophone (Precision Acoustics, Dorchester, UK). The piezoelectric unfocused single element transducer with a diameter of 20 mm (Precision Acoustics) operating at 1.5 MHz was placed at the bottom of a water tank, 8 cm below a cell culture chamber frame. The water surface was another 12 cm above the frame and heated to 37 °C. When exposing cells to US, the cell culture chamber was mounted in the frame and moved over the transducer for 80 s to expose the whole cell culture chamber surface, which resulted in a total exposure of approximately 5 s for each area of the cell culture chamber [14,25]. For USMB treatment control, untreated cells were used.

After US exposure, CTG-treated cells were washed carefully with PBS and incubated for another 2 h in EV-depleted serum-containing medium. For BSA FITC-treated cells, we first incubated these cells for 1 h before they were washed carefully with PBS and incubated for another 2 h. After incubation, the conditioned medium was harvested and centrifuged at 300× g for 10 min at room temperature (RT) to remove detached cells and large cellular debris. Conditioned medium containing EVs was collected, snap-frozen in liquid nitrogen and stored at −80 °C for EV measurements. Attached cells in the cell culture chamber were detached using trypsin-EDTA solution (Sigma-Aldrich). After serum-containing medium was added, cells were pelleted by centrifuging at 250× g for 3 min at RT. To wash cells, cold PBS was added and cells were pelleted again. Finally, cells were re-suspended in 300 µL PBS containing 0.5% BSA and used for flow cytometry measurement.

4.4. Flow Cytometry Measurement

The cell suspension was mixed with 5 µL of 10 µg/mL propidium iodide (PI) (Fisher Scientific) and incubated for 5 min. Up to 10,000 events were measured using BD FACScanto II (Becton Dickinson, CA, USA) and the fluorescent intensity of CTG or BSA FITC together with PI was monitored.

For EV measurement using flow cytometry, conditioned medium containing EVs was thawed quickly at 37 °C. We captured EVs using immuno-magnetic beads and measured these EV-bead complexes using BD FACScanto II according to our previously reported method [14]. Using 96-well round-bottom plate 70 µL conditioned medium containing EVs was mixed with 10 µL ExoCap magnetic capture beads CD9 or CD63 (JSR Life Sciences, Leuven, Belgium) to obtain end concentration of 6×10^4 beads per sample. This mixture was incubated overnight at 4 °C with gentle agitation. On the next day, the magnetic plate separator was used to hold EV-bead complexes during washing steps. The supernatant was removed and 100 µL 0.5% BSA-containing PBS (0.45 µm filtered) was added followed by gentle agitation to wash EV-bead complexes for 5 min at RT. After placing the plate on top of the magnetic plate separator, the supernatant was removed. Hundred microliter of diluted mouse anti-human CD9, mouse anti-CD63, or the corresponding mouse IgG1 isotype control coupled to Alexa Fluor 647 were added to the respective wells (see Supplementary Table S1 for the dilutions and manufacturer). This mixture was incubated at RT in the dark for 30 min with gentle agitation. Lastly, the plate was again placed on top of the magnetic plate separator and the antibody/isotype control solution was removed. The plate was washed once with 100 µL 0.5% BSA-containing PBS per well. Samples containing EVs attached to the beads were re-suspended in 250 µL 0.5% BSA/PBS and measured using FACS canto-II. Two independent experiments were performed and from each experiment, samples were measured in triplicate to assess the levels of CD9 and CD63.

The concentration of EVs exposing CD9 or CD63, and EVs carrying CTG or BSA FITC were measured using the A60-Micro flow cytometer (Apogee Flow Systems, Hertfordshire, UK). This flow cytometer enables the measurement of biological particles down to about 100 nm diameter by light scatter [26]. Twenty microliter of conditioned medium containing EVs was incubated with 2.5 µL of mouse-anti human CD9 coupled to PE and 2.5 µL of mouse-anti human CD63 coupled to Alexa Fluor 647. As negative controls, mouse IgG1 isotype controls coupled to PE and to Alexa Fluor 647 were used (please see Supplementary Table S1 for the dilutions of antibodies/isotype controls and their manufacturer). The mixture of samples with antibodies or IgG1 isotype controls were incubated for 15 min and diluted to 225 µL before being measured with flowrate 3.01 µL/ min for 120 s.

4.5. Immunogold Electron Microscopy

To investigate whether BSA FITC was carried by EVs after USMB, immunogold electron microscopy was performed as described previously [14,27]. EVs from conditioned medium collected from USMB-treated HUVEC in the presence of BSA FITC or non-conjugated BSA were measured. A thin layer of carbon on the 100 mesh formvar-carbon-coated copper grids (Electron Microscopy Sciences, Hatfield, PA, USA) was evaporated using a carbon-vacuum evaporator according to the manufacturer's instructions (Edwards Auto 306, West Sussex, UK) just before sample application. Grids were floated directly on top of 10 µL of cell supernatant containing EVs and incubated for 7 min at RT. The grids were washed three times using PBS (0.22 µm filtered). Next, the grids were incubated in a blocking solution (Aurion, Wageningen, The Netherlands) for 30 min at RT followed by washing three times with 0.1% BSA-c (Aurion). For double immuno-labelling, the grids were incubated overnight at 4 °C in a mixture of 20 µL of mouse anti-human primary antibody (anti-CD9 or anti-CD63 antibody). For negative controls, mouse IgG1 isotype control was used. Unbound antibodies were removed from the grids in six washing steps by placing the grids on top of 0.1% BSA-c solution. Afterwards, the grids were incubated with 10 µL goat anti mouse IgG secondary antibody labelled with 6-nm gold particles

(Aurion) for 1 h at RT. Grids were washed six times with 0.1% BSA-c before incubation with 10 µL mouse anti-FITC labelled with 10-nm gold particles for 1 h at RT. Dilutions of the antibodies, isotype control and immunogold particles can be found in Supplementary Table S1. Grids were washed again six times with 0.1% BSA-c, followed by three times washing with PBS. To fix the labelled sample, the grid was incubated for 5 min with 2% glutaraldehyde (Sigma-Aldrich) and washed six times with milli-Q water. Next, the grids were transferred to 0.4% uranyl acetate in 2% methyl cellulose and incubated for 10 min. Excess solution on the grids was removed by blotting the grid at a 45° angle once from the side of the grid with filter paper. Grids were imaged using a Tecnai 12 electron microscope (FEI, Fisher Scientific) operated at 80 kV. Images were recorded at 60,000x magnification and processed using ImageJ [28]. The presence of a 6-nm gold particle on the EV surface indicated the presence of CD9 or CD63 on EV surface, whereas the presence of a 10-nm gold particle indicated the presence of BSA FITC in EV.

4.6. EV Isolation and Concentration

Before the EV isolation, the Amicon® ultra centrifugal filter 100 kDa (Merck Millipore) was washed with EV-depleted serum-containing medium by centrifuging at 4000× g for 30 min. The eluate was thrown. Next, 4 mL of supernatant containing EV with CTG, BSA FITC, or Cre recombinase which was collected after USMB treatment on HUVEC cells was added to the filtration device and centrifuged at 4000× g for 30 min. The eluate was thrown and the filter was washed once with EV-depleted serum-containing medium followed by centrifuging at 4000× g for 30 min. Finally, the EV concentrate was collected and the same medium was added up to get 750 µL EV suspension. As negative controls, the supernatant containing EVs without model drug that was generated at the same USMB condition was used.

4.7. Uptake Assay

Prior to the uptake assay, 70,000 cells (FaDu, MDA-MB231, or T47D reporter cells) were plated in the 8-chambers Millicell® EZ slides (Merck Millipore) and incubated overnight. From 750 µL EV suspension, 500 µL was added to the cells (100% concentration). The rest of this EV suspension was added to cells in another chamber (50% concentration) and 250 µL EV-depleted serum-containing medium was added to fill up the chamber. We also performed a nanoparticle tracking analysis (NTA) to estimate the concentration of EVs added for co-culturing [29] (Supplementary Procedure S1). Cells were co-cultured with EVs and measured at time points 0, 2 and 4 h using a fluorescent microscope (Nikon Ti2-U from Nikon Instruments Europe BV, Amsterdam, The Netherlands; EVOS FL from Fisher scientific). At 4 h-time point cells were washed with PBS and followed by acid wash buffer (0.5 M NaCl, 0.2 M acetic acid) to remove EVs which were on the cell surface and not taken up. Cells were washed once more with PBS before fixing with 4% paraformaldehyde (Sigma-Aldrich) or harvesting them for further analysis. For fluorescence microscopy measurement, fixed cells were stained with 50 nM LysoTraker™ Red DND-99 (LTRD) (Fisher Scientific) to stain the cell lysosomal compartment and one drop of Fluoroshield with DAPI (Sigma-Aldrich) to stain the cell nuclei; and imaged using a confocal microscope (TCS SP5 X, Leica Microsystems B.V., Amsterdam, The Netherlands). For flow cytometry measurement, cells were detached using trypsin-EDTA solution. After serum containing-medium was added, cells were pelleted by centrifuging at 250× g for 3 min at RT. The supernatant was carefully removed and cells were finally re-suspended in 300 µL PBS containing 0.5% BSA for flow cytometry measurement using BD FACScanto II. The uptake of CTG, BSA FITC and Cre recombinase by cells was measured at wavelength 530/30 nm.

4.8. RT-PCR

To detect Cre recombinase gene expression in T47D reporter cells, RT-PCR was performed. T47D receptor cells after 4 h of co-culturing with EV containing Cre recombinase were harvested. The cell pellet was dissolved in 1 mL Trizol (Fisher Scientific) per 1 million cells. The cell lysate was incubated at RT for 10–20 min. This lysate could be frozen at −20 °C prior to RNA isolation. For RNA isolation, chloroform (Sigma) was added to the cell lysate at a dilution of 1:5. The mixture was shaken vigorously for 15 s and then incubated for 2 min at RT. Next, this mixture was centrifuged for 15 min at 12,000× g at 4 °C. The upper aqueous phase was collected and 1 µL of GlycoBlue (Fisher Scientific) was added. Isopropanol (Merck Millipore) at a dilution of 1:2 was added to each sample and vortexed thoroughly. The sample was incubated for 10 min at RT and then centrifuged for 10 min at 12,000× g at 4 °C. The supernatant was carefully removed and the pellet was resuspended in 80% ethanol (Merck Millipore) at the same volume as the cell lysate. Next, the sample was centrifuged for 5 min at 7500× g at 4 °C. The supernatant was carefully removed and the pellet was air-dried for 10–15 min at RT. RNA was reconstituted in 20 µL nuclease-free water (Fisher Scientific) and quantified by Nanodrop (DeNovix Inc., Wilmington, DE, USA). The cDNA was prepared using Superscript 4 (Fisher Scientific) according to the manufacturer's instructions. The cDNA was amplified using a PCR with Cre-specific primers (forward primer: 5′ GCCTGCATTACCGGTCGATGC 3′; reverse primer: 5′ GTGGCAGATGGC GCGGCAACA 3′) [15]. Thermal cycle conditions used for all reactions were as follows: 5 min at 95 °C, followed by 40 cycles consisting of denaturation for 15 s at 95 °C, annealing for 30 s at 58 °C and extension for 1 min at 72 °C. PCR reactions were concluded with incubation for 7 min at 72 °C to complete the extension of all synthesised products. PCR products were then visualised on a 1.5% TAE agarose gel (Roche Diagnostics, Manneheim, Germany).

4.9. Statistical Analysis

Statistical analysis was performed using GraphPad Prism 8 (La Jolla, CA, USA). ANOVA (one-way) followed by Tukey's multiple comparison tests were used to analyse and define significant differences between samples (untreated, 0.6, 0.7 and 0.8 MPa). Differences were considered significant when p-values were <0.05.

Supplementary Materials: Supplementary materials can be found at http://www.mdpi.com/1422-0067/21/8/3024/s1.

Author Contributions: Conceptualisation, Y.Y., R.M.S. and C.T.M.; methodology, Y.Y., R.M.S. and C.T.M.; formal analysis, Y.Y., B.B. and K.M.G.v.d.W.-J.; investigation, Y.Y., B.B. and K.M.G.v.d.W.-J.; writing—original draft preparation, Y.Y.; writing—review and editing, Y.Y., B.B., R.M.S. and C.T.M.; supervision, Y.Y. and C.T.M.; project administration, Y.Y.; funding acquisition, Y.Y. All authors have read and agreed to the published version of the manuscript.

Funding: The work was supported by the Focused Ultrasound Foundation (Y.Y., High Risk personal grant).

Acknowledgments: Authors acknowledge technical support given by Roel Deckers (ultrasound setup) from Imaging Division, University Medical Center Utrecht, Utrecht, the Netherlands and George Posthuma (transmission electron microscopy) from Cell Microscopy Center, Cell Biology Department, University Medical Center Utrecht, The Netherlands. This work was funded by Focused Ultrasound Foundation (High Risk Track grant, YY).

Conflicts of Interest: The authors declare no conflict of interest. The funders had no role in the design of the study; in the collection, analyses, or interpretation of data; in the writing of the manuscript, or in the decision to publish the results.

References

1. Balachandran, B.; Yuana, Y. Extracellular vesicles-based drug delivery system for cancer treatment. *Cogent Med.* **2019**, *6*, 1–23. [CrossRef]
2. Liu, D.; Yang, F.; Xiong, F.; Gu, N. The Smart Drug Delivery System and Its Clinical Potential. *Theranostics* **2016**, *6*, 1306–1323. [CrossRef] [PubMed]
3. Yuana, Y.; Sturk, A.; Nieuwland, R. Extracellular vesicles in physiological and pathological conditions. *Blood Rev.* **2013**, *27*, 31–39. [CrossRef] [PubMed]
4. Walker, S.; Busatto, S.; Pham, A.; Tian, M.; Suh, A.; Carson, K.; Quintero, A.; Lafrence, M.; Malik, H.; Santana, M.X.; et al. Extracellular vesicle-based drug delivery systems for cancer treatment. *Theranostics* **2019**, *9*, 8001–8017. [CrossRef] [PubMed]
5. Tang, K.; Zhang, Y.; Zhang, H.; Xu, P.; Liu, J.; Ma, J.; Lv, M.; Li, D.; Katirai, F.; Shen, G.X.; et al. Delivery of chemotherapeutic drugs in tumour cell-derived microparticles. *Nat. Commun.* **2012**, *3*, 1282. [CrossRef]

6. Van der Meel, R.; Fens, M.H.; Vader, P.; van Solinge, W.W.; Eniola-Adefeso, O.; Schiffelers, R.M. Extracellular vesicles as drug delivery systems: Lessons from the liposome field. *J. Control Release* **2014**, *195*, 72–85. [CrossRef]
7. Fais, S.; O'Driscoll, L.; Borras, F.E.; Buzas, E.; Camussi, G.; Cappello, F.; Carvalho, J.; Cordeiro da Silva, A.; Del Portillo, H.; El Andaloussi, S.; et al. Evidence-Based Clinical Use of Nanoscale Extracellular Vesicles in Nanomedicine. *ACS Nano.* **2016**, *10*, 3886–3899. [CrossRef]
8. Mitragotri, S. Healing sound: The use of ultrasound in drug delivery and other therapeutic applications. *Nat. Rev. Drug Discov.* **2005**, *4*, 255–260. [CrossRef]
9. Sennoga, C.A.; Kanbar, E.; Auboire, L.; Dujardin, P.A.; Fouan, D.; Escoffre, J.M.; Bouakaz, A. Microbubble-mediated ultrasound drug-delivery and therapeutic monitoring. *Expert Opin. Drug Deliv.* **2016**, 1–13. [CrossRef]
10. Bouakaz, A.; Zeghimi, A.; Doinikov, A.A. Sonoporation: Concept and Mechanisms. In *Therapeutic Ultrasound*; Escoffre, J.-M., Bouakaz, A., Eds.; Springer International Publishing: Cham, Switzerland, 2016; pp. 175–189. ISBN 978-3-319-22536-4.
11. Lentacker, I.; De Cock, I.; Deckers, R.; De Smedt, S.C.; Moonen, C.T. Understanding ultrasound induced sonoporation: Definitions and underlying mechanisms. *Adv. Drug Deliv. Rev.* **2014**, *72*, 49–64. [CrossRef]
12. Suzuki, R.; Klibanov, A.L. Co-administration of Microbubbles and Drugs in Ultrasound-Assisted Drug Delivery: Comparison with Drug-Carrying Particles. *Adv. Exp. Med. Biol.* **2016**, *880*, 205–220. [PubMed]
13. Zhao, Y.Z.; Du, L.N.; Lu, C.T.; Jin, Y.G.; Ge, S.P. Potential and problems in ultrasound-responsive drug delivery systems. *Int. J. Nanomedicine* **2013**, *8*, 1621–1633. [PubMed]
14. Yuana, Y.; Jiang, L.; Lammertink, B.H.A.; Vader, P.; Deckers, R.; Bos, C.; Schiffelers, R.M.; Moonen, C.T. Microbubbles-Assisted Ultrasound Triggers the Release of Extracellular Vesicles. *Int. J. Mol. Sci.* **2017**, *18*, 1610. [CrossRef] [PubMed]
15. Zomer, A.; Maynard, C.; Verweij, F.J.; Kamermans, A.; Schafer, R.; Beerling, E.; Schiffelers, R.M.; de Wit, E.; Berenguer, J.; Ellenbroek, S.I.; et al. In Vivo imaging reveals extracellular vesicle-mediated phenocopying of metastatic behavior. *Cell* **2015**, *161*, 1046–1057. [CrossRef] [PubMed]
16. Lammertink, B.; Deckers, R.; Storm, G.; Moonen, C.; Bos, C. Duration of ultrasound-mediated enhanced plasma membrane permeability. *Int. J. Pharm.* **2015**, *482*, 92–98. [CrossRef] [PubMed]
17. Donahue, N.D.; Acar, H.; Wilhelm, S. Concepts of nanoparticle cellular uptake, intracellular trafficking, and kinetics in nanomedicine. *Adv. Drug Deliv. Rev.* **2019**, *143*, 68–96. [CrossRef]
18. Hessvik, N.P.; Llorente, A. Current knowledge on exosome biogenesis and release. *Cell. Mol. Life Sci.* **2018**, *75*, 193–208. [CrossRef]
19. Ortega, F.G.; Roefs, M.T.; de Miguel Perez, D.; Kooijmans, S.A.; de Jong, O.G.; Sluijter, J.P.; Schiffelers, R.M.; Vader, P. Interfering with endolysosomal trafficking enhances release of bioactive exosomes. *Nanomed. Nanotechnol. Biol. Med.* **2019**, *20*, 1–12. [CrossRef]
20. Safaei, R.; Larson, B.J.; Cheng, T.C.; Gibson, M.A.; Otani, S.; Naerdemann, W.; Howell, S.B. Abnormal lysosomal trafficking and enhanced exosomal export of cisplatin in drug-resistant human ovarian carcinoma cells. *Mol. Cancer Ther.* **2005**, *4*, 1595–1604. [CrossRef]
21. Van Niel, G.; D'Angelo, G.; Raposo, G. Shedding light on the cell biology of extracellular vesicles. *Nat. Rev. Mol. Cell Biol.* **2018**, *19*, 213–228. [CrossRef]
22. Lázaro-Ibáñez, E.; Neuvonen, M.; Takatalo, M.; Thanigai Arasu, U.; Capasso, C.; Cerullo, V.; Rhim, J.S.; Rilla, K.; Yliperttula, M.; Siljander, P.R.M. Metastatic state of parent cells influences the uptake and functionality of prostate cancer cell-derived extracellular vesicles. *J. Extracell. Vesicles* **2017**, *6*, 1–12. [CrossRef] [PubMed]
23. Schneider, M. Characteristics of SonoVuetrade mark. *Echocardiography* **1999**, *16*, 743–746. [CrossRef]
24. Marwaha, R.; Sharma, M. DQ-Red BSA Trafficking Assay in Cultured Cells to Assess Cargo Delivery to Lysosomes. *Bio-Protocol* **2017**, *7*, 1–12. [CrossRef] [PubMed]
25. Lammertink, B.H.A.; Bos, C.; van der Wurff-Jacobs, K.M.; Storm, G.; Moonen, C.T.; Deckers, R. Increase of intracellular cisplatin levels and radiosensitization by ultrasound in combination with microbubbles. *J. Control. Release* **2016**, *238*, 157–165. [CrossRef] [PubMed]
26. Van der Pol, E.; Coumans, F.A.; Grootemaat, A.E.; Gardiner, C.; Sargent, I.L.; Harrison, P.; Sturk, A.; van Leeuwen, T.G.; Nieuwland, R. Particle size distribution of exosomes and microvesicles determined by transmission electron microscopy, flow cytometry, nanoparticle tracking analysis, and resistive pulse sensing. *J. Thromb. Haemost* **2014**, *12*, 1182–1192. [CrossRef] [PubMed]

27. Cizmar, P.; Yuana, Y. Detection and Characterization of Extracellular Vesicles by Transmission and Cryo-Transmission Electron Microscopy. *Methods Mol. Biol.* **2017**, *1660*, 221–232.
28. Schneider, C.A.; Rasband, W.S.; Eliceiri, K.W. NIH Image to ImageJ: 25 years of image analysis. *Nat. Methods* **2012**, *9*, 671–675. [CrossRef]
29. Van der Pol, E.; Coumans, F.; Varga, Z.; Krumrey, M.; Nieuwland, R. Innovation in detection of microparticles and exosomes. *J. Thromb. Haemost.* **2013**, *11*, 36–45. [CrossRef] [PubMed]

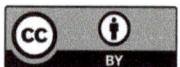

© 2020 by the authors. Licensee MDPI, Basel, Switzerland. This article is an open access article distributed under the terms and conditions of the Creative Commons Attribution (CC BY) license (http://creativecommons.org/licenses/by/4.0/).

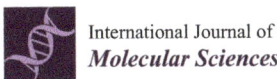

Review

Extracellular Vesicles in the Development of Cancer Therapeutics

Haoyao Sun [1,2], Stephanie Burrola [1], Jinchang Wu [2,3],* and Wei-Qun Ding [1],*

1. Department of Pathology, University of Oklahoma Health Science Center, Oklahoma City, OK 73104, USA; haoyao-sun@ouhsc.edu (H.S.); Stephanie-Burrola@ouhsc.edu (S.B.)
2. Department of Radiation Oncology, The Affiliated Suzhou Hospital of Nanjing Medical University, Suzhou 215001, China
3. Section of Oncology, The Second Affiliated Hospital of Xuzhou Medical University, Xuzhou 221006, China
* Correspondence: dr.wjinchang@gmail.com (J.W.); weiqun-ding@ouhsc.edu (W.-Q.D.); Tel.: +86-1377-604-8328 (J.W.); +1-405-271-1605 (W.-Q.D.)

Received: 5 August 2020; Accepted: 19 August 2020; Published: 24 August 2020

Abstract: Extracellular vesicles (EVs) are small lipid bilayer-delimited nanoparticles released from all types of cells examined thus far. Several groups of EVs, including exosomes, microvesicles, and apoptotic bodies, have been identified according to their size and biogenesis. With extensive investigations on EVs over the last decade, it is now recognized that EVs play a pleiotropic role in various physiological processes as well as pathological conditions through mediating intercellular communication. Most notably, EVs have been shown to be involved in cancer initiation and progression and EV signaling in cancer are viewed as potential therapeutic targets. Furthermore, as membrane nanoparticles, EVs are natural products with some of them, such as tumor exosomes, possessing tumor homing propensity, thus leading to strategies utilizing EVs as drug carriers to effectively deliver cancer therapeutics. In this review, we summarize recent reports on exploring EVs signaling as potential therapeutic targets in cancer as well as on developing EVs as therapeutic delivery carriers for cancer therapy. Findings from preclinical studies are primarily discussed, with early phase clinical trials reviewed. We hope to provide readers updated information on the development of EVs as cancer therapeutic targets or therapeutic carriers.

Keywords: extracellular vesicle; microvesicle; exosome; cancer therapeutic; drug carrier

1. Introduction

Extracellular vesicles (EVs) are a generic term referring to several groups of small lipid bilayer-delimited particles generated through various cellular processes and released from all types of cells investigated thus far. These membrane vesicles, including microvesicles (also known as microparticles or ectosomes), exosomes, and apoptotic bodies, all lack a functional nucleus and are unable to replicate themselves. They are constantly released from cells and are involved in a variety of physiological as well as pathological processes. The initial discovery of EVs can be tracked back to 1946 when ultracentrifugation pellets were found to be associated with the activation of platelets and procoagulant properties in human plasma [1]. In the 1980s, EVs released by reticulocytes were captured by electronic microscopy and were considered "waste disposals" to remove waste materials during red blood cell maturation [2,3]. However, EV-mediated transfer of genetic and cellular materials between different cell types was recognized in the late 2000s by several research groups [4–8], thus establishing EVs as messengers for intercellular communication with biological consequences.

Among all the EVs described, exosomes are defined by their small sizes (40–120 nm) and endocytic origin and are most extensively characterized over the years. In the context of cancer, it has been demonstrated that exosomes play a pivotal role in the tumor microenvironment by mediating intercellular communication among cancer cells and stromal cells, thereby promoting tumor proliferation, metastasis, and chemo-resistance [9]. The contribution of exosomal signaling to tumor progression has led to the development of therapeutic strategies targeting various steps of the exosomal signaling processes (see Section 2). On the other hand, since exosomes are endogenously produced and can be transferred among various types of cells, the potential of using these small vesicles as vehicles for drug delivery has been actively explored (see Section 3). In this review, we will focus on recent work in the development of cancer therapeutics targeting EV-mediated cellular processes or utilizing EVs as vehicles for drug delivery. Furthermore, we will discuss the clinical trials that are ongoing or completed using naturally produced EVs as cancer therapeutic vehicles. A simplified view of general aspects of EVs is provided at the first section of this review.

2. EV Cargos and Functions

2.1. EV Nomenclature

EVs were initially called platelet dust, as they were vesicles derived from platelets. In the 1970s, the term "extracellular vesicles" was used to describe calcifying globules in epiphyseal cartilage that were observed by histochemical staining [10]. Since then, the nomenclature of EVs has significantly evolved and EVs are now named primarily according to their sizes and biogenesis processes or the way of release [11]. It is well accepted that there are three main subgroups of EVs that have been identified thus far: (a) exosomes, (b) microvesicles (MVs, also named microparticles/ectosomes), and (c) apoptotic bodies [12]. The most researched EVs are exosomes, which were firstly termed in the 1980s as a group of vesicles ranging from 40 to 120 nm in diameter, formed by the invagination of the multi-vesicular bodies (MVBs) during the late endosome formation [2,3,13]. Differing from exosomes, MVs are larger membrane vesicles (up to 1000 nm in diameter) which are produced by direct budding from cellular membranes, whereas apoptotic bodies are even larger vesicles with 800–5000 nm in diameter and formed during programmed cell death [14,15]. Recently, a smaller group of non-membranous nanoparticles termed "exomeres" (~35 nm) was also reported, which is likely to be generated through a unique cellular process [16]. The overlap in sizes of different EV groups and the difficulty in separating individual EV groups by current isolation techniques have hindered our understanding of their biogenesis, molecular compositions, biodistributions, and functions. For this reason, the International Society for Extracellular Vesicles (ISEV) provided guidelines on the terminology and minimum requirements for defining EV populations in experimental research in 2014, which was updated in 2018 (MISEV2018) [17]. Most notably, instead of using the terms exosomes or MVs, the guidelines urge authors to name EV subtypes based on their physical characteristics, such as size or density, with ranges being defined, biochemical compositions, and the experimental conditions or cell of origin. In accordance with this recommendation, exosomes are considered small EVs (sEVs), which is the term we used interchangeably with exosomes, wherever appropriate, throughout this review.

2.2. EV Surface Markers and Cargos

EVs carry various biomolecules including proteins, RNA, DNA, and lipids. Each group of biomolecules in EVs is often heterogeneous, primarily relating to different EV types, experimental conditions, and their cellular origins [11]. The most characterized EV components are EV proteins and RNAs, especially small RNAs [18]. EV surface protein markers have been critically examined in order to establish specific markers for validating isolated EVs. The MISEV2018 guidelines provide several groups of protein markers in evaluating isolated EVs as well as minimal requirements in experimental data presentation when it comes to EV isolation and characterization [17].

It has come to a consensus that sEVs stably express specific transmembrane proteins such as tetraspanins (most notably CD63, CD9, CD81), Major Histocompatibility Complex (MHC) class I proteins (such as HLA-A/B/C), transferrin receptor, LAMP1/2, and others. These membrane proteins, especially tetraspanins, are frequently applied to validate isolated sEVs. In addition, cytosolic proteins can also be specific markers for sEVs, including Alix, TSG-101, flotillins-1/2, annexins, and heat shock proteins, among others. Cell- or tissue-specific EV markers have also been reported, such as TSPAN8 and EPCAM (epithelial cell), CD37 and CD53 (leukocytes), PECAM1 (endothelial cells), and ERBB2 (breast cancer). Given the heterogeneity of EVs, it is recommended that at least one membrane protein marker, one cytosolic protein marker, and one non-EV protein marker have to be used to validate the isolated sEVs from large EVs [16,17]. It has been recognized that proteins from the nucleus, mitochondria, endoplasmic reticulum, and the Golgi complex are mostly absent in sEVs, which can serve as negative control markers for these vesicles [19]. Enormous efforts have been placed on profiling proteomes of sEVs and the comprehensive databases of sEV proteins can be found at: Vesiclepedia [15], EVpedia [20], and ExoCarta [21].

sEVs contain various RNA species. However, most studies demonstrated that small non-coding RNAs, such as microRNAs, are the major RNA species contained in sEVs, although the presence of mRNA, rRNA, and tRNA in sEVs was also reported [22,23]. Typically, sEVs may contain hundreds of microRNA species in various quantities that play important roles in intercellular communication [7,23–25]. Both coding and non-coding RNAs seem to be functional through transferring from host cells to the recipient cells [26–28]. Specific RNA profiles of sEVs derived from different biofluids or tissues are categorized by several databases, including: Exobase [29], exRNA Atlas [30], and miRandola [31].

DNA in sEVs has also been described, with DNA fragments originating either from the nucleus or from the mitochondria. It seems that all genome DNA are represented randomly in sEVs, which eliminates the possibility of selective DNA packaging [32–34]. While cancer cell-derived sEVs may contain more genomic DNA than that from non-cancer cells [34], whether and how sEV DNA contributes to intercellular communications in the tumor microenvironment, thereby affecting tumor progression, remains to be determined.

2.3. EV Functions

It has long been known that cell-to-cell communication is a strategy utilized to facilitate physiological and pathological processes in various organisms. However, the EV-mediated intercellular communication was only recognized in recent years [7,23]. The double-layer lipid membrane of EVs protects inside contents, allowing transfer of EV materials to surrounding cells or to distal organs via the circulatory system. Most notably, sEVs have been considered potent vehicles to mediate intercellular communication [11]. By transferring signaling molecules among different cell types, sEVs have been shown to play pleiotropic roles in regulating cellular and physiological processes. This includes participating in hemostasis by enhancing coagulation, regulating both innate and acquired immune responses, involvement in pregnancy and embryonic development, as well as other physiological events [35–44].

In addition to mediating intercellular communication, EVs may function as waste disposals to remove unwanted cellular materials. In fact, sEVs were first observed to facilitate reticulocyte maturation via cargo disposing [2,3]. In supporting this function of sEVs, several recent studies revealed the cross-regulation of the EV pathway and lysosomal degradation pathway [45]. Two established lysosome inhibitors, chloroquine and bafilomycin A1, were shown to enhance sEV release [46–48], suggesting that sEVs may act as an alternate pathway for cell component degradation and clearance. The involvement of sEVs in cellular homeostasis is further supported by the findings showing that ubiquitin and ubiquitinated proteins are present in sEVs [49], along with selective lipids and other soluble cellular components [50,51].

The role of sEVs in pathological processes has been evident, especially in cancer. Cancer progression is a dysregulated and uncontrolled pathological process [52]. It is well described that cancer-derived sEVs promote tumor development [53–55] by acting at different stages of cancer progression [56] through various mechanisms. Evidence is provided to indicate that cancer sEVs are involved in enhancing tumorigenesis of epithelial cells [53,57], sustaining tumor angiogenesis [58,59], promoting tumor growth [60,61], facilitating cancer cell invasion and metastasis [54,55,62,63], and contributing to chemo-resistance [64,65] and immunosuppression [66,67]. These important findings of the tumor-promoting effects of cancer sEVs lead to new cancer therapeutic opportunities that aim at targeting cancer exosomal signaling processes, as discussed below.

3. EVs as Potential Therapeutic Targets in Cancer

Given the growing evidence of sEVs' involvement in cancer progression, several strategies have been tested or envisioned to target various steps of the sEVs signaling in order to block their tumor promoting effect. These include targeting cancer sEV biogenesis and release, blocking sEV uptake by recipient cells, eliminating circulating cancer sEVs, and removing specific components from sEVs that contribute to cancer pathogenesis [68–70].

3.1. Suppressing sEV Biogenesis and Release

At the cellular level, sEVs are derived from the endosomal pathway. The invagination of endosomal membranes generates intraluminal vesicles inside of the endosome, forming MVBs. These vesicles are released by cells upon fusion of the endosome with the cellular plasma membrane and the released vesicles are termed exosomes or sEVs [71,72]. The process of forming sEVs and releasing them from cells requires a coordinated effort by various cytoplasmic proteins. This includes endosomal sorting complexes required for transport (ESCRT) and tetraspanins necessary for intraluminal vesicle formation, sphingomyelinase to generate ceramides vital for intraluminal vesicles' formation and sorting, and Rab27a and Rab27b critical for cellular endosomal trafficking [55,71,73]. In an early effort to suppress sEVs' biogenesis, GW4869, a sphingomyelinase inhibitor, was used, which reduced ceramide generation and inhibited sEV formation [74]. Furthermore, attenuation of neutral sphingomyelinase 2 (nSMase2) in breast cancer cells by a knockdown approach reduced sEV formation and attenuated sEV-associated miR-210 transfer, leading to the suppression of cancer cell metastasis in vitro and in a xenograft mouse model [75]. However, the role of nSMase2 in sEV formation and secretion from other cultured cancer cell lines remains unclear [76,77], compromising this approach of targeting sEV biogenesis. Other potential strategies in targeting sEV biogenesis that have been tested or envisioned include the use of Amiloride, an anti-hypotension drug, which reduced sEV yields by blocking membrane-associated heat shock protein 72 (HSP72) in a STAT3-dependent manner in myeloid-derived suppressor cells [78]; inhibiting the syndecan-syntenin-Alix signaling process, since the syndecan heparan sulphate proteoglycans and their cytoplasmic adaptor syntenin, along with Alix and ESCRT, control the formation of sEVs [79]; and targeting cellular molecules, such as Rab27a/b [70,73,80], Rab11, Rab35 [81,82], TSG101, and TSAP6 [70], which are either related to sEV formation or trafficking and secretion from cancer cells. Using a high-throughput screening approach, a recent study identifies that manumycin-A (MA), a natural microbial metabolite, inhibits sEV biogenesis and secretion via the Ras/Raf/ERK1/2 signaling in castration-resistant prostate cancer cells but not in normal prostate epithelial cells [83], indicating a new compound that may serve as a cancer therapeutic via inhibiting sEV biogenesis and secretion. In another high-throughput screening study, miR-26a was identified as being involved in sEV secretion from prostate cancer cells [84], suggesting a new molecular target for suppressing cancer sEV secretion.

3.2. Preventing EV Uptake

Several sEV uptake mechanisms have been recently proposed (Figure 1), including sEV membrane direct fusion with plasma membrane, thereby releasing sEV contents to recipient cells [85,86], and receptor-mediated endocytosis [87], clathrin- and caveolin-mediated endocytosis [88,89], phagocytosis [90], and macropinocytosis [88,91]. Detailed regulation of each of the pathways and their proportional contributions to sEV uptake remains to be further elucidated. It seems reasonable to assume that the uptake to a large extent depends on sEV surface protein compositions and the type of cells in which the sEVs are internalized. Furthermore, irrespective of the uptake pathways, internalized materials will be processed via the endosomal/lysosomal pathway [92]. While limiting cancer sEV uptake by recipient cells is a potential strategy to block cancer sEV signaling and attenuate cancer sEVs' tumor-promoting effect, few studies have been published to support this strategy. Nevertheless, evidence has been provided to indicate that it is feasible to modulate the sEV uptake process in order to attenuate the sEV-induced effect in the recipient cells. Some examples include the following. Autophagy inhibitors such as chloroquine, bafilomycin A, and monensin, were shown to significantly inhibit sEV internalization into microglia, likely through altering vacuolar acidification [91]. Two potent PI3K inhibitors, Wortmannin and LY294002, concentration-dependently inhibited sEV uptake by macrophages, indicating that PI3K is essential for sEV phagocytosis [90]. Disruption of the actin cytoskeleton using Cytochalasin D or Lantrunculin A inhibited sEV uptake by Human Umbilical Vein Cells (HUVECs), confirming that an intact cytoskeleton facilitates sEV internalization [93]. Chlorpromazine, which blocks clathrin-mediated endocytosis, inhibited sEV uptake by ovarian cancer cells [94] and endothelial cells [95], and heparin dose-dependently inhibited sEV uptake by glioblastoma (GBM) cells [96] and bone marrow stromal cells [97]. These findings reinforce the notion that targeting the uptake of cancer sEVs is a promising strategy in the development of new cancer therapeutics, and future efforts should focus on small molecules capable of inhibiting cancer sEV uptake and suppressing tumor progression.

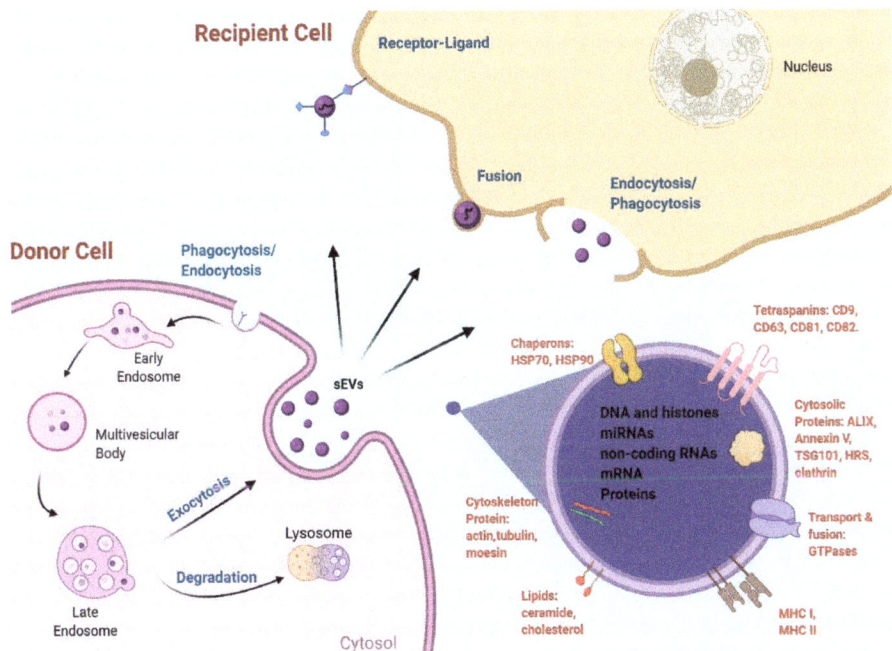

Figure 1. sEV biogenesis, release, uptake, and contents. Created with BioRender.com.

3.3. Eliminating Circulating Cancer sEVs

The transfer of cancer sEVs through the circulatory system to distal organs has been reported to promote tumor metastasis via various mechanisms, most notably by forming pre-metastatic niches in the distal organs [55,62,98]. Considering that most cancer deaths are due to metastatic disease, eliminating circulating cancer sEVs is presumably a great strategy to prevent cancer metastasis, thereby reducing cancer mortality. The idea of "cleaning" the blood to prevent cancer metastasis has been tested many years ago. In the late 1980s, using a continuous whole blood UltraPheresis procedure, plasma fractions with molecular weight less than 150 kDa were removed from patients with metastatic cancer, which reduced tumor size and improved patient immune response and Karnofsky Performance Status [99]. While this technique did not consider removing blood sEVs at the time, it inspired others to develop new devices to remove cancer sEVs from patient plasma [64]. For instance, Hemopurifier®, an affinity-based purifier developed by Aethlon Medical Inc. (San Diego, CA, USA), has been shown to selectively capture viral particles (which have similar size as sEVs) in the plasmas of individuals infected with Hepatitis C and Human Immunodeficiency Virus (HIV) [100,101], and this device is being modified and tested for removal of Her2-positive breast cancer exosomes from patient plasma ([64], https://grantome.com/grant/NIH/R43-CA232977-01). Moreover, a phase I clinical trial using Hemopurifier® in conjunction with pembrolizumab (Keytruda) in patients with advanced head and neck cancer has been recently approved by the Food and Drug Administration (FDA) (NCT04453046).

In line with the strategy of eliminating circulating cancer sEVs, a recent report demonstrated, in a xenograft nude mouse model, that treatment of the mice with human anti-CD9 and anti-CD63 antibodies (intravenous injection) disrupts cancer sEVs in the circulation and suppresses the pulmonary metastasis of implanted human breast cancer cells, yet, has no effect on primary tumor growth of the implants or metastatic ability of the cells in vitro [102]. These findings support the strategy to suppress cancer metastasis via inhibiting the pro-metastatic functions of cancer-derived sEVs using antibodies against their surface proteins. In addition, an innovative design of aptamer-functionalized nanoparticles was shown to eliminate blood oncogenic sEVs into the small intestine, and attenuate oncogenic sEV-induced lung metastasis in mice [103]. This technology utilized positively charged mesoporous silica nanoparticles equipped with Epidermal Growth Factor Receptor (EGFR)-targeting aptamers specifically recognizing and binding the negatively charged oncogenic sEVs and towing them from blood to bile duct for elimination. This interesting study proves that it is feasible to remove oncogenic sEVs selectively from the blood stream, thereby reducing tumor metastatic potential. Further investigations are warranted along this line of research.

3.4. Targeting Specific sEV Cargo Components

Specific sEV components that mediate sEVs' tumor-promoting activity are obvious potential cancer therapeutic targets. Some of the targets have been recently explored in order to develop new cancer therapeutics. As discussed above, antibodies against human CD9 and CD63, two well-established sEV surface markers [17], were shown to disrupt oncogenic sEVs and inhibit tumor metastasis in a breast cancer xenograft nude mouse model [102]. However, this experiment strategy of targeting human CD9 and CD63 is only applicable in a xenograft nude mouse model for selectively eliminating human cancer sEVs from the blood, since CD9 and CD63 are expressed in sEVs released from both noncancerous and cancerous cells in humans. Targeting of cancer-specific sEV components will be preferred to achieve a cancer-specific effect. In this context, a recent report demonstrated that cytoskeleton-associated protein 4 (CKAP4), a novel Dickkopf1 (DKK1) receptor, was selectively contained in sEVs from pancreatic ductal adenocarcinoma (PDAC) cells, not in sEVs from normal cells. Various anti-CKAP4 antibodies were then utilized to block the interaction of DKK1 with sEV-associated CKAP4, resulting in an inhibition of the proliferation and migration of PDAC cells and a prolonged survival of PDAC xenograft nude mice [104], supporting further development of this targeting strategy.

In another report, miR-365 in macrophage-derived sEVs was found to significantly decrease the sensitivity of PDAC cells to gemcitabine, and a miR-365 antagonist was able to reverse the gemcitabine resistance of PDAC cells in vitro and in vivo [105], thus suggesting that targeting miR-365 in macrophage-derived sEVs renders PDAC cells more sensitive to gemcitabine. Similarly, miR-155 was found in PDAC cell-derived sEVs that mediates transfer of the gemcitabine resistance traits from resistant PDAC cells to sensitive PDAC cells, conferring gemcitabine resistance of PDAC cells. Targeting miR-155 or the exosome secretion of PDAC cells effectively attenuated the gemcitabine resistance in PDAC cell lines and in xenograft nude mice [106]. Other cancer sEV-associated microRNAs, such as miR-21 and miR-1246, have also been found to be selectively enriched in cancer sEVs and considered as therapeutic targets [107,108]. Since cancer sEVs selectively encapsulate certain microRNA species [25,109–111], targeting cancer sEV-associated microRNAs will continue to be an attractive strategy for the development of new cancer therapeutics.

Immune checkpoint protein inhibitors, such as PD1/PD-L1 inhibitors, are novel cancer therapeutic targets which have revolutionized cancer therapy with great efficacy, even for those cancer patients whom standard therapy has failed [112]. However, only 10%–30% of patients responded to checkpoint inhibitor therapy [113]. The immune escape is partially due to the fact that tumor-derived sEVs contain PD-L1, a PD1 ligand, which binds to PD1 on the surface of T cells and suppresses T cell activation [66,67]. The sEV PD-L1 level was thus suggested to be a prognostic marker for anti-PD1 therapy response [114], and blocking sEV PD-L1 has been proposed to overcome the resistance to anti-PD-1/PD-L1 antibody therapy [115]. Indeed, anti-PD-L1 antibodies were shown to block sEV PD-L1, induce systemic anti-tumor immunity, and suppress tumor growth in a syngeneic colorectal cancer model [67].

New oncogenic components in cancer sEVs are continuously being identified which may contribute to tumor progression or chemo-resistance [116,117]. Efforts on targeting these sEV-associated oncogenic molecules for cancer therapeutic development are expected to expand.

4. EVs as Drug Carriers in Cancer Treatment

Compared to artificial drug vehicles, such as liposomes, EVs are favored drug carriers [118] because of their autologous nature that would prevent undesired immunogenicity and toxicity [119,120]. sEVs also possess high capacity of homing toward tumor cells when compared to liposomes [62,121], implying that sEVs are more efficient in delivering drugs for cancer therapy. Furthermore, studies have shown that sEVs are stable membrane vesicles under different pH values, temperatures, or freeze–thaw cycles [122], and these properties can be further enhanced by surface modification [123], supporting their potential compliance with good manufacturing practices (GMPs) in future clinical use. In addition, as nano-sized particles, sEVs were shown to be able to cross the blood–brain barrier and the tumor vasculature via enhanced permeability and retention (EPR), thereby potentially increasing accumulation of nanoparticles in brain tumors [124–126].

Diverse techniques have been practiced to encapsulate cancer therapeutics by sEVs in order to develop more efficient tumor-targeting vehicles. Here, we review the sEV loading strategies reported in recent literature.

4.1. EV Sources and Loading Efficiency

Based on the heterogeneity of sEVs derived from various biological sources [18], it is safe to assume that the source of the sEVs may relate to their drug loading efficiency and their therapeutic efficacy. Indeed, experimental evidence has been provided to show that drug loading efficiency of sEVs derived from pancreatic stellate cells (PSCs), pancreatic cancer cells (PCCs), and macrophages significantly differ when doxorubicin was simply incubated with the sEVs, with those from PCCs being most efficient. However, the doxorubicin-loaded macrophage sEVs are most effective in killing cancer cells, indicating that higher loading capacity does not equal to high anticancer activity of the drug-loaded sEVs [127]. This implies that both the biological source of the sEVs and the drug loading efficiency need to be evaluated when sEVs are applied as drug carriers for cancer therapy. In line with this concept, sEVs derived from mesenchymal stem cells (MSCs) are considered good carriers for drug delivery because they possess low immunogenicity [9,128] and are well tolerated in mice [129] and humans [130]. Both a miR-9 inhibitor and the chemo drug paclitaxel have been successfully incorporated into sEVs derived from MSCs which inhibited tumor cell growth [131,132]. However, allogeneic MSCs may also be able to transfer immunogenic proteins, such as MHC molecules, via secreted EVs, which might cause immunological responses [133]. Furthermore, the immunogenicity of MSCs-derived EVs varies, depending on experimental conditions by which the

EVs are produced [134]. Future efforts are required to closely monitor immunologic responses post administration of MSCs-derived EVs and develop uniform procedures in preparing MSCs-derived EVs. In addition to MSCs, sEVs from immature dendritic cells or self-derived dendritic cells were also considered, possessing low immunogenicity and used to encapsulate siRNA or doxorubicin for therapeutic applications [135,136]. Interestingly, cancer cell-derived sEVs were shown to have unique targeting abilities homing to tumorous microenvironments [137]. sEVs from HeLa and patient ascites were shown to deliver heterologous siRNAs to HeLa cells and cause cell death [138]. Autologous sEVs were found to be safe and effective in delivering gemcitabine for pancreatic cancer therapy in experimental model systems [139]. These results show that cancer cell-derived sEVs are promising carriers for effective delivery of chemotherapeutic drugs or nucleotides. Given the tumor-promoting activity of cancer-derived sEVs [53–55], the safety and long-term effect of these membrane vesicles as drug-delivery carriers needs to be carefully evaluated.

4.2. Loading Therapeutics into sEVs via Donor Cells

Efficient loading of cancer therapeutics into a given sEV population can be critical when it comes to drug efficacy. In this context, one loading strategy that has been described in packaging cancer therapeutics into sEVs is to load cancer therapeutics into sEVs via donor cells, which is in contrast to directly loading therapeutics into isolated sEVs. In this case, microRNAs have been most often loaded into sEVs via the donor cells. For example, adipose tissue-derived MSCs were transfected with a miR-122 expression plasmid to overexpress this microRNA and the sEVs derived from these cells were highly enriched in miR-122. An intra-tumor injection of miR-122-enriched sEVs significantly increased the efficacy of Sorafenib on inhibiting hepatocellular carcinoma in a xenograft nude mouse model [140]. Functional delivery of miR-21 derived from glioma cells to the surrounding microglia led to downregulation of specific miR-21 mRNA target genes [141]; likewise, sEVs from primary glioma cells, stably expressing miR-302-367, were shown to enrich in miR-302-367 by internalizing neighboring glioblastoma cells, and altering tumor development in vivo [142], and overexpression of miR-146b in marrow stromal cells generated sEVs with high miR-146b content, which significantly reduced glioma xenograft growth in rats [143]. More studies have been reported in testing the strategy of loading microRNA inhibitors or mimics into sEVs via the donor cells for therapeutic applications, as was recently reviewed [144].

An interesting study demonstrated that the chemotherapeutic paclitaxel (PTX) could be added directly to the culture of MSCs to generate sEVs that are highly associated with PTX and significantly suppress cancer cell proliferation [132]. However, this strategy of loading chemotherapeutics into sEVs has been less explored, likely because of the loading efficiency, considering the potential metalizing of PTX in treated cells. Instead, direct loading of chemotherapeutics and microRNA/siRNAs into the isolated sEVs has been widely adapted for testing sEVs as drug carriers for therapeutic delivery.

4.3. Loading Therapeutics into Isolated sEVs

The lipid-bilayer membrane structure of sEVs favors encapsulating hydrophobic compounds and molecules, which may directly integrate into the sEVs without disturbing their membrane barrier. In contrast, hydrophilic compounds and molecules require permeabilization of the bilayer membrane in order to be incorporated into the sEVs [145,146]. Various approaches have been proposed to load hydrophobic and hydrophilic drugs or biological molecules into sEVs. The most common approaches include opening up the pores in lipid membranes by physic forces, such as electroporation, sonication, freeze and thaw cycles, and extrusion, and by chemical means, such as using transfection reagents. The pros and cons of these methods for membrane permeabilization and cargo loading has been reviewed elsewhere [147]. Therefore, we will only briefly discuss these loading approaches in the following.

Direct incubation of therapeutics with sEVs at given temperatures and durations is a simple strategy for loading drugs into sEVs. The loading efficiency mainly relies on the concentration of the drugs or molecules and their hydrophobicity. A proper loading can usually be achieved for hydrophobic compounds without disturbing the integrity of the sEV membrane [132]. Nevertheless, the loading efficiency is often lower compared to other loading approaches.

Electroporation has been a method widely used to introduce DNA or RNA into mammalian cells [148,149], and is often applied for drug or nucleotide loading into sEVs [150,151]. The desired sEVs will be co-incubated with the therapeutics and exposed to certain volts of electric fields to open up the pores of the sEV membrane to allow the therapeutics to enter into the permeabilized sEVs. This method has been preferentially applied when incorporating nucleic acids like siRNA, mRNA, DNA, and microRNA, into sEVs [152]. Its loading efficiency is usually higher than incubation [139]. However, the main drawback of this method is the risk of damaging the EV membranes that may cause aggregation of sEVs and precipitation of nucleic acids.

Sonication uses ultrasound energy transmitted through a sonicating probe that reduces the rigidity of sEV membranes, thus allowing more therapeutic molecules to be incorporated into sEVs. For example, PTX was loaded into sEVs more efficiently by sonication than electroporation and incubation [139]. However, the sonicating probe produces consistent heat during the sonication and the operation has to be done on ice, with intervals between strokes [153]. There is no doubt that sonication may compromise the membrane integrity of sEVs, with the therapeutics occasionally being attached to the outer membrane of the sEV, which affects the drug distribution in vivo [139].

The freeze and thaw approach takes advantage of the formation of ice crystals that temporarily disrupt the sEV membrane, allowing therapeutic compounds to enter into the sEVs prior to membrane reconstitution [154]. This method shows lower cargo loading compared to sonication- and extrusion-based methods [155]. One to three cycles of freeze and thaw were usually performed during drug incorporation, which may accelerate the degradation and aggregation of the sEVs [122,156].

Extrusion utilizes a lipid syringe extruder with pore sizes between 100 and 400 nm, which break the sEV membrane physically and then mix with therapeutics. This method possesses high loading efficiency when compared to freeze and thaw, sonication, and saponin treatment [155,157]. One can imagine that the extrusion approach may cause damage of the sEV membranes as it does by sonication and electroporation.

Saponin treatment and the use of common transfection reagents, such as cationic lipids, have also been applied to load exogenous materials into sEVs. It was demonstrated to be an effective approach for sEV encapsulation of therapeutic drugs when compared to electroporation [155]. While we would expect more studies using the transfection approach for sEV loading, especially for loading of nucleic acids, the chemical transfection reagent itself will need to be removed prior to delivering the sEVs to target cells [157].

Through the above-mentioned approaches, multiple therapeutic agents in the forms of DNA, microRNA, siRNA, porphyrins, proteins (catalase, stress-induced heat shock proteins), and chemotherapeutics (curcumin, paclitaxel, docetaxel, gemcitabine) have been successfully loaded into sEVs and tested for their therapeutic value [158–161]. Nonetheless, it remains to be determined which approaches are most appropriate for loading specific agents into desired sEVs.

5. Clinical Trials Testing sEVs as Cancer Therapeutic Carriers

The potential of sEVs to serve as cancer therapeutic carriers and the promising results from preclinical studies have led to clinical trials aimed to develop sEV-based cancer therapy. We searched ClinicalTrials.gov and Pubmed.gov on 7 July 2020 and found 12 clinical trials testing sEVs as potential cancer therapeutics or therapeutic carriers, with 8 of them being registered in ClinicalTrials.gov (Table 1). Some of the clinical trials have reported their end results and others are still ongoing [162]. These clinical trials can be categorized according to their biological source of sEVs that are used as therapeutic carriers, as discussed below. Note that these clinical trials are mostly in early stages, and the definitive therapeutic value of sEVs for cancer therapy has yet to be determined.

Table 1. Clinical trials of EV-based cancer therapy.

Disease	Drug	EV Source	Phase, n of Patients	Status	Reference
Malignant Pleural Effusion	Methotrexate	Autologous Tumor-Derived Microparticles	Phase 2, n = 90	Recruiting	NCT02657460 [1] Guo, M. [163]
	Methotrexate	Microparticles	N/A, n = 248	Recruiting	NCT04131231 [1]
	Chemotherapeutic Drugs	Tumor Cell- Derived Microparticles	Phase 2, n = 30	Unknown	NCT01854866 [1] Tang, K. [164]
	Cisplatin	Tumor Cell- Derived Microparticles	N/A, n = 6	Completed	Ma, J. [165]
Metastatic Pancreatic Cancer	KRAS [2] G12D siRNA	MSC [3]-Derived Exosomes	Phase 1, n = 28	Recruiting	NCT03608631 [1] Kamerkar, S. [166]
Head and Neck Cancer	Grape Extract	Plant Exosomes	Phase 1, n = 60	Active, Not Recruiting	NCT01668849 [1]
	Hemopurifier Pembro-lizumab	Blood-Derived Exosomes	N/A, n = 12	Not Yet Recruiting	NCT04453046 [1]
Colorectal Cancer	Curcumin	Plant Exosomes	Phase 1, n = 7	Active, Not Recruiting	NCT01294072 [1]
	GM-CSF [4]	AEX [5]	Phase 1, n = 40	Completed	Dai, S. [167]
Non-Small Cell Lung Cancer	Antigens	Tumor Dex2 [6]	Phase 2, n = 41	Completed	NCT01159288 [1] Besse, B. [168]
	MAGE[7] Tumor Antigens	Autologous DEX [6]	Phase 1, n = 13	Completed	Morse, M.A. [169]
Metastatic Melanoma	MAGE[7] 3 Peptides	Autologous DEX [6]	Phase 1, n = 15	Completed	Escudier, B. [170]

[1] The NCT# refers to a registered National Clinical Trial (NCT) which can be found at Clinicaltrials.gov, [2] Kirsten Rat Sarcoma (KRAS), [3] Mesenchymal Stem Cells (MSC), [4] Granulocyte- Macrophage Colony-Stimulating Factor (GM-CSF), [5] Ascites- Derived Exosomes (AEX), [6] Dendritic Cell- Derived Exosomes (DEX), [7] Melanoma Antigens (MAGE).

5.1. Clinical Trials Using Dendritic Cell-Derived sEVs (DEX)

In 2005, two phase I clinical trials were reported using autologous DEX as immune stimulants, one for patients with metastatic melanoma, and another for patients with non-small cell lung cancer (NSCLC) [169,170]. Similar procedures were used in isolating sEVs from patients and loading MAGE-3 antigens to the sEVs for these trials. In the metastatic melanoma trial, 15 patients were included and received a 4-week outpatient vaccination course with antigen-loaded DEX given intradermally (1/10th) and subcutaneously (9/10th) per week for 4 weeks. There was no major toxicity being observed and some patients showed partial response and tumor repression. This is the first study to show the feasibility and safety of DEX-based vaccination in melanoma patients. In the NSCLC trial, 13 patients were enrolled, with 9 completing the therapy. The antigen-loaded DEX was given, intradermally (1/10th) and subcutaneously (9/10th), 4 times at weekly intervals. Similar to the melanoma trial, no major toxicity was observed during a 24-month follow up, and immune activation and stability of disease was observed in some patients with advanced NSCLC. The success of this phase I trial led to a phase II clinical trial for NSCLC in France (NCT01159288). In the phase II trial, DEX was upgraded from the first-generation interferon gamma-free DEX (IFN-γ-free DEX) to a second generation (IFN-γ-DEX) in order to enhance DEX-induced T cell responses. Twenty-four patients were recruited, and the results confirmed that DEX boosts antitumor immunity in patients with advanced NSCLC with outstanding safety [168]. Together, these clinical trials indicate a potential safe immunotherapy using DEX in metastatic melanoma and NSCLC, and an enhanced efficacy of DEX when administered in combination with IFN-γ.

5.2. Clinical Trials Using Ascites-Derived sEVs (AEX)

In 2008, a phase I study using autologous AEX combined with granulocyte-macrophage colony-stimulating factor (GM-CSF) for colorectal cancer was completed [167]. Forty patients with advanced colorectal cancer were included in the study and randomly assigned to AEX alone or AEX plus GM-CSF groups. Patients received 4 subcutaneous immunizations at weekly intervals. Results showed that both groups of patients tolerated the treatment well and AEX plus GM-CSF rather than

AEX alone induces beneficial antitumor cytotoxic T lymphocyte (CTL) response. These findings suggest that the immunotherapy of colorectal cancer with AEX in combination with GM-CSF is feasible and safe, and may be applied for immunotherapy of colorectal cancer.

5.3. Clinical Trials Using Tumor Cell-Derived EVs

A preclinical study has confirmed the feasibility of using apoptotic tumor cells induced by chemotherapeutic drugs to produce drug-packaging EVs [164]. Several anti-cancer drugs, including methotrexate, doxorubicin, and cisplatin, were shown to be packaged into EVs released by tumor cells, such as the mouse hepatocarcinoma tumor cell line H22 or the human ovarian cancer A2780. These drug-containing EVs effectively killed tumor cells in murine models without typical side effects, such as hair and/or weight loss or liver and/or kidney function impairment. Inspired by these preclinical results, three clinical trials were consecutively registered to test the effects of chemotherapeutic packed EVs in cancer patients (NCT01854866, NCT02657460, and NCT04131231). Whereas findings from two of the trials remain to be reported, one of the trials published their results in 2019 [163], showing that autologous tumor EVs packed with methotrexate symptomatically improved 10 of 11 lung cancer patients with malignant pleural effusion. The methotrexate-packed EVs activated antitumor effector cells including CTLs and TH1 in the pleural microenvironment and only caused mild (grades 1 to 2) adverse events.

Tumor EVs packed with chemotherapeutics also contributed to reverse drug resistance of malignant cells. Intrathoracic injection of cisplatin-packed tumor EVs in three end-stage lung cancer patients eliminated 95% of tumor cells in the malignant fluids and ameliorated patient symptoms. These therapeutic effects were absent in another three patients with intrathoracic injection of cisplatin alone [165].

5.4. Clinical Trials Using Plant-Derived sEVs

sEVs derived from plants are unquestionably safer than those from tumor cells. Grapefruits were found to yield higher sEVs (2.21 g/kg raw material) than grapes, tomatoes, bovine milk, or ginger [171]. Grapefruit-derived nanovectors (GNVs) were demonstrated to transport chemotherapeutic agents, siRNA, DNA expression vectors, and proteins to different kinds of cells. Co-delivery of folic acid and PTX by GNVs showed a therapeutic benefit in a mouse model of colon cancer [172]. These preclinical results led to a phase I clinical study investigating the efficacy of plant sEVs conjugated with curcumin that was orally delivered to patients with colon cancer (NCT01294072). Another phase I clinical trial was designed to evaluate the ability of plant sEVs to prevent oral mucositis during chemo-radiation of head and neck cancer (NCT01668849), which will shed light on the potential of using plant sEVs to alleviate side effects during cancer therapy.

5.5. Clinical Trials Using Normal Fibroblast-Like Mesenchymal Cell-Derived EVs

A preclinical study has demonstrated that sEVs, derived from fibroblast-like mesenchymal cells and loaded with siRNA or shRNA targeting KRAS mutation (KrasG12D), are significantly more effective than other drug carriers in inhibiting pancreatic ductal adenocarcinoma (PDAC) progression in vitro and in vivo [166]. Following the report, this research group initiated a phase I clinical trial (NCT03608631) aimed at testing this approach in patients with stage IV PDAC bearing the KrasG12D mutation. They will also evaluate median progression-free survival (PFS) and median overall survival (OS) as secondary objectives.

6. Conclusions

Research on EVs in cancer has been intensified over the last decade. The involvement of EVs, especially sEVs, in promoting cancer progression through intercellular communication is well recognized. This leads to efforts focusing on targeting EV signaling or utilizing EVs as drug carriers to develop novel cancer therapeutics. In this review, we have summarized recent progress in the development of EVs as cancer therapeutics, both in preclinical studies and clinical trials. Clearly, most of the studies reported on targeting sEV signaling, such as EV microRNA signaling, are at preclinical stages, and clinical trials are primarily related to developing EVs as therapeutic carriers at relatively early phases. This indicates that, on one hand, significant progress has been made in understanding how to better target EV signaling for the development of cancer therapeutics and the safety of delivering EVs into humans as therapeutic carriers, and on the other hand, clinical efficacy of EVs as therapeutic targets or therapeutic carriers remains to be determined. Compared to targeting EV signaling, utilizing EVs as therapeutic carriers seems to be a more practical strategy in therapeutic development and has advanced from preclinical studies to clinical trials. This is likely due to the fact that targeting cancer-specific EV signaling remains a challenge, as clear distinction of cancer EVs from healthy EVs has not been firmly established, and the heterogeneity of EVs is well recognized, which renders it difficult in specific targeting of EV signaling. In addition, current technology in EV isolation and validation needs to be improved, which also limits the effort in exploring EV signaling in cancer. Ongoing EV research needs to focus on these challenges in order to establish clinically applicable therapeutics targeting EV signaling in cancer. There are also challenges in the development of EVs as therapeutic carriers [173], including production and purification of EVs on an industrial scale, potential EV contamination with virus [100,174], and long-term side effects of tumor-derived EVs when they are applied as therapeutic carriers. However, these challenges are mostly technological, not conceptual, and hopefully can be overcome with concentrated effort. It is expected that EVs as therapeutic targets or delivery carriers may soon open up new avenues in clinical management of malignant diseases.

Author Contributions: H.S. searched the literature and drafted the manuscript. S.B. helped with drafting the manuscript and prepared the figure and table. J.W. conceived of and participated in drafting the manuscript. W.-Q.D. conceived of and finalized the manuscript. All authors have read and approved the final manuscript.

Funding: This study was supported in part by grants from the National Cancer Institute (CA235208-01), the Presbyterian Health Foundation, and the Peggy and Charles Stephenson Cancer Center.

Acknowledgments: We thank the Department of Pathology at the University of Oklahoma Health Sciences Center for administrative support.

Conflicts of Interest: The authors declare no conflict of interest. The funders had no role in the design of the study; in the collection, analyses, or interpretation of data; in the writing of the manuscript, or in the decision to publish the results.

Abbreviations

EV	Extracellular Vesicle
MV	Microvesicle
ISEV	International Society for Extracellular Vesicles
sEV	Small Extracellular Vesicle
MHC	Major Histocompatibility Complex
EPCAM	Epithelial Cell Adhesion Molecule
PECAM1	Platelet Endothelial Cell Adhesion Molecule 1
ERBB2	Erb-B2 Receptor Tyrosine Kinase 2
ESCRT	Endosomal Sorting Complexes Required for Transport
nSMase2	Neutral sphingomyelinase 2
HSP72	Heat-Shock Protein 72
STAT-3	Signal Transducer and Activator of Transcription 3
MA	Manumycin-A
PI3K	Phosphatidylinositol 3-Kinase
HUVEC	Human Umbilical Vein Endothelial Cell
GBM	Glioblastoma
CKAP4	Cytoskeleton-Associated Protein 4

DKK1	Dickkopf1
PDAC	Pancreatic Ductal Adenocarcinoma
PD1	Programmed Cell Death Protein 1
PD-L1	Programmed Death-Ligand 1
GMP	Good Manufacturing Practice
EPR	Enhanced Permeability and Retention
PSC	Pancreatic Stellate Cell
MSC	Mesenchymal Stem Cells
HeLa	Henrietta Lacks Cells
PTX	Paclitaxel
KRAS	Kirsten Rat Sarcoma
DEX	Dendrite Cell- Derived Exosomes
NSCLC	Non-Small Cell Lung Cancer
MAGE-3	Melanoma-Associated Antigen 3
IFN-γ-free DEX	Interferon Gamma-free Exosomes
IFN-γ-DEX	Interferon Gamma-containing Exosomes
AEX	Ascites-Derived Exosomes
GM-CSF	Granulocyte-Macrophage Colony-Stimulating Factor
CTL	Cytotoxic T Lymphocyte
TH1	T-cell Helper 1
GNV	Grapefruit-Derived Nanovectors
PFS	Progression-Free Survival
OS	Overall Survival

References

1. Chargaff, E.; West, R. The biological significance of the thromboplastic protein of blood. *J. Biol. Chem.* **1946**, *166*, 189–197. [PubMed]
2. Harding, C.; Heuser, J.; Stahl, P. Receptor-mediated endocytosis of transferrin and recycling of the transferrin receptor in rat reticulocytes. *J. Cell Biol.* **1983**, *97*, 329–339. [CrossRef] [PubMed]
3. Pan, B.T.; Teng, K.; Wu, C.; Adam, M.; Johnstone, R.M. Electron microscopic evidence for externalization of the transferrin receptor in vesicular form in sheep reticulocytes. *J. Cell Biol.* **1985**, *101*, 942–948. [CrossRef] [PubMed]
4. Baj-Krzyworzeka, M.; Szatanek, R.; Weglarczyk, K.; Baran, J.; Urbanowicz, B.; Branski, P.; Ratajczak, M.Z.; Zembala, M. Tumour-derived microvesicles carry several surface determinants and mRNA of tumour cells and transfer some of these determinants to monocytes. *Cancer Immunol. Immun.* **2006**, *55*, 808–818. [CrossRef] [PubMed]
5. Ratajczak, J.; Wysoczynski, M.; Hayek, F.; Janowska-Wieczorek, A.; Ratajczak, M.Z. Membrane-derived microvesicles: Important and underappreciated mediators of cell-to-cell communication. *Leukemia* **2006**, *20*, 1487–1495. [CrossRef]
6. Aliotta, J.M.; Sanchez-Guijo, F.M.; Dooner, G.J.; Johnson, K.W.; Dooner, M.S.; Greer, K.A.; Greer, D.; Pimentel, J.; Kolankiewicz, L.M.; Puente, N.; et al. Alteration of marrow cell gene expression, protein production, and engraftment into lung by lung-derived microvesicles: A novel mechanism for phenotype modulation. *Stem Cells* **2007**, *25*, 2245–2256. [CrossRef]
7. Valadi, H.; Ekstrom, K.; Bossios, A.; Sjostrand, M.; Lee, J.J.; Lotvall, J.O. Exosome-mediated transfer of mRNAs and microRNAs is a novel mechanism of genetic exchange between cells. *Nat. Cell Biol.* **2007**, *9*, 654–659. [CrossRef]
8. Skog, J.; Wurdinger, T.; van Rijn, S.; Meijer, D.H.; Gainche, L.; Sena-Esteves, M.; Curry, W.T., Jr.; Carter, B.S.; Krichevsky, A.M.; Breakefield, X.O. Glioblastoma microvesicles transport RNA and proteins that promote tumour growth and provide diagnostic biomarkers. *Nat. Cell Biol.* **2008**, *10*, 1470–1476. [CrossRef]
9. Kalluri, R.; LeBleu, V.S. The biology, function, and biomedical applications of exosomes. *Science* **2020**, *367*. [CrossRef]
10. Bonucci, E. Fine structure and histochemistry of "calcifying globules" in epiphyseal cartilage. *Z. Zellforsch. Mikrosk. Anat.* **1970**, *103*, 192–217. [CrossRef]

11. Yanez-Mo, M.; Siljander, P.R.; Andreu, Z.; Zavec, A.B.; Borras, F.E.; Buzas, E.I.; Buzas, K.; Casal, E.; Cappello, F.; Carvalho, J.; et al. Biological properties of extracellular vesicles and their physiological functions. *J. Extracell. Vesicles* **2015**, *4*, 27066. [CrossRef] [PubMed]
12. Gould, S.J.; Raposo, G. As we wait: Coping with an imperfect nomenclature for extracellular vesicles. *J. Extracell. Vesicles* **2013**, *2*. [CrossRef] [PubMed]
13. Hessvik, N.P.; Llorente, A. Current knowledge on exosome biogenesis and release. *Cell Mol. Life Sci.* **2018**, *75*, 193–208. [CrossRef]
14. Crescitelli, R.; Lasser, C.; Szabo, T.G.; Kittel, A.; Eldh, M.; Dianzani, I.; Buzas, E.I.; Lotvall, J. Distinct RNA profiles in subpopulations of extracellular vesicles: Apoptotic bodies, microvesicles and exosomes. *J. Extracell. Vesicles* **2013**, *2*. [CrossRef] [PubMed]
15. Kalra, H.; Simpson, R.J.; Ji, H.; Aikawa, E.; Altevogt, P.; Askenase, P.; Bond, V.C.; Borras, F.E.; Breakefield, X.; Budnik, V.; et al. Vesiclepedia: A compendium for extracellular vesicles with continuous community annotation. *Plos Biol.* **2012**, *10*, e1001450. [CrossRef] [PubMed]
16. Zhang, H.; Freitas, D.; Kim, H.S.; Fabijanic, K.; Li, Z.; Chen, H.; Mark, M.T.; Molina, H.; Martin, A.B.; Bojmar, L.; et al. Identification of distinct nanoparticles and subsets of extracellular vesicles by asymmetric flow field-flow fractionation. *Nat. Cell Biol.* **2018**, *20*, 332–343. [CrossRef]
17. Thery, C.; Witwer, K.W.; Aikawa, E.; Alcaraz, M.J.; Anderson, J.D.; Andriantsitohaina, R.; Antoniou, A.; Arab, T.; Archer, F.; Atkin-Smith, G.K.; et al. Minimal information for studies of extracellular vesicles 2018 (MISEV2018): A position statement of the International Society for Extracellular Vesicles and update of the MISEV2014 guidelines. *J. Extracell. Vesicles* **2018**, *7*, 1535750. [CrossRef]
18. Wortzel, I.; Dror, S.; Kenific, C.M.; Lyden, D. Exosome-Mediated Metastasis: Communication from a Distance. *Dev. Cell* **2019**, *49*, 347–360. [CrossRef]
19. Charoenviriyakul, C.; Takahashi, Y.; Morishita, M.; Matsumoto, A.; Nishikawa, M.; Takakura, Y. Cell type-specific and common characteristics of exosomes derived from mouse cell lines: Yield, physicochemical properties, and pharmacokinetics. *Eur. J. Pharm. Sci.* **2017**, *96*, 316–322. [CrossRef]
20. Kim, D.K.; Kang, B.; Kim, O.Y.; Choi, D.S.; Lee, J.; Kim, S.R.; Go, G.; Yoon, Y.J.; Kim, J.H.; Jang, S.C.; et al. EVpedia: An integrated database of high-throughput data for systemic analyses of extracellular vesicles. *J. Extracell. Vesicles* **2013**, *2*. [CrossRef]
21. Simpson, R.J.; Kalra, H.; Mathivanan, S. ExoCarta as a resource for exosomal research. *J. Extracell. Vesicles* **2012**, *1*. [CrossRef] [PubMed]
22. Wei, Z.; Batagov, A.O.; Schinelli, S.; Wang, J.; Wang, Y.; El Fatimy, R.; Rabinovsky, R.; Balaj, L.; Chen, C.C.; Hochberg, F.; et al. Coding and noncoding landscape of extracellular RNA released by human glioma stem cells. *Nat. Commun.* **2017**, *8*, 1145. [CrossRef] [PubMed]
23. Hannafon, B.N.; Ding, W.Q. Intercellular Communication by Exosome-Derived microRNAs in Cancer. *Int. J. Mol. Sci.* **2013**, *14*, 14240–14269. [CrossRef] [PubMed]
24. Ratajczak, J.; Miekus, K.; Kucia, M.; Zhang, J.; Reca, R.; Dvorak, P.; Ratajczak, M.Z. Embryonic stem cell-derived microvesicles reprogram hematopoietic progenitors: Evidence for horizontal transfer of mRNA and protein delivery. *Leukemia* **2006**, *20*, 847–856. [CrossRef]
25. Hannafon, B.N.; Carpenter, K.J.; Berry, W.L.; Janknecht, R.; Dooley, W.C.; Ding, W.Q. Exosome-mediated microRNA signaling from breast cancer cells is altered by the anti-angiogenesis agent docosahexaenoic acid (DHA). *Mol. Cancer* **2015**, *14*, 133. [CrossRef]
26. Pegtel, D.M.; Cosmopoulos, K.; Thorley-Lawson, D.A.; van Eijndhoven, M.A.; Hopmans, E.S.; Lindenberg, J.L.; de Gruijl, T.D.; Wurdinger, T.; Middeldorp, J.M. Functional delivery of viral miRNAs via exosomes. *Proc. Natl. Acad. Sci. USA* **2010**, *107*, 6328–6333. [CrossRef]
27. Montecalvo, A.; Larregina, A.T.; Shufesky, W.J.; Stolz, D.B.; Sullivan, M.L.; Karlsson, J.M.; Baty, C.J.; Gibson, G.A.; Erdos, G.; Wang, Z.; et al. Mechanism of transfer of functional microRNAs between mouse dendritic cells via exosomes. *Blood* **2012**, *119*, 756–766. [CrossRef]
28. Ismail, N.; Wang, Y.; Dakhlallah, D.; Moldovan, L.; Agarwal, K.; Batte, K.; Shah, P.; Wisler, J.; Eubank, T.D.; Tridandapani, S.; et al. Macrophage microvesicles induce macrophage differentiation and miR-223 transfer. *Blood* **2013**, *121*, 984–995. [CrossRef]
29. Li, S.; Li, Y.; Chen, B.; Zhao, J.; Yu, S.; Tang, Y.; Zheng, Q.; Li, Y.; Wang, P.; He, X.; et al. exoRBase: A database of circRNA, lncRNA and mRNA in human blood exosomes. *Nucleic Acids Res.* **2018**, *46*, D106–D112. [CrossRef]

30. Murillo, O.D.; Thistlethwaite, W.; Rozowsky, J.; Subramanian, S.L.; Lucero, R.; Shah, N.; Jackson, A.R.; Srinivasan, S.; Chung, A.; Laurent, C.D.; et al. exRNA Atlas Analysis Reveals Distinct Extracellular RNA Cargo Types and Their Carriers Present across Human Biofluids. *Cell* **2019**, *117*, 463–477.e415. [CrossRef]
31. Russo, F.; Di Bella, S.; Vannini, F.; Berti, G.; Scoyni, F.; Cook, H.V.; Santos, A.; Nigita, G.; Bonnici, V.; Lagana, A.; et al. miRandola 2017: A curated knowledge base of non-invasive biomarkers. *Nucleic Acids Res.* **2018**, *46*, D354–D359. [CrossRef] [PubMed]
32. Kahlert, C.; Melo, S.A.; Protopopov, A.; Tang, J.; Seth, S.; Koch, M.; Zhang, J.; Weitz, J.; Chin, L.; Futreal, A.; et al. Identification of double-stranded genomic DNA spanning all chromosomes with mutated KRAS and p53 DNA in the serum exosomes of patients with pancreatic cancer. *J. Biol. Chem.* **2014**, *289*, 3869–3875. [CrossRef] [PubMed]
33. Sansone, P.; Savini, C.; Kurelac, I.; Chang, Q.; Amato, L.B.; Strillacci, A.; Stepanova, A.; Iommarini, L.; Mastroleo, C.; Daly, L.; et al. Packaging and transfer of mitochondrial DNA via exosomes regulate escape from dormancy in hormonal therapy-resistant breast cancer. *Proc. Natl. Acad. Sci. USA* **2017**, *114*, E9066–E9075. [CrossRef] [PubMed]
34. Thakur, B.K.; Zhang, H.; Becker, A.; Matei, I.; Huang, Y.; Costa-Silva, B.; Zheng, Y.; Hoshino, A.; Brazier, H.; Xiang, J.; et al. Double-stranded DNA in exosomes: A novel biomarker in cancer detection. *Cell Res.* **2014**, *24*, 766–769. [CrossRef] [PubMed]
35. Magnette, A.; Chatelain, M.; Chatelain, B.; Ten Cate, H.; Mullier, F. Pre-analytical issues in the haemostasis laboratory: Guidance for the clinical laboratories. *Thromb. J.* **2016**, *14*, 49. [CrossRef] [PubMed]
36. Carayon, K.; Chaoui, K.; Ronzier, E.; Lazar, I.; Bertrand-Michel, J.; Roques, V.; Balor, S.; Terce, F.; Lopez, A.; Salome, L.; et al. Proteolipidic composition of exosomes changes during reticulocyte maturation. *J. Biol. Chem.* **2011**, *286*, 34426–34439. [CrossRef] [PubMed]
37. Gasser, O.; Schifferli, J.A. Activated polymorphonuclear neutrophils disseminate anti-inflammatory microparticles by ectocytosis. *Blood* **2004**, *104*, 2543–2548. [CrossRef]
38. Montecalvo, A.; Shufesky, W.J.; Stolz, D.B.; Sullivan, M.G.; Wang, Z.; Divito, S.J.; Papworth, G.D.; Watkins, S.C.; Robbins, P.D.; Larregina, A.T.; et al. Exosomes as a short-range mechanism to spread alloantigen between dendritic cells during T cell allorecognition. *J. Immunol.* **2008**, *180*, 3081–3090. [CrossRef]
39. Mincheva-Nilsson, L.; Baranov, V. Placenta-derived exosomes and syncytiotrophoblast microparticles and their role in human reproduction: Immune modulation for pregnancy success. *Am. J. Reprod. Immunol.* **2014**, *72*, 440–457. [CrossRef]
40. Lakkaraju, A.; Rodriguez-Boulan, E. Itinerant exosomes: Emerging roles in cell and tissue polarity. *Trends Cell Biol.* **2008**, *18*, 199–209. [CrossRef]
41. Quesenberry, P.J.; Aliotta, J.M. The paradoxical dynamism of marrow stem cells: Considerations of stem cells, niches, and microvesicles. *Stem Cell Rev.* **2008**, *4*, 137–147. [CrossRef] [PubMed]
42. Nahar, N.N.; Missana, L.R.; Garimella, R.; Tague, S.E.; Anderson, H.C. Matrix vesicles are carriers of bone morphogenetic proteins (BMPs), vascular endothelial growth factor (VEGF), and noncollagenous matrix proteins. *J. Bone Min. Metab.* **2008**, *26*, 514–519. [CrossRef] [PubMed]
43. Shirakami, Y.; Lee, S.A.; Clugston, R.D.; Blaner, W.S. Hepatic metabolism of retinoids and disease associations. *Biochim. Biophys. Acta* **2012**, *1821*, 124–136. [CrossRef] [PubMed]
44. Lai, C.P.; Breakefield, X.O. Role of exosomes/microvesicles in the nervous system and use in emerging therapies. *Front. Physiol.* **2012**, *3*, 228. [CrossRef] [PubMed]
45. Guo, H.; Chitiprolu, M.; Roncevic, L.; Javalet, C.; Hemming, F.J.; Trung, M.T.; Meng, L.; Latreille, E.; Tanese de Souza, C.; McCulloch, D.; et al. Atg5 Disassociates the V1V0-ATPase to Promote Exosome Production and Tumor Metastasis Independent of Canonical Macroautophagy. *Dev. Cell* **2017**, *43*, 716–730 e717. [CrossRef]
46. Villarroya-Beltri, C.; Baixauli, F.; Mittelbrunn, M.; Fernandez-Delgado, I.; Torralba, D.; Moreno-Gonzalo, O.; Baldanta, S.; Enrich, C.; Guerra, S.; Sanchez-Madrid, F. ISGylation controls exosome secretion by promoting lysosomal degradation of MVB proteins. *Nat. Commun.* **2016**, *7*, 13588. [CrossRef]
47. Ilie, A.; Gao, A.Y.L.; Boucher, A.; Park, J.; Berghuis, A.M.; Hoffer, M.J.V.; Hilhorst-Hofstee, Y.; McKinney, R.A.; Orlowski, J. A potential gain-of-function variant of SLC9A6 leads to endosomal alkalinization and neuronal atrophy associated with Christianson Syndrome. *Neurobiol. Dis.* **2019**, *121*, 187–204. [CrossRef]
48. Edgar, J.R.; Manna, P.T.; Nishimura, S.; Banting, G.; Robinson, M.S. Tetherin is an exosomal tether. *Elife* **2016**, *5*. [CrossRef]

49. Putz, U.; Howitt, J.; Lackovic, J.; Foot, N.; Kumar, S.; Silke, J.; Tan, S.S. Nedd4 family-interacting protein 1 (Ndfip1) is required for the exosomal secretion of Nedd4 family proteins. *J. Biol. Chem.* **2008**, *283*, 32621–32627. [CrossRef]
50. Phillips, M.C. Molecular mechanisms of cellular cholesterol efflux. *J. Biol. Chem.* **2014**, *289*, 24020–24029. [CrossRef]
51. Amzallag, N.; Passer, B.J.; Allanic, D.; Segura, E.; Thery, C.; Goud, B.; Amson, R.; Telerman, A. TSAP6 facilitates the secretion of translationally controlled tumor protein/histamine-releasing factor via a nonclassical pathway. *J. Biol. Chem.* **2004**, *279*, 46104–46112. [CrossRef] [PubMed]
52. Hanahan, D.; Weinberg, R.A. Hallmarks of cancer: The next generation. *Cell* **2011**, *144*, 646–674. [CrossRef] [PubMed]
53. Melo, S.A.; Sugimoto, H.; O'Connell, J.T.; Kato, N.; Villanueva, A.; Vidal, A.; Qiu, L.; Vitkin, E.; Perelman, L.T.; Melo, C.A.; et al. Cancer exosomes perform cell-independent microRNA biogenesis and promote tumorigenesis. *Cancer Cell* **2014**, *26*, 707–721. [CrossRef]
54. Costa-Silva, B.; Aiello, N.M.; Ocean, A.J.; Singh, S.; Zhang, H.; Thakur, B.K.; Becker, A.; Hoshino, A.; Mark, M.T.; Molina, H.; et al. Pancreatic cancer exosomes initiate pre-metastatic niche formation in the liver. *Nat. Cell Biol.* **2015**, *17*, 816–826. [CrossRef] [PubMed]
55. Peinado, H.; Aleckovic, M.; Lavotshkin, S.; Matei, I.; Costa-Silva, B.; Moreno-Bueno, G.; Hergueta-Redondo, M.; Williams, C.; Garcia-Santos, G.; Ghajar, C.; et al. Melanoma exosomes educate bone marrow progenitor cells toward a pro-metastatic phenotype through MET. *Nat. Med.* **2012**, *18*, 883–891. [CrossRef] [PubMed]
56. Xavier, C.P.R.; Caires, H.R.; Barbosa, M.A.G.; Bergantim, R.; Guimaraes, J.E.; Vasconcelos, M.H. The Role of Extracellular Vesicles in the Hallmarks of Cancer and Drug Resistance. *Cells* **2020**, *9*, 1141. [CrossRef]
57. Antonyak, M.A.; Li, B.; Boroughs, L.K.; Johnson, J.L.; Druso, J.E.; Bryant, K.L.; Holowka, D.A.; Cerione, R.A. Cancer cell-derived microvesicles induce transformation by transferring tissue transglutaminase and fibronectin to recipient cells. *Proc. Natl. Acad. Sci. USA* **2011**, *108*, 4852–4857. [CrossRef]
58. Sato, S.; Vasaikar, S.; Eskaros, A.; Kim, Y.; Lewis, J.S.; Zhang, B.; Zijlstra, A.; Weaver, A.M. EPHB2 carried on small extracellular vesicles induces tumor angiogenesis via activation of ephrin reverse signaling. *Jci Insight* **2019**, *4*. [CrossRef]
59. Bao, L.; You, B.; Shi, S.; Shan, Y.; Zhang, Q.; Yue, H.; Zhang, J.; Zhang, W.; Shi, Y.; Liu, Y.; et al. Metastasis-associated miR-23a from nasopharyngeal carcinoma-derived exosomes mediates angiogenesis by repressing a novel target gene TSGA10. *Oncogene* **2018**, *37*, 2873–2889. [CrossRef]
60. Pavlyukov, M.S.; Yu, H.; Bastola, S.; Minata, M.; Shender, V.O.; Lee, Y.; Zhang, S.; Wang, J.; Komarova, S.; Wang, J.; et al. Apoptotic Cell-Derived Extracellular Vesicles Promote Malignancy of Glioblastoma Via Intercellular Transfer of Splicing Factors. *Cancer Cell* **2018**, *34*, 119–135 e110. [CrossRef]
61. Setti, M.; Osti, D.; Richichi, C.; Ortensi, B.; Del Bene, M.; Fornasari, L.; Beznoussenko, G.; Mironov, A.; Rappa, G.; Cuomo, A.; et al. Extracellular vesicle-mediated transfer of CLIC1 protein is a novel mechanism for the regulation of glioblastoma growth. *Oncotarget* **2015**, *6*, 31413–31427. [CrossRef] [PubMed]
62. Hoshino, A.; Costa-Silva, B.; Shen, T.L.; Rodrigues, G.; Hashimoto, A.; Tesic Mark, M.; Molina, H.; Kohsaka, S.; Di Giannatale, A.; Ceder, S.; et al. Tumour exosome integrins determine organotropic metastasis. *Nature* **2015**, *527*, 329–335. [CrossRef] [PubMed]
63. Wang, X.; Luo, G.; Zhang, K.; Cao, J.; Huang, C.; Jiang, T.; Liu, B.; Su, L.; Qiu, Z. Hypoxic Tumor-Derived Exosomal miR-301a Mediates M2 Macrophage Polarization via PTEN/PI3Kgamma to Promote Pancreatic Cancer Metastasis. *Cancer Res.* **2018**, *78*, 4586–4598. [CrossRef] [PubMed]
64. Marleau, A.M.; Chen, C.S.; Joyce, J.A.; Tullis, R.H. Exosome removal as a therapeutic adjuvant in cancer. *J. Transl. Med.* **2012**, *10*, 134. [CrossRef] [PubMed]
65. Shedden, K.; Xie, X.T.; Chandaroy, P.; Chang, Y.T.; Rosania, G.R. Expulsion of small molecules in vesicles shed by cancer cells: Association with gene expression and chemosensitivity profiles. *Cancer Res.* **2003**, *63*, 4331–4337.
66. Chen, G.; Huang, A.C.; Zhang, W.; Zhang, G.; Wu, M.; Xu, W.; Yu, Z.; Yang, J.; Wang, B.; Sun, H.; et al. Exosomal PD-L1 contributes to immunosuppression and is associated with anti-PD-1 response. *Nature* **2018**, *560*, 382–386. [CrossRef]

67. Poggio, M.; Hu, T.; Pai, C.C.; Chu, B.; Belair, C.D.; Chang, A.; Montabana, E.; Lang, U.E.; Fu, Q.; Fong, L.; et al. Suppression of Exosomal PD-L1 Induces Systemic Anti-tumor Immunity and Memory. *Cell* **2019**, *177*, 414–427 e413. [CrossRef]
68. Andaloussi, S.E.L.; Mager, I.; Breakefield, X.O.; Wood, M.J. Extracellular vesicles: Biology and emerging therapeutic opportunities. *Nat. Rev. Drug Discov.* **2013**, *12*, 347–357. [CrossRef]
69. Urabe, F.; Kosaka, N.; Ito, K.; Kimura, T.; Egawa, S.; Ochiya, T. Extracellular vesicles as biomarkers and therapeutic targets for cancer. *Am. J. Physiol. Cell Physiol.* **2020**, *318*, C29–C39. [CrossRef]
70. Yamamoto, T.; Kosaka, N.; Ochiya, T. Latest advances in extracellular vesicles: From bench to bedside. *Sci. Technol. Adv. Mater.* **2019**, *20*, 746–757. [CrossRef]
71. D'Souza-Schorey, C.; Schorey, J.S. Regulation and mechanisms of extracellular vesicle biogenesis and secretion. *Essays Biochem.* **2018**, *62*, 125–133. [CrossRef] [PubMed]
72. Mathieu, M.; Martin-Jaular, L.; Lavieu, G.; Thery, C. Specificities of secretion and uptake of exosomes and other extracellular vesicles for cell-to-cell communication. *Nat. Cell Biol.* **2019**, *21*, 9–17. [CrossRef] [PubMed]
73. Ostrowski, M.; Carmo, N.B.; Krumeich, S.; Fanget, I.; Raposo, G.; Savina, A.; Moita, C.F.; Schauer, K.; Hume, A.N.; Freitas, R.P.; et al. Rab27a and Rab27b control different steps of the exosome secretion pathway. *Nat. Cell Biol.* **2010**, *12*, 19–30, sup pp. 11–13. [CrossRef] [PubMed]
74. Middleton, R.C.; Rogers, R.G.; De Couto, G.; Tseliou, E.; Luther, K.; Holewinski, R.; Soetkamp, D.; Van Eyk, J.E.; Antes, T.J.; Marban, E. Newt cells secrete extracellular vesicles with therapeutic bioactivity in mammalian cardiomyocytes. *J. Extracell. Vesicles* **2018**, *7*, 1456888. [CrossRef] [PubMed]
75. Kosaka, N.; Iguchi, H.; Hagiwara, K.; Yoshioka, Y.; Takeshita, F.; Ochiya, T. Neutral sphingomyelinase 2 (nSMase2)-dependent exosomal transfer of angiogenic microRNAs regulate cancer cell metastasis. *J. Biol. Chem.* **2013**, *288*, 10849–10859. [CrossRef]
76. Phuyal, S.; Hessvik, N.P.; Skotland, T.; Sandvig, K.; Llorente, A. Regulation of exosome release by glycosphingolipids and flotillins. *Febs J.* **2014**, *281*, 2214–2227. [CrossRef]
77. Yuyama, K.; Sun, H.; Mitsutake, S.; Igarashi, Y. Sphingolipid-modulated exosome secretion promotes clearance of amyloid-beta by microglia. *J. Biol. Chem.* **2012**, *287*, 10977–10989. [CrossRef]
78. Chalmin, F.; Ladoire, S.; Mignot, G.; Vincent, J.; Bruchard, M.; Remy-Martin, J.P.; Boireau, W.; Rouleau, A.; Simon, B.; Lanneau, D.; et al. Membrane-associated Hsp72 from tumor-derived exosomes mediates STAT3-dependent immunosuppressive function of mouse and human myeloid-derived suppressor cells. *J. Clin. Investig.* **2010**, *120*, 457–471. [CrossRef]
79. Baietti, M.F.; Zhang, Z.; Mortier, E.; Melchior, A.; Degeest, G.; Geeraerts, A.; Ivarsson, Y.; Depoortere, F.; Coomans, C.; Vermeiren, E.; et al. Syndecan-syntenin-ALIX regulates the biogenesis of exosomes. *Nat. Cell Biol.* **2012**, *14*, 677–685. [CrossRef]
80. Bobrie, A.; Krumeich, S.; Reyal, F.; Recchi, C.; Moita, L.F.; Seabra, M.C.; Ostrowski, M.; Thery, C. Rab27a supports exosome-dependent and -independent mechanisms that modify the tumor microenvironment and can promote tumor progression. *Cancer Res.* **2012**, *72*, 4920–4930. [CrossRef]
81. Savina, A.; Fader, C.M.; Damiani, M.T.; Colombo, M.I. Rab11 promotes docking and fusion of multivesicular bodies in a calcium-dependent manner. *Traffic* **2005**, *6*, 131–143. [CrossRef] [PubMed]
82. Hsu, C.; Morohashi, Y.; Yoshimura, S.; Manrique-Hoyos, N.; Jung, S.; Lauterbach, M.A.; Bakhti, M.; Gronborg, M.; Mobius, W.; Rhee, J.; et al. Regulation of exosome secretion by Rab35 and its GTPase-activating proteins TBC1D10A-C. *J. Cell Biol.* **2010**, *189*, 223–232. [CrossRef] [PubMed]
83. Datta, A.; Kim, H.; Lal, M.; McGee, L.; Johnson, A.; Moustafa, A.A.; Jones, J.C.; Mondal, D.; Ferrer, M.; Abdel-Mageed, A.B. Manumycin A suppresses exosome biogenesis and secretion via targeted inhibition of Ras/Raf/ERK1/2 signaling and hnRNP H1 in castration-resistant prostate cancer cells. *Cancer Lett.* **2017**, *408*, 73–81. [CrossRef] [PubMed]
84. Duffy, M.J.; Sturgeon, C.; Lamerz, R.; Haglund, C.; Holubec, V.L.; Klapdor, R.; Nicolini, A.; Topolcan, O.; Heinemann, V. Tumor markers in pancreatic cancer: A European Group on Tumor Markers (EGTM) status report. *Ann. Oncol.* **2010**, *21*, 441–447. [CrossRef] [PubMed]
85. Parolini, I.; Federici, C.; Raggi, C.; Lugini, L.; Palleschi, S.; De Milito, A.; Coscia, C.; Iessi, E.; Logozzi, M.; Molinari, A.; et al. Microenvironmental pH is a key factor for exosome traffic in tumor cells. *J. Biol. Chem.* **2009**, *284*, 34211–34222. [CrossRef]
86. Jahn, R.; Lang, T.; Sudhof, T.C. Membrane fusion. *Cell* **2003**, *112*, 519–533. [CrossRef]

87. Gonda, A.; Kabagwira, J.; Senthil, G.N.; Wall, N.R. Internalization of Exosomes through Receptor-Mediated Endocytosis. *Mol Cancer Res.* **2019**, *17*, 337–347. [CrossRef]
88. Tian, T.; Zhu, Y.L.; Zhou, Y.Y.; Liang, G.F.; Wang, Y.Y.; Hu, F.H.; Xiao, Z.D. Exosome uptake through clathrin-mediated endocytosis and macropinocytosis and mediating miR-21 delivery. *J. Biol. Chem.* **2014**, *289*, 22258–22267. [CrossRef]
89. Nanbo, A.; Kawanishi, E.; Yoshida, R.; Yoshiyama, H. Exosomes derived from Epstein-Barr virus-infected cells are internalized via caveola-dependent endocytosis and promote phenotypic modulation in target cells. *J. Virol.* **2013**, *87*, 10334–10347. [CrossRef]
90. Feng, D.; Zhao, W.L.; Ye, Y.Y.; Bai, X.C.; Liu, R.Q.; Chang, L.F.; Zhou, Q.; Sui, S.F. Cellular internalization of exosomes occurs through phagocytosis. *Traffic* **2010**, *11*, 675–687. [CrossRef]
91. Fitzner, D.; Schnaars, M.; van Rossum, D.; Krishnamoorthy, G.; Dibaj, P.; Bakhti, M.; Regen, T.; Hanisch, U.K.; Simons, M. Selective transfer of exosomes from oligodendrocytes to microglia by macropinocytosis. *J. Cell Sci.* **2011**, *124*, 447–458. [CrossRef] [PubMed]
92. Mulcahy, L.A.; Pink, R.C.; Carter, D.R. Routes and mechanisms of extracellular vesicle uptake. *J. Extracell. Vesicles* **2014**, *3*. [CrossRef] [PubMed]
93. Svensson, K.J.; Christianson, H.C.; Wittrup, A.; Bourseau-Guilmain, E.; Lindqvist, E.; Svensson, L.M.; Morgelin, M.; Belting, M. Exosome uptake depends on ERK1/2-heat shock protein 27 signaling and lipid Raft-mediated endocytosis negatively regulated by caveolin-1. *J. Biol. Chem.* **2013**, *288*, 17713–17724. [CrossRef] [PubMed]
94. Escrevente, C.; Keller, S.; Altevogt, P.; Costa, J. Interaction and uptake of exosomes by ovarian cancer cells. *BMC Cancer* **2011**, *11*, 108. [CrossRef]
95. Banizs, A.B.; Huang, T.; Nakamoto, R.K.; Shi, W.; He, J. Endocytosis Pathways of Endothelial Cell Derived Exosomes. *Mol. Pharm.* **2018**, *15*, 5585–5590. [CrossRef]
96. Christianson, H.C.; Svensson, K.J.; van Kuppevelt, T.H.; Li, J.P.; Belting, M. Cancer cell exosomes depend on cell-surface heparan sulfate proteoglycans for their internalization and functional activity. *Proc. Natl. Acad. Sci. USA* **2013**, *110*, 17380–17385. [CrossRef]
97. Zheng, Y.; Tu, C.; Zhang, J.; Wang, J. Inhibition of multiple myelomaderived exosomes uptake suppresses the functional response in bone marrow stromal cell. *Int. J. Oncol.* **2019**, *54*, 1061–1070. [CrossRef]
98. Fong, M.Y.; Zhou, W.; Liu, L.; Alontaga, A.Y.; Chandra, M.; Ashby, J.; Chow, A.; O'Connor, S.T.; Li, S.; Chin, A.R.; et al. Breast-cancer-secreted miR-122 reprograms glucose metabolism in premetastatic niche to promote metastasis. *Nat. Cell Biol.* **2015**, *17*, 183–194. [CrossRef]
99. Lentz, M.R. Continuous whole blood UltraPheresis procedure in patients with metastatic cancer. *J. Biol. Response Mod.* **1989**, *8*, 511–527.
100. Tullis, R.H.; Duffin, R.P.; Handley, H.H.; Sodhi, P.; Menon, J.; Joyce, J.A.; Kher, V. Reduction of hepatitis C virus using lectin affinity plasmapheresis in dialysis patients. *Blood Purif.* **2009**, *27*, 64–69. [CrossRef]
101. Tullis, R.H.; Duffin, R.P.; Zech, M.; Ambrus, J.L. Affinity hemodialysis for antiviral therapy. II. Removal of HIV-1 viral proteins from cell culture supernatants and whole blood. *Blood Purif.* **2003**, *21*, 58–63. [CrossRef] [PubMed]
102. Nishida-Aoki, N.; Tominaga, N.; Takeshita, F.; Sonoda, H.; Yoshioka, Y.; Ochiya, T. Disruption of Circulating Extracellular Vesicles as a Novel Therapeutic Strategy against Cancer Metastasis. *Mol. Ther.* **2017**, *25*, 181–191. [CrossRef] [PubMed]
103. Xie, X.; Nie, H.; Zhou, Y.; Lian, S.; Mei, H.; Lu, Y.; Dong, H.; Li, F.; Li, T.; Li, B.; et al. Eliminating blood oncogenic exosomes into the small intestine with aptamer-functionalized nanoparticles. *Nat. Commun.* **2019**, *10*, 5476. [CrossRef] [PubMed]
104. Kimura, H.; Yamamoto, H.; Harada, T.; Fumoto, K.; Osugi, Y.; Sada, R.; Maehara, N.; Hikita, H.; Mori, S.; Eguchi, H.; et al. CKAP4, a DKK1 Receptor, Is a Biomarker in Exosomes Derived from Pancreatic Cancer and a Molecular Target for Therapy. *Clin. Cancer Res.* **2019**, *25*, 1936–1947. [CrossRef]
105. Binenbaum, Y.; Fridman, E.; Yaari, Z.; Milman, N.; Schroeder, A.; Ben David, G.; Shlomi, T.; Gil, Z. Transfer of miRNA in Macrophage-Derived Exosomes Induces Drug Resistance in Pancreatic Adenocarcinoma. *Cancer Res.* **2018**, *78*, 5287–5299. [CrossRef]
106. Mikamori, M.; Yamada, D.; Eguchi, H.; Hasegawa, S.; Kishimoto, T.; Tomimaru, Y.; Asaoka, T.; Noda, T.; Wada, H.; Kawamoto, K.; et al. MicroRNA-155 Controls Exosome Synthesis and Promotes Gemcitabine Resistance in Pancreatic Ductal Adenocarcinoma. *Sci. Rep.* **2017**, *7*, 42339. [CrossRef]

107. Li, X.J.; Ren, Z.J.; Tang, J.H.; Yu, Q. Exosomal MicroRNA MiR-1246 Promotes Cell Proliferation, Invasion and Drug Resistance by Targeting CCNG2 in Breast Cancer. *Cell Physiol. Biochem.* **2017**, *44*, 1741–1748. [CrossRef]
108. Chen, J.H.; Wu, A.T.H.; Bamodu, O.A.; Yadav, V.K.; Chao, T.Y.; Tzeng, Y.M.; Mukhopadhyay, D.; Hsiao, M.; Lee, J.C. Ovatodiolide Suppresses Oral Cancer Malignancy by Down-Regulating Exosomal Mir-21/STAT3/beta-Catenin Cargo and Preventing Oncogenic Transformation of Normal Gingival Fibroblasts. *Cancers* **2019**, *12*, 56. [CrossRef]
109. Hannafon, B.N.; Trigoso, Y.D.; Calloway, C.L.; Zhao, Y.D.; Lum, D.H.; Welm, A.L.; Zhao, Z.J.; Blick, K.E.; Dooley, W.C.; Ding, W.Q. Plasma exosome microRNAs are indicative of breast cancer. *Breast Cancer Res.* **2016**, *18*, 90. [CrossRef]
110. Xu, Y.F.; Hannafon, B.N.; Khatri, U.; Gin, A.; Ding, W.Q. The origin of exosomal miR-1246 in human cancer cells. *Rna Biol.* **2019**, *16*, 770–784. [CrossRef] [PubMed]
111. Xu, Y.F.; Hannafon, B.N.; Zhao, Y.D.; Postier, R.G.; Ding, W.Q. Plasma exosome miR-196a and miR-1246 are potential indicators of localized pancreatic cancer. *Oncotarget* **2017**, *8*, 77028–77040. [CrossRef] [PubMed]
112. Chen, D.S.; Mellman, I. Oncology meets immunology: The cancer-immunity cycle. *Immunity* **2013**, *39*, 1–10. [CrossRef] [PubMed]
113. Page, D.B.; Postow, M.A.; Callahan, M.K.; Allison, J.P.; Wolchok, J.D. Immune modulation in cancer with antibodies. *Annu. Rev. Med.* **2014**, *65*, 185–202. [CrossRef] [PubMed]
114. Zhang, C.; Fan, Y.; Che, X.; Zhang, M.; Li, Z.; Li, C.; Wang, S.; Wen, T.; Hou, K.; Shao, X.; et al. Anti-PD-1 Therapy Response Predicted by the Combination of Exosomal PD-L1 and CD28. *Front. Oncol.* **2020**, *10*, 760. [CrossRef]
115. Xie, F.; Xu, M.; Lu, J.; Mao, L.; Wang, S. The role of exosomal PD-L1 in tumor progression and immunotherapy. *Mol. Cancer* **2019**, *18*, 146. [CrossRef]
116. Dong, H.; Wang, W.; Chen, R.; Zhang, Y.; Zou, K.; Ye, M.; He, X.; Zhang, F.; Han, J. Exosome-mediated transfer of lncRNASNHG14 promotes trastuzumab chemoresistance in breast cancer. *Int. J. Oncol.* **2018**, *53*, 1013–1026. [CrossRef]
117. Milman, N.; Ginini, L.; Gil, Z. Exosomes and their role in tumorigenesis and anticancer drug resistance. *Drug Resist. Updat* **2019**, *45*, 1–12. [CrossRef]
118. Elsharkasy, O.M.; Nordin, J.Z.; Hagey, D.W.; de Jong, O.G.; Schiffelers, R.M.; Andaloussi, S.E.; Vader, P. Extracellular vesicles as drug delivery systems: Why and how? *Adv. Drug Deliv. Rev.* **2020**, in press. [CrossRef]
119. Bastos, N.; Ruivo, C.F.; da Silva, S.; Melo, S.A. Exosomes in cancer: Use them or target them? *Semin Cell Dev. Biol.* **2018**, *78*, 13–21. [CrossRef]
120. Ohno, S.; Drummen, G.P.; Kuroda, M. Focus on Extracellular Vesicles: Development of Extracellular Vesicle-Based Therapeutic Systems. *Int. J. Mol. Sci.* **2016**, *17*, 172. [CrossRef]
121. Smyth, T.J.; Redzic, J.S.; Graner, M.W.; Anchordoquy, T.J. Examination of the specificity of tumor cell derived exosomes with tumor cells in vitro. *Biochim. Biophys. Acta* **2014**, *1838*, 2954–2965. [CrossRef] [PubMed]
122. Cheng, Y.; Zeng, Q.; Han, Q.; Xia, W. Effect of pH, temperature and freezing-thawing on quantity changes and cellular uptake of exosomes. *Protein. Cell* **2019**, *10*, 295–299. [CrossRef]
123. Luan, X.; Sansanaphongpricha, K.; Myers, I.; Chen, H.; Yuan, H.; Sun, D. Engineering exosomes as refined biological nanoplatforms for drug delivery. *Acta Pharm. Sin.* **2017**, *38*, 754–763. [CrossRef] [PubMed]
124. Zhuang, X.; Xiang, X.; Grizzle, W.; Sun, D.; Zhang, S.; Axtell, R.C.; Ju, S.; Mu, J.; Zhang, L.; Steinman, L.; et al. Treatment of brain inflammatory diseases by delivering exosome encapsulated anti-inflammatory drugs from the nasal region to the brain. *Mol. Ther.* **2011**, *19*, 1769–1779. [CrossRef]
125. Wolfram, J.; Ferrari, M. Clinical Cancer Nanomedicine. *Nano Today* **2019**, *25*, 85–98. [CrossRef] [PubMed]
126. Li, X.; Tsibouklis, J.; Weng, T.; Zhang, B.; Yin, G.; Feng, G.; Cui, Y.; Savina, I.N.; Mikhalovska, L.I.; Sandeman, S.R.; et al. Nano carriers for drug transport across the blood-brain barrier. *J. Drug Target.* **2017**, *25*, 17–28. [CrossRef] [PubMed]
127. Kanchanapally, R.; Deshmukh, S.K.; Chavva, S.R.; Tyagi, N.; Srivastava, S.K.; Patel, G.K.; Singh, A.P.; Singh, S. Drug-loaded exosomal preparations from different cell types exhibit distinctive loading capability, yield, and antitumor efficacies: A comparative analysis. *Int. J. Nanomed.* **2019**, *14*, 531–541. [CrossRef] [PubMed]
128. Borrelli, D.A.; Yankson, K.; Shukla, N.; Vilanilam, G.; Ticer, T.; Wolfram, J. Extracellular vesicle therapeutics for liver disease. *J. Control. Release* **2018**, *273*, 86–98. [CrossRef]

129. Mendt, M.; Kamerkar, S.; Sugimoto, H.; McAndrews, K.M.; Wu, C.C.; Gagea, M.; Yang, S.; Blanko, E.V.R.; Peng, Q.; Ma, X.; et al. Generation and testing of clinical-grade exosomes for pancreatic cancer. *JCI Insight* **2018**, *3*. [CrossRef]
130. Kordelas, L.; Rebmann, V.; Ludwig, A.K.; Radtke, S.; Ruesing, J.; Doeppner, T.R.; Epple, M.; Horn, P.A.; Beelen, D.W.; Giebel, B. MSC-derived exosomes: A novel tool to treat therapy-refractory graft-versus-host disease. *Leukemia* **2014**, *28*, 970–973. [CrossRef]
131. Munoz, J.L.; Bliss, S.A.; Greco, S.J.; Ramkissoon, S.H.; Ligon, K.L.; Rameshwar, P. Delivery of Functional Anti-miR-9 by Mesenchymal Stem Cell-derived Exosomes to Glioblastoma Multiforme Cells Conferred Chemosensitivity. *Mol. Nucleic Acids* **2013**, *2*, e126. [CrossRef] [PubMed]
132. Pascucci, L.; Cocce, V.; Bonomi, A.; Ami, D.; Ceccarelli, P.; Ciusani, E.; Vigano, L.; Locatelli, A.; Sisto, F.; Doglia, S.M.; et al. Paclitaxel is incorporated by mesenchymal stromal cells and released in exosomes that inhibit in vitro tumor growth: A new approach for drug delivery. *J. Control. Release* **2014**, *192*, 262–270. [CrossRef] [PubMed]
133. Lohan, P.; Treacy, O.; Griffin, M.D.; Ritter, T.; Ryan, A.E. Anti-Donor Immune Responses Elicited by Allogeneic Mesenchymal Stem Cells and Their Extracellular Vesicles: Are We Still Learning? *Front. Immunol.* **2017**, *8*, 1626. [CrossRef] [PubMed]
134. Kilpinen, L.; Impola, U.; Sankkila, L.; Ritamo, I.; Aatonen, M.; Kilpinen, S.; Tuimala, J.; Valmu, L.; Levijoki, J.; Finckenberg, P.; et al. Extracellular membrane vesicles from umbilical cord blood-derived MSC protect against ischemic acute kidney injury, a feature that is lost after inflammatory conditioning. *J. Extracell. Vesicles* **2013**, *2*. [CrossRef] [PubMed]
135. Alvarez-Erviti, L.; Seow, Y.; Yin, H.; Betts, C.; Lakhal, S.; Wood, M.J. Delivery of siRNA to the mouse brain by systemic injection of targeted exosomes. *Nat. Biotechnol.* **2011**, *29*, 341–345. [CrossRef]
136. Tian, Y.; Li, S.; Song, J.; Ji, T.; Zhu, M.; Anderson, G.J.; Wei, J.; Nie, G. A doxorubicin delivery platform using engineered natural membrane vesicle exosomes for targeted tumor therapy. *Biomaterials* **2014**, *35*, 2383–2390. [CrossRef]
137. Kharaziha, P.; Ceder, S.; Li, Q.; Panaretakis, T. Tumor cell-derived exosomes: A message in a bottle. *Biochim. Biophys. Acta* **2012**, *1826*, 103–111. [CrossRef]
138. Shtam, T.A.; Kovalev, R.A.; Varfolomeeva, E.Y.; Makarov, E.M.; Kil, Y.V.; Filatov, M.V. Exosomes are natural carriers of exogenous siRNA to human cells in vitro. *Cell Commun. Signal.* **2013**, *11*, 88. [CrossRef]
139. Becker, A.; Thakur, B.K.; Weiss, J.M.; Kim, H.S.; Peinado, H.; Lyden, D. Extracellular Vesicles in Cancer: Cell-to-Cell Mediators of Metastasis. *Cancer Cell* **2016**, *30*, 836–848. [CrossRef]
140. Lou, G.; Song, X.; Yang, F.; Wu, S.; Wang, J.; Chen, Z.; Liu, Y. Exosomes derived from miR-122-modified adipose tissue-derived MSCs increase chemosensitivity of hepatocellular carcinoma. *J. Hematol. Oncol.* **2015**, *8*, 122. [CrossRef]
141. Abels, E.R.; Maas, S.L.N.; Nieland, L.; Wei, Z.; Cheah, P.S.; Tai, E.; Kolsteeg, C.J.; Dusoswa, S.A.; Ting, D.T.; Hickman, S.; et al. Glioblastoma-Associated Microglia Reprogramming Is Mediated by Functional Transfer of Extracellular miR-21. *Cell Rep.* **2019**, *28*, 3105–3119 e3107. [CrossRef] [PubMed]
142. Fareh, M.; Almairac, F.; Turchi, L.; Burel-Vandenbos, F.; Paquis, P.; Fontaine, D.; Lacas-Gervais, S.; Junier, M.P.; Chneiweiss, H.; Virolle, T. Cell-based therapy using miR-302-367 expressing cells represses glioblastoma growth. *Cell Death Dis.* **2017**, *8*, e2713. [CrossRef] [PubMed]
143. Katakowski, M.; Buller, B.; Zheng, X.; Lu, Y.; Rogers, T.; Osobamiro, O.; Shu, W.; Jiang, F.; Chopp, M. Exosomes from marrow stromal cells expressing miR-146b inhibit glioma growth. *Cancer Lett.* **2013**, *335*, 201–204. [CrossRef] [PubMed]
144. O'Brien, K.; Breyne, K.; Ughetto, S.; Laurent, L.C.; Breakefield, X.O. RNA delivery by extracellular vesicles in mammalian cells and its applications. *Nat. Rev. Mol. Cell Biol.* **2020**. [CrossRef]
145. Fuhrmann, G.; Serio, A.; Mazo, M.; Nair, R.; Stevens, M.M. Active loading into extracellular vesicles significantly improves the cellular uptake and photodynamic effect of porphyrins. *J. Control. Release* **2015**, *205*, 35–44. [CrossRef]
146. O'Loughlin, A.J.; Mager, I.; de Jong, O.G.; Varela, M.A.; Schiffelers, R.M.; El Andaloussi, S.; Wood, M.J.A.; Vader, P. Functional Delivery of Lipid-Conjugated siRNA by Extracellular Vesicles. *Mol. Ther.* **2017**, *25*, 1580–1587. [CrossRef]

147. Srivastava, A.; Amreddy, N.; Pareek, V.; Chinnappan, M.; Ahmed, R.; Mehta, M.; Razaq, M.; Munshi, A.; Ramesh, R. Progress in extracellular vesicle biology and their application in cancer medicine. *Wiley Interdiscip Rev. Nanomed. Nanobiotechnol.* **2020**, *12*, e1621. [CrossRef]
148. Potter, H. Transfection by electroporation. *Curr. Protoc. Mol. Biol.* **2003**. [CrossRef]
149. Bak, R.O.; Dever, D.P.; Porteus, M.H. CRISPR/Cas9 genome editing in human hematopoietic stem cells. *Nat. Protoc.* **2018**, *13*, 358–376. [CrossRef]
150. Hood, J.L.; Scott, M.J.; Wickline, S.A. Maximizing exosome colloidal stability following electroporation. *Anal. Biochem.* **2014**, *448*, 41–49. [CrossRef]
151. Liu, C.; Su, C. Design strategies and application progress of therapeutic exosomes. *Theranostics* **2019**, *9*, 1015–1028. [CrossRef] [PubMed]
152. Asadirad, A.; Hashemi, S.M.; Baghaei, K.; Ghanbarian, H.; Mortaz, E.; Zali, M.R.; Amani, D. Phenotypical and functional evaluation of dendritic cells after exosomal delivery of miRNA-155. *Life Sci.* **2019**, *219*, 152–162. [CrossRef] [PubMed]
153. Li, Y.J.; Wu, J.Y.; Wang, J.M.; Hu, X.B.; Cai, J.X.; Xiang, D.X. Gemcitabine loaded autologous exosomes for effective and safe chemotherapy of pancreatic cancer. *Acta Biomater.* **2020**, *101*, 519–530. [CrossRef] [PubMed]
154. Sato, Y.T.; Umezaki, K.; Sawada, S.; Mukai, S.A.; Sasaki, Y.; Harada, N.; Shiku, H.; Akiyoshi, K. Engineering hybrid exosomes by membrane fusion with liposomes. *Sci. Rep.* **2016**, *6*, 21933. [CrossRef] [PubMed]
155. Haney, M.J.; Klyachko, N.L.; Zhao, Y.; Gupta, R.; Plotnikova, E.G.; He, Z.; Patel, T.; Piroyan, A.; Sokolsky, M.; Kabanov, A.V.; et al. Exosomes as drug delivery vehicles for Parkinson's disease therapy. *J. Control. Release* **2015**, *207*, 18–30. [CrossRef]
156. Goh, W.J.; Lee, C.K.; Zou, S.; Woon, E.C.; Czarny, B.; Pastorin, G. Doxorubicin-loaded cell-derived nanovesicles: An alternative targeted approach for anti-tumor therapy. *Int. J. Nanomed.* **2017**, *12*, 2759–2767. [CrossRef]
157. Kalimuthu, S.; Gangadaran, P.; Rajendran, R.L.; Zhu, L.; Oh, J.M.; Lee, H.W.; Gopal, A.; Baek, S.H.; Jeong, S.Y.; Lee, S.W.; et al. A New Approach for Loading Anticancer Drugs Into Mesenchymal Stem Cell-Derived Exosome Mimetics for Cancer Therapy. *Front. Pharm.* **2018**, *9*, 1116. [CrossRef]
158. Bunggulawa, E.J.; Wang, W.; Yin, T.; Wang, N.; Durkan, C.; Wang, Y.; Wang, G. Recent advancements in the use of exosomes as drug delivery systems. *J. Nanobiotechnol.* **2018**, *16*, 81. [CrossRef] [PubMed]
159. Rahbarghazi, R.; Jabbari, N.; Sani, N.A.; Asghari, R.; Salimi, L.; Kalashani, S.A.; Feghhi, M.; Etemadi, T.; Akbariazar, E.; Mahmoudi, M.; et al. Tumor-derived extracellular vesicles: Reliable tools for Cancer diagnosis and clinical applications. *Cell Commun. Signal.* **2019**, *17*, 73. [CrossRef] [PubMed]
160. Zhang, Y.F.; Shi, J.B.; Li, C. Small extracellular vesicle loading systems in cancer therapy: Current status and the way forward. *Cytotherapy* **2019**, *21*, 1122–1136. [CrossRef]
161. Walker, S.; Busatto, S.; Pham, A.; Tian, M.; Suh, A.; Carson, K.; Quintero, A.; Lafrence, M.; Malik, H.; Santana, M.X.; et al. Extracellular vesicle-based drug delivery systems for cancer treatment. *Theranostics* **2019**, *9*, 8001–8017. [CrossRef] [PubMed]
162. Chen, Y.S.; Lin, E.Y.; Chiou, T.W.; Harn, H.J. Exosomes in clinical trial and their production in compliance with good manufacturing practice. *Tzu-Chi Med. J.* **2019**, *32*, 113–120. [CrossRef]
163. Guo, M.; Wu, F.; Hu, G.; Chen, L.; Xu, J.; Xu, P.; Wang, X.; Li, Y.; Liu, S.; Zhang, S.; et al. Autologous tumor cell-derived microparticle-based targeted chemotherapy in lung cancer patients with malignant pleural effusion. *Sci. Transl. Med.* **2019**, *11*. [CrossRef]
164. Tang, K.; Zhang, Y.; Zhang, H.; Xu, P.; Liu, J.; Ma, J.; Lv, M.; Li, D.; Katirai, F.; Shen, G.X.; et al. Delivery of chemotherapeutic drugs in tumour cell-derived microparticles. *Nat. Commun.* **2012**, *3*, 1282. [CrossRef]
165. Ma, J.; Zhang, Y.; Tang, K.; Zhang, H.; Yin, X.; Li, Y.; Xu, P.; Sun, Y.; Ma, R.; Ji, T.; et al. Reversing drug resistance of soft tumor-repopulating cells by tumor cell-derived chemotherapeutic microparticles. *Cell Res.* **2016**, *26*, 713–727. [CrossRef]
166. Kamerkar, S.; LeBleu, V.S.; Sugimoto, H.; Yang, S.; Ruivo, C.F.; Melo, S.A.; Lee, J.J.; Kalluri, R. Exosomes facilitate therapeutic targeting of oncogenic KRAS in pancreatic cancer. *Nature* **2017**, *546*, 498–503. [CrossRef]
167. Dai, S.; Wei, D.; Wu, Z.; Zhou, X.; Wei, X.; Huang, H.; Li, G. Phase I clinical trial of autologous ascites-derived exosomes combined with GM-CSF for colorectal cancer. *Mol. Ther.* **2008**, *16*, 782–790. [CrossRef]
168. Besse, B.; Charrier, M.; Lapierre, V.; Dansin, E.; Lantz, O.; Planchard, D.; Le Chevalier, T.; Livartoski, A.; Barlesi, F.; Laplanche, A.; et al. Dendritic cell-derived exosomes as maintenance immunotherapy after first line chemotherapy in NSCLC. *Oncoimmunology* **2016**, *5*, e1071008. [CrossRef]

169. Morse, M.A.; Garst, J.; Osada, T.; Khan, S.; Hobeika, A.; Clay, T.M.; Valente, N.; Shreeniwas, R.; Sutton, M.A.; Delcayre, A.; et al. A phase I study of dexosome immunotherapy in patients with advanced non-small cell lung cancer. *J. Transl. Med.* **2005**, *3*, 9. [CrossRef]
170. Escudier, B.; Dorval, T.; Chaput, N.; Andre, F.; Caby, M.P.; Novault, S.; Flament, C.; Leboulaire, C.; Borg, C.; Amigorena, S.; et al. Vaccination of metastatic melanoma patients with autologous dendritic cell (DC) derived-exosomes: Results of thefirst phase I clinical trial. *J. Transl. Med.* **2005**, *3*, 10. [CrossRef]
171. Somiya, M.; Yoshioka, Y.; Ochiya, T. Drug delivery application of extracellular vesicles; insight into production, drug loading, targeting, and pharmacokinetics. *Aims Bioeng.* **2017**, *4*, 73–92. [CrossRef]
172. Wang, Q.; Zhuang, X.; Mu, J.; Deng, Z.B.; Jiang, H.; Zhang, L.; Xiang, X.; Wang, B.; Yan, J.; Miller, D.; et al. Delivery of therapeutic agents by nanoparticles made of grapefruit-derived lipids. *Nat. Commun.* **2013**, *4*, 1867. [CrossRef] [PubMed]
173. Burnouf, T.; Agrahari, V.; Agrahari, V. Extracellular Vesicles As Nanomedicine: Hopes And Hurdles In Clinical Translation. *Int. J. Nanomed.* **2019**, *14*, 8847–8859. [CrossRef] [PubMed]
174. Agrahari, V.; Agrahari, V.; Burnouf, P.A.; Chew, C.H.; Burnouf, T. Extracellular Microvesicles as New Industrial Therapeutic Frontiers. *Trends Biotechnol.* **2019**, *37*, 707–729. [CrossRef] [PubMed]

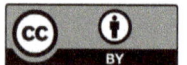

© 2020 by the authors. Licensee MDPI, Basel, Switzerland. This article is an open access article distributed under the terms and conditions of the Creative Commons Attribution (CC BY) license (http://creativecommons.org/licenses/by/4.0/).

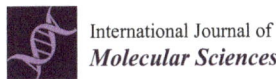

International Journal of
Molecular Sciences

Review

More than Nutrition: Therapeutic Potential of Breast Milk-Derived Exosomes in Cancer

Ki-Uk Kim [1], Wan-Hoon Kim [1], Chi Hwan Jeong [1], Dae Yong Yi [2,3,*] and Hyeyoung Min [1,*]

[1] College of Pharmacy, Chung-Ang University, Seoul 06974, Korea; hakiukah@cau.ac.kr (K.-U.K.); vessel37@cau.ac.kr (W.-H.K.); tolast12@cau.ac.kr (C.H.J.)
[2] Department of Pediatrics, Chung-Ang University College of Medicine, Seoul 06974, Korea
[3] Department of Pediatrics, Chung-Ang University Hospital, Seoul 06973, Korea
[*] Correspondence: meltemp2@cau.ac.kr (D.Y.Y.); hymin@cau.ac.kr (H.M.); Tel.: +82-2-820-5618 (H.M.); Fax: +82-2-816-7338 (H.M.)

Received: 28 August 2020; Accepted: 2 October 2020; Published: 3 October 2020

Abstract: Human breast milk (HBM) is an irreplaceable source of nutrition for early infant growth and development. Breast-fed children are known to have a low prevalence and reduced risk of various diseases, such as necrotizing enterocolitis, gastroenteritis, acute lymphocytic leukemia, and acute myeloid leukemia. In recent years, HBM has been found to contain a microbiome, extracellular vesicles or exosomes, and microRNAs, as well as nutritional components and non-nutritional proteins, including immunoregulatory proteins, hormones, and growth factors. Especially, the milk-derived exosomes exert various physiological and therapeutic function in cell proliferation, inflammation, immunomodulation, and cancer, which are mainly attributed to their cargo molecules such as proteins and microRNAs. The exosomal miRNAs are protected from enzymatic digestion and acidic conditions, and play a critical role in immune regulation and cancer. In addition, the milk-derived exosomes are developed as drug carriers for delivering small molecules and siRNA to tumor sites. In this review, we examined the various components of HBM and their therapeutic potential, in particular of exosomes and microRNAs, towards cancer.

Keywords: human milk; nutrient; microbiota; exosomes; microRNAs; cancer

---

1. Introduction

Human breast milk (HBM) is an irreplaceable source of nutrition for early infant growth and development. For this reason, the World Health Organization and the American Academy of Pediatrics recommend exclusive breastfeeding for at least 6 months and to continue breastfeeding until the age of 2 years [1–3]. It is widely known that HBM provides advantages for cognition and development in the short and long term [3,4]. Breast-fed children are known to have a low prevalence of necrotizing enterocolitis (NEC), gastroenteritis, otitis media, respiratory diseases, and acute diseases, as well as obesity, inflammatory bowel disease, and diabetes [3,5,6]. In addition, breastfeeding for more than 6 months reduces the risk of acute lymphocytic leukemia and acute myeloid leukemia, and there is evidence of reduced morbidity associated with lymphoma and other tumors [3,5–7]. Furthermore, breastfeeding mothers show various short-term benefits and long-term positive effects on cardiovascular disease, diabetes, and bone density [5]. In particular, breastfeeding is known to lower the risk of breast and ovarian cancer.

Although various multinational companies are conducting research to develop breast milk replacements, it has not yet been possible to completely replace breast milk by any method [8]. This is because HBM contains various ingredients that have not yet been identified, so it is difficult to artificially reproduce them. HBM contains not only nutritional components, such as macronutrients and micronutrients, but also various non-nutritional proteins or cellular components, including immune components, hormones, and growth factors [9–11]. In recent years, studies on HBM components, such as human milk oligosaccharides (HMOs) and fatty acids, have been actively conducted. The HBM components that have not been well appreciated in the past, such as the microbiome, extracellular vesicles (EVs) or exosomes, and microRNAs (miRNAs), are being examined, assisted by the development of various testing techniques [11–13]. Some of these components consistently show no considerable differences between regions and races, such as protein components and with regard to the energy content. However, there are differences according to the diet or weight of the breastfeeding mother in components such as vitamin A, vitamin D, water-soluble vitamins, and the composition of fatty acids, and also in other components according to the underlying condition of the breastfeeding mother [3,11,12]. In addition, the maturation, colonization, and immunity acquisition of immature intestinal mucosa are obtained through breastfeeding, and the incidence of various diseases is lower in breastfed infants than that in formula-fed infants. Considering these aspects, the HBM components, such as the immune components and exosomes, would be helpful in predicting and treating diseases in actual clinical practice.

In this article, we examined the various well-known components of HBM and those that are currently being studied, focusing on exosomes. In addition, we described how these ingredients affect the health of children and breastfeeding mothers and especially their potential use in diseases such as cancer.

2. Human Breast Milk Components

2.1. Nutritional Components (Macronutrients and Micronutrients)

As already known, HBM is mainly composed of macronutrients such as carbohydrates, proteins, and fats, along with 87–88% water [11]. Among them, carbohydrates are the most important component in HBM and play a critical role in infant nutrition. Although lactose is a major carbohydrate constituent of HBM, HMOs, which have recently been attracting attention, are unique components of HBM and are the third largest constituent of HBM. HMOs play a prebiotic role that affect the development of intestinal colonization and gut microbiota immediately after birth, directly affecting immunity, and also play a role in the production of short chain fatty acids [14,15]. The proteins in HBM are composed of various peptides along with a mixture of casein and whey. These proteins play an essential role in growth and development by being involved in the functionalization and organization of cells in the human body [11]. As HBM is known to play an essential role in the development of the early human immune system, whey proteins, such as alpha-lactalbumin, lactoferrin, and secretory IgA, play an important role in the immune system and have antibacterial properties [10,16,17]. Fat accounts for 50% of the total nutrition supplied by HBM, is the second largest macronutrient, and plays an important role in the development of the nervous system [18]. Fat in HBM varies according to the maternal diet and body weight during pregnancy, so there are large regional differences [18].

In addition, HBM contains various vitamins and micronutrients, such as iron, calcium, zinc, and copper. Although most of these micronutrients are sufficiently contained in breast milk, vitamin D or vitamin K may require supplementation if exclusively breastfeeding due to insufficiencies [19,20]. The nutrient content of HBM varies depending on whether it is colostrum or mature milk, and the ratio changes as lactation progresses. In addition, HBM fed to premature infants may have different components from that fed to mature infants [11].

2.2. Non-Nutritional Components and Clinical Applications

In addition to the nutrient components, HBM contains various non-nutritional components, bioactive proteins, and peptides. HBM is known to contain various hormones, such as parathyroid hormone, insulin, and leptin, but their functions are not fully understood [11]. However, the roles of many growth factors are well known. Epidermal growth factors play a crucial role in the maturation and healing of intestinal mucosa, and neuronal growth factors are known to be necessary for the development of the enteric nervous system and immature intestine in newborns [10,11]. Moreover, the insulin-like growth factor superfamily and vascular endothelial growth factor regulate erythropoiesis and angiogenesis, respectively [10,11].

Considering the development of the immune system through breastfeeding, the formation of a functional microbial community through colonization of microorganisms in the intestinal tract, and the low disease incidence in breast-fed infants, various components of HBM have been studied for their applicability in the clinic and infection [21]. Attempts have been made to use lactoferrin to treat colon cancer, advanced stage non-small-cell lung carcinoma, newly diagnosed lung cancer, and breast cancer in connection with regulating cellular growth and differentiation, playing an important role in immune response [22–26]. Another immune component, alpha-lactalbumin, is known as HAMLET (human alpha-lactalbumin made lethal to tumor cells) for its clinical applicability in oncologic diseases. Through the intratumoral administration of HAMLET, damage to the intact brain in human glioblastoma is minimized and tumor cell apoptosis is induced [27]. The effects of alpha-lactalbumin on apoptosis and resolution have also been confirmed in human skin papilloma and bladder cancer [28,29]. The transforming growth factor β (TGF-β) contained in milk acts on immunomodulation and cell proliferation and differentiation, particularly in pediatric Crohn's disease, and is used for enteral nutrition [21].

2.3. Microbiomes and Their Derived Extracellular Vesicles

Until the 20th century, HBM was considered sterile, and bacterial species identified in HBM were believed to be due to contamination or infection. However, it was known to some researchers that HBM also contains commensal bacteria, and rich and diverse communities have been identified by new testing techniques such as Next Generation Sequencing [30–32]. Through these advanced techniques, *Staphylococcus* and *Streptococcus* were found to be the predominant core genera in HBM, despite differences in regions and test techniques [11]. In addition, Togo et al. confirmed the diversity of human milk microbiota through a systematic review and identified commonly found species: *Staphylococcus aureus, Staphylococcus epidermidis, Streptococcus agalactiae, Cutibacterium acnes, Enterococcus faecalis, Bifidobacterium breve, Escherichia coli, Streptococcus sanguinis, Lactobacillus gasseri,* and *Salmonella enterica* [33].

The origin of the HBM microbiota remains unknown. The possibility of contamination of the skin or oral cavity cannot yet be ruled out. In fact, Ramsay et al. confirmed milk-ejection reflux from the mouth of the infant to mammary ducts during breastfeeding through ultrasound [34]. However, an introduction of microbiota from an endogenous origin, such as glands, rather than contamination is possible, since anaerobic gut-associated microbiota has been identified in breast milk. The maternal gut microbiota may be absorbed through the maternal intestinal epithelium and present in the mammary glands [35,36]. It is thought that these HBM microbes act as prebiotics with HMOs and indirectly affect the infant gut and various extra-intestinal environments [37–40]. Through many studies conducted so far, vertical transmission of HBM microbiota has been shown to play an important role in the initial formation of infant gut microbiota. It is already known that there is a difference between the stool microbiota of the infant and adulthood periods in breast-fed and non-breast-fed individuals, and a role for HBM microbiota in human health is possible, as it is associated with a low incidence of various diseases such as infectious diseases and allergies in breast-fed infants [41,42].

In addition to these microbiomes, HBM was also found to contain EVs of bacterial origin [12]. EVs are nanometer-sized membrane vesicles that have various bioactive functions in intercellular communication. EVs were generally classified into exosomes (endocytic pathway), microvesicles (plasma membrane), and apoptotic bodies (plasma membrane) according to their cargos, biogenesis, and size [43]. Bacterial origin EVs are present in a variety of body fluids such as blood, urine, and stool, but their role in breast milk remains unknown. At the genus level, HBM bacteria and bacterial EVs show a significant difference. It is believed that bacterial origin EVs act on the host receptor to move bioactive molecules to host cells or to move the EVs themselves to host cells to play a role in infant gut colonization and immunity [12].

3. Breast Milk-Derived Exosomes

Exosomes are small membranous extracellular vesicles secreted by most eukaryotic cells into surrounding body fluids, such as blood, saliva, urine, cerebrospinal fluid, lymphatic fluid, and amniotic fluid [44–46]. These vesicles are 40~100 nm in diameter and are involved in cell–cell communication by transporting the bioactive cargo molecules, including DNAs, mRNAs, microRNAs, lipids, and proteins, derived from the cells of origin to the target cells. Exosomes are also present in breast milk, and the diverse health benefits of breastfeeding are attributed to exosomes, as well as to well-known immunoregulatory components such as lactoferrin, lactalbumin, lysozyme, and sIgA [47,48].

Exosomes were first extracted from human colostrum and breast milk and characterized in 2007 [47], and subsequent studies have reported the isolation and characterization of milk exosomes from cows, camels, buffalos, pigs, sheep, and pigeons [49–55]. Milk exosomes are secreted by mammary gland epithelial cells and also released from milk fat globules during lactation [56]. Higher concentrations of exosomes were detected in early milk collected at day 3–8 postpartum than in mature milk collected at 2 months, whereas no significant differences were found in the expression of marker proteins, such as the tetraspanins CD63, CD81, and the scavenger receptor CD36, between early and mature milk [57].

3.1. The Role of Milk Exosomes in Cell Proliferation and Inflammation

Studies have reported that milk exosomes function in regulating cell proliferation and inflammation. Hock et al. showed that rat milk-derived exosomes promote the viability and proliferation of intestinal epithelial cells and intestinal stem cell activity [58], supporting the previous observations that HBM reduces the incidence of NEC in infants [59–62]. Consistently, Martin et al. have also reported that human milk-derived exosomes protect intestinal epithelial cells from cell death upon exposure to oxidative stress [63]. Furthermore, a neonatal mouse intestinal organoid model and experimental NEC in C57BL/6 mouse pups supported the protective activities of HBM exosomes by decreasing inflammation and intestinal damage [64]. A reduction in intestinal damage has also been observed by exosomes derived from pasteurized breast milk and raw breast milk, indicating that milk exosomes are resistant to the pasteurization process. In addition, an increasing number of studies have reported the protective effects of milk exosomes in various in vitro and in vivo NEC models, confirming the critical role of exosomes in the prevention of NEC development in premature infants [65,66].

The anti-inflammatory effects of bovine milk-derived exosomes have also been shown in IL-1Ra(-/-) and collagen-induced arthritis mouse models [67]. When administered orally by oral gavage or drinking water, milk exosomes delay the onset of arthritis and reduce the swelling of ankle joints, cartilage depletion, and bone marrow inflammation. In addition, the circulating levels of MCP-1, IL-6, and anti-collagen IgG$_{2a}$ declined, accompanied by a decrease in mRNA expression of T-bet (Th1) and ROR-γT (Th17) in the primary splenocytes. These results suggest the therapeutic potential of milk exosomes in the treatment of autoimmune and inflammatory diseases.

3.2. Immunomodulatory Function of Milk Exosomes

Breast milk exosomes also show immunomodulatory effects. The Gabrielsson group demonstrated that HBM-derived exosomes inhibit CD3-induced production of IL-2, IFN-γ, and TNF-α in peripheral blood mononuclear cells (PBMCs), while increasing the number of FoxP3$^+$ CD4$^+$ CD25$^+$ regulatory T cells in PBMCs [47]. They also reported that MUC-1 expressed on HBM-derived exosomes binds to DC-SIGN on monocyte-derived dendritic cells (MDDCs) and blocks HIV-1 infection and viral transfer from MDDCs to CD4$^+$ T cells [68]. In addition, human milk exosomes possess different phenotypes, depending upon maternal sensitization and lifestyle, and differentially influence allergy development in children [57]. For example, exosomes derived from mothers with an anthroposophic lifestyle are associated with a lower prevalence of allergic sensitization than those from non-anthroposophic mothers. Cow milk-derived exosomes upregulate CD69 expression in NK cells and IFN-γ production in NK cells and γδ T cells in the presence of IL-2 and IL-12 [69]. Furthermore, bovine milk exosomes induce proliferation of macrophages and RAW264.7 cells and protect macrophages against cisplatin-induced cell death [70]. These data suggest that milk exosomes potentially influence the immune system.

A proteomic analysis has been performed to compare the exosomal protein contents between bovine colostrum and mature milk (mid-lactation period) [71]. The results revealed that exosomes from colostrum are highly enriched in proteins implicated in the innate immune response, inflammatory response, acute-phase response, platelet activation, cell growth, and complement activation, whereas proteins implicated in transport and apoptosis are enriched in exosomes from mature milk [71]. A further proteomic analysis of bovine milk exosomes also reported that exosomal proteins map to the Kyoto Encyclopedia of Genes and Genomes (KEGG) pathways with immunological functions such as Fc gamma receptor-mediated phagocytosis, antigen processing and presentation, T cell receptor signaling, B cell receptor signaling, and NK cell-mediated cytotoxicity [72]. Proteome studies supported the immunoregulatory function of milk exosomes and suggested the importance of colostrum in immune defense and immune system development during the early period after birth.

3.3. Milk Exosomes and Cancer

The chemopreventive effects of breast milk have been well studied in childhood leukemia and lymphoma [73–77]. Martin et al. performed a systemic review and meta-analysis and showed that ever having been breast-fed is inversely associated with the incidence of acute lymphoblastic leukemia, Hodgkin's disease, and neuroblastoma in childhood [78]. Similarly, a recent meta-analysis and systemic review reported that 14–19% of all childhood leukemia cases might be prevented by breastfeeding for 6 months or more, whereas breastfeeding for a short duration or non-breastfeeding may be associated with a slightly increased risk of acute childhood leukemia [7,79]. Given the severity and detrimental effects of these illnesses, any factor lowering the risk of childhood cancer would be useful.

Reif et al. reported that HBM-derived exosomes promote the proliferation of normal colon epithelial cells without affecting the growth of colonic cancer cells [80]. Although this study does not show the direct antitumor effects of human milk exosomes, it suggests the beneficial function of human milk exosomes through differential effects on normal cells compared to cancer cells. Bovine milk-derived exosomes have revealed their intrinsic antitumor activity by inhibiting the proliferation of various types of cancers, such as lung, prostate, colon, pancreatic, breast, and ovarian cancers [81]. Treatment of cancer cells with 50 μg/mL exosomal proteins for 72 h reduces cell growth by 8–47% as assessed by MTT assay, suggesting the benefit of exosomes as delivery vehicles for anticancer drugs. In addition, camel milk and its components have also been shown to exert antitumor effects in human hepatoma (HepG2), human breast cancer cells (MCF7), and murine hepatoma (Hepa 1c1c7) [82,83]. Camel milk inhibits cell growth and induces apoptosis by activating caspase-3 and death receptor DR4 and accumulates intracellular reactive oxygen species in HepG2 and MCF7 cells [83]. Badawy et al. demonstrated that camel milk and its exosomes inhibit the proliferation of MCF7 cells, accompanied by a decrease in MCF7 migration, as measured by a wound-healing assay [53]. In tumor-bearing rats, oral or local (in the tumor tissue) administration of camel milk and its exosomes significantly reduces tumor weight and progression by inducing apoptosis and inhibiting oxidative stress, inflammation, angiogenesis, and metastasis. Moreover, the numbers of CD4$^+$, CD8$^+$, and NKT1.1$^+$ T cells increase in the spleen following treatment with camel milk and its exosomes. Although exosomes show better overall antitumor effects, the increase in the numbers of splenic T cells is more potent in milk-treated rats, suggesting that camel milk possesses more immune-stimulating constituents than exosomes.

In contrast, breast milk exosomes may negatively influence some type of cancers. TGF-β isolated from breast milk exosomes promotes the proliferation of breast cancer cells and epithelial–mesenchymal transition (EMT), as demonstrated by changes in the actin cytoskeletal structure and loss of E-cadherin expression [84]. Since epithelial cells acquire migratory and invasive properties during EMT, TGF-β in exosomes may lead to the transformation of normal cells and a change in breast cancer cells into a more aggressive and invasive tumor.

4. Breast Milk-Derived Exosomal MicroRNAs

MicroRNAs are endogenous small non-coding RNA molecules that are 19~24 bp in length [85–87]. miRNAs interact with the 3′ untranslated region (UTR) of target mRNAs and control gene expression post-transcriptionally. Ample studies have reported the function of miRNAs in diverse biological processes, such as proliferation, differentiation, cell cycle, and cell death [88,89], and dysregulated miRNAs are implicated in the development and progression of many human diseases [90,91]. In relation to cancer, miRNAs may function as tumor suppressor genes or oncogenes, and accordingly, aberrantly expressed miRNAs in particular types of cancer have been suggested as useful biomarkers for cancer diagnostics and therapeutic targets [92–95].

HBM is highly enriched in miRNAs, with more than 1400 identified miRNAs [96–100]. Breast milk miRNAs are thought to originate from the mammary epithelium and are present in the cells, skimmed fractions, and lipid fractions of breast milk [98]. More miRNAs are detected in the cell and lipid fractions of breast milk than the skimmed milk fraction, suggesting the importance of cell and lipid fractions in the analysis of breast milk miRNAs [96,100]. Exosomes are mostly present in the skimmed milk fraction, and exosomal miRNAs are often reported within breast milk miRNA if it has not been specifically mentioned that exosomes were isolated from milk before miRNA extraction.

Studies have reported that milk exosomes protect exosomal miRNAs from enzymatic, chemical, or mechanical degradation. When exposed to acidic conditions that mimic gastric and pancreatic digestion, milk exosomes prevent the degradation of vulnerable miRNAs [101]. Commercial bovine milk also protects miRNAs from acidic environments and RNase treatment, safely delivering miRNAs into the digestive tract [102]. Subsequently, milk exosomes are taken up by intestinal epithelial cells by endocytosis and moved into systemic circulation [103,104]. In addition, studies have shown that milk exosomes containing miRNAs are absorbed into macrophages, PBMCs, and kidney cells, and regulate gene expression in the target cells [67,105]. For example, upon incubation of normal intestinal CRL 1831 cells, K562 leukemia cells, and Lim 1215 colon cancer cells with milk exosomes, the expression of miR-148a-3p, the most abundant miRNA in breast milk, is increased accompanied by a decrease in the expression of DNA methyltransferase1 (DNMT1), a target of miR-148a-3p [106]. Although the composition of breast milk and miRNAs vary depending on the maternal health and nutrition status and lactation stage [107,108], miR-148a-3p is highly expressed in breast milk and conserved across mammalian species, and other highly expressed miRNAs, such as miR-320, miR-375, and miR-99, are also frequently found in different species [106].

4.1. Immune-Regulating miRNAs

Exosomal miRNAs contribute to the physiological and therapeutic functions of milk exosomes. Several studies have reported that breast milk is rich in immune-regulating miRNAs, such as miR-125b, miR-146b, miR-155, miR-181a, and miR-181b [108–110]. These miRNAs are known to regulate B cell, T cell, and monocyte development, and control the innate immune response and cytokine production (Table 1). Zhou et al. demonstrated that immune-regulating miRNAs are abundant in milk exosomes [99]. Among the 453 pre-miRNAs detected in milk exosomes, 59 pre-miRNAs were immune related, based on annotation in the Pathway Central database. For example, miR-30b-5p promotes cellular invasion by directly targeting GalNAc transferase and immunosuppression by increasing IL-10 [111], whereas miR-182-5p promotes helper T cell-mediated immune response upon induction by IL-2 [112]. Other frequently found immune-related exosomal miRNAs are miR-148a-3p, miR-146a, miR-146b-5p, miR-200a-3p, and miR-29a-3p [99,106,113]. These immune-regulating miRNAs may be transferred into the infant body during breastfeeding and function in the development of the immune system [99]. Future studies extending beyond in silico analysis are needed to elucidate the mechanisms by which individual miRNAs control immune responses in infants.

Table 1. Immune-regulating miRNAs in milk.

miRNA	Immune Function	Reference
miR-17 and miR-92 cluster	B-cell, T-cell, and monocyte development	[108]
miR-29a-3p	Suppression of immune responses to intracellular pathogens by targeting IFN-γ	[99]
miR-30b-5p	Promotion of cellular invasion by directly targeting GalNAc transferase, immunosuppression by increasing IL-10	[99,111]
miR-106	Regulation of IL-10 production	[113]
miR-125b	Negative regulation of TNF-α production, activation, and sensitivity	[108]
miR-146b-5p	Negative regulation of the innate immune response by targeting NF-κB signaling, control of TLR and cytokine signaling	[108,109]
miR-150	Control of B cell differentiation, pre- and pro-B cell formation or function	[109]
miR-155	T- and B-cell maturation, the innate immune response	[108,109]
miR-181a, miR-181b	B-cell differentiation, CD4+ T-cell sensitivity and selection	[108,109,113]
miR-182-5p	Promotion of helper T cell-mediated immune responses upon induction by IL-2	[99,112]
miR-223	Neutrophil proliferation and activation	[108,109]
miR-451	Regulation of Macrophage migration inhibitory factor (MIF)	[113]
let-7i	Toll-like receptor 4 expression in human cholangiocytes	[108]

IFN-γ, interferon- γ; GalNAc, N-acetylgalactosamine; IL, interleukin; NF-κB, nuclear factor kappa-light-chain-enhancer of activated B cells.

4.2. Tumor-Associated miRNAs

In addition to immune-regulating miRNAs, milk exosomes also contain tumor-suppressive or oncogenic miRNAs (oncomiRs) [114]. miR-148a-3p has been shown to function as a tumor suppressor by targeting DNMT1, ERBB3, and ROCK1, which are all involved in the development, proliferation, and metastasis of tumors [106,115–117]. Given that miR-148a-3p is highly expressed in breast milk but less expressed in leukemia, miR-148a-3p in breast milk may be able to protect infants against childhood leukemia [79,118,119].

In contrast, some well-known oncomiRs, such as the miR-21, miR-155, miR-223, and miR-17-92 clusters, have been found in breast milk [120]. Of note, Melnik suggested that miRNA-21-5p, a highly expressed miRNA in human and cow milk, is one of the major environmental factors eliciting melanomagenesis through exosomal transfer of miRNAs [99,121]. miR-21-5p downregulates the expression of tumor suppressor genes, such as PTEN (phosphatase and tensin homolog), Sprouty1 and Sprouty2, and PDCD4 (programmed cell death protein 4), thereby promoting the initiation and progression of malignant melanoma [122–124]. It has been proposed that an exogenous supply of exosomal miR-21 through breastfeeding or milk consumption may enhance oncogenic miR-21 signaling and lead to the transition of benign melanocytes to malignant melanoma [121]. Additionally, miR-155, an oncomiR that enhances STAT3 expression by targeting SOCS1 (suppressor of cytokine signaling 1) and facilitates STAT3-mediated tumorigenesis, is also found in exosomes derived from bovine colostrum, implying the association of milk exosomal miR-155 with tumorigenesis [113,125,126].

Nonetheless, studies that provide a direct evidence of the role of breast milk miRNAs in the prevention or development of cancer are limited. Most studies reporting the function of milk exosomal miRNAs are in silico analyses accompanied by Gene Ontology and KEGG pathway analyses. Further investigations merging in silico analysis and in vitro and/or in vivo experimental validation are required to determine any significant association between breast milk miRNAs and cancer.

5. Breast Milk-Derived Exosomes as Natural Carriers for Drug Delivery

As natural carriers of endogenous biomolecules, exosomes have remarkable advantages over other drug delivery vehicles. Exosomes are biocompatible and low in toxicity and immunogenicity and have long circulating half-lives [44,45]. Furthermore, they can cross many biological barriers such as the blood–brain barrier and cytoplasmic membrane [127]. Accordingly, numerous exosome-based delivery systems have been developed for targeted drug delivery by transporting small molecules, proteins, and small interfering RNA (siRNA) to target tissues. In particular, milk exosomes possess unique benefits compared with those of other origins [128,129]. Milk exosomes can be obtained from bovine milk enabling low-cost and mass production and show cross-species tolerance [128]. Moreover, milk exosomes are stable in acidic environments and can be absorbed from the digestive tract in humans, suggesting the potential use of milk exosomes as oral delivery vehicles of drugs that are conventionally administered intravenously [130]. With additional modification for target-specific drug delivery, milk exosomes have been widely investigated as promising carriers to transport diverse biomolecules and chemotherapeutic agents.

5.1. Delivery of Small Molecules

Milk exosomes have been shown to deliver natural compounds isolated from plant resources, such as celastrol, anthocyanidin, and curcumin [81,131,132]. When loaded onto cow milk-derived exosomes, curcumin with poor oral bioavailability is taken up and shows enhanced antiproliferative effects compared with free curcumin in Caco-2 cells [131]. Exosomal formulation of anthocyanidin (ExoAnthos) also exerts greater antiproliferative effects than that of free Anthos in lung, breast, ovarian, colon, pancreatic, and prostate cancers in vitro, and has higher antitumor efficacy in mice bearing A549 xenografts upon oral administration [81]. In addition to the improvement in oral bioavailability, ExoAnthos is well tolerated with no systemic toxicity, as determined by biochemical and hematological parameters. Similarly, celastrol encapsulated in milk exosomes inhibits the proliferation of the non-small-cell lung carcinoma cell lines A549 and H1299 in vitro, and shows greater antitumor effects in vivo without toxicity than that of free celastrol [132].

Agrawal et al. demonstrated that paclitaxel-loaded milk exosomes (ExoPACs) inhibit the growth of human lung tumor in athymic nude mice bearing A549 xenografts [133]. The ExoPACs are highly stable in simulated gastrointestinal fluids and under cold storage conditions at −80 °C for 1 month, allowing oral delivery of paclitaxel. Furthermore, oral administration of ExoPACs maintains the number and function of immune cells with reduced systemic and tissue toxicity in mice compared with intravenous administration of the drug, indicating the safety and efficacy of drug-loaded milk exosomes. Considering the discomfort and inconvenience of the intravenous route, the use of milk exosomes would be beneficial for the oral delivery of chemotherapeutic agents with low oral bioavailability.

5.2. Delivery of Nucleic Acid

Since the discovery of RNA interference mediated by siRNA, siRNAs have attracted much attention as a new generation of therapeutics based on nucleic acid. Despite the promising therapeutic potential of silencing gene expression in a sequence-specific manner, siRNAs have some intrinsic undruggable properties [134,135]. They are readily degraded by nuclease in serum and tissue and cleared by renal excretion or phagocytes in the reticuloendothelial system (RES). Negatively charged siRNAs are not easily taken up by cells due to electrostatic repulsion, and endosomal escape is required for siRNAs to reach mRNA targets, once internalized. To overcome the obstacles that limit the safe and effective application of siRNAs, the chemical modification of their nucleotide components, including ribose, phosphate, and base, as well as the special siRNA delivery systems, such as polymeric nanoparticles and liposomes, have been extensively investigated [134,135].

In addition to the oral delivery of small molecule drugs, milk exosomes have also been used for the delivery of siRNAs. siRNAs were loaded onto milk exosomes by electroporation and chemical transfection, and their gene silencing activities were tested in multiple cancers in vitro [129]. The siRNA-loaded exosomes are resistant to RNase and taken up by cancer cells accompanied by silencing of the target genes. Exo-siKRAS (siRNA against KRAS-loaded exosomes) suppresses the proliferation of A549 in vitro and exhibits antitumor effects in A549 tumor-bearing mice upon intravenous administration.

Similarly, siRNAs against *bcl-2*, an oncogene that inhibits apoptosis and promotes proliferation, were loaded onto milk exosomes using an ultrasonic approach, and their antitumor activity was tested in vitro and in vivo [136]. The results demonstrated that exosiBcl-2 (siRNA against *bcl-2*-loaded exosomes) inhibits *bcl-2* expression followed by an increase in apoptosis and a decrease in cell growth, migration, and invasion of cancer cells in vitro. An in vivo study also confirmed that intravenous administration of exosiBcl-2 suppresses tumor growth in xenograft nude mice. In view of the advantages of milk exosomes over other siRNA delivery vehicles, future studies are expected to establish optimal methods for siRNA loading, surface functionalization, and administration routes to attain effective antitumor therapies.

5.3. Targeted Dug Delivery

Despite excellent biocompatibility and low toxicity, exosomes from bovine milk may require further modification for targeted drug delivery. Folate receptors are highly expressed on many types of tumor cells, and accordingly, folic acid (FA)-conjugated milk exosomes have been generated for enhanced delivery of siRNAs to tumor sites [129]. FA-functionalized milk exosomes show higher accumulation in tumor tissue than non-FA milk exosomes and significantly inhibit tumor growth in vivo.

CD44, a receptor for hyaluronic acid, is overexpressed in some types of cancer such as pancreatic, lung, ovarian, and breast cancer [137]. For targeted cancer therapy, attempts have been made to generate conjugates of membrane incorporating molecule DSPE-PEG$_{200}$ and Hyaluronan (HA), a CD44-specific ligand, which are then self-assembled into the phospholipid bilayer of milk exosomes [138]. The resulting HA-incorporated milk exosomes (HA-mExo) expose the HA ligand on the surface of the exosomes and are loaded with doxorubicin to obtain HA-mExo-Dox, a doxorubicin-loaded milk exosome with an HA ligand. The results showed that HA-mExo-Dox selectively delivers doxorubicin to CD44-overexpressing cancer cells and exerts enhanced antitumor activity.

Another example of a tumor-targeting ligand is iRGD (CRGDK/RGPD/EC), a 9-amino acid cyclic peptide that binds to $\alpha v \beta 3$ and $\alpha v \beta 5$ integrin on the endothelial cells of tumor vessels to promote transcytosis across tumor vasculature [139]. After translocation, the iRGD ligand is cleaved by an endogenous protease to yield a CRGDK/R peptide that serves as a ligand for the neuropilin-1 receptor to activate the transport of co-administered anticancer drugs into tumors [140]. When iRGD peptides are incorporated into milk exosomes, the oral administration of iRGD exosomes exhibits an increase in penetration and accumulation into tumors compared with intravenously administered control exosomes [130]. In contrast, the accumulation of iRGD exosomes in other organs, such as liver, heart, lung, and spleen, is decreased. Considering the increased tumor accumulation and decreased systemic distribution, iRGD exosomes might be used as promising delivery vehicles for chemotherapeutic agents with a high antitumor efficacy and decreased off-target effects.

In addition, a milk exosome-based pH and light-sensitive drug carrier has been developed for targeting an acidic and hypoxic tumor microenvironment (TME) [141]. Given that most solid tumors exhibit a pH from 6.5 to 7.4, milk exosomes are conjugated to doxorubicin by a pH-sensitive imine bond, which gets cleaved and releases doxorubicin in an acidic TME. Furthermore, photodynamic therapy is introduced by encapsulating photosensitizer-chlorin e6 (Ce6) and the anthracene endoperoxide derivative (EPT1) within milk exosomes. Upon exposure to 808 nm near-infrared light, Ce6 releases plasmonic heat that generates singlet oxygen from EPT1 and corrects hypoxia in TME. This Exo@Dox-EPT1 nanocarrier shows enhanced antitumor effects and biocompatibility with less cardiotoxicity caused by doxorubicin in an in vitro and in vivo mouse model of oral squamous cell carcinoma.

6. Conclusions

With the significant advancements in technology analyzing nucleic acids, proteins, and microbiota, HBM and animal-derived milk are now known to contain distinct bioactive molecules along with renowned nutritional components, and their therapeutic roles are becoming appreciated. In particular, milk-derived exosomes have gathered much attention owing to their intrinsic antitumor activities.

The milk exosomes modulate immune function and suppress the proliferation of various cancer cells in vitro and in vivo, and their chemotherapeutic function is mainly due to the exosomal miRNAs with immunoregulatory and tumor-suppressive activities. The milk exosomes can also serve as oral delivery vehicles for chemotherapeutic agents and siRNAs, and further modification of the exosomes with a tumor-targeting ligand enables the targeted delivery of drugs to the tumor sites.

Given the physiological activity, safety, biocompatibility, and drug delivery potential, the application of milk exosomes in cancer therapeutics are innumerable. Future studies are required to demonstrate how individual bioactive components within exosomes exert biological function, including antitumor activity, and to clarify any possible unwanted effects upon exosome treatment. In addition, it would be important to establish a cost effective and standardized method to isolate, purify, and manipulate exosomes from milk to ensure the quality of the exosomes for clinical and industrial implementation.

Author Contributions: Conceptualization, D.Y.Y. and H.M.; original draft preparation, K.-U.K., W.-H.K., C.H.J., D.Y.Y. and H.M.; editing, K.-U.K., D.Y.Y. and H.M.; funding acquisition, D.Y.Y. and H.M.; supervision, D.Y.Y. and H.M. All authors have read and agreed to the published version of the manuscript.

Funding: This work was supported by the Chung-Ang University Graduate Research Scholarship in 2019 (K.-U.K.) and National Research Foundation of Korea (NRF) grant funded by the Korea government (Ministry of Science and ICT, no. NRF-2019R1F1A1059569).

Conflicts of Interest: The authors declare no conflict of interest.

Abbreviations

HBM	human breast milk
NEC	necrotizing enterocolitis
HMOs	human milk oligosaccharides
EVs	extracellular vesicles
TGF-β	transforming growth factor β
TME	tumor microenvironment

References

1. Section on Breastfeeding. Breastfeeding and the Use of Human Milk. *Pediatrics* **2012**, *129*, e827–e841. [CrossRef]
2. Gartner, L.M.; Morton, J.; Lawrence, R.A.; Naylor, A.J.; O'Hare, D.; Schanler, R.J.; Eidelman, A.I. Breastfeeding and the use of human milk. *Pediatrics* **2005**, *115*, 496–506. [CrossRef]
3. Agostoni, C.; Braegger, C.; Decsi, T.; Kolacek, S.; Koletzko, B.; Michaelsen, K.F.; Mihatsch, W.; Moreno, L.A.; Puntis, J.; Shamir, R.; et al. Breast-feeding: A commentary by the ESPGHAN Committee on Nutrition. *J. Pediatr. Gastroenterol. Nutr.* **2009**, *49*, 112–125. [CrossRef]
4. Bernard, J.Y.; De Agostini, M.; Forhan, A.; Alfaiate, T.; Bonet, M.; Champion, V.; Kaminski, M.; de Lauzon-Guillain, B.; Charles, M.A.; Heude, B.; et al. Breastfeeding duration and cognitive development at 2 and 3 years of age in the EDEN mother-child cohort. *J. Pediatr.* **2013**, *163*, 36–42. [CrossRef] [PubMed]
5. van Rossum, C.T.M.; Buchner, F.L.; Hoekstra, J. *Quantification of Health Effects of Breastfeeding—Review of the Literature and Model Simulation*; RIVM: Bilthoven, The Netherlands, 2006; pp. 19–21.
6. Ip, S.; Chung, M.; Raman, G.; Chew, P.; Magula, N.; DeVine, D.; Trikalinos, T.; Lau, J. Breastfeeding and maternal and infant health outcomes in developed countries. *Evid Rep. Technol. Assess. (Full Rep.)* **2007**, *153*, 1–186.
7. Güngör, D.; Nadaud, P.; Dreibelbis, C.; LaPergola, C.C.; Wong, Y.P.; Terry, N.; Abrams, S.A.; Beker, L.; Jacobovits, T.; Järvinen, K.M.; et al. Infant milk-feeding practices and childhood leukemia: A systematic review. *Am. J. Clin. Nutr.* **2019**, *109*, 757S–771S. [CrossRef] [PubMed]
8. Koletzko, B.; Baker, S.; Cleghorn, G.; Neto, U.F.; Gopalan, S.; Hernell, O.; Hock, Q.S.; Jirapinyo, P.; Lonnerdal, B.; Pencharz, P.; et al. Global standard for the composition of infant formula: Recommendations of an ESPGHAN coordinated international expert group. *J. Pediatr. Gastroenterol. Nutr.* **2005**, *41*, 584–599. [CrossRef] [PubMed]

9. Kim, M.H.; Shim, K.S.; Yi, D.Y.; Lim, I.S.; Chae, S.A.; Yun, S.W.; Lee, N.M.; Kim, S.Y.; Kim, S. Macronutrient Analysis of Human Milk according to Storage and Processing in Korean Mother. *Pediatr. Gastroenterol. Hepatol. Nutr.* **2019**, *22*, 262–269. [CrossRef]
10. Ballard, O.; Morrow, A.L. Human milk composition: Nutrients and bioactive factors. *Pediatr. Clin. N. Am.* **2013**, *60*, 49–74. [CrossRef]
11. Kim, S.Y.; Yi, D.Y. Components of human breast milk: From macronutrient to microbiome and microRNA. *Clin. Exp. Pediatr.* **2020**, *63*, 301–309. [CrossRef]
12. Kim, S.Y.; Yi, D.Y. Analysis of the human breast milk microbiome and bacterial extracellular vesicles in healthy mothers. *Exp. Mol. Med.* **2020**. [CrossRef] [PubMed]
13. Hegar, B.; Wibowo, Y.; Basrowi, R.W.; Ranuh, R.G.; Sudarmo, S.M.; Munasir, Z.; Widodo, A.D.; Kadim, M.; Suryawan, A.; Diana, N.R.; et al. The Role of Two Human Milk Oligosaccharides, 2'-Fucosyllactose and Lacto-N-Neotetraose, in Infant Nutrition. *Pediatr. Gastroenterol. Hepatol. Nutr.* **2019**, *22*, 330–340. [CrossRef] [PubMed]
14. Walker, A.W.; Ince, J.; Duncan, S.H.; Webster, L.M.; Holtrop, G.; Ze, X.; Brown, D.; Stares, M.D.; Scott, P.; Bergerat, A.; et al. Dominant and diet-responsive groups of bacteria within the human colonic microbiota. *ISME J.* **2011**, *5*, 220–230. [CrossRef] [PubMed]
15. Plaza-Díaz, J.; Fontana, L.; Gil, A. Human Milk Oligosaccharides and Immune System Development. *Nutrients* **2018**, *10*, 1038. [CrossRef] [PubMed]
16. Lönnerdal, B.; Woodhouse, L.R.; Glazier, C. Compartmentalization and quantitation of protein in human milk. *J. Nutr.* **1987**, *117*, 1385–1395. [CrossRef]
17. Lönnerdal, B.; Lien, E.L. Nutritional and physiologic significance of alpha-lactalbumin in infants. *Nutr. Rev.* **2003**, *61*, 295–305. [CrossRef]
18. Martin, C.R.; Ling, P.R.; Blackburn, G.L. Review of Infant Feeding: Key Features of Breast Milk and Infant Formula. *Nutrients* **2016**, *8*, 279. [CrossRef]
19. Perrine, C.G.; Sharma, A.J.; Jefferds, M.E.; Serdula, M.K.; Scanlon, K.S. Adherence to vitamin D recommendations among US infants. *Pediatrics* **2010**, *125*, 627–632. [CrossRef]
20. Committee on Fetus and Newborn. Controversies concerning vitamin K and the newborn. American Academy of Pediatrics Committee on Fetus and Newborn. *Pediatrics* **2003**, *112*, 191–192. [CrossRef]
21. Hill, D.R.; Newburg, D.S. Clinical applications of bioactive milk components. *Nutr. Rev.* **2015**, *73*, 463–476. [CrossRef]
22. Parodi, P.W. A role for milk proteins and their peptides in cancer prevention. *Curr. Pharm. Des.* **2007**, *13*, 813–828. [CrossRef] [PubMed]
23. Kozu, T.; Iinuma, G.; Ohashi, Y.; Saito, Y.; Akasu, T.; Saito, D.; Alexander, D.B.; Iigo, M.; Kakizoe, T.; Tsuda, H. Effect of orally administered bovine lactoferrin on the growth of adenomatous colorectal polyps in a randomized, placebo-controlled clinical trial. *Cancer Prev. Res.* **2009**, *2*, 975–983. [CrossRef] [PubMed]
24. Parikh, P.M.; Vaid, A.; Advani, S.H.; Digumarti, R.; Madhavan, J.; Nag, S.; Bapna, A.; Sekhon, J.S.; Patil, S.; Ismail, P.M.; et al. Randomized, double-blind, placebo-controlled phase II study of single-agent oral talactoferrin in patients with locally advanced or metastatic non-small-cell lung cancer that progressed after chemotherapy. *J. Clin. Oncol.* **2011**, *29*, 4129–4136. [CrossRef] [PubMed]
25. Digumarti, R.; Wang, Y.; Raman, G.; Doval, D.C.; Advani, S.H.; Julka, P.K.; Parikh, P.M.; Patil, S.; Nag, S.; Madhavan, J.; et al. A randomized, double-blind, placebo-controlled, phase II study of oral talactoferrin in combination with carboplatin and paclitaxel in previously untreated locally advanced or metastatic non-small cell lung cancer. *J. Thorac. Oncol.* **2011**, *6*, 1098–1103. [CrossRef]
26. Sun, X.; Jiang, R.; Przepiorski, A.; Reddy, S.; Palmano, K.P.; Krissansen, G.W. "Iron-saturated" bovine lactoferrin improves the chemotherapeutic effects of tamoxifen in the treatment of basal-like breast cancer in mice. *BMC Cancer* **2012**, *12*, 591. [CrossRef]
27. Fischer, W.; Gustafsson, L.; Mossberg, A.K.; Gronli, J.; Mork, S.; Bjerkvig, R.; Svanborg, C. Human alpha-lactalbumin made lethal to tumor cells (HAMLET) kills human glioblastoma cells in brain xenografts by an apoptosis-like mechanism and prolongs survival. *Cancer Res.* **2004**, *64*, 2105–2112. [CrossRef] [PubMed]
28. Mossberg, A.K.; Hun Mok, K.; Morozova-Roche, L.A.; Svanborg, C. Structure and function of human α-lactalbumin made lethal to tumor cells (HAMLET)-type complexes. *FEBS J.* **2010**, *277*, 4614–4625. [CrossRef]

29. Gustafsson, L.; Aits, S.; Onnerfjord, P.; Trulsson, M.; Storm, P.; Svanborg, C. Changes in proteasome structure and function caused by HAMLET in tumor cells. *PLoS ONE* **2009**, *4*, e5229. [CrossRef]
30. Heikkilä, M.P.; Saris, P.E. Inhibition of Staphylococcus aureus by the commensal bacteria of human milk. *J. Appl. Microbiol.* **2003**, *95*, 471–478. [CrossRef]
31. Hunt, K.M.; Foster, J.A.; Forney, L.J.; Schütte, U.M.; Beck, D.L.; Abdo, Z.; Fox, L.K.; Williams, J.E.; McGuire, M.K.; McGuire, M.A. Characterization of the diversity and temporal stability of bacterial communities in human milk. *PLoS ONE* **2011**, *6*, e21313. [CrossRef]
32. Fitzstevens, J.L.; Smith, K.C.; Hagadorn, J.I.; Caimano, M.J.; Matson, A.P.; Brownell, E.A. Systematic Review of the Human Milk Microbiota. *Nutr. Clin. Pract.* **2017**, *32*, 354–364. [CrossRef] [PubMed]
33. Togo, A.; Dufour, J.C.; Lagier, J.C.; Dubourg, G.; Raoult, D.; Million, M. Repertoire of human breast and milk microbiota: A systematic review. *Future Microbiol.* **2019**, *14*, 623–641. [CrossRef] [PubMed]
34. Ramsay, D.T.; Kent, J.C.; Owens, R.A.; Hartmann, P.E. Ultrasound imaging of milk ejection in the breast of lactating women. *Pediatrics* **2004**, *113*, 361–367. [CrossRef] [PubMed]
35. Civardi, E.; Garofoli, F.; Tzialla, C.; Paolillo, P.; Bollani, L.; Stronati, M. Microorganisms in human milk: Lights and shadows. *J. Matern. Fetal Neonatal. Med.* **2013**, *26* (Suppl. S2), 30–34. [CrossRef]
36. Rodríguez, J.M. The origin of human milk bacteria: Is there a bacterial entero-mammary pathway during late pregnancy and lactation? *Adv. Nutr.* **2014**, *5*, 779–784. [CrossRef] [PubMed]
37. Gomez-Llorente, C.; Plaza-Diaz, J.; Aguilera, M.; Muñoz-Quezada, S.; Bermudez-Brito, M.; Peso-Echarri, P.; Martinez-Silla, R.; Vasallo-Morillas, M.I.; Campaña-Martin, L.; Vives-Piñera, I.; et al. Three main factors define changes in fecal microbiota associated with feeding modality in infants. *J. Pediatr. Gastroenterol. Nutr.* **2013**, *57*, 461–466. [CrossRef] [PubMed]
38. Martín, V.; Maldonado-Barragán, A.; Moles, L.; Rodriguez-Baños, M.; Campo, R.D.; Fernández, L.; Rodríguez, J.M.; Jiménez, E. Sharing of bacterial strains between breast milk and infant feces. *J. Hum. Lact.* **2012**, *28*, 36–44. [CrossRef]
39. Coppa, G.V.; Bruni, S.; Morelli, L.; Soldi, S.; Gabrielli, O. The first prebiotics in humans: Human milk oligosaccharides. *J. Clin. Gastroenterol.* **2004**, *38*, S80–S83. [CrossRef]
40. Oozeer, R.; van Limpt, K.; Ludwig, T.; Ben Amor, K.; Martin, R.; Wind, R.D.; Boehm, G.; Knol, J. Intestinal microbiology in early life: Specific prebiotics can have similar functionalities as human-milk oligosaccharides. *Am. J. Clin. Nutr.* **2013**, *98*, 561S–571S. [CrossRef]
41. Zimmermann, P.; Curtis, N. Factors Influencing the Intestinal Microbiome During the First Year of Life. *Pediatr. Infect. Dis. J.* **2018**, *37*, e315–e335. [CrossRef]
42. Moossavi, S.; Sepehri, S.; Robertson, B.; Bode, L.; Goruk, S.; Field, C.J.; Lix, L.M.; de Souza, R.J.; Becker, A.B.; Mandhane, P.J.; et al. Composition and Variation of the Human Milk Microbiota Are Influenced by Maternal and Early-Life Factors. *Cell Host Microbe* **2019**, *25*, 324–335. [CrossRef] [PubMed]
43. Yoo, J.Y.; Rho, M.; You, Y.A.; Kwon, E.J.; Kim, M.H.; Kym, S.; Jee, Y.K.; Kim, Y.K.; Kim, Y.J. 16S rRNA gene-based metagenomic analysis reveals differences in bacteria-derived extracellular vesicles in the urine of pregnant and non-pregnant women. *Exp. Mol. Med.* **2016**, *48*, e208. [CrossRef] [PubMed]
44. Rashed, M.H.; Bayraktar, E.; Helal, G.K.; Abd-Ellah, M.F.; Amero, P.; Chavez-Reyes, A.; Rodriguez-Aguayo, C. Exosomes: From Garbage Bins to Promising Therapeutic Targets. *Int. J. Mol. Sci.* **2017**, *18*, 538. [CrossRef] [PubMed]
45. Hessvik, N.P.; Llorente, A. Current knowledge on exosome biogenesis and release. *Cell Mol. Life Sci.* **2018**, *75*, 193–208. [CrossRef]
46. Vlassov, A.V.; Magdaleno, S.; Setterquist, R.; Conrad, R. Exosomes: Current knowledge of their composition, biological functions, and diagnostic and therapeutic potentials. *Biochim. Biophys. Acta* **2012**, *1820*, 940–948. [CrossRef]
47. Admyre, C.; Johansson, S.M.; Qazi, K.R.; Filén, J.J.; Lahesmaa, R.; Norman, M.; Neve, E.P.; Scheynius, A.; Gabrielsson, S. Exosomes with immune modulatory features are present in human breast milk. *J. Immunol.* **2007**, *179*, 1969–1978. [CrossRef]
48. Galley, J.D.; Besner, G.E. The Therapeutic Potential of Breast Milk-Derived Extracellular Vesicles. *Nutrients* **2020**, *12*, 745. [CrossRef]
49. Hata, T.; Murakami, K.; Nakatani, H.; Yamamoto, Y.; Matsuda, T.; Aoki, N. Isolation of bovine milk-derived microvesicles carrying mRNAs and microRNAs. *Biochem. Biophys. Res. Commun.* **2010**, *396*, 528–533. [CrossRef]

50. Gu, Y.; Li, M.; Wang, T.; Liang, Y.; Zhong, Z.; Wang, X.; Zhou, Q.; Chen, L.; Lang, Q.; He, Z.; et al. Lactation-related microRNA expression profiles of porcine breast milk exosomes. *PLoS ONE* **2012**, *7*, e43691. [CrossRef]
51. Chen, Z.; Xie, Y.; Luo, J.; Chen, T.; Xi, Q.; Zhang, Y.; Sun, J. Milk exosome-derived miRNAs from water buffalo are implicated in immune response and metabolism process. *BMC Vet. Res.* **2020**, *16*, 123. [CrossRef]
52. Baddela, V.S.; Nayan, V.; Rani, P.; Onteru, S.K.; Singh, D. Physicochemical Biomolecular Insights into Buffalo Milk-Derived Nanovesicles. *Appl. Biochem. Biotechnol.* **2016**, *178*, 544–557. [CrossRef]
53. Badawy, A.A.; El-Magd, M.A.; AlSadrah, S.A. Therapeutic Effect of Camel Milk and Its Exosomes on MCF7 Cells In Vitro and In Vivo. *Integr. Cancer Ther.* **2018**, *17*, 1235–1246. [CrossRef] [PubMed]
54. Ma, Y.; Feng, S.; Wang, X.; Qazi, I.H.; Long, K.; Luo, Y.; Li, G.; Ning, C.; Wang, Y.; Hu, S.; et al. Exploration of exosomal microRNA expression profiles in pigeon 'Milk' during the lactation period. *BMC Genom.* **2018**, *19*, 828. [CrossRef] [PubMed]
55. Quan, S.; Nan, X.; Wang, K.; Jiang, L.; Yao, J.; Xiong, B. Characterization of Sheep Milk Extracellular Vesicle-miRNA by Sequencing and Comparison with Cow Milk. *Animals* **2020**, *10*, 331. [CrossRef]
56. Gallier, S.; Vocking, K.; Post, J.A.; Van De Heijning, B.; Acton, D.; Van Der Beek, E.M.; Van Baalen, T. A novel infant milk formula concept: Mimicking the human milk fat globule structure. *Colloids Surf. B Biointerfaces* **2015**, *136*, 329–339. [CrossRef] [PubMed]
57. Torregrosa Paredes, P.; Gutzeit, C.; Johansson, S.; Admyre, C.; Stenius, F.; Alm, J.; Scheynius, A.; Gabrielsson, S. Differences in exosome populations in human breast milk in relation to allergic sensitization and lifestyle. *Allergy* **2014**, *69*, 463–471. [CrossRef] [PubMed]
58. Hock, A.; Miyake, H.; Li, B.; Lee, C.; Ermini, L.; Koike, Y.; Chen, Y.; Määttänen, P.; Zani, A.; Pierro, A. Breast milk-derived exosomes promote intestinal epithelial cell growth. *J. Pediatr. Surg.* **2017**, *52*, 755–759. [CrossRef]
59. Maffei, D.; Schanler, R.J. Human milk is the feeding strategy to prevent necrotizing enterocolitis! *Semin. Perinatol.* **2017**, *41*, 36–40. [CrossRef]
60. Cortez, J.; Makker, K.; Kraemer, D.F.; Neu, J.; Sharma, R.; Hudak, M.L. Maternal milk feedings reduce sepsis, necrotizing enterocolitis and improve outcomes of premature infants. *J. Perinatol.* **2018**, *38*, 71–74. [CrossRef]
61. O'Connor, D.L.; Gibbins, S.; Kiss, A.; Bando, N.; Brennan-Donnan, J.; Ng, E.; Campbell, D.M.; Vaz, S.; Fusch, C.; Asztalos, E.; et al. Effect of Supplemental Donor Human Milk Compared with Preterm Formula on Neurodevelopment of Very Low-Birth-Weight Infants at 18 Months: A Randomized Clinical Trial. *JAMA* **2016**, *316*, 1897–1905. [CrossRef]
62. Quigley, M.; Embleton, N.D.; McGuire, W. Formula versus donor breast milk for feeding preterm or low birth weight infants. *Cochrane Database Syst. Rev.* **2018**, *6*, CD002971. [CrossRef] [PubMed]
63. Martin, C.; Patel, M.; Williams, S.; Arora, H.; Sims, B. Human breast milk-derived exosomes attenuate cell death in intestinal epithelial cells. *Innate Immun.* **2018**, *24*, 278–284. [CrossRef] [PubMed]
64. Miyake, H.; Lee, C.; Chusilp, S.; Bhalla, M.; Li, B.; Pitino, M.; Seo, S.; O'Connor, D.L.; Pierro, A. Human breast milk exosomes attenuate intestinal damage. *Pediatr. Surg. Int.* **2020**, *36*, 155–163. [CrossRef] [PubMed]
65. Wang, X.; Yan, X.; Zhang, L.; Cai, J.; Zhou, Y.; Liu, H.; Hu, Y.; Chen, W.; Xu, S.; Liu, P.; et al. Identification and Peptidomic Profiling of Exosomes in Preterm Human Milk: Insights Into Necrotizing Enterocolitis Prevention. *Mol. Nutr. Food Res.* **2019**, *63*, e1801247. [CrossRef] [PubMed]
66. Li, B.; Hock, A.; Wu, R.Y.; Minich, A.; Botts, S.R.; Lee, C.; Antounians, L.; Miyake, H.; Koike, Y.; Chen, Y.; et al. Bovine milk-derived exosomes enhance goblet cell activity and prevent the development of experimental necrotizing enterocolitis. *PLoS ONE* **2019**, *14*, e0211431. [CrossRef] [PubMed]
67. Arntz, O.J.; Pieters, B.C.; Oliveira, M.C.; Broeren, M.G.; Bennink, M.B.; de Vries, M.; van Lent, P.L.; Koenders, M.I.; van den Berg, W.B.; van der Kraan, P.M.; et al. Oral administration of bovine milk derived extracellular vesicles attenuates arthritis in two mouse models. *Mol. Nutr. Food Res.* **2015**, *59*, 1701–1712. [CrossRef]
68. Näslund, T.I.; Paquin-Proulx, D.; Paredes, P.T.; Vallhov, H.; Sandberg, J.K.; Gabrielsson, S. Exosomes from breast milk inhibit HIV-1 infection of dendritic cells and subsequent viral transfer to CD4+ T cells. *Aids* **2014**, *28*, 171–180. [CrossRef]
69. Komine-Aizawa, S.; Ito, S.; Aizawa, S.; Namiki, T.; Hayakawa, S. Cow milk exosomes activate NK cells and $\gamma\delta$T cells in human PBMCs in vitro. *Immunol. Med.* **2020**, 1–10. [CrossRef]

70. Matic, S.; D'Souza, D.H.; Wu, T.; Pangloli, P.; Dia, V.P. Bovine Milk Exosomes Affect Proliferation and Protect Macrophages against Cisplatin-Induced Cytotoxicity. *Immunol. Investig.* **2020**, 1–15. [CrossRef]
71. Samuel, M.; Chisanga, D.; Liem, M.; Keerthikumar, S.; Anand, S.; Ang, C.S.; Adda, C.G.; Versteegen, E.; Jois, M.; Mathivanan, S. Bovine milk-derived exosomes from colostrum are enriched with proteins implicated in immune response and growth. *Sci. Rep.* **2017**, *7*, 5933. [CrossRef]
72. Reinhardt, T.A.; Lippolis, J.D.; Nonnecke, B.J.; Sacco, R.E. Bovine milk exosome proteome. *J. Proteomics* **2012**, *75*, 1486–1492. [CrossRef]
73. Amitay, E.; Keinan-Boker, L. Breastfeeding and childhood leukemia and lymphoma. *Harefuah* **2014**, *153*, 273–279. [PubMed]
74. Amitay, E.L.; Dubnov Raz, G.; Keinan-Boker, L. Breastfeeding, Other Early Life Exposures and Childhood Leukemia and Lymphoma. *Nutr. Cancer* **2016**, *68*, 968–977. [CrossRef]
75. Küçükçongar, A.; Oğuz, A.; Pınarlı, F.G.; Karadeniz, C.; Okur, A.; Kaya, Z.; Çelik, B. Breastfeeding and Childhood Cancer: Is Breastfeeding Preventative to Childhood Cancer? *Pediatr. Hematol. Oncol.* **2015**, *32*, 374–381. [PubMed]
76. Mathur, G.P.; Gupta, N.; Mathur, S.; Gupta, V.; Pradhan, S.; Dwivedi, J.N.; Tripathi, B.N.; Kushwaha, K.P.; Sathy, N.; Modi, U.J. Breastfeeding and childhood cancer. *Indian Pediatr.* **1993**, *30*, 651–657.
77. Shu, X.O.; Clemens, J.; Zheng, W.; Ying, D.M.; Ji, B.T.; Jin, F. Infant breastfeeding and the risk of childhood lymphoma and leukaemia. *Int. J. Epidemiol.* **1995**, *24*, 27–32. [CrossRef] [PubMed]
78. Martin, R.M.; Gunnell, D.; Owen, C.G.; Smith, G.D. Breast-feeding and childhood cancer: A systematic review with metaanalysis. *Int. J. Cancer* **2005**, *117*, 1020–1031. [CrossRef]
79. Amitay, E.L.; Keinan-Boker, L. Breastfeeding and Childhood Leukemia Incidence: A Meta-analysis and Systematic Review. *JAMA Pediatr.* **2015**, *169*, e151025. [CrossRef] [PubMed]
80. Reif, S.; Elbaum Shiff, Y.; Golan-Gerstl, R. Milk-derived exosomes (MDEs) have a different biological effect on normal fetal colon epithelial cells compared to colon tumor cells in a miRNA-dependent manner. *J. Transl. Med.* **2019**, *17*, 325. [CrossRef]
81. Munagala, R.; Aqil, F.; Jeyabalan, J.; Agrawal, A.K.; Mudd, A.M.; Kyakulaga, A.H.; Singh, I.P.; Vadhanam, M.V.; Gupta, R.C. Exosomal formulation of anthocyanidins against multiple cancer types. *Cancer Lett.* **2017**, *393*, 94–102. [CrossRef]
82. Korashy, H.M.; El Gendy, M.A.; Alhaider, A.A.; El-Kadi, A.O. Camel milk modulates the expression of aryl hydrocarbon receptor-regulated genes, Cyp1a1, Nqo1, and Gsta1, in murine hepatoma Hepa 1c1c7 cells. *J. Biomed. Biotechnol.* **2012**, *2012*, 782642. [CrossRef] [PubMed]
83. Korashy, H.M.; Maayah, Z.H.; Abd-Allah, A.R.; El-Kadi, A.O.; Alhaider, A.A. Camel milk triggers apoptotic signaling pathways in human hepatoma HepG2 and breast cancer MCF7 cell lines through transcriptional mechanism. *J. Biomed. Biotechnol.* **2012**, *2012*, 593195. [CrossRef] [PubMed]
84. Qin, W.; Tsukasaki, Y.; Dasgupta, S.; Mukhopadhyay, N.; Ikebe, M.; Sauter, E.R. Exosomes in Human Breast Milk Promote EMT. *Clin. Cancer Res.* **2016**, *22*, 4517–4524. [CrossRef]
85. Bartel, D.P.; Chen, C.Z. Micromanagers of gene expression: The potentially widespread influence of metazoan microRNAs. *Nat. Rev. Genet.* **2004**, *5*, 396–400. [CrossRef] [PubMed]
86. Bartel, D.P. MicroRNAs: Genomics, biogenesis, mechanism, and function. *Cell* **2004**, *116*, 281–297. [CrossRef]
87. Friedman, R.C.; Farh, K.K.; Burge, C.B.; Bartel, D.P. Most mammalian mRNAs are conserved targets of microRNAs. *Genome Res.* **2009**, *19*, 92–105. [CrossRef]
88. Ambros, V. MicroRNA pathways in flies and worms: Growth, death, fat, stress, and timing. *Cell* **2003**, *113*, 673–676. [CrossRef]
89. Carrington, J.C.; Ambros, V. Role of microRNAs in plant and animal development. *Science* **2003**, *301*, 336–338. [CrossRef]
90. Chang, T.C.; Mendell, J.T. microRNAs in vertebrate physiology and human disease. *Annu. Rev. Genom. Hum. Genet.* **2007**, *8*, 215–239. [CrossRef]
91. Bushati, N.; Cohen, S.M. microRNA functions. *Annu. Rev. Cell Dev. Biol.* **2007**, *23*, 175–205. [CrossRef]
92. Mollaei, H.; Safaralizadeh, R.; Rostami, Z. MicroRNA replacement therapy in cancer. *J. Cell Physiol.* **2019**, *234*, 12369–12384. [CrossRef] [PubMed]
93. Rupaimoole, R.; Slack, F.J. MicroRNA therapeutics: Towards a new era for the management of cancer and other diseases. *Nat. Rev. Drug Discov.* **2017**, *16*, 203–222. [CrossRef] [PubMed]

94. Garzon, R.; Calin, G.A.; Croce, C.M. MicroRNAs in Cancer. *Annu. Rev. Med.* **2009**, *60*, 167–179. [CrossRef] [PubMed]
95. Ling, H.; Fabbri, M.; Calin, G.A. MicroRNAs and other non-coding RNAs as targets for anticancer drug development. *Nat. Rev. Drug Discov.* **2013**, *12*, 847–865. [CrossRef] [PubMed]
96. Alsaweed, M.; Hepworth, A.R.; Lefèvre, C.; Hartmann, P.E.; Geddes, D.T.; Hassiotou, F. Human Milk MicroRNA and Total RNA Differ Depending on Milk Fractionation. *J. Cell Biochem.* **2015**, *116*, 2397–2407. [CrossRef]
97. Alsaweed, M.; Lai, C.T.; Hartmann, P.E.; Geddes, D.T.; Kakulas, F. Human milk miRNAs primarily originate from the mammary gland resulting in unique miRNA profiles of fractionated milk. *Sci. Rep.* **2016**, *6*, 20680. [CrossRef]
98. Alsaweed, M.; Hartmann, P.E.; Geddes, D.T.; Kakulas, F. MicroRNAs in Breastmilk and the Lactating Breast: Potential Immunoprotectors and Developmental Regulators for the Infant and the Mother. *Int. J. Environ. Res. Public Health* **2015**, *12*, 13981–14020. [CrossRef]
99. Zhou, Q.; Li, M.; Wang, X.; Li, Q.; Wang, T.; Zhu, Q.; Zhou, X.; Gao, X.; Li, X. Immune-related microRNAs are abundant in breast milk exosomes. *Int. J. Biol. Sci.* **2012**, *8*, 118–123. [CrossRef]
100. Munch, E.M.; Harris, R.A.; Mohammad, M.; Benham, A.L.; Pejerrey, S.M.; Showalter, L.; Hu, M.; Shope, C.D.; Maningat, P.D.; Gunaratne, P.H.; et al. Transcriptome profiling of microRNA by Next-Gen deep sequencing reveals known and novel miRNA species in the lipid fraction of human breast milk. *PLoS ONE* **2013**, *8*, e50564. [CrossRef]
101. Lönnerdal, B. Human Milk MicroRNAs/Exosomes: Composition and Biological Effects. *Nestle Nutr. Inst. Workshop Ser.* **2019**, *90*, 83–92. [CrossRef]
102. Izumi, H.; Kosaka, N.; Shimizu, T.; Sekine, K.; Ochiya, T.; Takase, M. Bovine milk contains microRNA and messenger RNA that are stable under degradative conditions. *J. Dairy Sci.* **2012**, *95*, 4831–4841. [CrossRef] [PubMed]
103. Liao, Y.; Du, X.; Li, J.; Lönnerdal, B. Human milk exosomes and their microRNAs survive digestion in vitro and are taken up by human intestinal cells. *Mol. Nutr. Food Res.* **2017**, *61*, 1700082. [CrossRef] [PubMed]
104. Kahn, S.; Liao, Y.; Du, X.; Xu, W.; Li, J.; Lönnerdal, B. Exosomal MicroRNAs in Milk from Mothers Delivering Preterm Infants Survive in Vitro Digestion and Are Taken Up by Human Intestinal Cells. *Mol. Nutr. Food Res.* **2018**, *62*, e1701050. [CrossRef] [PubMed]
105. Zempleni, J.; Aguilar-Lozano, A.; Sadri, M.; Sukreet, S.; Manca, S.; Wu, D.; Zhou, F.; Mutai, E. Biological Activities of Extracellular Vesicles and Their Cargos from Bovine and Human Milk in Humans and Implications for Infants. *J. Nutr.* **2017**, *147*, 3–10. [CrossRef]
106. Golan-Gerstl, R.; Elbaum Shiff, Y.; Moshayoff, V.; Schecter, D.; Leshkowitz, D.; Reif, S. Characterization and biological function of milk-derived miRNAs. *Mol. Nutr. Food Res.* **2017**, *61*, 1700009. [CrossRef]
107. Nojiri, K.; Kobayashi, S.; Higurashi, S.; Takahashi, T.; Tsujimori, Y.; Ueno, H.M.; Watanabe-Matsuhashi, S.; Toba, Y.; Yamamura, J.; Nakano, T.; et al. Maternal Health and Nutrition Status, Human Milk Composition, and Growth and Development of Infants and Children: A Prospective Japanese Human Milk Study Protocol. *Int. J. Environ. Res. Public Health* **2020**, *17*, 1869. [CrossRef]
108. Kosaka, N.; Izumi, H.; Sekine, K.; Ochiya, T. microRNA as a new immune-regulatory agent in breast milk. *Silence* **2010**, *1*, 7. [CrossRef]
109. Na, R.S.; E, G.X.; Sun, W.; Sun, X.W.; Qiu, X.Y.; Chen, L.P.; Huang, Y.F. Expressional analysis of immune-related miRNAs in breast milk. *Genet. Mol. Res.* **2015**, *14*, 11371–11376. [CrossRef]
110. Chen, X.; Gao, C.; Li, H.; Huang, L.; Sun, Q.; Dong, Y.; Tian, C.; Gao, S.; Dong, H.; Guan, D.; et al. Identification and characterization of microRNAs in raw milk during different periods of lactation, commercial fluid, and powdered milk products. *Cell Res.* **2010**, *20*, 1128–1137. [CrossRef]
111. Gaziel-Sovran, A.; Segura, M.F.; Di Micco, R.; Collins, M.K.; Hanniford, D.; Vega-Saenz de Miera, E.; Rakus, J.F.; Dankert, J.F.; Shang, S.; Kerbel, R.S.; et al. miR-30b/30d regulation of GalNAc transferases enhances invasion and immunosuppression during metastasis. *Cancer Cell* **2011**, *20*, 104–118. [CrossRef]
112. Stittrich, A.B.; Haftmann, C.; Sgouroudis, E.; Kühl, A.A.; Hegazy, A.N.; Panse, I.; Riedel, R.; Flossdorf, M.; Dong, J.; Fuhrmann, F.; et al. The microRNA miR-182 is induced by IL-2 and promotes clonal expansion of activated helper T lymphocytes. *Nat. Immunol.* **2010**, *11*, 1057–1062. [CrossRef] [PubMed]
113. Sun, Q.; Chen, X.; Yu, J.; Zen, K.; Zhang, C.Y.; Li, L. Immune modulatory function of abundant immune-related microRNAs in microvesicles from bovine colostrum. *Protein Cell* **2013**, *4*, 197–210. [CrossRef]

114. Melnik, B.C.; Schmitz, G. Exosomes of pasteurized milk: Potential pathogens of Western diseases. *J. Transl. Med.* **2019**, *17*, 3. [CrossRef] [PubMed]
115. Long, X.R.; He, Y.; Huang, C.; Li, J. MicroRNA-148a is silenced by hypermethylation and interacts with DNA methyltransferase 1 in hepatocellular carcinogenesis. *Int. J. Oncol.* **2014**, *44*, 1915–1922. [CrossRef] [PubMed]
116. Li, J.; Song, Y.; Wang, Y.; Luo, J.; Yu, W. MicroRNA-148a suppresses epithelial-to-mesenchymal transition by targeting ROCK1 in non-small cell lung cancer cells. *Mol. Cell Biochem.* **2013**, *380*, 277–282. [CrossRef]
117. Yu, J.; Li, Q.; Xu, Q.; Liu, L.; Jiang, B. MiR-148a inhibits angiogenesis by targeting ERBB3. *J. Biomed. Res.* **2011**, *25*, 170–177. [CrossRef]
118. Zhang, H.; Luo, X.Q.; Zhang, P.; Huang, L.B.; Zheng, Y.S.; Wu, J.; Zhou, H.; Qu, L.H.; Xu, L.; Chen, Y.Q. MicroRNA patterns associated with clinical prognostic parameters and CNS relapse prediction in pediatric acute leukemia. *PLoS ONE* **2009**, *4*, e7826. [CrossRef]
119. de Oliveira, J.C.; Brassesco, M.S.; Scrideli, C.A.; Tone, L.G.; Narendran, A. MicroRNA expression and activity in pediatric acute lymphoblastic leukemia (ALL). *Pediatr. Blood Cancer* **2012**, *59*, 599–604. [CrossRef]
120. Tomé-Carneiro, J.; Fernández-Alonso, N.; Tomás-Zapico, C.; Visioli, F.; Iglesias-Gutierrez, E.; Dávalos, A. Breast milk microRNAs harsh journey towards potential effects in infant development and maturation. Lipid encapsulation can help. *Pharmacol. Res.* **2018**, *132*, 21–32. [CrossRef]
121. Melnik, B.C. MiR-21: An environmental driver of malignant melanoma? *J. Transl. Med.* **2015**, *13*, 202. [CrossRef]
122. Meng, F.; Henson, R.; Wehbe-Janek, H.; Ghoshal, K.; Jacob, S.T.; Patel, T. MicroRNA-21 regulates expression of the PTEN tumor suppressor gene in human hepatocellular cancer. *Gastroenterology* **2007**, *133*, 647–658. [CrossRef] [PubMed]
123. Sayed, D.; Rane, S.; Lypowy, J.; He, M.; Chen, I.Y.; Vashistha, H.; Yan, L.; Malhotra, A.; Vatner, D.; Abdellatif, M. MicroRNA-21 targets Sprouty2 and promotes cellular outgrowths. *Mol. Biol. Cell* **2008**, *19*, 3272–3282. [CrossRef] [PubMed]
124. Asangani, I.A.; Rasheed, S.A.; Nikolova, D.A.; Leupold, J.H.; Colburn, N.H.; Post, S.; Allgayer, H. MicroRNA-21 (miR-21) post-transcriptionally downregulates tumor suppressor Pdcd4 and stimulates invasion, intravasation and metastasis in colorectal cancer. *Oncogene* **2008**, *27*, 2128–2136. [CrossRef] [PubMed]
125. Cao, Q.; Li, Y.Y.; He, W.F.; Zhang, Z.Z.; Zhou, Q.; Liu, X.; Shen, Y.; Huang, T.T. Interplay between microRNAs and the STAT3 signaling pathway in human cancers. *Physiol. Genom.* **2013**, *45*, 1206–1214. [CrossRef]
126. Huang, C.; Li, H.; Wu, W.; Jiang, T.; Qiu, Z. Regulation of miR-155 affects pancreatic cancer cell invasiveness and migration by modulating the STAT3 signaling pathway through SOCS1. *Oncol. Rep.* **2013**, *30*, 1223–1230. [CrossRef]
127. Ha, D.; Yang, N.; Nadithe, V. Exosomes as therapeutic drug carriers and delivery vehicles across biological membranes: Current perspectives and future challenges. *Acta Pharm. Sin. B* **2016**, *6*, 287–296. [CrossRef]
128. Munagala, R.; Aqil, F.; Jeyabalan, J.; Gupta, R.C. Bovine milk-derived exosomes for drug delivery. *Cancer Lett.* **2016**, *371*, 48–61. [CrossRef]
129. Aqil, F.; Munagala, R.; Jeyabalan, J.; Agrawal, A.K.; Kyakulaga, A.H.; Wilcher, S.A.; Gupta, R.C. Milk exosomes—Natural nanoparticles for siRNA delivery. *Cancer Lett.* **2019**, *449*, 186–195. [CrossRef]
130. Betker, J.L.; Angle, B.M.; Graner, M.W.; Anchordoquy, T.J. The Potential of Exosomes from Cow Milk for Oral Delivery. *J. Pharm. Sci.* **2019**, *108*, 1496–1505. [CrossRef]
131. Carobolante, G.; Mantaj, J.; Ferrari, E.; Vllasaliu, D. Cow Milk and Intestinal Epithelial Cell-derived Extracellular Vesicles as Systems for Enhancing Oral Drug Delivery. *Pharmaceutics* **2020**, *12*, 226. [CrossRef]
132. Aqil, F.; Kausar, H.; Agrawal, A.K.; Jeyabalan, J.; Kyakulaga, A.H.; Munagala, R.; Gupta, R. Exosomal formulation enhances therapeutic response of celastrol against lung cancer. *Exp. Mol. Pathol.* **2016**, *101*, 12–21. [CrossRef] [PubMed]
133. Agrawal, A.K.; Aqil, F.; Jeyabalan, J.; Spencer, W.A.; Beck, J.; Gachuki, B.W.; Alhakeem, S.S.; Oben, K.; Munagala, R.; Bondada, S.; et al. Milk-derived exosomes for oral delivery of paclitaxel. *Nanomedicine* **2017**, *13*, 1627–1636. [CrossRef] [PubMed]
134. Dong, Y.; Siegwart, D.J.; Anderson, D.G. Strategies, design, and chemistry in siRNA delivery systems. *Adv. Drug Deliv. Rev.* **2019**, *144*, 133–147. [CrossRef] [PubMed]
135. Das, M.; Musetti, S.; Huang, L. RNA Interference-Based Cancer Drugs: The Roadblocks, and the "Delivery" of the Promise. *Nucleic Acid Ther.* **2019**, *29*, 61–66. [CrossRef] [PubMed]

136. Tao, H.; Xu, H.; Zuo, L.; Li, C.; Qiao, G.; Guo, M.; Zheng, L.; Leitgeb, M.; Lin, X. Exosomes-coated bcl-2 siRNA inhibits the growth of digestive system tumors both in vitro and in vivo. *Int. J. Biol. Macromol.* **2020**, *161*, 470–480. [CrossRef]
137. Naor, D.; Nedvetzki, S.; Golan, I.; Melnik, L.; Faitelson, Y. CD44 in cancer. *Crit. Rev. Clin. Lab. Sci.* **2002**, *39*, 527–579. [CrossRef]
138. Li, D.; Yao, S.; Zhou, Z.; Shi, J.; Huang, Z.; Wu, Z. Hyaluronan decoration of milk exosomes directs tumor-specific delivery of doxorubicin. *Carbohydr. Res.* **2020**, *493*, 108032. [CrossRef]
139. Sugahara, K.N.; Teesalu, T.; Karmali, P.P.; Kotamraju, V.R.; Agemy, L.; Greenwald, D.R.; Ruoslahti, E. Coadministration of a tumor-penetrating peptide enhances the efficacy of cancer drugs. *Science* **2010**, *328*, 1031–1035. [CrossRef]
140. Teesalu, T.; Sugahara, K.N.; Kotamraju, V.R.; Ruoslahti, E. C-end rule peptides mediate neuropilin-1-dependent cell, vascular, and tissue penetration. *Proc. Natl. Acad. Sci. USA* **2009**, *106*, 16157–16162. [CrossRef]
141. Zhang, Q.; Xiao, Q.; Yin, H.; Xia, C.; Pu, Y.; He, Z.; Hu, Q.; Wang, J.; Wang, Y. Milk-exosome based pH/light sensitive drug system to enhance anticancer activity against oral squamous cell carcinoma. *RSC Adv.* **2020**, *10*, 28314–28323. [CrossRef]

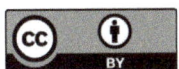

© 2020 by the authors. Licensee MDPI, Basel, Switzerland. This article is an open access article distributed under the terms and conditions of the Creative Commons Attribution (CC BY) license (http://creativecommons.org/licenses/by/4.0/).

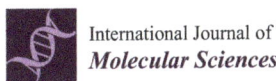

Review

The Biological Function and Therapeutic Potential of Exosomes in Cancer: Exosomes as Efficient Nanocommunicators for Cancer Therapy

Jeong Uk Choi [1], In-Kyu Park [2], Yong-Kyu Lee [3] and Seung Rim Hwang [4,5,*]

1. College of Pharmacy, Chonnam National University, 77 Yongbong-ro, Buk-gu, Gwangju 61186, Korea; cju0667@jnu.ac.kr
2. Department of Biomedical Sciences, Chonnam National University Medical School, 322 Seoyang-ro, Hwasun 58128, Korea; pik96@jnu.ac.kr
3. Department of Chemical and Biological Engineering, Korea National University of Transportation, 50 Daehak-ro, Chungju, Chungbuk 27469, Korea; leeyk@ut.ac.kr
4. College of Pharmacy, Chosun University, 309 Pilmun-daero, Dong-gu, Gwangju 61452, Korea
5. Department of Biomedical Sciences, Graduate School, Chosun University, 309 Pilmun-daero, Dong-gu, Gwangju 61452, Korea
* Correspondence: srhwang@chosun.ac.kr; Tel.: +82-62-230-6365

Received: 29 August 2020; Accepted: 3 October 2020; Published: 5 October 2020

Abstract: Cancer therapeutics must be delivered to their targets for improving efficacy and reducing toxicity, though they encounter physiological barriers in the tumor microenvironment. They also face limitations associated with genetic instability and dynamic changes of surface proteins in cancer cells. Nanosized exosomes generated from the endosomal compartment, however, transfer their cargo to the recipient cells and mediate the intercellular communication, which affects malignancy progression, tumor immunity, and chemoresistance. In this review, we give an overview of exosomes' biological aspects and therapeutic potential as diagnostic biomarkers and drug delivery vehicles for oncotherapy. Furthermore, we discuss whether exosomes could contribute to personalized cancer immunotherapy drug design as efficient nanocommunicators.

Keywords: exosome; cancer; nanocommunicator; diagnostic biomarker; drug delivery vehicle; personalized cancer immunotherapy

---

1. Introduction

Oncology drugs constitute the largest therapeutics section approved by the Center for Drug Evaluation and Research, a division of the United States Food and Drug Administration [1]. Once cancer metastasizes from the primary tumor to new sites at the time of detection, the survival rate of cancer patients decreases substantially, posing a threat to overall health [2]. In recent times, an early diagnosis of cancer via timely screening using liquid biopsy tools such as circulating tumor cells (CTCs) or circulating tumor DNA (ctDNA) as well as extracellular vesicles (EVs) has received attention, and the survival rate of cancer patients has increased with the development of treatment strategies [3,4].

Anticancer drug approval trends have changed since cancer chemotherapeutic agents were first developed in the 1940s. Cancer chemotherapeutics show efficacy as well as side effects as they not only interfere with the growth or division of cancer cells but also normal cells. Cancer cells even evade anticancer drugs by mediating a cellular efflux of drugs or by reducing target gene expression. They not only receive external signals but also transmit signals to form new blood vessels in cancer tissues. EVs secreted by cancer cells transfer signals for cancer progression and metastasis [5].

As technical limitations associated with cancer chemotherapy have been recognized, and the understanding of cancer biology has improved, the paradigm of research and development has shifted towards targeted therapy using monoclonal antibodies and small molecules that target the signaling process of cancer cells. Recently, synthetic small molecules such as a FGFR (fibroblast growth factor receptor) inhibitor (erdafitinib; Janssen Pharmaceutica, Beerse, Belgium), CSF1R (colony-stimulating factor-1 receptor)/RTK (receptor tyrosine kinase)/FLT3 (FMS-like tyrosine kinase 3) inhibitor (pexidartinib; Daiichi Sankyo, Tokyo, Japan), and exportin 1 inhibitor (selinexor; Karyopharm Therapeutics, Newton, MA, USA), and biologics such as an antibody-drug conjugate (ADC) targeting nectin-4 (enfortumab vedotin; Astellas Pharma, Tokyo, Japan), and ADC targeting CD79B (polatuzumab vedotin; Genentech/Roche, South San Francisco, CA, USA) have been approved. Interestingly, entrectinib (Genentech/Roche) simultaneously targets c-ROS oncogene 1 (ROS1), ALK (anaplastic lymphoma kinase) RTKs, and tropomyosin receptor kinase proteins encoded by neurotrophic tyrosine receptor kinase (NTRK) genes; it was approved as a biomarker-based treatment for ROS1-positive and NTRK fusion-positive cancer. In the same vein, engineered EVs that carry small interfering RNA (siRNA) or short hairpin RNA specifically targeting oncogenic KRAS mutation showed their therapeutic potential in pancreatic ductal adenocarcinoma mouse models [6].

Despite the remarkable performance of targeted anticancer drugs, limitations have been associated with the targeting of markers on the cancer cell surface, because cancer cells are genetically unstable, and surface proteins in cancer cells change dynamically during disease progression [7]. The necessity of developing new therapeutic approaches has emerged due to the genetic heterogeneity between cancer cells and drug resistance mechanisms [8]. Since 2010, cancer immunotherapy drugs including CTLA4 (cytotoxic T-lymphocyte-associated protein 4) inhibitors, PD-1 (programmed cell death protein 1) inhibitors, PD-L1 (programmed cell death ligand 1) inhibitors, and CAR (chimeric antigen receptor)-T cell therapy have received a lot of attention. As cancer cells proliferate by evading the immune system, cancer immunotherapy drugs interfere with the evasion mechanism or stimulate immune cells to attack tumor cells [9].

However, cancer therapeutics encounter barriers against transport to target sites owing to the elevated levels of solid stress, vascular network formation, interstitial fluid pressure, and density of extracellular matrix (ECM) in the tumor microenvironment [10]. Nanocarriers can enhance the permeability and retention of their cargo drugs in solid tumor tissues. Certain cancer therapeutics need to be delivered to intracellular targets such as the cytosol or nucleus to elicit their proper action [11]. Interestingly, nanosized EVs called exosomes, transfer their cargo nucleic acids and proteins to the recipient cells via the cellular uptake of vesicles; this contributes to the intercellular communication between tumor cells and bone marrow stromal cells. Recurrent mutations or specific alterations of niches within hematopoietic cells of the bone marrow regulating the production of blood and immune cells play roles in malignancy progression and chemoresistance [12]. In that exosomes orchestrate immune cells in the tumor microenvironment through cell-to-cell signaling, they have been tested for cancer immunotherapy in clinical trials. Dendritic cell (DC)-derived exosomes (DEXs) showed modest efficacy in patients with metastatic melanoma and non-small cell lung cancer (NSCLC) [13,14]. Autologous tumor-derived exosomes (TEXs) in combination with the GM-CSF (granulocyte-macrophage colony-stimulating factor) could induce antitumor T lymphocyte response in colorectal cancer [15]. TEXs can also provide diagnostic biomarkers, because they circulate in biological fluids and the exosomal components enclosed in lipid membrane vesicles reflect the characteristics of the cells of origin in the tumor tissue.

In this review, we aimed to provide a comprehensive overview of the biological aspects and potential therapeutic applications of exosomes in cancer. Here, we also discuss whether exosomes could contribute to personalized cancer immunotherapy drug design as efficient nanocommunicators.

2. Biologic Aspects of Exosomes and Cancer

2.1. Exosome Biogenesis

Cells release EVs enclosed in lipid membranes into the extracellular environment. Exosomes, microvesicles (MVs)/microparticles, and apoptotic bodies form a subgroup of EVs. They have been defined by their biogenesis, size, or constituent molecules. The process of exosome biogenesis starts with endocytic membrane transport through which the cell surface proteins can be recycled [16]. The perimeter membrane of endocytic vesicles buds inward during endosome maturation from the early endosome to the late endosome [17]. Further invagination of the endosomal membrane into the endosomal compartment forms intraluminal vesicles (ILVs) in the multivesicular body (MVB). Subsequently, the MVB is either fused with the lysosome for degradation or release its contents in the form of exosomes by merging with the plasma membrane [18]. This process of exosome formation is different from that of MV/microparticle formation that takes place via outward budding directly from the plasma membrane (Figure 1) [18].

The most well-known mechanism for packaging receptors internalized from the cell surface and other exosomal cargo proteins in the late endosome membrane depend on the endosomal sorting complex required for transport (ESCRT) machinery [19]. Cytosolic protein complexes composed of ESCRT-0, ESCRT-I, ESCRT-II, and ESCRT–III, together with accessory proteins, participate in binding ubiquitinated cargo and sculpting MVB vesicles [20]. The addition of a regulatory ubiquitin protein to the substrate is a reversible post-translational modification catalyzed by a ubiquitin-activating enzyme, ubiquitin-conjugating enzyme, and ubiquitin ligase [21]. Even though it is debatable whether the contents of MVBs are released into the extracellular medium or enter the lysosome under certain circumstances, the tagging of misfolded or damaged proteins with ubiquitin plays a role in maintaining intracellular protein levels for cell cycle regulation and is also associated with the oncogenic processes [22]. For example, mutations in genes encoding components for ubiquitin ligase activity lead to the development of renal cell carcinoma and breast cancer [23,24].

Alternatively, ESCRT-independent pathways are supported by MVB formation even in the depletion of key subunits of ESCRTs [25]. Sphingolipids and cholesterol that are enriched in detergent-resistant membrane domains may be involved in ubiquitin-independent protein sorting [26]. The sphingolipid ceramide also triggers the formation of ILVs in the late endosome that are destined for secretion as exosomes [27]. Observation of human lymphoblastoid cells via immunoelectron microscopy demonstrated low cholesterol labeling in the lysosome but high cholesterol labeling in the MVB and exosomes [28]. Despite the possibility of ubiquitin-independent exosomal cargo sorting, certain ESCRT components are involved in exosome formation. Apoptosis-linked gene 2-interacting protein X (ALIX), an ESCRT accessory protein, contributes to the sorting of transferrin receptor into the late endosome membrane and interacts with syntenin-linking syndecan-mediated signaling [29,30]. Hepatocyte growth factor-regulated tyrosine kinase substrate (HRS), an ESCRT-0 protein, is related to exosomal secretion and antigen-presenting activity in DCs [31].

The pathways of packaging RNAs into exosomes are still unclear. Specific linear sequence motifs that are shared by exosomal RNAs may function as cis-acting elements that target RNAs to exosomes [32]. GW-bodies containing protein components of RNA-induced silencing complex congregate with the endosome and MVB, where microRNA (miRNAs) are enriched. The exosome-like vesicles secreted by MVBs are rich in GW182, which modulates miRNA loading or gene silencing [33].

2.2. Exosome–Cell Interaction and Biodistribution of Exosomes

After being secreted by the original cell into the extracellular space, exosomes circulate in body fluids or are distributed into the tissue ECM [34,35]. Owing to their nanosize, they even penetrate the nasal mucosa and bypass the blood-brain barrier [36]. Labeling and tracking exosomes using fluorescence or bioluminescence helps us understand exosome–cell interaction and the biodistribution of exosomes [37].

Exosomes with lipid bilayer structures can be taken up into the recipient cell via membrane fusion, clathrin-mediated endocytosis, caveolin-dependent endocytosis, macropinocytosis, or phagocytosis, leading to the delivery of exosomal contents to the cytosolic space of the recipient cell (Figure 2) [38–41]. Exosomal cargo is then released by the acidification of the endo/lysosome compartment in the recipient cell [42]. Receptor-ligand interactions between cell surface receptors and exosomal ligands may also occur based on specific cell types, and mediate antigen presentation, cell signaling, the release of soluble factor, disease progression, and immune surveillance [43].

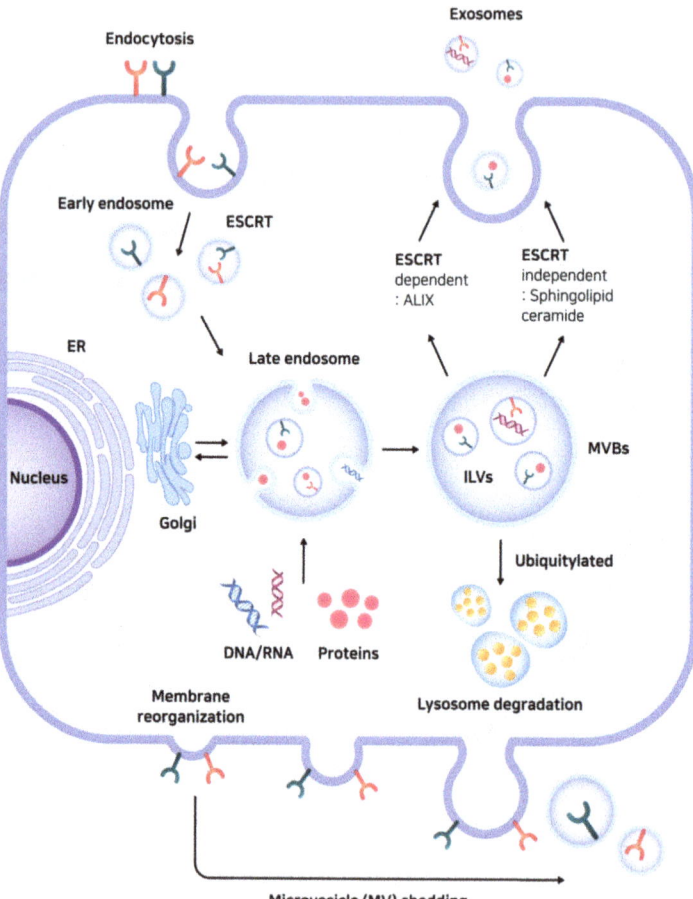

Figure 1. The process of exosome biogenesis. The perimeter membrane of endocytic vesicles buds inward during endosome maturation from the early endosome to the late endosome. Further invagination of the endosomal membrane forms intraluminal vesicles (ILVs) in the multivesicular body (MVB). Subsequently, the MVB is fused with the lysosome or release its contents in the form of exosomes (top right). This process of exosome biogenesis is different from that of microvesicle (MV) shedding (bottom). Receptors internalized from the cell surface and other exosomal cargo proteins are packed in the late endosome either by endosomal sorting complex required for transport (ESCRT)-dependent or ESCRT-independent pathway. ER: endoplasmic reticulum; ILV: intraluminal vesicle; MVB: multivesicular body; MV: microvesicle; ESCRT: endosomal sorting complex required for transport; ALIX: apoptosis-linked gene 2-interacting protein X.

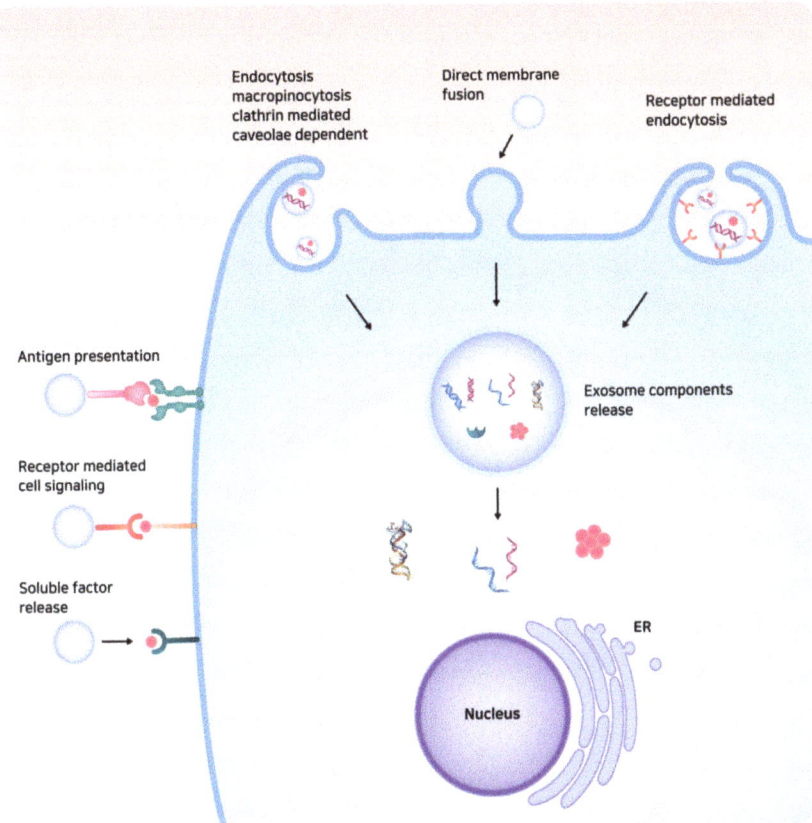

Figure 2. The illustration of exosome–cell interaction. Exosomes can be taken up into the recipient cell via direct membrane fusion or endocytosis, leading to the delivery of exosomal contents such as DNAs, messenger RNAs, long non-coding RNAs, enzymes, and signaling peptides or proteins to the cytosolic space of the recipient cell. Receptor-ligand interactions between cell surface receptors and exosomal ligands may also occur.

The diverse functions of exosomes are governed by the delivery of exosomal components, including lipids, nucleic acids, and proteins such as tetraspanins, adhesion molecules, antigen-presenting molecules, transmembrane receptors, MVB formation proteins, membrane trafficking proteins, cytoskeletal proteins, enzymes, signaling proteins, and heat shock proteins (Figure 3) [44]. Finally, clearance of exosomes from the body might take place via the liver, spleen, and kidneys with the mononuclear phagocytic system [45].

2.3. The Biological Functions of Exosomes in Cancer

Exosomes function as unique intercellular communicators and debris managers for cellular homeostasis [46]. Delivery of exosomal cargo mediates cell motility, immune responses, and reprogramming of the tumor microenvironment. Whether exosomes promote cancer progression and escape from immunosurveillance depends on the type of the cells of origin and malignancy at the time of exosome release [47,48]. TEXs have autocrine and paracrine roles in cancer progression [49]. At the site of the primary lesion, they carry fibronectin and proteinases, including membrane type 1-matrix metalloproteinase (MMP) and MMP2, and facilitate adhesion and invasiveness of cancer cells [50]. Delivery of miRNAs via TEXs transforms fibroblasts into cancer-associated fibroblasts (CAFs) [51–53]. Meanwhile, fibroblast-derived exosomes have been reported to stimulate directional movements of breast cancer cells, which is dependent on Wnt-planar cell polarity signaling [54]. Exosomes secreted from CAFs are rich in disintegrin and metalloproteinase domain-containing protein 10, which can enhance cancer cell motility via Notch receptor activation and the GTPase RhoA signalling [55]. Adipocyte-derived exosomes have been shown to increase migration and invasion of melanoma cells via fatty acid oxidation [56].

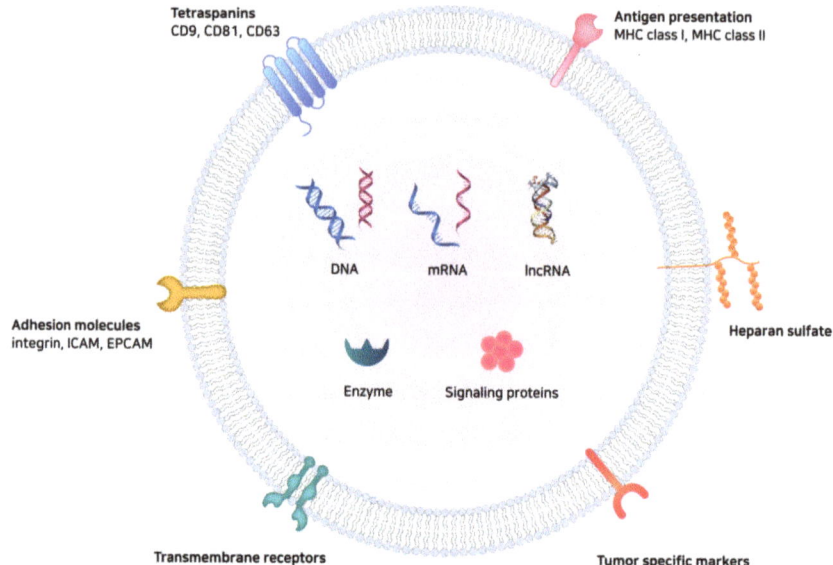

Figure 3. The illustration of exosomal components. The diverse functions of exosomes are governed by the delivery of exosomal cargo proteins and nucleic acids to the recipient cells. Exosomal components include lipids, nucleic acids, tetraspanins, adhesion molecules, antigen-presenting molecules, transmembrane receptors, MVB formation proteins, membrane trafficking proteins, enzymes, signaling proteins, etc. mRNA: messenger RNAs; lncRNA: long non-coding RNA; ICAM: intercellular adhesion molecule; EpCAM: epithelial cell adhesion molecule; MHC: major histocompatibility complex.

Exosomes also regulate angiogenesis and vascular permeability [57]. A mucin-type podoplanin glycoprotein, which is upregulated in certain types of cancer and incorporated into exosomes, reprograms exosomal proteins and promotes lymphangiogenesis [58]. Uptake of leukemia-derived exosomes containing miR-92a by endothelial cells enhanced endothelial tube formation [59]. Exosomes released by metastatic tumor cells led to endothelial hyperpermeability contrary to the exosomes released by non-metastatic tumor cells [60]. Under hypoxia, miR-23a upregulation in TEXs leads to the accumulation of hypoxia-inducible factor-1 α, enhancing angiogenesis, and inhibits tight junction protein ZO-1, increasing vascular permeability [61].

After the intravasation of tumor cells, TEXs traveling through the bloodstream develop "pre-metastatic niches" by modifying microenvironments in distant target organs and affecting organ-specific stromal cells [62]. Exosomes from highly metastatic melanomas reprogrammed bone marrow progenitor cells, resulting in exosome-mediated tyrosine-protein kinase Met signaling [63]. Uptake of exosomes derived from pancreatic ductal adenocarcinomas by Kupffer cells induced transforming growth factor-β secretion and fibronectin production, which initiated liver pre-metastatic niche formation [64]. Specific integrin expression patterns on TEXs were shown to correlate with the localization of TEXs and organotropic metastasis [65]. Targeting the exosomal integrin $\alpha_6\beta_4$ was associated with lung metastasis, whereas targeting the exosomal integrin $\alpha_v\beta_5$ was associated with liver metastasis. TEXs can also enter sentinel lymph nodes and influence lymph node distribution of cancer cells, which is driven by synchronized molecular signals that affect tumor metastasis [66]. Meanwhile, reports indicate that exosomes from non-metastatic cells inhibit metastasis. Exosomes isolated from non-metastatic patient sera suppressed experimental lung metastasis by increasing the number of patrolling monocytes in the lungs and inducing macrophage differentiation, leading to immune surveillance in the pre-metastatic niche [67].

As TEXs contain immunosuppressive ligands as well as immunostimulatory tumor-associated antigens (TAAs), they can play roles in mediating tumor immunity [68]. Binding immune-inhibitory ligands of TEXs to T cell receptors and IL-2 receptors leads to tolerogenic signals [69]. TEXs also induce apoptosis of $CD8^+$ T lymphocytes and differentiation of myeloid precursor cells and regulatory T cells. They can also inhibit the cytotoxic functions of natural killer (NK) cells via downregulation of NK group 2D, an NK-activating receptor that recognizes ligands on the surface of malignant cells as well as TEXs [70]. Meanwhile, DEXs pulsed with tumor peptides activate cytotoxic T lymphocytes [71]. Mast cell-derived exosomes associated with antigens induce maturation of DCs. Antigen presentation by DCs activates B and T cells [72].

Exosomes have also been reported to mediate cancer chemoresistance by cargo transfer [73]. Exosomes derived from drug-resistant breast cancer cells modulated the cell cycle and drug-induced apoptosis, which might be dependent on selective miRNA patterns [73]. Restoration of miR-151a via exosomes derived from temozolomide (TMZ)-resistant glioblastoma multiforme enhances chemosensitivity to TMZ, whereas miR-151a loss drives TMZ resistance [74]. In cisplatin-resistant tumor cells, acidic pH in the extracellular microenvironment reduces cisplatin uptake into tumor cells and increases cisplatin levels eliminated via TEXs [75]. Exosomes isolated from fibroblast-derived conditioned medium prime cancer stem cells and promote chemoresistance in colorectal cancer [76]. Transfer of exosomal RNA from stromal to breast cancer cells activates signal transducer and activator of transcription 1 and NOTCH3 signaling, which regulate the expansion of chemoresistant cancer cells [77].

3. Potential Therapeutic Applications of Exosomes in Cancer

3.1. Exosomes as Diagnostic Biomarkers for Cancer

3.1.1. Identification Techniques of Exosomes in Liquid Biopsy

As exosomes have the potential to be used as prognostic biomarkers, isolation and identification of exosomes and their contents are also critical issues. For exosome isolation/purification, various methods have been evaluated. The most common method is differential centrifugation at $300\times g$ for 10 min, $2000\times g$ for 10 min, and $10,000\times g$ for 30 min, followed by ultracentrifugation at $100,000\times g$ for 2 h. For higher purity of exosomes, gradient centrifugation using sucrose can also be used [78]. An immuno-isolation method using antibody-coated magnetic beads can also be used to obtain higher purity and recovery rates. Rapid surface protein characterization using flow cytometry provides additional benefits with this method [79]. However, only specific types of exosomes can be isolated using this method, which can be considered as one of the limitations of this method. Currently, exosome extraction kits such as the ExoSpin™ Exosome purification Kit (Cell Guidance Systems LLC; St. Louis, MO, USA) and Total Exosome Isolation Kit™ (Life Technologies; Waltham, MA, USA) are also available. Typically, these kits use polymers such as polyethylene glycol with centrifugation to induce exosome sedimentation [80]. Microfluidic technology enables rapid and precise isolation/purification of exosomes with a very small volume of samples using a micro-electromechanical system [81]. Turbidimetry-enabled particle purification liquid chromatography based on the size exclusion principle also has been proven superior in purification of EVs in biofluids [82]. Using biosensors is another technique to determine exosomes with higher sensitivity and automated analysis [83]. For identification of exosome contents, general methods such as polymerase chain reaction (PCR), next-generation sequencing (NGS), and proteomics can be used.

3.1.2. Applications of Exosomes as Diagnostic Biomarkers for Cancer

Liquid biopsy tools such as CTCs, ctDNA, and exosomes have advantages in non-invasive diagnosis and prognosis over traditional tissue biopsy strategies. Prognostic potential of CTCs has been already tested for monitoring epithelium-originating tumors in clinical trials [84]. However, CTCs shed from the primary tumor are found as only a few CTCs per mL of blood among millions of erythrocytes or leukocytes, and CTC enrichment techniques are needed for their detection [85]. Fragmented DNA shed from tumor cells may reflect the genetic signature of tumors [86]. Analysis of ctDNA in blood is challenging because there is a small fraction of ctDNA among cell-free DNAs from leukocytes in the blood sample [87]. In addition, the heterogeneity of tumor cells makes determining tumor-specific mutation in the ctDNA sample difficult.

Compared to the limited amounts of CTCs or ctDNA in the bloodstream, exosomes can be detected not only in blood but also in urine, cerebrospinal fluid, or lymphatic exudate [88,89]. Exosomes can be actively involved in cellular communication by delivering various signaling molecules. They serve as effective carriers, as the lipid bilayer can protect the contents and directly deliver them to the target cells. Exosome contents include nucleic acids, enzymes, and various signaling proteins. The contents can vary depending on the cells of origin. Therefore, the identification of exosomal contents can provide important clues regarding the cells of origin, which makes them ideal biomarkers for the diagnosis of diseases such as cancer, infection, metabolic, and neurodegenerative disorders [90,91].

As exosomes and their contents released from cancer cells display unique properties, many attempts have been made to use TEXs as cancer diagnostic biomarkers (Table 1) [92]. TEXs play important roles in facilitating tumor growth and are involved in every step of cancer development, including angiogenesis, proliferation, metastasis, and fostering the tumor microenvironment by delivering relevant genes, growth factors, and cell signaling molecules [93–95]. For example, exosomes isolated from urine samples can be used to diagnose prostate cancer, bladder cancer, and glioblastoma. Typically, exosomal proteins related to epidermal growth factor receptor (EGFR) pathways (resistin, α-subunit of Gs protein, retinoic acid-induced protein 3, EGFR variant III, etc.) are present at diagnostic levels and hence, can be used as reliable biomarkers [96–98]. Prostate-specific antigen, survivin, and prostate cancer antigen 3 in exosomal contents can be also used for detecting prostate cancer [97,99,100]. Nucleic acids present in cancer exosomes, including miRNA, messenger RNA (mRNA), and long non-coding RNA (lncRNA), can also be used as diagnostic markers. For example, unique nucleic acids from exosomes have been identified in patients with glioblastoma [98]. Specific lncRNA, LINC00152, was also identified in gastric cancer-derived exosomes, which makes it a useful diagnostic biomarker [101]. miRNAs such as miR-21, -141, -200a, etc. can be detected in ovarian cancer patients, and miR-17-3p, -21, etc. were identified in lung cancer patients [102,103]. The genetic mutation in cancer patients is detectable by using exosome samples instead of CTCs or ctDNA. Exosomal RNA/DNA demonstrated the diagnostic value for KRAS mutation in pancreatic cancer and EGFR mutation in NSCLC [104–106]. BRAF mutation in EVs from lymphatic exudate of melanoma patients was reported to be useful for the prognosis [107]. Therefore, identification of unique exosomal contents corresponding to various types of cancers can help develop reliable diagnostic biomarkers (Figure 4).

3.2. Exosomes as Drug Delivery Vehicles for Oncotherapy

Exosomes are attractive nanovehicles for targeting cancer (Figure 4). As exosomes originate from endogenous cells, they possess low immunogenicity and thus induce low toxicity and side effects [108]. Exosomes are stable under physiological conditions. Owing to the presence of a lipid bilayer, they can protect the contents from the immune system and various enzymes. Furthermore, they demonstrate a homing capability by cell/tissue tropism with a longer circulation period, and can also cross the blood-brain barrier [109]. Unlike liposomes or other synthetic drug delivery nanoparticles, exosomes have characteristic membrane proteins and lipids that promote efficient targeting of exosomes to the recipient cell [110]. Exosomes can also enhance the delivery of contents as they can be directly fused or internalized into target cells. CD47, an integrin-associated protein upregulated in mesenchymal stem cells (MSCs), interacts with signal-regulatory protein, which helps inhibition of phagocytosis [111]. Thus, exosomes derived from fibroblast-like MSCs show the enhanced retention in the circulation in mice [6]. As the average size of exosomes ranges from 30 to 200 nm, passive targeting of exosomes to tumor tissue with enhanced permeability and retention effect can also be expected. With these benefits, a number of clinical and preclinical trials have been conducted to utilize exosomes as delivery vehicles.

Table 1. Applications of exosomes as diagnostic biomarkers for cancer.

Exosome Contents	Associated Molecule	Target Disease	Reference
Proteins	Resistin, α-subunit of Gs protein, retinoic acid-induced protein 3	Prostate, bladder cancer	[96,97]
	Epidermal growth factor receptor (EGFR) variant III	Glioblastoma	[98]
	Prostate-specific antigen, survivin, prostate cancer antigen 3	Prostate cancer	[97,99,100]
RNAs	lncRNA, LINC00152	Gastric cancer	[101]
	miR-21, miR-141, miR-200a	Ovarian cancer	[102]
	miR-17-3p, miR-21	Non-small cell lung cancer (NSCLC)	[103]
DNAs	Mutant KRAS	Pancreatic cancer	[104]
	EGFR T790M mutation	NSCLC	[105]
	Mutant KRAS, TP53	Pancreatic cancer	[106]
	BRAF^{V600E} mutation	Melanoma	[107]

EGFR: epidermal growth factor receptor; NSCLC: non-small cell lung cancer.

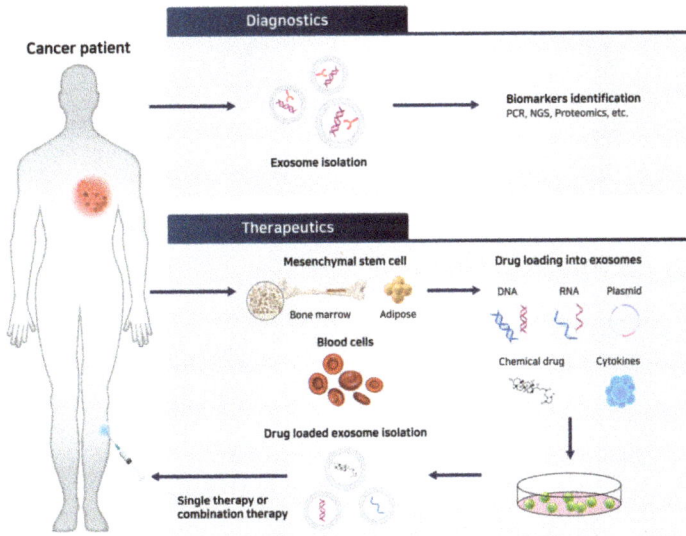

Figure 4. Potential therapeutic applications of exosomes in cancer. As exosomal components reflect the characteristics of the cells of origin, many attempts have been made to use tumor-derived exosomes (TEXs) as cancer diagnostic biomarkers. For identification of exosome contents, general methods such as polymerase chain reaction (PCR), next-generation sequencing (NGS), and proteomics can be used. Exosomes also have therapeutic potential as nanovehicles for drug delivery and personalized cancer immunotherapy. TEX: tumor-derived exosome; PCR: polymerase chain reaction; NGS: next-generation sequencing.

3.2.1. Methods for Loading Drugs into Exosomes

A number of studies have demonstrated that drug-loaded exosomes show better outcomes in inhibiting cancers, but the methods for loading drugs into exosomes also need to be explored further because they are closely related to the stability and loading efficiency of the drugs. To date, there are three types of drug loading methods for exosomes: exogenous loading, endogenous loading, and liposome fusion loading [108]. Exogenous loading refers to the method that directly entraps the drugs inside an isolated exosome with simple incubation, sonication, electroporation, repeated freeze/thaw, and extrusion [112]. Simple incubation can be easily used, but the average loading efficiency of paclitaxel into EVs was below 10%. Sonication can elevate the average loading efficiency up to 28.29%, but affecting the loading amount of hydrophobic drugs by altering the membrane of the exosome is an issue [113]. Typically, the exogenous loading method is advantageous in maintaining the aqueous stability of drug-loaded exosomes over one month at 4 °C and 37 °C, but it is limited by relatively low loading efficiency. Endogenous loading refers to a method that entraps desired molecules in exosomes by modifying the cells of origin before the isolation of exosomes. For instance, treating host cells with chemical drugs, such as paclitaxel, can induce the release of exosomes loaded with paclitaxel [114]. For protein or gene delivery, host cells can be transfected with desired genes, which facilitates the release of exosomes with desired proteins or genes [115]. Although the endogenous loading method demonstrates a relatively high loading efficiency, it is difficult to quantify the amount of content inside the exosome and maintain high purity. Exosomes used in membrane protein engineering approaches protect their cargo proteins, but can be degraded by proteinase [116]. The liposome fusion method uses the hybridization of drug-loaded liposomes and exosomes by the freeze/melting process. This fusion method exhibits higher loading efficiency, especially for loading large plasmids, including CRISPR-Cas9 expressing vectors [117]. However, it is unclear whether this hybridized liposome-exosome can maintain the unique properties of exosomes [118]. Hence, further comprehensive evaluation of parameters such as targetability, half-life, and side effects for hybridized liposome-exosome is required.

3.2.2. Delivering Chemical Drugs via Exosomes for Oncotherapy

As many of chemical drugs can act after being internalized into cancer cells, they need to diffuse through the cell membrane to exert cytotoxicity, which is one of the factors reducing the efficacy of drugs [108]. In this aspect, exosomes can be potential candidates for delivering chemical drugs directly into the target cells. Many trials have been conducted to deliver chemical drugs such as paclitaxel, doxorubicin, cisplatin, and curcumin by packaging into exosomes for the treatment of various cancers (Table 2). For instance, paclitaxel-loaded exosomes isolated from MSCs, macrophages, and prostate cancer cells enhanced antitumor efficacy against pancreatic, breast, prostate, and Lewis lung carcinomas both in in vitro and in vivo studies [113,114,119,120]. Similarly, doxorubicin-loaded exosomes were also examined either by using the mechanical extrusion method to obtain higher drug loading efficiency [121] or surface engineering of exosomes to enhance targetability [122] for the treatment of colon and breast cancers, respectively. Treatment with cisplatin-loaded exosomes could prolong the survival rate of mice with ovarian cancer compared to the free cisplatin-treated group [123]. Pancreatic cancer-derived exosomes containing curcumin also effectively induced apoptosis in pancreatic cancer cells [124]. These studies show that by using exosomes as delivery vehicles, chemical drugs can be delivered more efficiently to target cells, which results in better outcomes.

Table 2. Exosomes as drug delivery vehicles for oncotherapy in preclinical studies.

Therapeutic Molecules	Exosome Origin	Targeted Disease	Reference
Chemical drugs			
Paclitaxel	Macrophage	Lewis lung carcinoma	[113]
	MSC	Pancreatic, breast cancer	[114,119]
	Prostate cancer cell	Prostate cancer	[120]
Droxorubicin	U937 RAW264.7	Colon cancer	[121]
	DCs expressing iRGD	Breast cancer	[122]
Cisplatin	Hepatocarcinoma cell	Hepatocarcinoma	[123]
Curcumin	Pancreatic cancer cell	Pancreatic cancer	[124]
Proteins			
TRIM3	Gastric cancer cell	Gastric cancer	[125]
CD-UPRT fusion protein	HEK293T	Schwannoma	[126]
TRAIL	K562	Lymphoma	[127]
MHC class I/peptide complex	DC	Breast cancer	[128]
HSP70	Myeloma cell	Myeloma	[129]
EGFR nanobodies	Myeloid leukemia cell	Epidermal carcinoma	[130]
SIRPα	Embryonic kidney cell	Colon cancer	[131]
miRNA			
miR-145-5p	MSC	Pancreatic cancer	[115]
Let-7a	HEK293T expressing GE11	Breast cancer with EGFR	[132]
miR-146b	MSC	Glioma	[133]
miR-122	MSC	Hepatocellular carcinoma	[134]
miR-335-5p	Stellate cell	Hepatocellular carcinoma	[135]
miR-379	MSC	Breast cancer	[136]
miR-25-3p inhibitor	Colorectal cancer cell	Colorectal cancer	[137]
siRNA			
PLK-1 siRNA	HEK293T + MSC	Bladder cancer	[138]
GRP78 siRNA	MSC	Hepatocellular carcinoma	[139]
HSP27 siRNA	Neuroblastoma cell	Neuroblastoma	[140]
mRNA			
Cas9 mRNA	Red blood cell	Breast cancer	[141]
PTEN mRNA	Mouse embryonic fibroblast serum	Glioma	[142]
ECRG4 mRNA	Neuroblastoma cell	Tongue carcinoma	[143]

MSC: mesenchymal stem cell; DC: dendritic cell; TRIM: tripartite motif-containing protein; CD: cytosine deaminase; UPRT: uracil phosphoribosyltransferase; TRAIL: TNF-related apoptosis-inducing ligand; MHC: major histocompatibility complex; HSP: heat shock protein; EGFR: epidermal growth factor receptor; SIRP: signal-regulatory protein; PLK: polo-like kinase; Cas: CRISPR associated protein; PTEN: phosphatase and tensin homolog; ECRG: esophageal cancer related gene.

3.2.3. Delivering Therapeutic Proteins via Exosomes for Oncotherapy

As the efficacy of many proteins is limited due to several barriers such as short half-life, low delivery rate, and induction of resistance, the use of appropriate delivery vehicles is one of the best ways to achieve successful protein drug therapies. As exosomes can protect the contents from various enzymes and the immune system, they can act as effective delivery vehicles for proteins. Proteins can be loaded either inside or on the surface of the exosome, based on the mechanism of action of the drugs. However, as therapeutic proteins are macromolecules, it is difficult to directly incorporate them into exosomes. Therefore, genetic modification of the cells of origin leading to the expression of therapeutic proteins in exosomes is usually preferred to prepare protein-loaded exosomes. Several preclinical studies regarding protein-loaded exosomes are summarized in Table 2. For example, the delivery of tripartite motif-containing protein 3 (TRIM3) using gastric cancer-derived exosomes successfully suppressed the proliferation, migration, and metastasis of gastric cancer [125]. Similarly, apoptosis-inducing proteins such as suicide-inducing fusion protein or TNF-related apoptosis-inducing ligand (TRAIL) were loaded into exosomes, and this method could elicit substantially reduced tumor growth in in vivo tumor models [126,127]. Some signaling-related proteins can be expressed on the surface of exosomes to improve tumor immunity, such as the major histocompatibility (MHC) class I/peptide complex [128]. In other studies, immunogenic proteins such as HSP70 were loaded onto exosomes, which resulted in enhanced antitumor T cell activity [129]. Some studies have shown that EGFR nanobodies anchored on exosomes via glycosylphosphatidylinositol (GPI) could bind to EGFR-expressing tumor cells with higher affinity [130].

3.2.4. Delivering RNA Drugs via Exosomes for Oncotherapy

Similar to therapeutic proteins, delivery vehicles are an essential component of successful gene therapy. Exosomes can protect genes from various enzymes, such as DNases and RNases, and can also directly deliver genes inside the cells, which enhances their therapeutic efficacy. Different types of RNAs such as mRNA, miRNA, and siRNA are promising candidates for the treatment of cancers. Studies on exosome RNA delivery are summarized in Table 2. miRNAs are non-coding RNAs involved in the regulation of gene expression. Pathophysiological conditions such as cancer are usually characterized by abnormal expression of certain types of miRNAs, which suggests that targeting miRNAs could be an effective way to treat cancer [144]. Treatment with exosomes overexpressing miR-122 showed substantially elevated chemosensitivity in hepatocellular carcinoma [134]. As the downregulation of miR-335-5p in both hepatocellular carcinoma and stellate cells acts as a pro-tumorigenic factor, delivery of miR-335-5p-overexpressing exosome exhibited substantial tumor shrinkage in an in vivo tumor model [135]. Similarly, treatment with miR-379-overexpressing exosomes significantly suppressed tumor growth in a T47D breast tumor model [136]. In addition, miR-145-5p overexpression inhibited the proliferation of pancreatic ductal adenocarcinoma and induced tumor cell apoptosis in an in vivo model [115]. In addition, specific miRNA inhibitors could act as potential drug candidates. For example, miR-25-3p is known to play an important role in facilitating colorectal cancer metastasis and promoting angiogenesis by targeting KLF (Kruppel-like factor)-2 and KLF-4, which implies that miR-25-3p can be a promising target for treating colorectal cancer. One study showed that treatment with exosomes loaded with miR-25-3p inhibitor considerably attenuated the tumor metastasis of colorectal cancer by balancing the level of miR-25-3p [137]. Silencing target genes using siRNA is another way to inhibit tumor growth. As overexpression of polo-like kinase (PLK)-1 is associated with the development of bladder cancer, one study showed that treatment with PLK-1 siRNA containing exosomes inhibited bladder cancer growth [138]. Similarly, as GRP78 overexpression is implicated in the growth and metastasis of hepatocellular carcinoma, treatment with GRP78 siRNA expressing exosomes resulted in an efficacious antitumor response in a sorafenib-resistant hepatocellular carcinoma model [139]. HSP27, a member of the heat-shock protein family, is known to promote neuron maturation and can be involved in the development of neuroblastoma. Treatment with Hsp27 siRNA-tagged exosome showed a significant reduction in tumor growth of the neuroblastoma cell line SH-SY5Y [140]. mRNA can be another candidate for anticancer therapy using exosome vehicles. Transferring CRISPR-associated protein (Cas) 9 mRNA-expressing exosomes from red blood cells induced miRNA inhibition and Cas9 genome editing effects in a breast cancer model [141]. Phosphatase and tensin homolog (PTEN) and esophageal cancer-related gene (ECRG) 4 are classified as tumor suppressors and are generally mutated in cancer cells. Therefore, treatment with exosomes expressing PTEN or ECRG4 mRNA could inhibit the growth of glioma cells [145] and tongue squamous cell carcinoma cells, respectively [143]. These studies show that depending on the target, different types of RNA therapeutics can be chosen, and the therapeutic efficacy of these drugs can be substantially enhanced by using exosomes as delivery vehicles.

3.3. Exosomes into Personalized Cancer Immunotherapy Drug Design (Single or in Combination)

Exosomes can be used as cell-free vaccines owing to the fact that exosomes derived from various donor cells, such as immune cells and cancer cells, are involved in fostering antitumor immunity [146]. DEXs can perform important immunostimulatory functions, as DCs that act as sentinel antigen-presenting cells play a crucial role in orchestrating cancer-specific adaptive immunity [147]. The surface of DEXs is characterized by various functional molecules for priming T cells such as MHC class I/II and costimulatory molecules including CD40, CD80, and CD86 [148]. This can foster antitumor immunity by inducing the activation of both innate and adaptive immunity. In several preclinical tests, treating DEXs could elicit antitumor effects and prolong the survival rate of tumor-bearing mice by expanding the repertoire of tumor-specific cytotoxic T cells as well as activating naïve T cells [149]. DEXs are also known to induce NK cell-mediated cytotoxicity to inhibit tumor growth [150]. In order to potentiate the efficacy of DEX as a therapeutic cancer vaccine, choosing an appropriate TAA and a relevant adjuvant is essential. To date, both for human and preclinical studies, only MHC class I/II binding peptides such as Epstein-Barr virus, melanoma-associated antigen, and melanoma antigen recognized by T cells-1 have been used for DEX vaccine [13,14,151]. However, the use of peptide-based DEX vaccine was not very effective in inducing antitumor effects due to modest activation of antitumor immune responses [152]. Several studies have reported that a more intense adaptive immune response can be induced with a DEX vaccine loaded with protein antigen [152,153]. This effect might be attributable to the presence of a broad range of epitopes with protein antigens, which might be more effective in activating various repertoires of tumor-specific cytotoxic T cells. These studies demonstrate the ability of personalized DEX vaccines based on patient tumor lysates. Therefore, a more potent DEX vaccine that can evoke strong antigen-specific responses can be manufactured with the loading of an allogenic protein antigen. Based on other studies, B cells are required to boost antitumor immunity, suggesting that epitopes, which activate B cells, are also needed for a successful DEX vaccine [152,153]. These results also provide a rationale for utilizing personalized protein antigens as cargo in DEX vaccines. General adjuvants such as interferon-γ and toll-like receptor agonists, including polyinosinic:polycytidylic acid and CpG oligodeoxynucleotides can be used to potentiate the efficacy of DEX vaccine. It is also known that the use of these adjuvants can result in the maturation of DCs and ultimately produce more immunogenic DEXs [154]. DEXs derived from mature DCs are known to express more costimulatory surface molecules including CD40, CD80, CD86, and intercellular adhesion molecule -1 and MHC class I/II [149]. Even though the DEX vaccine seems to show promising outcomes, several challenges remain until it can be widely used in clinics, as the research on this therapy is still at an early stage. For example, it is not clear whether the mass production of personalized DEX vaccine possessing a homogenous quality is available. At present, there are no clear guidelines regarding the production of exosome-based therapeutics. Proper storage, maintenance of stability, and route of administration for exosomes are also the issues to be considered [155].

Besides, CAR exosomes derived from effector CAR-T cells showed cytotoxic effects on cancer cells [156]. Intravenous injection of CAR exosomes into a mouse xenograft model exerted potent tumor growth inhibition. A combination of exosomal therapy with other immunotherapies such as immune-checkpoint blockers, cytokines, adoptive T cell transfer, and cancer vaccines might be a good way to elicit synergistic anticancer effects. For the combined utilization of CAR exosomes and CAR-T cells, further clinical/preclinical studies are required, and the clinically applicable scheme should be proposed.

4. Conclusions and Future Perspectives

Recently, cancer therapeutics has made great strides, and various clinical trials for targeted cancer therapy or immunotherapy have been conducted singly or in combination. However, there remains an unmet need, because only a few types of cancer patients are restrictedly responsive to current immune checkpoint blockers. In order to elevate response rate for personalized immunotherapy, prognostic biomarkers need to be established. As mentioned above, exosomal components can be used as diagnostic biomarkers in liquid biopsy, nanovehicles for delivery of anticancer drugs, and mediators between cells affecting tumor immunity. Detection of marker proteins or nucleic acids in circulating exosomes shows potential for predicting patients' clinical response [157]. "TEXs-on-chip" techniques using patient-derived tumor spheroids obtained from liquid biopsy will be applicable in the near future.

In that vaccinating autologous exosomes obtained from patients can avoid allograft reaction and carry tumor antigens, patient-derived exosomes have received attention as good candidates for personalized immunotherapy. Using bone marrow aspirate from patients, MSCs are isolated and expanded ex vivo, and then large scale of MSCs engineered with anticancer genes can be transplanted to patients for personalized treatment [158]. As exosomes released from MSCs acquire tropism toward tumor locations and the corresponding receptors with the original MSC, they would mediate anticancer activity [159]. Engineering techniques for enhancing therapeutic efficacy of these cell-free vaccines are needed for the development of innovative personalized immunotherapy.

Author Contributions: Conceptualization, J.U.C. and S.R.H.; methodology and validation, I.-K.P.; investigation, J.U.C.; writing—Original draft preparation, J.U.C.; writing—Review and editing, S.R.H.; visualization, Y.-K.L.; supervision, I.-K.P.; funding acquisition, Y.-K.L. and S.R.H. All authors have read and agreed to the published version of the manuscript.

Funding: This research was supported by the National Research Foundation of Korea (NRF) grant funded by the Ministry of Science and ICT (grant numbers NRF-2019R1F1A1057702, NRF-2019R1A4A1024116 and NRF-2018R1D1A1A09083269).

Acknowledgments: The authors acknowledge KB BIOMED Inc. for administrative and technical support.

Conflicts of Interest: The authors declare no conflict of interest.

Abbreviations

ADC	Antibody-drug conjugate
ALIX	Apoptosis-linked gene 2-interacting protein X
ALK	Anaplastic lymphoma kinase
CAF	Cancer-associated fibroblasts
CAR	Chimeric antigen receptor
Cas	CRISPR-associated protein
CD	Cytosine deaminase
CSF1R	Colony-stimulating factor-1 receptor
CTC	Circulating-tumor cell
ctDNA	Circulating tumor DNA
CTLA4	Cytotoxic T-lymphocyte-associated protein 4
DC	Dendritic cell
DEX	Dendritic cell-derived exosome
ECM	Extracellular matrix
ECRG	Esophageal cancer-related gene
EGFR	Epidermal growth factor receptor
EpCAM	Epithelial cell adhesion molecule
ER	Endoplasmic reticulum
ESCRT	Endosomal sorting complex required for transport
EV	Extracellular vesicle
FGFR	Fibroblast growth factor receptor
FLT3	FMS-like tyrosine kinase 3
GM-CSF	Granulocyte-macrophage colony-stimulating factor
GPI	Glycosylphosphatidylinositol
HRS	Hepatocyte growth factor-regulated tyrosine kinase substrate
HSP	Heat shock protein
ICAM	Intercellular adhesion molecule
ILV	Intraluminal vesicle
KLF	Kruppel-like factor
lncRNA	Long non-coding RNA
MHC	Major histocompatibility complex
miRNA	MicroRNA
MMP	Matrix metalloproteinase
mRNA	Messenger RNA
MSC	Mesenchymal stem cell
MV	Microvesicle
MVB	Multivesicular body

NGS	Next-generation sequencing
NK	Natural killer
NSCLC	Non-small cell lung cancer
NTRK	Neurotrophic tyrosine receptor kinase
PCR	Polymerase chain reaction
PD-1	Programmed cell death protein 1
PD-L1	Programmed cell death ligand 1
PLK	Polo-like kinase
PTEN	Phosphatase and tensin homolog
ROS1	C-ros oncogene 1
RTK	Receptor tyrosine kinase
siRNA	Small interfering RNA
SIRP	Signal-regulatory protein
TAA	Tumor-associated antigen
TEX	Tumor-derived exosome
TMZ	Temozolomide
TRAIL	TNF-related apoptosis-inducing ligand
TRIM	Tripartite motif-containing protein
UPRT	Uracil phosphoribosyltransferase

References

1. Mullard, A. 2019 FDA drug approvals. *Nat. Rev. Drug Discov.* **2020**, *19*, 79–84. [CrossRef] [PubMed]
2. Zhang, Y.; Li, M.; Gao, X.; Chen, Y.; Liu, T. Nanotechnology in cancer diagnosis: Progress, challenges and opportunities. *J. Hematol. Oncol.* **2019**, *12*, 137. [CrossRef] [PubMed]
3. Jeon, S.M.; Kwon, J.W.; Choi, S.H.; Park, H.Y. Economic burden of lung cancer: A retrospective cohort study in South Korea, 2002-2015. *PLoS ONE* **2019**, *14*, e0212878. [CrossRef] [PubMed]
4. Yang, Y.; Miller, C.R.; Lopez-Beltran, A.; Montironi, R.; Cheng, M.; Zhang, S.; Koch, M.O.; Kaimakliotis, H.Z.; Cheng, L. Liquid Biopsies in the Management of Bladder Cancer: Next-Generation Biomarkers for Diagnosis, Surveillance, and Treatment-Response Prediction. *Crit. Rev. Oncog.* **2017**, *22*, 389–401. [CrossRef]
5. Melo, S.A.; Sugimoto, H.; O'Connell, J.T.; Kato, N.; Villanueva, A.; Vidal, A.; Qiu, L.; Vitkin, E.; Perelman, L.T.; Melo, C.A.; et al. Cancer exosomes perform cell-independent microRNA biogenesis and promote tumorigenesis. *Cancer Cell* **2014**, *26*, 707–721. [CrossRef]
6. Kamerkar, S.; LeBleu, V.S.; Sugimoto, H.; Yang, S.; Ruivo, C.F.; Melo, S.A.; Lee, J.J.; Kalluri, R. Exosomes facilitate therapeutic targeting of oncogenic KRAS in pancreatic cancer. *Nature* **2017**, *546*, 498–503. [CrossRef]
7. Jan, M.; Majeti, R. Clonal evolution of acute leukemia genomes. *Oncogene* **2013**, *32*, 135–140. [CrossRef]
8. Turner, N.C.; Reis-Filho, J.S. Genetic heterogeneity and cancer drug resistance. *Lancet. Oncol.* **2012**, *13*, e178–e185. [CrossRef]
9. Waldmann, T.A. Immunotherapy: Past, present and future. *Nat. Med.* **2003**, *9*, 269–277. [CrossRef]
10. Chauhan, V.P.; Stylianopoulos, T.; Boucher, Y.; Jain, R.K. Delivery of molecular and nanoscale medicine to tumors: Transport barriers and strategies. *Annu. Rev. Chem. Biomol. Eng.* **2011**, *2*, 281–298. [CrossRef]
11. Au, J.L.; Yeung, B.Z.; Wientjes, M.G.; Lu, Z.; Wientjes, M.G. Delivery of cancer therapeutics to extracellular and intracellular targets: Determinants, barriers, challenges and opportunities. *Adv. Drug. Deliv. Rev.* **2016**, *97*, 280–301. [CrossRef] [PubMed]
12. Mendez-Ferrer, S.; Bonnet, D.; Steensma, D.P.; Hasserjian, R.P.; Ghobrial, I.M.; Gribben, J.G.; Andreeff, M.; Krause, D.S. Bone marrow niches in haematological malignancies. *Nat. Rev. Cancer* **2020**, *20*, 285–298. [CrossRef] [PubMed]
13. Escudier, B.; Dorval, T.; Chaput, N.; Andre, F.; Caby, M.P.; Novault, S.; Flament, C.; Leboulaire, C.; Borg, C.; Amigorena, S.; et al. Vaccination of metastatic melanoma patients with autologous dendritic cell (DC) derived-exosomes: Results of the first phase I clinical trial. *J Transl. Med.* **2005**, *3*, 10. [CrossRef] [PubMed]
14. Morse, M.A.; Garst, J.; Osada, T.; Khan, S.; Hobeika, A.; Clay, T.M.; Valente, N.; Shreeniwas, R.; Sutton, M.A.; Delcayre, A.; et al. A phase I study of dexosome immunotherapy in patients with advanced non-small cell lung cancer. *J. Transl. Med.* **2005**, *3*, 9. [CrossRef] [PubMed]
15. Dai, S.; Wei, D.; Wu, Z.; Zhou, X.; Wei, X.; Huang, H.; Li, G. Phase I clinical trial of autologous ascites-derived exosomes combined with GM-CSF for colorectal cancer. *Mol. Ther.* **2008**, *16*, 782–790. [CrossRef] [PubMed]

16. Hessvik, N.P.; Llorente, A. Current knowledge on exosome biogenesis and release. *Cell Mol. Life Sci.* **2018**, *75*, 193–208. [CrossRef]
17. Huotari, J.; Helenius, A. Endosome maturation. *EMBO J.* **2011**, *30*, 3481–3500. [CrossRef]
18. Raposo, G.; Stoorvogel, W. Extracellular vesicles: Exosomes, microvesicles, and friends. *J. Cell Biol.* **2013**, *200*, 373–383. [CrossRef]
19. Wollert, T.; Hurley, J.H. Molecular mechanism of multivesicular body biogenesis by ESCRT complexes. *Nature* **2010**, *464*, 864–869. [CrossRef]
20. Henne, W.M.; Stenmark, H.; Emr, S.D. Molecular mechanisms of the membrane sculpting ESCRT pathway. *Cold Spring Harb. Perspect. Biol.* **2013**, *5*, a016766. [CrossRef]
21. Glickman, M.H.; Ciechanover, A. The ubiquitin-proteasome proteolytic pathway: Destruction for the sake of construction. *Physiol. Rev.* **2002**, *82*, 373–428. [CrossRef]
22. Mani, A.; Gelmann, E.P. The ubiquitin-proteasome pathway and its role in cancer. *J. Clin. Oncol.* **2005**, *23*, 4776–4789. [CrossRef]
23. Clifford, S.C.; Cockman, M.E.; Smallwood, A.C.; Mole, D.R.; Woodward, E.R.; Maxwell, P.H.; Ratcliffe, P.J.; Maher, E.R. Contrasting effects on HIF-1alpha regulation by disease-causing pVHL mutations correlate with patterns of tumourigenesis in von Hippel-Lindau disease. *Hum. Mol. Genet.* **2001**, *10*, 1029–1038. [CrossRef]
24. Hashizume, R.; Fukuda, M.; Maeda, I.; Nishikawa, H.; Oyake, D.; Yabuki, Y.; Ogata, H.; Ohta, T. The RING heterodimer BRCA1-BARD1 is a ubiquitin ligase inactivated by a breast cancer-derived mutation. *J. Biol. Chem.* **2001**, *276*, 14537–14540. [CrossRef] [PubMed]
25. Stuffers, S.; Sem Wegner, C.; Stenmark, H.; Brech, A. Multivesicular endosome biogenesis in the absence of ESCRTs. *Traffic* **2009**, *10*, 925–937. [CrossRef] [PubMed]
26. Wubbolts, R.; Leckie, R.S.; Veenhuizen, P.T.; Schwarzmann, G.; Mobius, W.; Hoernschemeyer, J.; Slot, J.W.; Geuze, H.J.; Stoorvogel, W. Proteomic and biochemical analyses of human B cell-derived exosomes. Potential implications for their function and multivesicular body formation. *J. Biol. Chem.* **2003**, *278*, 10963–10972. [CrossRef]
27. Trajkovic, K.; Hsu, C.; Chiantia, S.; Rajendran, L.; Wenzel, D.; Wieland, F.; Schwille, P.; Brugger, B.; Simons, M. Ceramide triggers budding of exosome vesicles into multivesicular endosomes. *Science* **2008**, *319*, 1244–1247. [CrossRef] [PubMed]
28. Mobius, W.; Ohno-Iwashita, Y.; van Donselaar, E.G.; Oorschot, V.M.; Shimada, Y.; Fujimoto, T.; Heijnen, H.F.; Geuze, H.J.; Slot, J.W. Immunoelectron microscopic localization of cholesterol using biotinylated and non-cytolytic perfringolysin O. *J. Histochem. Cytochem.* **2002**, *50*, 43–55. [CrossRef]
29. Baietti, M.F.; Zhang, Z.; Mortier, E.; Melchior, A.; Degeest, G.; Geeraerts, A.; Ivarsson, Y.; Depoortere, F.; Coomans, C.; Vermeiren, E.; et al. Syndecan-syntenin-ALIX regulates the biogenesis of exosomes. *Nat. Cell Biol.* **2012**, *14*, 677–685. [CrossRef]
30. Geminard, C.; De Gassart, A.; Blanc, L.; Vidal, M. Degradation of AP2 during reticulocyte maturation enhances binding of hsc70 and Alix to a common site on TFR for sorting into exosomes. *Traffic* **2004**, *5*, 181–193. [CrossRef]
31. Tamai, K.; Tanaka, N.; Nakano, T.; Kakazu, E.; Kondo, Y.; Inoue, J.; Shiina, M.; Fukushima, K.; Hoshino, T.; Sano, K.; et al. Exosome secretion of dendritic cells is regulated by Hrs, an ESCRT-0 protein. *Biochem. Biophys. Res. Commun.* **2010**, *399*, 384–390. [CrossRef] [PubMed]
32. Batagov, A.O.; Kuznetsov, V.A.; Kurochkin, I.V. Identification of nucleotide patterns enriched in secreted RNAs as putative cis-acting elements targeting them to exosome nano-vesicles. *BMC Genomics.* **2011**, *12*, S3–S18. [CrossRef] [PubMed]
33. Gibbings, D.J.; Ciaudo, C.; Erhardt, M.; Voinnet, O. Multivesicular bodies associate with components of miRNA effector complexes and modulate miRNA activity. *Nat. Cell. Biol.* **2009**, *11*, 1143–1149. [CrossRef] [PubMed]
34. Spaull, R.; McPherson, B.; Gialeli, A.; Clayton, A.; Uney, J.; Heep, A.; Cordero-Llana, O. Exosomes populate the cerebrospinal fluid of preterm infants with post-haemorrhagic hydrocephalus. *Int J. Dev. Neurosci.* **2019**, *73*, 59–65. [CrossRef] [PubMed]
35. Huleihel, L.; Hussey, G.S.; Naranjo, J.D.; Zhang, L.; Dziki, J.L.; Turner, N.J.; Stolz, D.B.; Badylak, S.F. Matrix-bound nanovesicles within ECM bioscaffolds. *Sci. Adv.* **2016**, *2*, e1600502. [CrossRef]

36. Zhuang, X.; Xiang, X.; Grizzle, W.; Sun, D.; Zhang, S.; Axtell, R.C.; Ju, S.; Mu, J.; Zhang, L.; Steinman, L. Treatment of brain inflammatory diseases by delivering exosome encapsulated anti-inflammatory drugs from the nasal region to the brain. *Mol. Ther.* **2011**, *19*, 1769–1779. [CrossRef]
37. Sung, B.H.; von Lersner, A.; Guerrero, J.; Krystofiak, E.S.; Inman, D.; Pelletier, R.; Zijlstra, A.; Ponik, S.M.; Weaver, A.M. A live cell reporter of exosome secretion and uptake reveals pathfinding behavior of migrating cells. *Nat. Commun.* **2020**, *11*, 2092. [CrossRef]
38. Tian, T.; Zhu, Y.L.; Zhou, Y.Y.; Liang, G.F.; Wang, Y.Y.; Hu, F.H.; Xiao, Z.D. Exosome uptake through clathrin—mediated endocytosis and macropinocytosis and mediating miR-21 delivery. *J. Biol. Chem.* **2014**, *289*, 22258–22267. [CrossRef]
39. Fitzner, D.; Schnaars, M.; van Rossum, D.; Krishnamoorthy, G.; Dibaj, P.; Bakhti, M.; Regen, T.; Hanisch, U.K.; Simons, M. Selective transfer of exosomes from oligodendrocytes to microglia by macropinocytosis. *J. Cell Sci.* **2011**, *124*, 447–458. [CrossRef]
40. Nanbo, A.; Kawanishi, E.; Yoshida, R.; Yoshiyama, H. Exosomes derived from Epstein-Barr virus-infected cells are internalized via caveola-dependent endocytosis and promote phenotypic modulation in target cells. *J. Virol.* **2013**, *87*, 10334–10347. [CrossRef]
41. Valapala, M.; Vishwanatha, J.K. Lipid raft endocytosis and exosomal transport facilitate extracellular trafficking of annexin A2. *J. Biol. Chem.* **2011**, *286*, 30911–30925. [CrossRef] [PubMed]
42. Bonsergent, E.; Lavieu, G. Content release of extracellular vesicles in a cell-free extract. *FEBS Lett.* **2019**, *593*, 1983–1992. [CrossRef] [PubMed]
43. Mincheva-Nilsson, L.; Baranov, V. Cancer exosomes and NKG2D receptor-ligand interactions: Impairing NKG2D-mediated cytotoxicity and anti-tumour immune surveillance. *Semin. Cancer Biol.* **2014**, *28*, 24–30. [CrossRef]
44. Thery, C.; Zitvogel, L.; Amigorena, S. Exosomes: Composition, biogenesis and function. *Nat. Rev. Immunol.* **2002**, *2*, 569–579. [CrossRef] [PubMed]
45. Imai, T.; Takahashi, Y.; Nishikawa, M.; Kato, K.; Morishita, M.; Yamashita, T.; Matsumoto, A.; Charoenviriyakul, C.; Takakura, Y. Macrophage-dependent clearance of systemically administered B16BL6-derived exosomes from the blood circulation in mice. *J. Extracell. Vesicles* **2015**, *4*, 26238. [CrossRef]
46. Maas, S.L.N.; Breakefield, X.O.; Weaver, A.M. Extracellular Vesicles: Unique Intercellular Delivery Vehicles. *Trends. Cell Biol.* **2017**, *27*, 172–188. [CrossRef] [PubMed]
47. Oushy, S.; Hellwinkel, J.E.; Wang, M.; Nguyen, G.J.; Gunaydin, D.; Harland, T.A.; Anchordoquy, T.J.; Graner, M.W. Glioblastoma multiforme-derived extracellular vesicles drive normal astrocytes towards a tumour-enhancing phenotype. *Philos. Trans. R. Soc. Lond. B. Biol. Sci.* **2018**, *373*, 200160477. [CrossRef]
48. Syn, N.; Wang, L.; Sethi, G.; Thiery, J.P.; Goh, B.C. Exosome-Mediated Metastasis: From Epithelial-Mesenchymal Transition to Escape from Immunosurveillance. *Trends. Pharmacol. Sci.* **2016**, *37*, 606–617. [CrossRef]
49. Sato, S.; Weaver, A.M. Extracellular vesicles: Important collaborators in cancer progression. *Essays. Biochem.* **2018**, *62*, 149–163.
50. Hoshino, D.; Kirkbride, K.C.; Costello, K.; Clark, E.S.; Sinha, S.; Grega-Larson, N.; Tyska, M.J.; Weaver, A.M. Exosome secretion is enhanced by invadopodia and drives invasive behavior. *Cell Rep.* **2013**, *5*, 1159–1168. [CrossRef]
51. Baroni, S.; Romero-Cordoba, S.; Plantamura, I.; Dugo, M.; D'ippolito, E.; Cataldo, A.; Cosentino, G.; Angeloni, V.; Rossini, A.; Daidone, M. Exosome-mediated delivery of miR-9 induces cancer-associated fibroblast-like properties in human breast fibroblasts. *Cell Death Dis.* **2016**, *7*, e2312. [CrossRef] [PubMed]
52. Webber, J.P.; Spary, L.K.; Sanders, A.J.; Chowdhury, R.; Jiang, W.G.; Steadman, R.; Wymant, J.; Jones, A.T.; Kynaston, H.; Mason, M.D.; et al. Differentiation of tumour-promoting stromal myofibroblasts by cancer exosomes. *Oncogene* **2015**, *34*, 290–302. [CrossRef] [PubMed]
53. Webber, J.; Steadman, R.; Mason, M.D.; Tabi, Z.; Clayton, A. Cancer exosomes trigger fibroblast to myofibroblast differentiation. *Cancer Res.* **2010**, *70*, 9621–9630. [CrossRef] [PubMed]
54. Luga, V.; Zhang, L.; Viloria-Petit, A.M.; Ogunjimi, A.A.; Inanlou, M.R.; Chiu, E.; Buchanan, M.; Hosein, A.N.; Basik, M.; Wrana, J.L. Exosomes mediate stromal mobilization of autocrine Wnt-PCP signaling in breast cancer cell migration. *Cell* **2012**, *151*, 1542–1556. [CrossRef] [PubMed]

55. Shimoda, M.; Principe, S.; Jackson, H.W.; Luga, V.; Fang, H.; Molyneux, S.D.; Shao, Y.W.; Aiken, A.; Waterhouse, P.D.; Karamboulas, C. Loss of the Timp gene family is sufficient for the acquisition of the CAF-like cell state. *Nat. Cell Biol.* **2014**, *16*, 889–901. [CrossRef] [PubMed]
56. Lazar, I.; Clement, E.; Dauvillier, S.; Milhas, D.; Ducoux-Petit, M.; LeGonidec, S.; Moro, C.; Soldan, V.; Dalle, S.; Balor, S. Adipocyte exosomes promote melanoma aggressiveness through fatty acid oxidation: A novel mechanism linking obesity and cancer. *Cancer Res.* **2016**, *76*, 4051–4057. [CrossRef] [PubMed]
57. Ribeiro, M.F.; Zhu, H.; Millard, R.W.; Fan, G.C. Exosomes Function in Pro- and Anti-Angiogenesis. *Curr. Angiogenes* **2013**, *2*, 54–59.
58. Carrasco-Ramírez, P.; Greening, D.W.; Andrés, G.; Gopal, S.K.; Martín-Villar, E.; Renart, J.; Simpson, R.J.; Quintanilla, M. Podoplanin is a component of extracellular vesicles that reprograms cell-derived exosomal proteins and modulates lymphatic vessel formation. *Oncotarget* **2016**, *7*, 16070. [CrossRef]
59. Umezu, T.; Ohyashiki, K.; Kuroda, M.; Ohyashiki, J. Leukemia cell to endothelial cell communication via exosomal miRNAs. *Oncogene* **2013**, *32*, 2747–2755. [CrossRef]
60. Schillaci, O.; Fontana, S.; Monteleone, F.; Taverna, S.; Di Bella, M.A.; Di Vizio, D.; Alessandro, R. Exosomes from metastatic cancer cells transfer amoeboid phenotype to non-metastatic cells and increase endothelial permeability: Their emerging role in tumor heterogeneity. *Sci. Rep.* **2017**, *7*, 1–15. [CrossRef]
61. Hsu, Y.L.; Hung, J.Y.; Chang, W.A.; Lin, Y.S.; Pan, Y.C.; Tsai, P.H.; Wu, C.Y.; Kuo, P.L. Hypoxic lung cancer-secreted exosomal miR-23a increased angiogenesis and vascular permeability by targeting prolyl hydroxylase and tight junction protein ZO-1. *Oncogene* **2017**, *36*, 4929–4942. [CrossRef] [PubMed]
62. Liu, Y.; Cao, X. Characteristics and Significance of the Pre-metastatic Niche. *Cancer Cell* **2016**, *30*, 668–681. [CrossRef] [PubMed]
63. Peinado, H.; Alečković, M.; Lavotshkin, S.; Matei, I.; Costa-Silva, B.; Moreno-Bueno, G.; Hergueta-Redondo, M.; Williams, C.; García-Santos, G.; Ghajar, C.M. Melanoma exosomes educate bone marrow progenitor cells toward a pro-metastatic phenotype through MET. *Nat. Med.* **2012**, *18*, 883–891. [CrossRef] [PubMed]
64. Costa-Silva, B.; Aiello, N.M.; Ocean, A.J.; Singh, S.; Zhang, H.; Thakur, B.K.; Becker, A.; Hoshino, A.; Mark, M.T.; Molina, H. Pancreatic cancer exosomes initiate pre-metastatic niche formation in the liver. *Nat. cell Biol.* **2015**, *17*, 816–826. [CrossRef]
65. Hoshino, A.; Costa-Silva, B.; Shen, T.-L.; Rodrigues, G.; Hashimoto, A.; Mark, M.T.; Molina, H.; Kohsaka, S.; Di Giannatale, A.; Ceder, S. Tumour exosome integrins determine organotropic metastasis. *Nature* **2015**, *527*, 329–335. [CrossRef]
66. Hood, J.L.; San, R.S.; Wickline, S.A. Exosomes released by melanoma cells prepare sentinel lymph nodes for tumor metastasis. *Cancer Res.* **2011**, *71*, 3792–3801. [CrossRef]
67. Plebanek, M.P.; Angeloni, N.L.; Vinokour, E.; Li, J.; Henkin, A.; Martinez-Marin, D.; Filleur, S.; Bhowmick, R.; Henkin, J.; Miller, S.D.; et al. Pre-metastatic cancer exosomes induce immune surveillance by patrolling monocytes at the metastatic niche. *Nat. Commun.* **2017**, *8*, 1319. [CrossRef]
68. Whiteside, T.L. Exosomes and tumor-mediated immune suppression. *J. Clin. Investig.* **2016**, *126*, 1216–1223. [CrossRef]
69. Clayton, A.; Mitchell, J.P.; Court, J.; Mason, M.D.; Tabi, Z. Human tumor-derived exosomes selectively impair lymphocyte responses to interleukin-2. *Cancer Res.* **2007**, *67*, 7458–7466. [CrossRef]
70. Clayton, A.; Mitchell, J.P.; Court, J.; Linnane, S.; Mason, M.D.; Tabi, Z. Human tumor-derived exosomes down-modulate NKG2D expression. *J. Immunol.* **2008**, *180*, 7249–7258. [CrossRef]
71. Zitvogel, L.; Regnault, A.; Lozier, A.; Wolfers, J.; Flament, C.; Tenza, D.; Ricciardi-Castagnoli, P.; Raposo, G.; Amigorena, S. Eradication of established murine tumors using a novel cell-free vaccine: Dendritic cell-derived exosomes. *Nat. Med.* **1998**, *4*, 594–600. [CrossRef] [PubMed]
72. Skokos, D.; Botros, H.G.; Demeure, C.; Morin, J.; Peronet, R.; Birkenmeier, G.; Boudaly, S.; Mecheri, S. Mast cell-derived exosomes induce phenotypic and functional maturation of dendritic cells and elicit specific immune responses in vivo. *J. Immunol.* **2003**, *170*, 3037–3045. [CrossRef] [PubMed]
73. Chen, W.X.; Liu, X.M.; Lv, M.M.; Chen, L.; Zhao, J.H.; Zhong, S.L.; Ji, M.H.; Hu, Q.; Luo, Z.; Wu, J.Z.; et al. Exosomes from drug-resistant breast cancer cells transmit chemoresistance by a horizontal transfer of microRNAs. *PLoS ONE* **2014**, *9*, e95240. [CrossRef] [PubMed]

74. Zeng, A.; Wei, Z.; Yan, W.; Yin, J.; Huang, X.; Zhou, X.; Li, R.; Shen, F.; Wu, W.; Wang, X. Exosomal transfer of miR-151a enhances chemosensitivity to temozolomide in drug-resistant glioblastoma. *Cancer Lett.* **2018**, *436*, 10–21. [CrossRef] [PubMed]
75. Federici, C.; Petrucci, F.; Caimi, S.; Cesolini, A.; Logozzi, M.; Borghi, M.; D'Ilio, S.; Lugini, L.; Violante, N.; Azzarito, T.; et al. Exosome release and low pH belong to a framework of resistance of human melanoma cells to cisplatin. *PLoS ONE* **2014**, *9*, e88193. [CrossRef] [PubMed]
76. Hu, Y.; Yan, C.; Mu, L.; Huang, K.; Li, X.; Tao, D.; Wu, Y.; Qin, J. Fibroblast-Derived Exosomes Contribute to Chemoresistance through Priming Cancer Stem Cells in Colorectal Cancer. *PLoS ONE* **2015**, *10*, e0125625. [CrossRef]
77. Boelens, M.C.; Wu, T.J.; Nabet, B.Y.; Xu, B.; Qiu, Y.; Yoon, T.; Azzam, D.J.; Twyman-Saint Victor, C.; Wiemann, B.Z.; Ishwaran, H.; et al. Exosome transfer from stromal to breast cancer cells regulates therapy resistance pathways. *Cell* **2014**, *159*, 499–513. [CrossRef]
78. Thery, C.; Amigorena, S.; Raposo, G.; Clayton, A. Isolation and characterization of exosomes from cell culture supernatants and biological fluids. *Curr. Protoc. Cell Biol.* **2006**, *30*, 3.22.1–3.22.29. [CrossRef]
79. Tauro, B.J.; Greening, D.W.; Mathias, R.A.; Ji, H.; Mathivanan, S.; Scott, A.M.; Simpson, R.J. Comparison of ultracentrifugation, density gradient separation, and immunoaffinity capture methods for isolating human colon cancer cell line LIM1863-derived exosomes. *Methods* **2012**, *56*, 293–304. [CrossRef]
80. Taylor, D.D.; Shah, S. Methods of isolating extracellular vesicles impact down-stream analyses of their cargoes. *Methods* **2015**, *87*, 3–10. [CrossRef]
81. Riahi, R.; Shaegh, S.A.; Ghaderi, M.; Zhang, Y.S.; Shin, S.R.; Aleman, J.; Massa, S.; Kim, D.; Dokmeci, M.R.; Khademhosseini, A. Automated microfluidic platform of bead-based electrochemical immunosensor integrated with bioreactor for continual monitoring of cell secreted biomarkers. *Sci. Rep.* **2016**, *6*, 24598. [CrossRef] [PubMed]
82. Kaddour, H.; Lyu, Y.; Shouman, N.; Mohan, M.; Okeoma, C.M. Development of Novel High-Resolution Size-Guided Turbidimetry-Enabled Particle Purification Liquid Chromatography (PPLC): Extracellular Vesicles and Membraneless Condensates in Focus. *Int. J. Mol. Sci* **2020**, *21*, 5361. [CrossRef] [PubMed]
83. Doldan, X.; Fagundez, P.; Cayota, A.; Laiz, J.; Tosar, J.P. Electrochemical Sandwich Immunosensor for Determination of Exosomes Based on Surface Marker-Mediated Signal Amplification. *Anal. Chem.* **2016**, *88*, 10466–10473. [CrossRef] [PubMed]
84. Miller, M.C.; Doyle, G.V.; Terstappen, L.W. Significance of Circulating Tumor Cells Detected by the CellSearch System in Patients with Metastatic Breast Colorectal and Prostate Cancer. *J. Oncol.* **2010**, *2010*, 617421. [CrossRef] [PubMed]
85. Yu, M.; Stott, S.; Toner, M.; Maheswaran, S.; Haber, D.A. Circulating tumor cells: Approaches to isolation and characterization. *J. Cell Biol.* **2011**, *192*, 373–382. [CrossRef]
86. Wan, J.C.M.; Massie, C.; Garcia-Corbacho, J.; Mouliere, F.; Brenton, J.D.; Caldas, C.; Pacey, S.; Baird, R.; Rosenfeld, N. Liquid biopsies come of age: Towards implementation of circulating tumour DNA. *Nat. Rev. Cancer* **2017**, *17*, 223–238. [CrossRef] [PubMed]
87. Heitzer, E.; Ulz, P.; Geigl, J.B. Circulating tumor DNA as a liquid biopsy for cancer. *Clin. Chem.* **2015**, *61*, 112–123. [CrossRef]
88. Figueroa, J.M.; Skog, J.; Akers, J.; Li, H.; Komotar, R.; Jensen, R.; Ringel, F.; Yang, I.; Kalkanis, S.; Thompson, R.; et al. Detection of wild-type EGFR amplification and EGFRvIII mutation in CSF-derived extracellular vesicles of glioblastoma patients. *Neuro. Oncol.* **2017**, *19*, 1494–1502. [CrossRef]
89. Pisitkun, T.; Shen, R.F.; Knepper, M.A. Identification and proteomic profiling of exosomes in human urine. *Proc. Natl. Acad. Sci. USA* **2004**, *101*, 13368–13373. [CrossRef]
90. Chung, I.M.; Rajakumar, G.; Venkidasamy, B.; Subramanian, U.; Thiruvengadam, M. Exosomes: Current use and future applications. *Clin. Chim. Acta.* **2020**, *500*, 226–232. [CrossRef]
91. Jalalian, S.H.; Ramezani, M.; Jalalian, S.A.; Abnous, K.; Taghdisi, S.M. Exosomes, new biomarkers in early cancer detection. *Anal. Biochem.* **2019**, *571*, 1–13. [CrossRef] [PubMed]
92. Logozzi, M.; De Milito, A.; Lugini, L.; Borghi, M.; Calabro, L.; Spada, M.; Perdicchio, M.; Marino, M.L.; Federici, C.; Iessi, E.; et al. High levels of exosomes expressing CD63 and caveolin-1 in plasma of melanoma patients. *PLoS ONE* **2009**, *4*, e5219. [CrossRef] [PubMed]

93. Qu, J.L.; Qu, X.J.; Zhao, M.F.; Teng, Y.E.; Zhang, Y.; Hou, K.Z.; Jiang, Y.H.; Yang, X.H.; Liu, Y.P. Gastric cancer exosomes promote tumour cell proliferation through PI3K/Akt and MAPK/ERK activation. *Dig. Liver. Dis.* **2009**, *41*, 875–880. [CrossRef] [PubMed]
94. Yang, L.; Wu, X.H.; Wang, D.; Luo, C.L.; Chen, L.X. Bladder cancer cell-derived exosomes inhibit tumor cell apoptosis and induce cell proliferation in vitro. *Mol. Med. Rep.* **2013**, *8*, 1272–1278. [CrossRef] [PubMed]
95. Sento, S.; Sasabe, E.; Yamamoto, T. Application of a Persistent Heparin Treatment Inhibits the Malignant Potential of Oral Squamous Carcinoma Cells Induced by Tumor Cell-Derived Exosomes. *PLoS ONE* **2016**, *11*, e0148454. [CrossRef] [PubMed]
96. Smalley, D.M.; Sheman, N.E.; Nelson, K.; Theodorescu, D. Isolation and identification of potential urinary microparticle biomarkers of bladder cancer. *J. Proteome Res.* **2008**, *7*, 2088–2096. [CrossRef]
97. Nilsson, J.; Skog, J.; Nordstrand, A.; Baranov, V.; Mincheva-Nilsson, L.; Breakefield, X.O.; Widmark, A. Prostate cancer-derived urine exosomes: A novel approach to biomarkers for prostate cancer. *Br. J. Cancer* **2009**, *100*, 1603–1607. [CrossRef]
98. Skog, J.; Wurdinger, T.; van Rijn, S.; Meijer, D.H.; Gainche, L.; Sena-Esteves, M.; Curry, W.T., Jr.; Carter, B.S.; Krichevsky, A.M.; Breakefield, X.O. Glioblastoma microvesicles transport RNA and proteins that promote tumour growth and provide diagnostic biomarkers. *Nat. Cell Biol.* **2008**, *10*, 1470–1476. [CrossRef]
99. Khan, S.; Jutzy, J.M.; Valenzuela, M.M.; Turay, D.; Aspe, J.R.; Ashok, A.; Mirshahidi, S.; Mercola, D.; Lilly, M.B.; Wall, N.R. Plasma-derived exosomal survivin, a plausible biomarker for early detection of prostate cancer. *PLoS ONE* **2012**, *7*, e46737. [CrossRef]
100. McKiernan, J.; Donovan, M.J.; Margolis, E.; Partin, A.; Carter, B.; Brown, G.; Torkler, P.; Noerholm, M.; Skog, J.; Shore, N.; et al. A Prospective Adaptive Utility Trial to Validate Performance of a Novel Urine Exosome Gene Expression Assay to Predict High-grade Prostate Cancer in Patients with Prostate-specific Antigen 2–10 ng/mL at Initial Biopsy. *Eur. Urol.* **2018**, *74*, 731–738. [CrossRef]
101. Li, Q.; Shao, Y.; Zhang, X.; Zheng, T.; Miao, M.; Qin, L.; Wang, B.; Ye, G.; Xiao, B.; Guo, J. Plasma long noncoding RNA protected by exosomes as a potential stable biomarker for gastric cancer. *Tumour. Biol.* **2015**, *36*, 2007–2012. [CrossRef] [PubMed]
102. Taylor, D.D.; Gercel-Taylor, C. MicroRNA signatures of tumor-derived exosomes as diagnostic biomarkers of ovarian cancer. *Gynecol. Oncol.* **2008**, *110*, 13–21. [CrossRef] [PubMed]
103. Rabinowits, G.; Gercel-Taylor, C.; Day, J.M.; Taylor, D.D.; Kloecker, G.H. Exosomal microRNA: A diagnostic marker for lung cancer. *Clin. Lung Cancer* **2009**, *10*, 42–46. [CrossRef] [PubMed]
104. Allenson, K.; Castillo, J.; San Lucas, F.A.; Scelo, G.; Kim, D.U.; Bernard, V.; Davis, G.; Kumar, T.; Katz, M.; Overman, M.J.; et al. High prevalence of mutant KRAS in circulating exosome-derived DNA from early-stage pancreatic cancer patients. *Ann. Oncol.* **2017**, *28*, 741–747. [CrossRef]
105. Castellanos-Rizaldos, E.; Grimm, D.G.; Tadigotla, V.; Hurley, J.; Healy, J.; Neal, P.L.; Sher, M.; Venkatesan, R.; Karlovich, C.; Raponi, M.; et al. Exosome-Based Detection of EGFR T790M in Plasma from Non-Small Cell Lung Cancer Patients. *Clin. Cancer Res.* **2018**, *24*, 2944–2950. [CrossRef]
106. Yang, S.; Che, S.P.; Kurywchak, P.; Tavormina, J.L.; Gansmo, L.B.; Correa de Sampaio, P.; Tachezy, M.; Bockhorn, M.; Gebauer, F.; Haltom, A.R.; et al. Detection of mutant KRAS and TP53 DNA in circulating exosomes from healthy individuals and patients with pancreatic cancer. *Cancer Biol. Ther.* **2017**, *18*, 158–165. [CrossRef]
107. Garcia-Silva, S.; Benito-Martin, A.; Sanchez-Redondo, S.; Hernandez-Barranco, A.; Ximenez-Embun, P.; Nogues, L.; Mazariegos, M.S.; Brinkmann, K.; Amor Lopez, A.; Meyer, L.; et al. Use of extracellular vesicles from lymphatic drainage as surrogate markers of melanoma progression and BRAF (V600E) mutation. *J. Exp. Med.* **2019**, *216*, 1061–1070. [CrossRef]
108. Zhao, X.; Wu, D.; Ma, X.; Wang, J.; Hou, W.; Zhang, W. Exosomes as drug carriers for cancer therapy and challenges regarding exosome uptake. *Biomed. Pharmacother.* **2020**, *128*, 110237. [CrossRef]
109. Hu, Q.; Su, H.; Li, J.; Lyon, C.; Tang, W.; Wan, M.; Hu, T.Y. Clinical applications of exosome membrane proteins. *Precis. Clin. Med.* **2020**, *3*, 54–66. [CrossRef]
110. Johnsen, K.B.; Gudbergsson, J.M.; Skov, M.N.; Pilgaard, L.; Moos, T.; Duroux, M. A comprehensive overview of exosomes as drug delivery vehicles—endogenous nanocarriers for targeted cancer therapy. *Biochim. Biophys. Acta.* **2014**, *1846*, 75–87. [CrossRef]

111. Jaiswal, S.; Jamieson, C.H.; Pang, W.W.; Park, C.Y.; Chao, M.P.; Majeti, R.; Traver, D.; van Rooijen, N.; Weissman, I.L. CD47 is upregulated on circulating hematopoietic stem cells and leukemia cells to avoid phagocytosis. *Cell* **2009**, *138*, 271–285. [CrossRef] [PubMed]
112. Haney, M.J.; Klyachko, N.L.; Zhao, Y.; Gupta, R.; Plotnikova, E.G.; He, Z.; Patel, T.; Piroyan, A.; Sokolsky, M.; Kabanov, A.V.; et al. Exosomes as drug delivery vehicles for Parkinson's disease therapy. *J. Control. Release* **2015**, *207*, 18–30. [CrossRef] [PubMed]
113. Kim, M.S.; Haney, M.J.; Zhao, Y.; Mahajan, V.; Deygen, I.; Klyachko, N.L.; Inskoe, E.; Piroyan, A.; Sokolsky, M.; Okolie, O.; et al. Development of exosome-encapsulated paclitaxel to overcome MDR in cancer cells. *Nanomedicine* **2016**, *12*, 655–664. [CrossRef] [PubMed]
114. Pascucci, L.; Cocce, V.; Bonomi, A.; Ami, D.; Ceccarelli, P.; Ciusani, E.; Vigano, L.; Locatelli, A.; Sisto, F.; Doglia, S.M.; et al. Paclitaxel is incorporated by mesenchymal stromal cells and released in exosomes that inhibit in vitro tumor growth: A new approach for drug delivery. *J. Control. Release* **2014**, *192*, 262–270. [CrossRef] [PubMed]
115. Ding, Y.; Cao, F.; Sun, H.; Wang, Y.; Liu, S.; Wu, Y.; Cui, Q.; Mei, W.; Li, F. Exosomes derived from human umbilical cord mesenchymal stromal cells deliver exogenous miR-145-5p to inhibit pancreatic ductal adenocarcinoma progression. *Cancer Lett.* **2019**, *442*, 351–361. [CrossRef]
116. Sterzenbach, U.; Putz, U.; Low, L.H.; Silke, J.; Tan, S.S.; Howitt, J. Engineered Exosomes as Vehicles for Biologically Active Proteins. *Mol. Ther.* **2017**, *25*, 1269–1278. [CrossRef]
117. Sato, Y.T.; Umezaki, K.; Sawada, S.; Mukai, S.A.; Sasaki, Y.; Harada, N.; Shiku, H.; Akiyoshi, K. Engineering hybrid exosomes by membrane fusion with liposomes. *Sci Rep.* **2016**, *6*, 21933. [CrossRef]
118. Lee, J.; Kim, J.; Jeong, M.; Lee, H.; Goh, U.; Kim, H.; Kim, B.; Park, J.H. Liposome-based engineering of cells to package hydrophobic compounds in membrane vesicles for tumor penetration. *Nano Lett.* **2015**, *15*, 2938–2944. [CrossRef]
119. Kalimuthu, S.; Gangadaran, P.; Rajendran, R.L.; Zhu, L.; Oh, J.M.; Lee, H.W.; Gopal, A.; Baek, S.H.; Jeong, S.Y.; Lee, S.W.; et al. A New Approach for Loading Anticancer Drugs Into Mesenchymal Stem Cell-Derived Exosome Mimetics for Cancer Therapy. *Front. Pharmacol.* **2018**, *9*, 1116. [CrossRef]
120. Saari, H.; Lázaro-Ibáñez, E.; Viitala, T.; Vuorimaa-Laukkanen, E.; Siljander, P.; Yliperttula, M. Microvesicle-and exosome-mediated drug delivery enhances the cytotoxicity of Paclitaxel in autologous prostate cancer cells. *J. Control. Release* **2015**, *220*, 727–737. [CrossRef]
121. Jang, S.C.; Kim, O.Y.; Yoon, C.M.; Choi, D.S.; Roh, T.Y.; Park, J.; Nilsson, J.; Lotvall, J.; Kim, Y.K.; Gho, Y.S. Bioinspired exosome-mimetic nanovesicles for targeted delivery of chemotherapeutics to malignant tumors. *ACS Nano* **2013**, *7*, 7698–7710. [CrossRef] [PubMed]
122. Tian, Y.; Li, S.; Song, J.; Ji, T.; Zhu, M.; Anderson, G.J.; Wei, J.; Nie, G. A doxorubicin delivery platform using engineered natural membrane vesicle exosomes for targeted tumor therapy. *Biomaterials* **2014**, *35*, 2383–2390. [CrossRef] [PubMed]
123. Tang, K.; Zhang, Y.; Zhang, H.; Xu, P.; Liu, J.; Ma, J.; Lv, M.; Li, D.; Katirai, F.; Shen, G.X.; et al. Delivery of chemotherapeutic drugs in tumour cell-derived microparticles. *Nat. Commun.* **2012**, *3*, 1282. [CrossRef] [PubMed]
124. Osterman, C.J.; Lynch, J.C.; Leaf, P.; Gonda, A.; Ferguson Bennit, H.R.; Griffiths, D.; Wall, N.R. Curcumin Modulates Pancreatic Adenocarcinoma Cell-Derived Exosomal Function. *PLoS ONE* **2015**, *10*, e0132845. [CrossRef] [PubMed]
125. Fu, H.; Yang, H.; Zhang, X.; Wang, B.; Mao, J.; Li, X.; Wang, M.; Zhang, B.; Sun, Z.; Qian, H.; et al. Exosomal TRIM3 is a novel marker and therapy target for gastric cancer. *J. Exp. Clin. Cancer Res.* **2018**, *37*, 162. [CrossRef] [PubMed]
126. Mizrak, A.; Bolukbasi, M.F.; Ozdener, G.B.; Brenner, G.J.; Madlener, S.; Erkan, E.P.; Strobel, T.; Breakefield, X.O.; Saydam, O. Genetically engineered microvesicles carrying suicide mRNA/protein inhibit schwannoma tumor growth. *Mol. Ther.* **2013**, *21*, 101–108. [CrossRef]
127. Rivoltini, L.; Chiodoni, C.; Squarcina, P.; Tortoreto, M.; Villa, A.; Vergani, B.; Burdek, M.; Botti, L.; Arioli, I.; Cova, A.; et al. TNF-Related Apoptosis-Inducing Ligand (TRAIL)-Armed Exosomes Deliver Proapoptotic Signals to Tumor Site. *Clin. Cancer Res.* **2016**, *22*, 3499–3512. [CrossRef]

128. Andre, F.; Chaput, N.; Schartz, N.E.; Flament, C.; Aubert, N.; Bernard, J.; Lemonnier, F.; Raposo, G.; Escudier, B.; Hsu, D.H.; et al. Exosomes as potent cell-free peptide-based vaccine. I. Dendritic cell-derived exosomes transfer functional MHC class I/peptide complexes to dendritic cells. *J. Immunol.* **2004**, *172*, 2126–2136. [CrossRef]
129. Xie, Y.; Bai, O.; Zhang, H.; Yuan, J.; Zong, S.; Chibbar, R.; Slattery, K.; Qureshi, M.; Wei, Y.; Deng, Y.; et al. Membrane-bound HSP70-engineered myeloma cell-derived exosomes stimulate more efficient CD8(+) CTL- and NK-mediated antitumour immunity than exosomes released from heat-shocked tumour cells expressing cytoplasmic HSP70. *J. Cell Mol. Med.* **2010**, *14*, 2655–2666. [CrossRef]
130. Kooijmans, S.A.; Aleza, C.G.; Roffler, S.R.; van Solinge, W.W.; Vader, P.; Schiffelers, R.M. Display of GPI-anchored anti-EGFR nanobodies on extracellular vesicles promotes tumour cell targeting. *J. Extracell. Vesicles* **2016**, *5*, 31053. [CrossRef]
131. Koh, E.; Lee, E.J.; Nam, G.H.; Hong, Y.; Cho, E.; Yang, Y.; Kim, I.S. Exosome-SIRPalpha, a CD47 blockade increases cancer cell phagocytosis. *Biomaterials* **2017**, *121*, 121–129. [CrossRef] [PubMed]
132. Ohno, S.; Takanashi, M.; Sudo, K.; Ueda, S.; Ishikawa, A.; Matsuyama, N.; Fujita, K.; Mizutani, T.; Ohgi, T.; Ochiya, T.; et al. Systemically injected exosomes targeted to EGFR deliver antitumor microRNA to breast cancer cells. *Mol. Ther.* **2013**, *21*, 185–191. [CrossRef]
133. Katakowski, M.; Buller, B.; Zheng, X.; Lu, Y.; Rogers, T.; Osobamiro, O.; Shu, W.; Jiang, F.; Chopp, M. Exosomes from marrow stromal cells expressing miR-146b inhibit glioma growth. *Cancer Lett.* **2013**, *335*, 201–204. [CrossRef] [PubMed]
134. Lou, G.; Song, X.; Yang, F.; Wu, S.; Wang, J.; Chen, Z.; Liu, Y. Exosomes derived from miR-122-modified adipose tissue-derived MSCs increase chemosensitivity of hepatocellular carcinoma. *J. Hematol. Oncol.* **2015**, *8*, 122. [CrossRef] [PubMed]
135. Wang, F.; Li, L.; Piontek, K.; Sakaguchi, M.; Selaru, F.M. Exosome miR-335 as a novel therapeutic strategy in hepatocellular carcinoma. *Hepatology* **2018**, *67*, 940–954. [CrossRef] [PubMed]
136. O'Brien, K.P.; Khan, S.; Gilligan, K.E.; Zafar, H.; Lalor, P.; Glynn, C.; O'Flatharta, C.; Ingoldsby, H.; Dockery, P.; De Bhulbh, A.; et al. Employing mesenchymal stem cells to support tumor-targeted delivery of extracellular vesicle (EV)-encapsulated microRNA-379. *Oncogene* **2018**, *37*, 2137–2149. [CrossRef] [PubMed]
137. Zeng, Z.; Li, Y.; Pan, Y.; Lan, X.; Song, F.; Sun, J.; Zhou, K.; Liu, X.; Ren, X.; Wang, F.; et al. Cancer-derived exosomal miR-25-3p promotes pre-metastatic niche formation by inducing vascular permeability and angiogenesis. *Nat. Commun.* **2018**, *9*, 5395. [CrossRef]
138. Greco, K.A.; Franzen, C.A.; Foreman, K.E.; Flanigan, R.C.; Kuo, P.C.; Gupta, G.N. PLK-1 Silencing in Bladder Cancer by siRNA Delivered With Exosomes. *Urology* **2016**, *91*, e1–e7. [CrossRef]
139. Li, H.; Yang, C.; Shi, Y.; Zhao, L. Exosomes derived from siRNA against GRP78 modified bone-marrow-derived mesenchymal stem cells suppress Sorafenib resistance in hepatocellular carcinoma. *J. Nanobiotechnol.* **2018**, *16*, 103. [CrossRef]
140. Shokrollahi, E.; Nourazarian, A.; Rahbarghazi, R.; Salimi, L.; Karbasforush, S.; Khaksar, M.; Salarinasab, S.; Abhari, A.; Heidarzadeh, M. Treatment of human neuroblastoma cell line SH-SY5Y with HSP27 siRNA tagged-exosomes decreased differentiation rate into mature neurons. *J. Cell Physiol.* **2019**, *234*, 21005–21013. [CrossRef]
141. Usman, W.M.; Pham, T.C.; Kwok, Y.Y.; Vu, L.T.; Ma, V.; Peng, B.; Chan, Y.S.; Wei, L.; Chin, S.M.; Azad, A.; et al. Efficient RNA drug delivery using red blood cell extracellular vesicles. *Nat. Commun.* **2018**, *9*, 2359. [CrossRef] [PubMed]
142. Yang, Z.; Shi, J.; Xie, J.; Wang, Y.; Sun, J.; Liu, T.; Zhao, Y.; Zhao, X.; Wang, X.; Ma, Y.; et al. Large-scale generation of functional mRNA-encapsulating exosomes via cellular nanoporation. *Nat. Biomed. Eng.* **2020**, *4*, 69–83. [CrossRef] [PubMed]
143. Mao, L.; Li, X.; Gong, S.; Yuan, H.; Jiang, Y.; Huang, W.; Sun, X.; Dang, X. Serum exosomes contain ECRG4 mRNA that suppresses tumor growth via inhibition of genes involved in inflammation, cell proliferation, and angiogenesis. *Cancer Gene Ther.* **2018**, *25*, 248–259. [CrossRef] [PubMed]
144. Ell, B.; Mercatali, L.; Ibrahim, T.; Campbell, N.; Schwarzenbach, H.; Pantel, K.; Amadori, D.; Kang, Y. Tumor-induced osteoclast miRNA changes as regulators and biomarkers of osteolytic bone metastasis. *Cancer Cell* **2013**, *24*, 542–556. [CrossRef] [PubMed]

145. Yang, L.; Zhang, L.; Lu, L.; Wang, Y. lncRNA UCA1 Increases Proliferation and Multidrug Resistance of Retinoblastoma Cells Through Downregulating miR-513a-5p. *DNA Cell Biol.* **2020**, *39*, 69–77. [CrossRef] [PubMed]
146. Syn, N.L.; Wang, L.; Chow, E.K.; Lim, C.T.; Goh, B.C. Exosomes in Cancer Nanomedicine and Immunotherapy: Prospects and Challenges. *Trends Biotechnol.* **2017**, *35*, 665–676. [CrossRef] [PubMed]
147. Munich, S.; Sobo-Vujanovic, A.; Buchser, W.J.; Beer-Stolz, D.; Vujanovic, N.L. Dendritic cell exosomes directly kill tumor cells and activate natural killer cells via TNF superfamily ligands. *Oncoimmunology* **2012**, *1*, 1074–1083. [CrossRef]
148. Viaud, S.; Terme, M.; Flament, C.; Taieb, J.; Andre, F.; Novault, S.; Escudier, B.; Robert, C.; Caillat-Zucman, S.; Tursz, T.; et al. Dendritic cell-derived exosomes promote natural killer cell activation and proliferation: A role for NKG2D ligands and IL-15Ralpha. *PLoS ONE* **2009**, *4*, e4942. [CrossRef]
149. Viaud, S.; Ploix, S.; Lapierre, V.; Thery, C.; Commere, P.H.; Tramalloni, D.; Gorrichon, K.; Virault-Rocroy, P.; Tursz, T.; Lantz, O.; et al. Updated technology to produce highly immunogenic dendritic cell-derived exosomes of clinical grade: A critical role of interferon-gamma. *J. Immunother.* **2011**, *34*, 65–75. [CrossRef]
150. Damo, M.; Wilson, D.S.; Simeoni, E.; Hubbell, J.A. TLR-3 stimulation improves anti-tumor immunity elicited by dendritic cell exosome-based vaccines in a murine model of melanoma. *Sci. Rep.* **2015**, *5*, 17622. [CrossRef]
151. Besse, B.; Charrier, M.; Lapierre, V.; Dansin, E.; Lantz, O.; Planchard, D.; Le Chevalier, T.; Livartoski, A.; Barlesi, F.; Laplanche, A.; et al. Dendritic cell-derived exosomes as maintenance immunotherapy after first line chemotherapy in NSCLC. *Oncoimmunology* **2016**, *5*, e1071008. [CrossRef] [PubMed]
152. Naslund, T.I.; Gehrmann, U.; Qazi, K.R.; Karlsson, M.C.; Gabrielsson, S. Dendritic cell-derived exosomes need to activate both T and B cells to induce antitumor immunity. *J. Immunol.* **2013**, *190*, 2712–2719. [CrossRef] [PubMed]
153. Hiltbrunner, S.; Larssen, P.; Eldh, M.; Martinez-Bravo, M.J.; Wagner, A.K.; Karlsson, M.C.; Gabrielsson, S. Exosomal cancer immunotherapy is independent of MHC molecules on exosomes. *Oncotarget* **2016**, *7*, 38707–38717. [CrossRef] [PubMed]
154. Pitt, J.M.; Andre, F.; Amigorena, S.; Soria, J.C.; Eggermont, A.; Kroemer, G.; Zitvogel, L. Dendritic cell-derived exosomes for cancer therapy. *J. Clin. Investig.* **2016**, *126*, 1224–1232. [CrossRef] [PubMed]
155. Srinivasan, S.; Vannberg, F.O.; Dixon, J.B. Lymphatic transport of exosomes as a rapid route of information dissemination to the lymph node. *Sci. Rep.* **2016**, *6*, 24436. [CrossRef] [PubMed]
156. Fu, W.; Lei, C.; Liu, S.; Cui, Y.; Wang, C.; Qian, K.; Li, T.; Shen, Y.; Fan, X.; Lin, F.; et al. CAR exosomes derived from effector CAR-T cells have potent antitumour effects and low toxicity. *Nat. Commun.* **2019**, *10*, 4355. [CrossRef]
157. Vafaizadeh, V.; Barekati, Z. Immuno-Oncology Biomarkers for Personalized Immunotherapy in Breast Cancer. *Front. Cell Dev. Biol.* **2020**, *8*, 162. [CrossRef]
158. Dai, L.J.; Moniri, M.R.; Zeng, Z.R.; Zhou, J.X.; Rayat, J.; Warnock, G.L. Potential implications of mesenchymal stem cells in cancer therapy. *Cancer Lett.* **2011**, *305*, 8–20. [CrossRef]
159. Kim, H.S.; Choi, D.Y.; Yun, S.J.; Choi, S.M.; Kang, J.W.; Jung, J.W.; Hwang, D.; Kim, K.P.; Kim, D.W. Proteomic analysis of microvesicles derived from human mesenchymal stem cells. *J. Proteome Res.* **2012**, *11*, 839–849. [CrossRef]

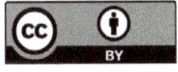

© 2020 by the authors. Licensee MDPI, Basel, Switzerland. This article is an open access article distributed under the terms and conditions of the Creative Commons Attribution (CC BY) license (http://creativecommons.org/licenses/by/4.0/).

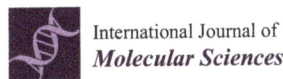

Review

Diagnostic and Therapeutic Applications of Exosomes in Cancer with a Special Focus on Head and Neck Squamous Cell Carcinoma (HNSCC)

Eliane Ebnoether [1,2] and Laurent Muller [1,2,*]

1 Department of Biomedicine, University of Basel, 4031 Basel, Switzerland; Eliane.Ebnoether@usb.ch
2 Department of Otorhinolaryngology, Head and Neck Surgery, University Hospital of Basel, 4051 Basel, Switzerland
* Correspondence: laurent.muller@usb.ch

Received: 18 May 2020; Accepted: 12 June 2020; Published: 18 June 2020

Abstract: Exosomes are nanovesicles part of a recently described intercellular communication system. Their properties seem promising as a biomarker in cancer research, where more sensitive monitoring and therapeutic applications are desperately needed. In the case of head and neck squamous cell carcinoma (HNSCC), overall survival often remains poor, although huge technological advancements in the treatment of this disease have been made. In the following review, diagnostic and therapeutic properties are highlighted and summarised. Impressive first results have been obtained but more research is needed to implement these innovative techniques into daily clinical routines.

Keywords: head and neck squamous cell carcinoma (HNSCC); exosomes; cancer; biomarker; diagnostic; therapy; liquid biopsy

1. Introduction

After the discovery of exosomes decades ago, they have moved into spotlight for various applications. Their potential as promising biomarkers, especially in cancer, has led to new research approaches making personalised medicine more reachable. In the field of head and neck cancer, biomarkers that simplify diagnosis and treatment are scarce.

Head and neck cancer is the sixth leading cancer by incidence worldwide with a poor five-year overall survival rate of 50% [1]. More than 90% are histologically head and neck squamous cell carcinoma (HNSCC). Although progress has been made and therapies have been enhanced, survival rate has not improved significantly. Eventually a lot of patients die due to metastasis and recurrences.

As diagnosis is tedious, needing a lot of clinical experience as well as resources, and the available therapies are toxic and have a huge impact on quality of life, validated biomarkers would support treatment stratification with improved outcome and reduced toxicity.

In this review, interaction within the immune system, potential diagnostic and therapeutic applications of exosomes with focus on HNSCC are highlighted. Changes of exosomal levels with cancer, under radiation and chemotherapy are discussed and therapeutic options like vaccination, immunomodulation and elimination are studied.

2. Intercellular Communication by Exosomes

The first descriptions of exosomes date back more than 30 years. In 1983, a study group discovered the "blebbing" of membranes from transferrin into red blood cells due to maturation of reticulocytes [2]. It was only later that the term exosome was born to describe this "blebbing".

Exosomes were largely dismissed as means of cellular waste and had fallen into oblivion for many decades. Things changed when their ability for intercellular communication, interaction with the immune system and possible use as a vector of drugs were identified [3]. To date, the exact definition of exosomes has led to a lot of discussions. Different types of vesicles, such as exosomes, extracellular vesicles (EVs) and microvesicles (MVs), have been used to describe similar properties intermixing. Up to now, differences between them and exact functions have not been universally defined [4]. The current opinion describes exosomes as double layered nanovesicles (30–50 nm) originating from the endosomal pathway, thus carrying, for example, tsg101 as a typical marker. They are released by all cell types of the body and are present in extracellular spaces and liquids (e.g., blood, saliva, urine) [5]. They can be directly visualised by electron microscopy (see Figure 1). As seen in Figure 1, differential centrifugation and size-exclusion chromatography, usually yields exosomes of different sizes. Typical surface markers are tetraspanins (CD9, CD63, CD81) and Rab proteins (Ras-related in brain) [6].

Exosomes could be compared to hemerodromes in ancient Greece. Pheidippides is said to be the first marathon runner and covered around 240 km in two days to ask for military support in the fight of Marathon. Exosomes are, like Pheidippides, a messenger system allowing intercellular communication. After this huge run, the hemerodrome Pheidippides is said to have collapsed and died [7]. This ancient story may compare to exosomes that are mostly used up after transmission of the message.

Cancer cells especially are thought to use this communication system avidly. As such, they are known to massively produce exosomes, called tumour-derived exosomes (TEX). During their formation, they acquire lipids, nucleic acids and proteins from the parental cell [8]. Thakur discovered in 2014 the representation of the whole cancer genomic DNA in exosomes [9]. TEX carry double-stranded DNA representing the entire genome and reflecting the mutational status of parental tumour cells. From our own results and that of others, we know that exosomes are able to interact with immune cells and assist in tumour immune escape [10,11]. TEX take part in the development, progression and response to treatment in cancer by alternating intercellular communication.

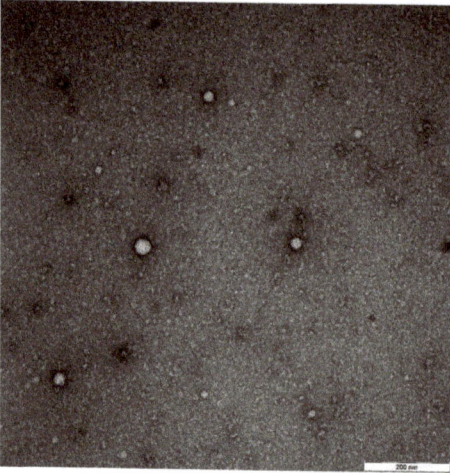

Figure 1. Representative electron microscopy picture by negative staining showing their typical appearance and size range. The exosomes were isolated as described previously from the plasma of a head and neck squamous cell carcinoma (HNSCC) patient [11].

Because of the described properties above, exosomes are ideal candidates to be used as biomarkers and for implementation in new cancer therapies.

3. Exosomes in Cancer

Exosomes have gained attention in various cancer types as possible biomarkers. In pancreatic cancer RNA, proteins and DNA in cancer-derived exosomes have been studied. Researchers found 3000 proteins secreted in exosomes derived from pancreatic cancer [12]. Epidermal growth factor receptor (EGFR) seemed to play an important role as binding leads to an increased activity of carcinogenesis signal transduction pathway and binding of associated ligands (EGF, TGF-alpha) is enhanced in most of pancreatic cancer types [13]. Through binding of EGF to EGFR tumour aggressiveness can increase and enhance cell proliferation, migration and probably metastasis [14]. In 2015, Melo et al. described glypican-1 (GPC1) as a specific surface marker for pancreatic cancer. It additionally was able to distinguish normal control subjects from subjects with benign pancreatic lesions [15].

Kahlert et al. assessed possible participation of genomic DNA in cancer-derived exosomes of patients with pancreatic ductal adenocarcinoma (PDAC). Fragments of genomic DNA could be harvested in exosomes and KRAS as well as p53 mutations were detected, giving an opportunity for profiling cancer. These findings underline their use to forecast prognosis and suited management [16].

In breast cancer, exosomal levels of CEA and CA 153 are linked with cancer progression [17,18]. The amount of miRNA in exosomes correlates with malignancy and prognosis [19,20]. A variety of miRNA have been studied and showed an association with breast tumour subtype as well as stage [21].

Concerning the most frequent cancer worldwide, the protein NY-ESO-1 was found to have a significant correlation with survival in lung cancer [22]. In non-small-cell lung cancer miRNA, miR-21 and miR-4257 in exosomes were upregulated in case of recurrence [23]. Decline in miR-51 and miR-373 in lung cancer patients was a factor of poor prognosis [24]. TEX also demonstrated a higher affinity to EGFR resulting in activation of Akt/protein kinase B pathway and overexpression of VEGF and finally augmented tumour vascularity [25]. Ueda et al. described CD91 as specific exosomal marker for lung adenocarcinoma. A panel of exosomal surface marker CD91, CD317 and EGFR was able to differentiate 75% of patients [26,27].

Studies of exosomes in patients with brain tumor showed that exosomes, depending on their cargo, can be used to analyse tumor mutations and predict outcomes of therapy [28]. Analysis of mRNA and total protein expression of patients with glioma after a vaccination trial could show a relation to immunopathological and clinical parameters [29].

Peinado et al. found in 2012 that the size distribution and number of exosomes did not alternate with clinical stage in patients with melanoma, though protein concentration showed a tumour-stage-dependent rise, being highest at the WHO IV stage compared to normal controls and other stages. Protein-poor exosomes in stage IV patients (< 50 µg/mL) showed a survival advantage [30]. Not only could changes in protein levels be detected, but also protein accumulation patterns. Exosomes marked with radioactive iodine-131 in breast-cancer-bearing mice concentrated in the field of the primary tumor as well as in the lung as a premetastastic niche. Moreover, after receiving cancer treatment radioactivity in lung cells diminished and cancer promoting factors declined (VEGFR2, ICAM-1, bFGF, KC, TNF-α, IL-6, IL-12, IL-10 and IL-13) showing a diminution of metastatic competency of the exosomes [31].

These findings implicate similar results. Although a good approach is made, a well-founded, stable biomarker in mentioned carcinomas has not been established up to now.

4. Diagnostic Application of Exosomes

4.1. Exosomal Blood Levels Correlate With Clinical Disease

To date, for diagnosis of HNSCC and many other cancers, we have to rely on clinical, histopathological and radiological findings. Often a biopsy in the operating room with possible side-effects is inevitable; however, a minimal tumour growth is needed for detection. Exosomes have moved into scope as possible biomarkers, showing early changes in cell properties in real time and being noninvasive.

Skog and his research group showed in 2008 a similar mutational pattern in blood exosomes and glioblastoma cells [32]. In breast cancer, a correlation between rising levels in CEA and CA 153 in exosomes and cancer progression could be shown [9,18,33]. In 2012, Peinado was able to demonstrate an increase in metastatic behaviour in advanced melanoma and exosomal levels in blood correlated well with disease stage [30].

Coming to HNSCC results are very sparse. Studies could show a disease-activity-dependent level of exosomes in HNSCC with advanced-stage tumours exhibiting an elevated level [34]. Other authors showed similar results [35]. Patients had higher exosomal levels in plasma compared to healthy controls. This is the first study describing action of exosomes in this kind of cancer [34]. Finally, the amount of exosomes almost doubled with progression of cancer stage [36].

Aggravated stress situations like inflammation as well as cancer both lead to an increase of exosomes as part of an enhanced intercellular communication, complicating the differentiation between both [37].

Exosomes produced by normal hematopoietic cells mediate antitumour responses and maintain homeostasis, whereas TEX profile changes during the course of disease and treatment. TEX are able to reprogram the bone marrow, cell differentiation migration and organise metastatic tumour spread. These results raised thoughts of a need to subcategorize exosomes as "immune-system-induced" and "tumour-induced", as functions differ [38]. The Whiteside group separated exosomes in $CD3^{positive}$-fractions (descending from T-lymphocytes) and $CD3^{negative}$-fractions. Hereby, the fraction of immune-derived and tumour-derived exosomes could be studied. In the course of disease, $CD3^{positive}$-exosomes alter their cargo and the ratio of $CD3^{negative}$-exosomes increases, being a marker for cancer progression [38,39]. Clinical response shows an association with found alternations in exosomal cargo.

It has therefore to be considered that TEX show immunosuppressive functions and interference with immune cells, and are used by cancer for tumour escape. A correlation with disease stage and activity could be shown [10,36].

4.2. Isolation of Exosomes

Exosomes can be obtained from many body fluids, such as urine, liquor, ascites, saliva or blood of patients [34,40,41]. However, the isolation process is still time-consuming [42–44]. Different research groups may use various isolation techniques, which makes their comparison difficult [45]. The international society for extracellular vesicles designed an online course to support with methods [46]. In 2013, a consensus paper for standardisation and isolation was released [47]. Our group uses initial differential centrifugation and size-exclusion chromatography by means of columns. If exosomes will be implicated in daily clinical routine, a standardised, time-saving procedure needs to be developed, which is less prone to errors. Our group is working at the moment on rapid bead-based capturing of exosomes for an easier isolation of exosomes, leading to a drastic time reduction and less vulnerability.

In the future, reproducible and reliable techniques are needed as monitoring tools in the clinical setting. Some starting points have been set but still more results are needed. A huge potential will be, as shown by Hong et al., the increased sensitivity of exosomes compared to standard diagnosis techniques [48,49].

4.3. Advantages and Drawbacks of Exosomal Applications

As mentioned above, diagnosis of HNSCC is still strenuous, invasive and linked with great medical expertise. Exosomes, as a potential new diagnostic tool, open up the era of liquid biopsy. As blood collection is a standard procedure in clinical settings, it would be easily applicable to the clinical routine. Further methods like flow cytometry, Western blot or electron microscopy are already established and can be used for continuative examinations. Together with circulating tumor DNA (ct DNA) and circulating tumor cells (CTC), a very sensitive panel for liquid biopsy can be built up, leading to presumably higher sensitivity and earlier diagnosis compared to biopsy or radiography. Initial promising results have been shown in colorectal cancer as well as breast cancer [50,51]. Scholer et al. showed appearance of ct DNA in patients postoperatively after colorectal cancer and detected relapse 9.4 months earlier than CT scan [52]. Compared to ct DNA and CTCs, exosomes seem to be of higher abundance and more stable, which makes them easier to apply into the busy clinical routine.

A persisting main drawback is the lack of standardisation of isolation techniques, which would be important for comparison of results. Besides, platelets in blood seem to secrete exosomes avidly. Already venepuncture and shear forces can lead to release of platelet-derived exosomes and falsification of data [47]. Another not negligible influencing factor is alteration of exosomal levels by infections and other diseases. Owing to the small size of exosomes ranging between 30–150 nm, direct analysis is difficult.

Summing up, the potential of exosomes as diagnostic markers in terms of liquid biopsy is great but prior to clinical application some questions have to be clarified.

4.4. Exosome Tropism and Building of a Premetastatic Niche

Biodistribution of TEX shows organ-specific colonisation due to exosomal integrins. Based on this organotropism TEX seem to prepare a premetastatic niche. Clinical results showed that profiles of integrin expression in plasma TEX could be prognostic factors to predict locations for future metastasis. Exosomal integrins are proposed to promote adhesion, trigger signalling pathways and inflammatory responses in target cells leading to educating the organ for expansion of metastatic cells [53]. Garofalo et al. could not support the theory of exosomal integrins responsible for building of the premetastatic niche in their work. They assume a special "receptor/ligand" combination on the exosomes responsible for exosome tropism [54].

Further studies are needed to focus on the mechanism underlying cancer tropism in exosomes as better understanding is important for use of exosome in delivery as theranostic agents and exosomal integrins as a probable diagnostic factor.

4.5. Exosomal Alterations with Active Therapy

Changes of plasmatic level of exosomes could not just be shown in cancer but also under active therapy. Patients who underwent surgery had a drastic reduction of plasmatic levels of $CD63^+$-exosomes, leading to the assumption, that the tumor mass is responsible for a high number of circulating exosomes. In contrast, exosomes containing Caveolin-1 (CAV-1) increased after surgery with the possible cause directed by inflammation [55]. According to Zorrilla et al. a lower level of exosomes prior and after surgery is linked with increased life expectancy in oral squamous cell carcinoma [55].

Interesting results were found by the group of Lisa Mutschelknaus. As radiation is a common therapy in HNSCC, they discovered a radiation-induced change in the exosomal cargo. It promoted AKT-dependent migration and motility in recipient cancer cells. The AKT pathway is one of the most frequently mutated oncogenic pathways [56–58]. The effect was dose-dependent and is an explanation for tumour immune escape and potential driving force for metastatic progression under radiation [59].

Our recent results showed a dramatic decrease of exosomal level seven weeks after primary, combined radio-chemotherapy of HNSCC patients (see Figure 2, results unpublished). This preliminary data demonstrates a positive correlation between clinical response and exosomal blood levels. Although more patients have to be analysed these encouraging results points toward their possible successful use to monitor the therapy.

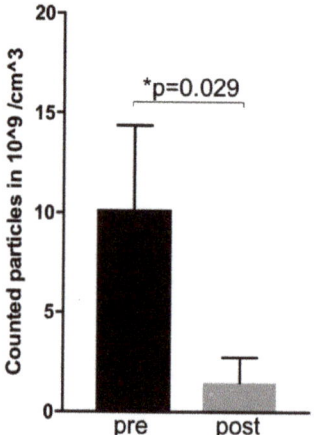

Figure 2. *Preliminary results:* Mean exosomal levels in blood of three patients with active HNSCC before (pre—week 0) and after (post—week 7) primary radio-chemotherapy. The exosomes were isolated as described before [11]. Measurements were performed by Zetaviewer (Particle Metrix, Duesseldorf, Germany). Statistical significance was calculated by a Student t-test.

5. Therapeutic Approaches Based On Exosomes

When it comes to therapeutic options, research results are even scarcer. At this point we want to express a warning. Since we are still very early in this research field and the biology behind exosomes is incompletely understood, the application of these new and innovative techniques, although of high research interest, may cause unforeseen harm to patients, and so experiments should be well planned.

5.1. Modulation Of Immune System

An imbalance of the immune system might lead to overaction of the inflammatory pathway. Inflammation gets induced through tissue damage or recognition of pathogens. Chronic inflammation has been associated with an increased risk of malignant cell transformation [60,61]. If progression of cancer takes place, different modulations within the immune system are required: apoptosis, proliferation and angiogenesis. The culmination of inflammatory mediators (Stat3, IL-6, TNF-alpha) guides to an immuno-suppression and following progression of cancer. Exosomes are able to participate in this regulation and alteration of immune players with either inhibiting or promoting action.

Exosomes isolated from malignant ascites of ovarian cancer modulated the function of monocytic cells [62]. Production and secretion of proinflammatory cytokines was induced, like interleukin, tumour necrosis factor alpha via TLR2 and 4, leading to an activated nuclear factor as well as signal transducer and activator of transcription (Stat3). The appearance of activated nuclear factor is often observed in cancer cells and results in a more aggressive phenotype with tissue invasion, metastasis and resistance to growth inhibition. [63] Communication between Stat3 and nuclear factor is important for regulation among inflammatory and cancer cells. Apoptosis, angiogenesis and tumour invasion is regulated making resistance towards immune surveillance possible [64].

Apoptosis, as one of the first steps for cancer progression, can be seen through activated T-cells via expression of death ligands (FasL [65] and TRAIL [66]), leading to an evasion of immune surveillance. Concluding modulation with release of FasL-positive exosomes is able to guide immune escape. A regulation of T-cell apoptosis was exemplary shown in human colorectal cancer [67]. Adding up impaired dendritic cell differentiation and suppression of natural killer cells has a similar effect [68,69]. In metastatic ovarian cancer, Yokoi et al. proved that cancer-derived exosomes induced apoptosis after uptake by mesothelial cells perforated the peritoneum resulting in peritoneal dissemination [70].

Concerning proliferation as an important modulation, exosomes derived from thrombin-activated platelets showed an exciting potential for survival, proliferation and chemotaxis of hematopoietic cells [71]. Besides they were capable of activating monocytes and B-cells [72].

Angiogenesis plays an important role during tumour growth, supplying oxygen and nutrition to the cancer and showing effect on an exosomal level [73].

The induction of angiogenesis has been described by various research groups. In 2008, a promotion of angiogenesis could be seen in exosomes secreted by glioblastoma cells [32]. In the same disease, Svensson et al. noted activation of PAR-2 also in vascular endothelial cells. They have arisen through induced angiogenesis after hypoxic treatment [74]. Later, mRNA of exosomes demonstrated proliferation of vascular endothelial cells [75]. An impact while studying renal cancer cell line was seen as CD105-positive exosomes led after affection of vascular endothelial cells to a promotion of growth. CD105-negative cells maintained no effect [76]. Subsequently, promotion of angiogenesis was shown in breast cancer, as miR-210 contained by exosomes seemed to have an impact on it and reversion by suppression of exosomes secretion stated the contrary [77]. Similar findings were reported by Li et al. in liver cancer cells [78].

The migration and invasion of cancer cells are subsequent important factors in metastasis. In colon carcinoma, a transfer of TEX induced a rise of cell proliferation and chemoresistance [79]. In melanoma cells of patients with advanced stages of carcinoma, bone marrow-derived cells were stimulated by exosomes forming a metastatic niche and leading to a prometastatic phenotype [30]. Also, HSP90alpha, as an exosomal surface marker, is able to activate plasminogen to lead to enhanced invasive capacity of tumor cells [80].

Exosomes were studied in relation to T- and NK-cells, as well as macrophages. Exosomes possess the ability of downregulating CD69 expression on $CD4^+$ T-cells and interfere with T-cell activation. Exosomes of cancer patients showed even higher immune suppression by decreased levels of CD69 expression. [34] These findings confirm results of other groups [11,81–83]. It is suspected that mRNA expression and the translation into inhibitory proteins gets enhanced by TEX.

When looking at $CD8^+$ T-cells, coincubation with TEX lets them undergo apoptosis [11].

TEX also exert effects on Treg-cells. The adenosine pathway is used by Treg-cells to operate suppression. A downregulation of mRNA coding for this pathway genes was shown in Treg-cells after coincubation with TEX. Also, TEX appear to activate resting Treg-cells through the increase of CD39 as well as CD73 production. Furthermore, calcium signalling is important for T-cell activation and T-cell-dependent immune responses. Incubation with TEX showed a calcium influx in T-cells, which was stronger than the response induced by dendritic cells [11].

The contribution of B-cells was, to date, not well respected. Results of our experiments could show a suppression of activated B-cells by TEX, which seems to be another way TEX may exert protumour effects (unpublished results).

The exact mechanism of immunomodulation through TEX is still unclear. An important part seems to be the uptake of small noncoding RNA (microRNA, miRNA), which leads to alteration of RNA expression and reprogramming of recipient cells [38]. This was, in particular, shown in immune cells, which take up exosomes as B-cells, monocytes and dendritic cells [82]. miRNA leads to destabilisation of RMA after binding and consecutive reduction of expression of the encoded protein [84]. Some of exosomes-mediated post-transcriptional alternations are associated with horizontal transfer of miRNA and oncogenic proteins from tumour cells to endothelial cells.

Exosomes having miRNA as their cargo are able to shape immune responses and seem responsible for protumorigenic functions in the recipient cells.

TEX signalling happens through receptor binding either on the vesicle surface or an internalisation by the recipient cell takes place. Our work could show that a direct surface interaction of exosomes with T-cells is sufficient to transfer signals. There is no internalisation needed as seen in phagocytic cells [11]. Internalisation and binding of TEX by B-cells and monocytes appeared to be time-dependent, dose-dependent and recipient cell type dependent.

Taken together, TEX take effect in antitumor immune functions and promotion of tumour progression leading to a gain or loss of function in recipient cells and being an option used by tumours as immune escape [30,38,85]. TEX play a dual part, having proinflammatory as well as anti-inflammatory properties. Exosomes of healthy donors did not induce immunosuppression [86].

5.2. Loaded Exosomes as Targeted Drug Delivery

Yang et al. showed that unmodified exosomes are able to cross the blood–brain barrier to some extent [87]. Brain exposure can, however, be increased by using certain brain-targeting ligands [88,89].

Exosomes can be modified using various techniques after isolation (exogenous loading): freeze–thaw cycles, incubation, sonication, electroporation and extrusion.

On the contrary, modification can also be made during the formation of exosomes (endogenous loading).

As a breakthrough, Batrakova managed to load exosomes exogenous with the chemotherapeutic agent paclitaxel as the drug-delivery technique. Therapy was, with respect to lung metastasis within mice and in vitro, a lot more successful, having effect even on multiresistant cells and reducing required medication 50 times [90]. Loading drugs into exosomes seems a powerful way of delivering anticancer drugs, but it may lead to increased toxicity, which has to be evaluated carefully.

Another study group loaded glioblastoma-derived exosomes with curcumin (an anti-inflammatory drug) and administered it intranasal to animals with encephalitis. It led to a clinical amelioration with induction of immune tolerance and apoptosis of activated immune cells [91].

Several groups studied the delivery of small interfering RNA (siRNA) into cells using exosomes loaded with electroporation. Some report functional siRNA, others were unsuccessful in proceeding with electroporation [89,92–94].

The endogenous approach uses direct transfection of RNA in interest cells, from which exosomes are later derived. Loading with miRNA and siRNA was possible and functional delivery was shown by various groups [94–98]. At the moment, limiting factors of this method are unknown alterations made to the exosome donor cell due to transfection leading to the changed cargo of exosomes. Besides, when conducting transfection, the produced side-products are copurified during isolation, features of exosomes can be changed leading to false-positive effects.

These are promising results for using exosomes as drug delivery vehicles and could be the solution to therapy-resistant cells as well as tumour immune escape.

A huge advantage, the possibility of exosomes to cross the blood–brain barrier, has to be highlighted; this leads to a higher bioavailability regarding the therapeutic use of exosomes if drugs of biologics are administered to them. Additionally, the toxicological effect is selective and targeted, reducing systemic effects compared to conventional free drugs.

However, research is in the fledgling stages and loading of the vesicles can be challenging, with probable alteration of exosomal membrane and function. Another known limitation is well known in cancer research, that once the successful research moves on from animal models to humans, the observed effects may be fading.

5.3. Modified Exosomes as Vaccinations

Already two decades ago, dendritic-cell derived exosomes were pulsed with tumour-cell peptides and injected in immune-competent mice. An immunogenic rejection of the tumour was obtained [99]. Due to promising results two clinical trials against melanoma and non-small-cell lung cancer were launched. Regrettably just a small number of patients benefitted from the vaccines.

Some years later, a phase I clinical trial was conducted in China. Extracellular vesicles (EV) from ascites of colorectal cancer patients were taken and combined with granulocyte-macrophage colony-stimulating factor (GM-CSF) to enhance antitumour dendritic cell activity. Patients benefited from GM-CSF combined with EV but not from EV alone [100].

The results show the successful use of exosomes to induce an antitumour immune response. From previous vaccination trials performed in cancer, it is known that the antitumour response is not enough to get rid of the cancer and new studies are being performed to combine immune-modulatory drugs with vaccines to increase their efficiency.

5.4. Engineered/Designer Exosomes

The first approaches for delivery drug technologies in the context of loading already existing exosomes have already been described above. This technology bears some problems like probable missing tissue specificity and immunogenic potential.

Alvarez-Erviti et al. engineered exosomes with self-derived immature dendritic cells to reduce immunogenicity and conducted them to express Lamp2b to realise tissue-specificity. Purified exosomes were loaded with siRNA by electroporation fused to a peptide important in the treatment of Alzheimer's disease and injected intravenously. Results showed specific delivery to the brain with a knockdown of mRNA and peptid by 60% [89].

Rashid et al. highlights further engineering of exosomes and their accumulated future hopes and problems. The perfect cell used to engineer exosomes should be nonimmunogenic, have an unlimited cell passage capacity without mutating, have an ability to produce itself abundantly and be easily modified. They believe to have found these potentials in HEK293-Tcells. Mice with metastatic breast cancer showed slower tumor growth after injection with engineered exosomes combined with a better survival compared to control.

Based on HEK293-Tcells, Kojima et al. even took it a step further and designed exosomes completely out of single components. Therapeutic catalase mRNA as cargo in exosomes showed attenuated neuroinflammation in Parkinson's disease as a positive results [101].

Designer exosomes are still in their fledgling stages but deliver promising results for further research as drug-delivering technologies.

5.5. Exosomes in Immune-Modulatory Therapies

Therapy in HNSCC has been mainly limited to surgery and radio-chemotherapy in the past few years. With growing understanding of the immune system and discovery of CTLA-4, PD-1, its inhibiting functions and suitable antibodies through James Allison and Tasuku Honjo check-point inhibition was found. Antibodies of CTLA-4 showed auspicious results in metastasised melanoma. PD-1 was further studied in HNSCC.

PD-L1 is found on the surface of many cell types being a membrane-bound ligand and upregulated in inflammation or malign situations. After binding to the PD-1 receptor on immune T-cells an activation of T-cells gets suppressed important to keep inflammatory responses regulated, being a checkpoint inhibitor. Tumor cells can adapt the mechanism to evade immune destruction [102]. After the discovery of Honjo, an immune-modulatory treatment with anti-PD-1 treatment was developed, showing some response in metastasised HNSCC. To date, it is the only FDA-approved immune-modulatory therapy with successful results.

One of the great drawbacks remains the poor response rate of 10–30% with anti-PD-1 treatment [103]. In 2017, isolated exosomes of patients with HNSCC could be shown to carry PD-L1 and PD-1 [36]. PD-L1-carrying exosomes correlate with clinical stage, disease activity and prognosis. Higher numbers of PD-L1^{positive} exosomes leads to poorer prognosis. In contrast, PD-1-containing exosomes did not match with the clinicopathological profile.

Plasma-derived exosomes in HNSCC showed biologically active PD-L1, which managed T-cell dysfunction. Anti-PD-1 was able to reverse this suppression. Maybe exosomal PD-L1, but not PD-1, is clinically relevant, possibly explaining reduced response rate with anti-PD-1 treatment and stratifying clinical responders from nonresponders. [104,105]. Besides, the membrane-bound form PD-L1 was also shown to be freely soluble in blood and other liquids (sPD-L1). Comparing exosome-bound PD-L1 and sPD-L1 levels in HNSCC, the soluble form did not correlate with clinicopathological findings. Results of other studies showed alternating results [106,107].

Exosomal PD-L1 recently moved into the spotlight as a possible therapeutic target, as suppression induces antitumour immunity and memory. Membrane-bound PD-L1 leads to diminished activity of T-cells in lymph nodes. Blocking of exosomal PD-L1 leads to a reversion and suppression of growth of local tumour cells.

Summing up, exosomal PD-L1 is an important regulator of tumour progression with the ability to suppress T-cell activation. Inhibition can lead to antitumour immunity [108].

5.6. Blocking/Elimination of Exosomes

A group from Massachusetts observed an interesting finding: incubation of glioma-cell derived exosomes with heparin led to a decreased transfer of exosomes between the parental and recipient cell [109,110]. The blockage happened on the surface and not internally. Further studies concerning the blocking of exosomes or removing them have, to our knowledge, not been conducted.

5.7. Challenges to Overcome Application of Exosomes

Exosomes may undergo morphological and functional changes during carcinogenesis, making them elusive for therapeutic applications. In peripheral blood, tumour-associated antigens (TAA) can be found also. Circulating anti-TAA antibodies appear years before clinical diagnosis and are present in all tumor types [111–113]. Despite vast research, no specific TAA has been found for HNSCC. Maybe a panel of expression markers will increase sensitivity and specificity.

6. Ongoing Clinical Trials with Exosomes in Cancer

In recent years, exosomes have risen to be a trending topic, and a lot of clinical trials have emerged. At the moment, there are 85 active studies listed (www.clinicaltrials.gov, 05 June 2020). Owing to the amount, we omit to list them all. Four studies are listed in the field of HNSCC and exosomes. Further details are mentioned in Figure 3.

Status	Study Title	Conditions	Interventions	Locations
Active, not recruiting	**Edible Plant Exosome** Ability to Prevent Oral Mucositis Associated With Chemoradiation Treatment of Head and Neck Cancer	- Head and Neck Cancer - Oral Mucositis	Dietary Supplement: Grape extract Drug: Lortab, Fentanyl patch, mouthwash	James Graham Brown Cancer Center Louisville, Kentucky, United States
Active, not recruiting Has results	**Metformin** Hydrochloride in Affecting Cytokines and **Exosomes** in Patients With Head and Neck Cancer	- Larynx - Lip - Oral Cavity - Pharynx	Radiation: External Beam Radiation Therapy Drug: Metformin Hydrochloride Other: Placebo	Sidney Kimmel Cancer Center at Thomas Jefferson University Philadelphia, Pennsylvania, United States
Recruiting	**Nivolumab and BMS986205** in Treating Patients With Stage II-IV Squamous Cell Cancer of the Head and Neck	- Lip - Oral Cavity Squamous Cell Carcinoma - Pharynx	Biological: Nivolumab Biological: IDO1 Inhibitor (BMS-986205) Procedure: Therapeutic Conventional Surgery Other: Questionnaire Administration	- Ohio State University Columbus, Ohio, United States - Sidney Kimmel Cancer Center at Thomas Jefferson University Philadelphia, Pennsylvania, United States
Recruiting	**Exosome Testing** as a Screening Modality for **Human Papillomavirus-Positive** Oropharyngeal Squamous Cell Carcinoma	- Oropharyngeal Cancer		University of New Mexico Cancer Center Albuquerque, New Mexico, United States

Figure 3. Ongoing clinical trials in cancer involving exosomes in HNSCC.

The first study investigates grape exosomes as a possible treatment of oral mucositis and examines production of cytokines and immune responses to tumour exosomal antigens and metabolic and molecular markers. The second study examines effects of metformin treatment during radiotherapy on mucositis and change in exosomes and cytokines. The third study is led by Brystol-Myers Squibb. A new biological is tested (BMS986205) for advanced-stage HNSCC. Exosomes are studied in a sidearm and do not belong to the direct treatment. The last study conducted by University of New Mexico analyses a prophylactical swab similar to the cervix PAP-swab and compares it with exosomal levels.

7. Conclusions

Since the discovery of exosomes some decades ago, an extended research occurred in this field. Regarding diagnostic possibilities there have been potential approaches, especially within monitoring of HNSCC shown for a follow-up marker (Figure 4). However, for implication in the clinical setting an amendment, stabilisation and standardisation of isolation techniques is needed. Moreover, techniques need to be quick and adequate to present a high sensitivity and specificity in clinical daily routine. There are already ongoing studies.

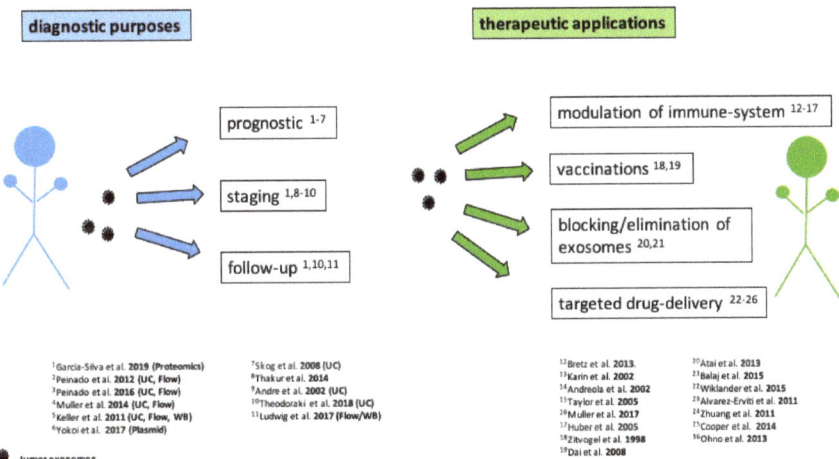

Figure 4. Applications of exosomes in cancer treatment. Isolation technique and method of analysis are written in brackets for the diagnostic purposes. Most research groups used size exclusion chromatography with ultracentrifugation (UC) or flow cytometry (Flow). Some used Western blotting (WB), plasmid transfection (Plasmid) or Fluorescence Activated Cell Sorting (FACS). List of papers consists of a selection.

As in the case of diagnosing recurrences, there is as a complicating factor the hazard of differentiation between recurrence and inflammation (e.g., as result to immunotherapy) as both show increase in exosomal levels and exosomes play a key role in both pathways. This factor aggravates the interpretation of immunotherapy either just being inflammation, tumor necrosis or active recurrence.

In respect of therapeutic options, a great need of action is required. Immunotherapy by PD-1/PD-L1 inhibitors showed already the right direction. A targeted-oriented therapy would be the aim.

Prevailing setbacks in work with exosomes is the not completely understood biology behind them. Therefore, application as targeted drug therapy is delicate as accurate changes and interactions are not known.

Summing up, exosomes seem promising agents to be used for diagnostic or therapeutic purposes in the future, but further studies, including of larger patient cohorts, are needed.

Author Contributions: E.E. wrote the original manuscript, revised and finalized the manuscript. L.M. provided supervision, reviewed and edited the original manuscript. All authors have read and agreed to the published version of the manuscript.

Funding: This work was supported by the "pro patient" grant (pp18–08) and Krebsliga beider Basel (Nr. 18-2016).

Conflicts of Interest: The authors declare no conflict of interest.

References

1. Bray, F.; Ferlay, J.; Soerjomataram, I.; Siegel, R.L.; Torre, L.A.; Jemal, A. Global cancer statistics 2018: GLOBOCAN estimates of incidence and mortality worldwide for 36 cancers in 185 countries. *CA Cancer J. Clin.* **2018**, *68*, 394–424. [CrossRef] [PubMed]
2. Harding, C.; Heuser, J.; Stahl, P. Receptor-mediated endocytosis of transferrin and recycling of the transferrin receptor in rat reticulocytes. *J. Cell Biol.* **1983**, *97*, 329–339. [CrossRef] [PubMed]
3. Raposo, G.; Nijman, H.W.; Stoorvogel, W.; Liejendekker, R.; Harding, C.V.; Melief, C.J.; Geuze, H.J. B lymphocytes secrete antigen-presenting vesicles. *J. Exp. Med.* **1996**, *183*, 1161–1172. [CrossRef] [PubMed]
4. Mathieu, M.; Martin-Jaular, L.; Lavieu, G.; Thery, C. Specificities of secretion and uptake of exosomes and other extracellular vesicles for cell-to-cell communication. *Nat. Cell Biol.* **2019**, *21*, 9–17. [CrossRef]
5. Keller, S.; Ridinger, J.; Rupp, A.K.; Janssen, J.W.; Altevogt, P. Body fluid derived exosomes as a novel template for clinical diagnostics. *J. Transl. Med.* **2011**, *9*, 86. [CrossRef]
6. Colombo, M.; Moita, C.; van Niel, G.; Kowal, J.; Vigneron, J.; Benaroch, P.; Manel, N.; Moita, L.F.; Thery, C.; Raposo, G. Analysis of ESCRT functions in exosome biogenesis, composition and secretion highlights the heterogeneity of extracellular vesicles. *J. Cell Sci.* **2013**, *126*, 5553–5565. [CrossRef]
7. TEOE, B. Battle of Marathon. In *Encylopaedia Britannica*; Encyclopaedia Britannica Inc.: Chicago, IL, USA, 1998.
8. Xin, T.; Greco, V.; Myung, P. Hardwiring stem cell communication through tissue structure. *Cell* **2016**, *164*, 1212–1225. [CrossRef]
9. Thakur, B.K.; Zhang, H.; Becker, A.; Matei, I.; Huang, Y.; Costa-Silva, B.; Zheng, Y.; Hoshino, A.; Brazier, H.; Xiang, J.; et al. Double-stranded DNA in exosomes: A novel biomarker in cancer detection. *Cell Res.* **2014**, *24*, 766–769. [CrossRef]
10. Muller, L.; Mitsuhashi, M.; Simms, P.; Gooding, W.E.; Whiteside, T.L. Tumor-derived exosomes regulate expression of immune function-related genes in human T cell subsets. *Sci. Rep.* **2016**, *6*, 20254. [CrossRef]
11. Muller, L.; Simms, P.; Hong, C.S.; Nishimura, M.I.; Jackson, E.K.; Watkins, S.C.; Whiteside, T.L. Human tumor-derived exosomes (TEX) regulate Treg functions via cell surface signaling rather than uptake mechanisms. *Oncoimmunology* **2017**, *6*, e1261243. [CrossRef]
12. Adamczyk, K.A.; Klein-Scory, S.; Tehrani, M.M.; Warnken, U.; Schmiegel, W.; Schnolzer, M.; Schwarte-Waldhoff, I. Characterization of soluble and exosomal forms of the EGFR released from pancreatic cancer cells. *Life Sci.* **2011**, *89*, 304–312. [CrossRef] [PubMed]
13. Bloomston, M.; Bhardwaj, A.; Ellison, E.C.; Frankel, W.L. Epidermal growth factor receptor expression in pancreatic carcinoma using tissue microarray technique. *Dig. Surg.* **2006**, *23*, 74–79. [CrossRef] [PubMed]
14. Nuzhat, Z.; Kinhal, V.; Sharma, S.; Rice, G.E.; Joshi, V.; Salomon, C. Tumour-derived exosomes as a signature of pancreatic cancer - liquid biopsies as indicators of tumour progression. *Oncotarget* **2017**, *8*, 17279–17291. [CrossRef] [PubMed]
15. Melo, S.A.; Luecke, L.B.; Kahlert, C.; Fernandez, A.F.; Gammon, S.T.; Kaye, J.; LeBleu, V.S.; Mittendorf, E.A.; Weitz, J.; Rahbari, N.; et al. Glypican-1 identifies cancer exosomes and detects early pancreatic cancer. *Nature* **2015**, *523*, 177–182. [CrossRef]
16. Kahlert, C.; Melo, S.A.; Protopopov, A.; Tang, J.; Seth, S.; Koch, M.; Zhang, J.; Weitz, J.; Chin, L.; Futreal, A.; et al. Identification of double-stranded genomic DNA spanning all chromosomes with mutated KRAS and p53 DNA in the serum exosomes of patients with pancreatic cancer. *J. Biol. Chem.* **2014**, *289*, 3869–3875. [CrossRef]
17. Dreyer, F.; Baur, A. Biogenesis and Functions of Exosomes and Extracellular Vesicles. *Methods Mol. Biol.* **2016**, *1448*, 201–216. [CrossRef]

18. Andre, F.; Schartz, N.E.; Movassagh, M.; Flament, C.; Pautier, P.; Morice, P.; Pomel, C.; Lhomme, C.; Escudier, B.; Le Chevalier, T.; et al. Malignant effusions and immunogenic tumour-derived exosomes. *Lancet* **2002**, *360*, 295–305. [CrossRef]
19. Tetta, C.; Ghigo, E.; Silengo, L.; Deregibus, M.C.; Camussi, G. Extracellular vesicles as an emerging mechanism of cell-to-cell communication. *Endocrine* **2013**, *44*, 11–19. [CrossRef]
20. Joyce, D.P.; Kerin, M.J.; Dwyer, R.M. Exosome-encapsulated microRNAs as circulating biomarkers for breast cancer. *Int. J. Cancer* **2016**, *139*, 1443–1448. [CrossRef]
21. Jia, Y.; Chen, Y.; Wang, Q.; Jayasinghe, U.; Luo, X.; Wei, Q.; Wang, J.; Xiong, H.; Chen, C.; Xu, B.; et al. Exosome: Emerging biomarker in breast cancer. *Oncotarget* **2017**, *8*, 41717–41733. [CrossRef]
22. Sandfeld-Paulsen, B.; Jakobsen, K.R.; Baek, R.; Folkersen, B.H.; Rasmussen, T.R.; Meldgaard, P.; Varming, K.; Jorgensen, M.M.; Sorensen, B.S. Exosomal proteins as diagnostic biomarkers in lung cancer. *J. Thorac. Oncol.* **2016**, *11*, 1701–1710. [CrossRef] [PubMed]
23. Dejima, H.; Iinuma, H.; Kanaoka, R.; Matsutani, N.; Kawamura, M. Exosomal microRNA in plasma as a non-invasive biomarker for the recurrence of non-small cell lung cancer. *Oncol. Lett.* **2017**, *13*, 1256–1263. [CrossRef]
24. Alipoor, S.D.; Adcock, I.M.; Garssen, J.; Mortaz, E.; Varahram, M.; Mirsaeidi, M.; Velayati, A. The roles of miRNAs as potential biomarkers in lung diseases. *Eur. J. Pharmacol.* **2016**, *791*, 395–404. [CrossRef] [PubMed]
25. Reclusa, P.; Sirera, R.; Araujo, A.; Giallombardo, M.; Valentino, A.; Sorber, L.; Bazo, I.G.; Pauwels, P.; Rolfo, C. Exosomes genetic cargo in lung cancer: A truly Pandora's box. *Transl. Lung Cancer Res.* **2016**, *5*, 483–491. [CrossRef] [PubMed]
26. Ueda, K.; Ishikawa, N.; Tatsuguchi, A.; Saichi, N.; Fujii, R.; Nakagawa, H. Antibody-coupled monolithic silica microtips for highthroughput molecular profiling of circulating exosomes. *Sci. Rep.* **2014**, *4*, 6232. [CrossRef] [PubMed]
27. Jakobsen, K.R.; Paulsen, B.S.; Baek, R.; Varming, K.; Sorensen, B.S.; Jorgensen, M.M. Exosomal proteins as potential diagnostic markers in advanced non-small cell lung carcinoma. *J. Extracell. Vesicles* **2015**, *4*, 26659. [CrossRef] [PubMed]
28. Redzic, J.S.; Ung, T.H.; Graner, M.W. Glioblastoma extracellular vesicles: Reservoirs of potential biomarkers. *Pharmgenomics Pers. Med.* **2014**, *7*, 65–77. [CrossRef]
29. Muller, L.; Muller-Haegele, S.; Mitsuhashi, M.; Gooding, W.; Okada, H.; Whiteside, T.L. Exosomes isolated from plasma of glioma patients enrolled in a vaccination trial reflect antitumor immune activity and might predict survival. *Oncoimmunology* **2015**, *4*, e1008347. [CrossRef]
30. Peinado, H.; Aleckovic, M.; Lavotshkin, S.; Matei, I.; Costa-Silva, B.; Moreno-Bueno, G.; Hergueta-Redondo, M.; Williams, C.; Garcia-Santos, G.; Ghajar, C.; et al. Melanoma exosomes educate bone marrow progenitor cells toward a pro-metastatic phenotype through MET. *Nat. Med.* **2012**, *18*, 883–891, corrected in *Nat. Med.* **2016**, *22*, 1502, doi:10.1038/nm1216-1502b. [CrossRef]
31. Rashid, M.H.; Borin, T.F.; Ara, R.; Angara, K.; Cai, J.; Achyut, B.R.; Liu, Y.; Arbab, A.S. Differential in vivo biodistribution of (131)I-labeled exosomes from diverse cellular origins and its implication for theranostic application. *Nanomedicine* **2019**, *21*, 102072. [CrossRef]
32. Skog, J.; Wurdinger, T.; van Rijn, S.; Meijer, D.H.; Gainche, L.; Sena-Esteves, M.; Curry, W.T., Jr.; Carter, B.S.; Krichevsky, A.M.; Breakefield, X.O. Glioblastoma microvesicles transport RNA and proteins that promote tumour growth and provide diagnostic biomarkers. *Nat. Cell Biol.* **2008**, *10*, 1470–1476. [CrossRef] [PubMed]
33. Garcia-Silva, S.; Benito-Martin, A.; Sanchez-Redondo, S.; Hernandez-Barranco, A.; Ximenez-Embun, P.; Nogues, L.; Mazariegos, M.S.; Brinkmann, K.; Amor Lopez, A.; Meyer, L.; et al. Use of extracellular vesicles from lymphatic drainage as surrogate markers of melanoma progression and BRAF (V600E) mutation. *J. Exp. Med.* **2019**, *216*, 1061–1070. [CrossRef] [PubMed]
34. Muller, L.; Hong, C.S.; Stolz, D.B.; Watkins, S.C.; Whiteside, T.L. Isolation of biologically-active exosomes from human plasma. *J. Immunol. Methods* **2014**, *411*, 55–65. [CrossRef] [PubMed]
35. Theodoraki, M.N.; Hoffmann, T.K.; Jackson, E.K.; Whiteside, T.L. Exosomes in HNSCC plasma as surrogate markers of tumour progression and immune competence. *Clin. Exp. Immunol.* **2018**, *194*, 67–78. [CrossRef]
36. Ludwig, S.; Floros, T.; Theodoraki, M.N.; Hong, C.S.; Jackson, E.K.; Lang, S.; Whiteside, T.L. Suppression of Lymphocyte Functions by Plasma Exosomes Correlates with Disease Activity in Patients with Head and Neck Cancer. *Clin. Cancer Res.* **2017**, *23*, 4843–4854. [CrossRef] [PubMed]

37. Isola, A.L.; Chen, S. Exosomes: The Messengers of Health and Disease. *Curr. Neuropharmacol.* **2017**, *15*, 157–165. [CrossRef]
38. Whiteside, T.L. Tumor-Derived Exosomes and Their Role in Cancer Progression. *Adv. Clin. Chem.* **2016**, *74*, 103–141. [CrossRef]
39. Theodoraki, M.N.; Hoffmann, T.K.; Whiteside, T.L. Separation of plasma-derived exosomes into CD3((+)) and CD3((-)) fractions allows for association of immune cell and tumour cell markers with disease activity in HNSCC patients. *Clin. Exp. Immunol.* **2018**, *192*, 271–283. [CrossRef]
40. Hong, C.S.; Funk, S.; Whiteside, T.L. Isolation of Biologically Active Exosomes from Plasma of Patients with Cancer. *Methods Mol. Biol.* **2017**, *1633*, 257–265. [CrossRef]
41. Nonaka, T.; Wong, D.T.W. Liquid Biopsy in Head and Neck Cancer: Promises and Challenges. *J. Dent. Res.* **2018**, *97*, 701–708. [CrossRef]
42. Whiteside, T.L. Extracellular vesicles isolation and their biomarker potential: Are we ready for testing? *Ann. Transl. Med.* **2017**, *5*, 54. [CrossRef] [PubMed]
43. Thery, C.; Amigorena, S.; Raposo, G.; Clayton, A. Isolation and characterization of exosomes from cell culture supernatants and biological fluids. *Curr. Protoc. Cell Biol.* **2006**, *3*, 3.22.1–3.22.29. [CrossRef] [PubMed]
44. Taylor, D.D.; Shah, S. Methods of isolating extracellular vesicles impact down-stream analyses of their cargoes. *Methods* **2015**, *87*, 3–10. [CrossRef]
45. Van Deun, J.; Mestdagh, P.; Sormunen, R.; Cocquyt, V.; Vermaelen, K.; Vandesompele, J.; Bracke, M.; De Wever, O.; Hendrix, A. The impact of disparate isolation methods for extracellular vesicles on downstream RNA profiling. *J. Extracell. Vesicles* **2014**, *3*. [CrossRef] [PubMed]
46. Lasser, C.; Thery, C.; Buzas, E.I.; Mathivanan, S.; Zhao, W.; Gho, Y.S.; Lotvall, J. The International Society for Extracellular Vesicles launches the first massive open online course on extracellular vesicles. *J. Extracell. Vesicles* **2016**, *5*, 34299. [CrossRef] [PubMed]
47. Witwer, K.W.; Buzas, E.I.; Bemis, L.T.; Bora, A.; Lasser, C.; Lotvall, J.; Nolte-'t Hoen, E.N.; Piper, M.G.; Sivaraman, S.; Skog, J.; et al. Standardization of sample collection, isolation and analysis methods in extracellular vesicle research. *J. Extracell. Vesicles* **2013**, *2*. [CrossRef] [PubMed]
48. Hong, C.S.; Danet-Desnoyers, G.; Shan, X.; Sharma, P.; Whiteside, T.L.; Boyiadzis, M. Human acute myeloid leukemia blast-derived exosomes in patient-derived xenograft mice mediate immune suppression. *Exp. Hematol.* **2019**, *76*, 60–66.e2. [CrossRef] [PubMed]
49. Hong, C.S.; Sharma, P.; Yerneni, S.S.; Simms, P.; Jackson, E.K.; Whiteside, T.L.; Boyiadzis, M. Circulating exosomes carrying an immunosuppressive cargo interfere with cellular immunotherapy in acute myeloid leukemia. *Sci. Rep.* **2017**, *7*, 14684. [CrossRef] [PubMed]
50. Jia, S.; Zhang, R.; Li, Z.; Li, J. Clinical and biological significance of circulating tumor cells, circulating tumor DNA, and exosomes as biomarkers in colorectal cancer. *Oncotarget* **2017**, *8*, 55632–55645. [CrossRef] [PubMed]
51. Alimirzaie, S.; Bagherzadeh, M.; Akbari, M.R. Liquid biopsy in breast cancer: A comprehensive review. *Clin. Genet.* **2019**, *95*, 643–660. [CrossRef]
52. Scholer, L.V.; Reinert, T.; Orntoft, M.W.; Kassentoft, C.G.; Arnadottir, S.S.; Vang, S.; Nordentoft, I.; Knudsen, M.; Lamy, P.; Andreasen, D.; et al. Clinical Implications of Monitoring Circulating Tumor DNA in Patients with Colorectal Cancer. *Clin. Cancer Res.* **2017**, *23*, 5437–5445. [CrossRef]
53. Hoshino, A.; Costa-Silva, B.; Shen, T.L.; Rodrigues, G.; Hashimoto, A.; Tesic Mark, M.; Molina, H.; Kohsaka, S.; Di Giannatale, A.; Ceder, S.; et al. Tumour exosome integrins determine organotropic metastasis. *Nature* **2015**, *527*, 329–335. [CrossRef] [PubMed]
54. Garofalo, M.; Villa, A.; Crescenti, D.; Marzagalli, M.; Kuryk, L.; Limonta, P.; Mazzaferro, V.; Ciana, P. Heterologous and cross-species tropism of cancer-derived extracellular vesicles. *Theranostics* **2019**, *9*, 5681–5693. [CrossRef] [PubMed]
55. Rodriguez Zorrilla, S.; Perez-Sayans, M.; Fais, S.; Logozzi, M.; Gallas Torreira, M.; Garcia Garcia, A. A Pilot Clinical Study on the Prognostic Relevance of Plasmatic Exosomes Levels in Oral Squamous Cell Carcinoma Patients. *Cancers* **2019**, *11*, 429. [CrossRef] [PubMed]
56. Knowles, J.A.; Golden, B.; Yan, L.; Carroll, W.R.; Helman, E.E.; Rosenthal, E.L. Disruption of the AKT pathway inhibits metastasis in an orthotopic model of head and neck squamous cell carcinoma. *Laryngoscope* **2011**, *121*, 2359–2365. [CrossRef] [PubMed]

57. Bussink, J.; van der Kogel, A.J.; Kaanders, J.H. Activation of the PI3-K/AKT pathway and implications for radioresistance mechanisms in head and neck cancer. *Lancet Oncol.* **2008**, *9*, 288–296. [CrossRef]
58. Liu, Q.; Turner, K.M.; Alfred Yung, W.K.; Chen, K.; Zhang, W. Role of AKT signaling in DNA repair and clinical response to cancer therapy. *Neuro Oncol.* **2014**, *16*, 1313–1323. [CrossRef]
59. Mutschelknaus, L.; Azimzadeh, O.; Heider, T.; Winkler, K.; Vetter, M.; Kell, R.; Tapio, S.; Merl-Pham, J.; Huber, S.M.; Edalat, L.; et al. Radiation alters the cargo of exosomes released from squamous head and neck cancer cells to promote migration of recipient cells. *Sci. Rep.* **2017**, *7*, 12423. [CrossRef]
60. Landskron, G.; De la Fuente, M.; Thuwajit, P.; Thuwajit, C.; Hermoso, M.A. Chronic inflammation and cytokines in the tumor microenvironment. *J. Immunol. Res.* **2014**, *2014*, 149185. [CrossRef]
61. Bermejo-Martin, J.F.; Martin-Loeches, I.; Bosinger, S. Inflammation and infection in critical care medicine. *Mediators Inflamm.* **2014**, *2014*, 456256. [CrossRef]
62. Bretz, N.P.; Ridinger, J.; Rupp, A.K.; Rimbach, K.; Keller, S.; Rupp, C.; Marme, F.; Umansky, L.; Umansky, V.; Eigenbrod, T.; et al. Body fluid exosomes promote secretion of inflammatory cytokines in monocytic cells via Toll-like receptor signaling. *J. Biol. Chem.* **2013**, *288*, 36691–36702. [CrossRef] [PubMed]
63. Karin, M.; Cao, Y.; Greten, F.R.; Li, Z.W. NF-kappaB in cancer: From innocent bystander to major culprit. *Nat. Rev. Cancer* **2002**, *2*, 301–310. [CrossRef] [PubMed]
64. Bromberg, J.; Darnell, J.E., Jr. The role of STATs in transcriptional control and their impact on cellular function. *Oncogene* **2000**, *19*, 2468–2473.. [CrossRef] [PubMed]
65. Andreola, G.; Rivoltini, L.; Castelli, C.; Huber, V.; Perego, P.; Deho, P.; Squarcina, P.; Accornero, P.; Lozupone, F.; Lugini, L.; et al. Induction of lymphocyte apoptosis by tumor cell secretion of FasL-bearing microvesicles. *J. Exp. Med.* **2002**, *195*, 1303–1316. [CrossRef]
66. Taylor, D.D.; Gercel-Taylor, C. Tumour-derived exosomes and their role in cancer-associated T-cell signalling defects. *Br. J. Cancer* **2005**, *92*, 305–311. [CrossRef] [PubMed]
67. Huber, V.; Fais, S.; Iero, M.; Lugini, L.; Canese, P.; Squarcina, P.; Zaccheddu, A.; Colone, M.; Arancia, G.; Gentile, M.; et al. Human colorectal cancer cells induce T-cell death through release of proapoptotic microvesicles: Role in immune escape. *Gastroenterology* **2005**, *128*, 1796–1804. [CrossRef]
68. Clayton, A.; Mason, M.D. Exosomes in tumour immunity. *Curr. Oncol.* **2009**, *16*, 46–49. [CrossRef]
69. Clayton, A.; Mitchell, J.P.; Court, J.; Mason, M.D.; Tabi, Z. Human tumor-derived exosomes selectively impair lymphocyte responses to interleukin-2. *Cancer Res.* **2007**, *67*, 7458–7466. [CrossRef]
70. Yokoi, A.; Yoshioka, Y.; Yamamoto, Y.; Ishikawa, M.; Ikeda, S.I.; Kato, T.; Kiyono, T.; Takeshita, F.; Kajiyama, H.; Kikkawa, F.; et al. Malignant extracellular vesicles carrying MMP1 mRNA facilitate peritoneal dissemination in ovarian cancer. *Nat. Commun.* **2017**, *8*, 14470. [CrossRef]
71. Baj-Krzyworzeka, M.; Majka, M.; Pratico, D.; Ratajczak, J.; Vilaire, G.; Kijowski, J.; Reca, R.; Janowska-Wieczorek, A.; Ratajczak, M.Z. Platelet-derived microparticles stimulate proliferation, survival, adhesion, and chemotaxis of hematopoietic cells. *Exp. Hematol.* **2002**, *30*, 450–459. [CrossRef]
72. Sprague, D.L.; Elzey, B.D.; Crist, S.A.; Waldschmidt, T.J.; Jensen, R.J.; Ratliff, T.L. Platelet-mediated modulation of adaptive immunity: Unique delivery of CD154 signal by platelet-derived membrane vesicles. *Blood* **2008**, *111*, 5028–5036. [CrossRef] [PubMed]
73. Folkman, J. Anti-angiogenesis: New concept for therapy of solid tumors. *Ann. Surg.* **1972**, *175*, 409–416. [CrossRef] [PubMed]
74. Svensson, K.J.; Kucharzewska, P.; Christianson, H.C.; Skold, S.; Lofstedt, T.; Johansson, M.C.; Morgelin, M.; Bengzon, J.; Ruf, W.; Belting, M. Hypoxia triggers a proangiogenic pathway involving cancer cell microvesicles and PAR-2-mediated heparin-binding EGF signaling in endothelial cells. *Proc. Natl. Acad. Sci. USA* **2011**, *108*, 13147–13152. [CrossRef] [PubMed]
75. Hong, B.S.; Cho, J.H.; Kim, H.; Choi, E.J.; Rho, S.; Kim, J.; Kim, J.H.; Choi, D.S.; Kim, Y.K.; Hwang, D.; et al. Colorectal cancer cell-derived microvesicles are enriched in cell cycle-related mRNAs that promote proliferation of endothelial cells. *BMC Genom.* **2009**, *10*, 556. [CrossRef]
76. Grange, C.; Tapparo, M.; Collino, F.; Vitillo, L.; Damasco, C.; Deregibus, M.C.; Tetta, C.; Bussolati, B.; Camussi, G. Microvesicles released from human renal cancer stem cells stimulate angiogenesis and formation of lung premetastatic niche. *Cancer Res.* **2011**, *71*, 5346–5356. [CrossRef]
77. Kosaka, N.; Iguchi, H.; Hagiwara, K.; Yoshioka, Y.; Takeshita, F.; Ochiya, T. Neutral sphingomyelinase 2 (nSMase2)-dependent exosomal transfer of angiogenic microRNAs regulate cancer cell metastasis. *J. Biol. Chem.* **2013**, *288*, 10849–10859. [CrossRef]

78. Li, R.; Wang, Y.; Zhang, X.; Feng, M.; Ma, J.; Li, J.; Yang, X.; Fang, F.; Xia, Q.; Zhang, Z.; et al. Exosome-mediated secretion of LOXL4 promotes hepatocellular carcinoma cell invasion and metastasis. *Mol. Cancer* **2019**, *18*, 18. [CrossRef]
79. Soldevilla, B.; Rodriguez, M.; San Millan, C.; Garcia, V.; Fernandez-Perianez, R.; Gil-Calderon, B.; Martin, P.; Garcia-Grande, A.; Silva, J.; Bonilla, F.; et al. Tumor-derived exosomes are enriched in DeltaNp73, which promotes oncogenic potential in acceptor cells and correlates with patient survival. *Hum. Mol. Genet.* **2014**, *23*, 467–478. [CrossRef]
80. McCready, J.; Sims, J.D.; Chan, D.; Jay, D.G. Secretion of extracellular hsp90alpha via exosomes increases cancer cell motility: A role for plasminogen activation. *BMC Cancer* **2010**, *10*, 294. [CrossRef]
81. Kim, J.W.; Wieckowski, E.; Taylor, D.D.; Reichert, T.E.; Watkins, S.; Whiteside, T.L. Fas ligand-positive membranous vesicles isolated from sera of patients with oral cancer induce apoptosis of activated T lymphocytes. *Clin. Cancer Res.* **2005**, *11*, 1010–1020.
82. Czystowska, M.; Han, J.; Szczepanski, M.J.; Szajnik, M.; Quadrini, K.; Brandwein, H.; Hadden, J.W.; Signorelli, K.; Whiteside, T.L. IRX-2, a novel immunotherapeutic, protects human T cells from tumor-induced cell death. *Cell Death Differ.* **2009**, *16*, 708–718. [CrossRef] [PubMed]
83. Wieckowski, E.U.; Visus, C.; Szajnik, M.; Szczepanski, M.J.; Storkus, W.J.; Whiteside, T.L. Tumor-derived microvesicles promote regulatory T cell expansion and induce apoptosis in tumor-reactive activated CD8+ T lymphocytes. *J. Immunol.* **2009**, *183*, 3720–3730. [CrossRef] [PubMed]
84. Fanini, F.; Fabbri, M. Cancer-derived exosomic microRNAs shape the immune system within the tumor microenvironment: State of the art. *Semin. Cell Dev. Biol.* **2017**, *67*, 23–28. [CrossRef]
85. Zhang, H.G.; Grizzle, W.E. Exosomes: A novel pathway of local and distant intercellular communication that facilitates the growth and metastasis of neoplastic lesions. *Am. J. Pathol.* **2014**, *184*, 28–41. [CrossRef] [PubMed]
86. Whiteside, T.L. Immune modulation of T-cell and NK (natural killer) cell activities by TEXs (tumour-derived exosomes). *Biochem. Soc. Trans.* **2013**, *41*, 245–251. [CrossRef] [PubMed]
87. Yang, T.; Martin, P.; Fogarty, B.; Brown, A.; Schurman, K.; Phipps, R.; Yin, V.P.; Lockman, P.; Bai, S. Exosome delivered anticancer drugs across the blood-brain barrier for brain cancer therapy in Danio rerio. *Pharm. Res.* **2015**, *32*, 2003–2014. [CrossRef]
88. Wiklander, O.P.; Nordin, J.Z.; O'Loughlin, A.; Gustafsson, Y.; Corso, G.; Mager, I.; Vader, P.; Lee, Y.; Sork, H.; Seow, Y.; et al. Extracellular vesicle in vivo biodistribution is determined by cell source, route of administration and targeting. *J. Extracell. Vesicles* **2015**, *4*, 26316. [CrossRef]
89. Alvarez-Erviti, L.; Seow, Y.; Yin, H.; Betts, C.; Lakhal, S.; Wood, M.J. Delivery of siRNA to the mouse brain by systemic injection of targeted exosomes. *Nat. Biotechnol.* **2011**, *29*, 341–345. [CrossRef]
90. Kim, M.S.; Haney, M.J.; Zhao, Y.; Mahajan, V.; Deygen, I.; Klyachko, N.L.; Inskoe, E.; Piroyan, A.; Sokolsky, M.; Okolie, O.; et al. Development of exosome-encapsulated paclitaxel to overcome MDR in cancer cells. *Nanomedicine* **2016**, *12*, 655–664. [CrossRef]
91. Zhuang, X.; Xiang, X.; Grizzle, W.; Sun, D.; Zhang, S.; Axtell, R.C.; Ju, S.; Mu, J.; Zhang, L.; Steinman, L.; et al. Treatment of brain inflammatory diseases by delivering exosome encapsulated anti-inflammatory drugs from the nasal region to the brain. *Mol. Ther.* **2011**, *19*, 1769–1779. [CrossRef]
92. Cooper, J.M.; Wiklander, P.B.; Nordin, J.Z.; Al-Shawi, R.; Wood, M.J.; Vithlani, M.; Schapira, A.H.; Simons, J.P.; El-Andaloussi, S.; Alvarez-Erviti, L. Systemic exosomal siRNA delivery reduced alpha-synuclein aggregates in brains of transgenic mice. *Mov. Disord.* **2014**, *29*, 1476–1485. [CrossRef] [PubMed]
93. Wahlgren, J.; De, L.K.T.; Brisslert, M.; Vaziri Sani, F.; Telemo, E.; Sunnerhagen, P.; Valadi, H. Plasma exosomes can deliver exogenous short interfering RNA to monocytes and lymphocytes. *Nucleic Acids Res.* **2012**, *40*, e130. [CrossRef]
94. Ohno, S.; Takanashi, M.; Sudo, K.; Ueda, S.; Ishikawa, A.; Matsuyama, N.; Fujita, K.; Mizutani, T.; Ohgi, T.; Ochiya, T.; et al. Systemically injected exosomes targeted to EGFR deliver antitumor microRNA to breast cancer cells. *Mol. Ther.* **2013**, *21*, 185–191. [CrossRef] [PubMed]
95. Kosaka, N.; Iguchi, H.; Yoshioka, Y.; Takeshita, F.; Matsuki, Y.; Ochiya, T. Secretory mechanisms and intercellular transfer of microRNAs in living cells. *J. Biol. Chem.* **2010**, *285*, 17442–17452. [CrossRef] [PubMed]
96. Zhou, Y.; Xiong, M.; Fang, L.; Jiang, L.; Wen, P.; Dai, C.; Zhang, C.Y.; Yang, J. miR-21-containing microvesicles from injured tubular epithelial cells promote tubular phenotype transition by targeting PTEN protein. *Am. J. Pathol.* **2013**, *183*, 1183–1196. [CrossRef]

97. Zhang, Y.; Liu, D.; Chen, X.; Li, J.; Li, L.; Bian, Z.; Sun, F.; Lu, J.; Yin, Y.; Cai, X.; et al. Secreted monocytic miR-150 enhances targeted endothelial cell migration. *Mol. Cell* **2010**, *39*, 133–144. [CrossRef]
98. Zhang, Y.; Li, L.; Yu, J.; Zhu, J.; Zhang, Y.; Li, X.; Gu, H.; Zhang, C.Y.; Zen, K. Microvesicle-mediated delivery of transforming growth factor beta1 siRNA for the suppression of tumor growth in mice. *Biomaterials* **2014**, *35*, 4390–4400. [CrossRef]
99. Zitvogel, L.; Regnault, A.; Lozier, A.; Wolfers, J.; Flament, C.; Tenza, D.; Ricciardi-Castagnoli, P.; Raposo, G.; Amigorena, S. Eradication of established murine tumors using a novel cell-free vaccine: Dendritic cell-derived exosomes. *Nat. Med.* **1998**, *4*, 594–600. [CrossRef]
100. Dai, S.; Wei, D.; Wu, Z.; Zhou, X.; Wei, X.; Huang, H.; Li, G. Phase I clinical trial of autologous ascites-derived exosomes combined with GM-CSF for colorectal cancer. *Mol. Ther.* **2008**, *16*, 782–790. [CrossRef]
101. Kojima, R.; Bojar, D.; Rizzi, G.; Hamri, G.C.; El-Baba, M.D.; Saxena, P.; Auslander, S.; Tan, K.R.; Fussenegger, M. Designer exosomes produced by implanted cells intracerebrally deliver therapeutic cargo for Parkinson's disease treatment. *Nat. Commun.* **2018**, *9*, 1305. [CrossRef]
102. Topalian, S.L.; Drake, C.G.; Pardoll, D.M. Immune checkpoint blockade: A common denominator approach to cancer therapy. *Cancer Cell* **2015**, *27*, 450–461. [CrossRef] [PubMed]
103. Page, D.B.; Postow, M.A.; Callahan, M.K.; Allison, J.P.; Wolchok, J.D. Immune modulation in cancer with antibodies. *Annu. Rev. Med.* **2014**, *65*, 185–202. [CrossRef] [PubMed]
104. Theodoraki, M.N.; Yerneni, S.S.; Hoffmann, T.K.; Gooding, W.E.; Whiteside, T.L. Clinical Significance of PD-L1(+) Exosomes in Plasma of Head and Neck Cancer Patients. *Clin. Cancer Res.* **2018**, *24*, 896–905. [CrossRef] [PubMed]
105. Chen, G.; Huang, A.C.; Zhang, W.; Zhang, G.; Wu, M.; Xu, W.; Yu, Z.; Yang, J.; Wang, B.; Sun, H.; et al. Exosomal PD-L1 contributes to immunosuppression and is associated with anti-PD-1 response. *Nature* **2018**, *560*, 382–386. [CrossRef]
106. Zhang, J.; Gao, J.; Li, Y.; Nie, J.; Dai, L.; Hu, W.; Chen, X.; Han, J.; Ma, X.; Tian, G.; et al. Circulating PD-L1 in NSCLC patients and the correlation between the level of PD-L1 expression and the clinical characteristics. *Thorac. Cancer* **2015**, *6*, 534–538. [CrossRef]
107. Okuma, Y.; Hosomi, Y.; Nakahara, Y.; Watanabe, K.; Sagawa, Y.; Homma, S. High plasma levels of soluble programmed cell death ligand 1 are prognostic for reduced survival in advanced lung cancer. *Lung Cancer* **2017**, *104*, 1–6. [CrossRef]
108. Poggio, M.; Hu, T.; Pai, C.C.; Chu, B.; Belair, C.D.; Chang, A.; Montabana, E.; Lang, U.E.; Fu, Q.; Fong, L.; et al. Suppression of Exosomal PD-L1 Induces Systemic Anti-tumor Immunity and Memory. *Cell* **2019**, *177*, 414–427.e13. [CrossRef]
109. Atai, N.A.; Balaj, L.; van Veen, H.; Breakefield, X.O.; Jarzyna, P.A.; Van Noorden, C.J.; Skog, J.; Maguire, C.A. Heparin blocks transfer of extracellular vesicles between donor and recipient cells. *J. Neurooncol.* **2013**, *115*, 343–351. [CrossRef]
110. Balaj, L.; Atai, N.A.; Chen, W.; Mu, D.; Tannous, B.A.; Breakefield, X.O.; Skog, J.; Maguire, C.A. Heparin affinity purification of extracellular vesicles. *Sci. Rep.* **2015**, *5*, 10266. [CrossRef]
111. Chapman, C.J.; Thorpe, A.J.; Murray, A.; Parsy-Kowalska, C.B.; Allen, J.; Stafford, K.M.; Chauhan, A.S.; Kite, T.A.; Maddison, P.; Robertson, J.F. Immunobiomarkers in small cell lung cancer: Potential early cancer signals. *Clin. Cancer Res.* **2011**, *17*, 1474–1480. [CrossRef]
112. Zhong, L.; Coe, S.P.; Stromberg, A.J.; Khattar, N.H.; Jett, J.R.; Hirschowitz, E.A. Profiling tumor-associated antibodies for early detection of non-small cell lung cancer. *J. Thorac. Oncol.* **2006**, *1*, 513–519. [CrossRef] [PubMed]
113. Li, G.; Miles, A.; Line, A.; Rees, R.C. Identification of tumour antigens by serological analysis of cDNA expression cloning. *Cancer Immunol. Immunother.* **2004**, *53*, 139–143. [CrossRef] [PubMed]

© 2020 by the authors. Licensee MDPI, Basel, Switzerland. This article is an open access article distributed under the terms and conditions of the Creative Commons Attribution (CC BY) license (http://creativecommons.org/licenses/by/4.0/).

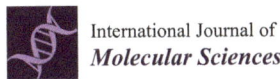

Review

Signaling of Tumor-Derived sEV Impacts Melanoma Progression

Aneta Zebrowska [1], Piotr Widlak [1], Theresa Whiteside [2,3] and Monika Pietrowska [1,*]

1. Maria Sklodowska-Curie National Research Institute of Oncology, Gliwice Branch, 44-100 Gliwice, Poland; aneta7zebrowska@gmail.com (A.Z.); piotr.widlak@io.gliwice.pl (P.W.)
2. UPMC Hillman Cancer Center, University of Pittsburgh, Pittsburgh, PA 15213, USA; whitesidetl@upmc.edu
3. Department of Pathology, University of Pittsburgh School of Medicine Pittsburgh, Pittsburgh, PA 15261, USA
* Correspondence: monika.pietrowska@io.gliwice.pl; Tel.: +48-32-278-9627

Received: 30 June 2020; Accepted: 15 July 2020; Published: 17 July 2020

Abstract: Small extracellular vesicles (sEV or exosomes) are nanovesicles (30–150 nm) released both in vivo and in vitro by most cell types. Tumor cells produce sEV called TEX and disperse them throughout all body fluids. TEX contain a cargo of proteins, lipids, and RNA that is similar but not identical to that of the "parent" producer cell (i.e., the cargo of exosomes released by melanoma cells is similar but not identical to exosomes released by melanocytes), possibly due to selective endosomal packaging. TEX and their role in cancer biology have been intensively investigated largely due to the possibility that TEX might serve as key component of a "liquid tumor biopsy." TEX are also involved in the crosstalk between cancer and immune cells and play a key role in the suppression of anti-tumor immune responses, thus contributing to the tumor progression. Most of the available information about the TEX molecular composition and functions has been gained using sEV isolated from supernatants of cancer cell lines. However, newer data linking plasma levels of TEX with cancer progression have focused attention on TEX in the patients' peripheral circulation as potential biomarkers of cancer diagnosis, development, activity, and response to therapy. Here, we consider the molecular cargo and functions of TEX as potential biomarkers of one of the most fatal malignancies—melanoma. Studies of TEX in plasma of patients with melanoma offer the possibility of an in-depth understanding of the melanoma biology and response to immune therapies. This review features melanoma cell-derived exosomes (MTEX) with special emphasis on exosome-mediated signaling between melanoma cells and the host immune system.

Keywords: small extracellular vesicles (sEV); tumor-derived exosomes (TEX); melanoma cell-derived exosomes (MTEX); proteomics; tumor microenvironment; biomarkers

1. Introduction

Small extracellular vesicles (sEV), also known as exosomes (EX), are virus-size (30–150 nm) membrane-bound vesicles released by different cell types under both normal and pathological conditions. They represent a subset of the heterogeneous group of extracellular vesicles (EV) that in addition to sEV include larger (250–1000 nm) microvesicles (MV, ectosomes) and the largest (>1000 nm) apoptotic bodies (AB). EV vary in size, biogenesis, release mechanisms, and biochemical properties. sEV or exosomes are formed in the endosomal network as intraluminal vesicles (ILV) within the multivesicular bodies (MVB) and are released to the extracellular space when MVBs fuse with the cellular plasma membrane. In contrast, MV are produced by outward budding ("blebbing") of the plasma membrane, while apoptotic bodies are released when cells undergo the programmed cell death [1–7]. At present, inconsistency in the EV nomenclature exists causing much confusion in the field, which extends to the methodology for sEV isolation and characterization. Currently, the most common vesicle isolation methods, including ultracentrifugation, do not adequately discriminate between various EV subsets. To ease confusion, a simplified nomenclature has been recently adopted in the literature that distinguishes small EV (i.e., <200 nm) and medium/large EV (>200 nm). The class of small EV consists mostly of exosomes, yet other types of EV, e.g., small MV, could also copurify with this fraction [8–11]. In this review, the terms "exosomes" (EX) and (small) extracellular vesicles (sEV) are used interchangeably for simplicity and to stay in line with the recent guidelines from International Society for Extracellular Vesicles (ISEV) [8].

Among various subsets of EV in body fluids of cancer patients, tumor-derived exosomes, called TEX, have attracted much attention as major mediators of intercellular communication in the tumor microenvironment (TME) and as potentially promising diagnostic, prognostic, and predictive biomarkers in cancer and other diseases. The knowledge of the molecular profiles and biology of TEX offers the possibility of a deeper understanding of pathological processes involved in cancer development and may provide important clinical information about disease activity and response to treatment. Today, TEX are considered as prime candidates for a liquid tumor biopsy, and much effort is being invested in validation of this concept. In this review, we summarize recent insights into the biology and composition of melanoma cell-derived exosomes (MTEX) and provide an up-to-date account of their pleiotropic role in melanoma progression and response to anti-melanoma therapies.

2. General Characteristics of sEV

sEV are produced and released by various cell types, including hematopoietic cells and a broad variety of normal or malignant tissue cells [5,7,12,13]. sEV can be isolated from supernatants of cultured cells or diverse body fluids, including blood, urine, saliva, breast milk, ascites effusions, bile, tears, nasal secretions, amniotic, synovial, cerebrospinal, lymphatic, and seminal fluids [5,7,10,14–23]. The molecular content of sEV is of special interest, as it reflects the nature of parental cells. sEV originating from different cell types share their general features, such as the structure of the bilayer lipid–protein membrane and key molecular components. Their molecular cargo consists of proteins (including cytoskeletal proteins, transmembrane proteins, tetraspanins, heat shock proteins, adhesion proteins, enzymes, immunocompetent proteins e.g., death receptor ligands: tumor necrosis factor ligand (FasL, CD95L or CD178) or TNF-related apoptosis-inducing ligand (TRAIL), check-point receptor ligands such as: programmed death-ligand 1 (PD-L1), inhibitory cytokines such as: interleukin 10 (IL-10), IL-6, TNF-α, IL-1β, and TGF-β1, prostaglandin E2, major histocompatibility molecules MHC-I and II, and tumor-associated antigens), nucleic acids (including DNA, RNA, miRNA, non-coding RNA), lipids, and low-molecular-weight metabolites (including alcohols, amides, amino acids, carboxylic acids, sugars). Proteomic analysis of exosome cargos revealed that some proteins are typical for most of these vesicles (including proteins such as Rab2, Rab7, flotillin, and annexin; cytoskeletal proteins, including actin, myosin, tubulin; or heat shock proteins, such as Hsc70 and Hsc90). Tetraspanins, such as CD9, CD63, CD81, CD83, along with housekeeping proteins, ALIX (programmed cell death 6-interacting protein) and TSG101 (tumor susceptibility gene 101 protein), are widely considered as exosome markers. However, in addition to the "common" set of components, sEV of different cellular origins may also carry proteins that are cell-type specific [8–12,24]. It has been shown in many studies that the molecular profile of TEX is distinct from that of sEV derived from non-malignant cells such as dendritic cells (DC), T cells, and others [6,7,11–13,25]. However, it should be noted that the discrimination of TEX from other types of sEV in patients' plasma using, e.g., tetraspanins as sEV-specific markers has been limited and currently, separation of TEX from total sEV in plasma has not been readily available or reliably performed.

sEV circulating in body fluids represent a complex mixture of vesicles released by many different cell types. The majority of studies of TEX present in body fluids of cancer patients are based on analyzes performed with a mixture of sEV derived from different normal or pathological cells. Separation of TEX from this mixture remains a challenge due to the lack of universal cancer-specific antigens that could be targeted for TEX isolation. Nevertheless, a few studies that used specific membrane markers for isolation of TEX from body fluids have been reported. Chondroitin sulfate proteoglycan 4 (CSPG4) was used for separation of melanoma-derived TEX, referred to as MTEX, from vesicles released by non-malignant cells [26–28]. Glypican 1 (GPC1) was used to isolate TEX from plasma of patients with pancreatic cancer [29], and prostate-specific membrane antigen (PSMA) was used to isolate TEX from plasma of prostate cancer patients [30]. CD34 antigen, a unique marker of AML blasts, was used to isolate TEX from the plasma of patients with acute myeloid leukemia [31]. Moreover, MAGE3/6 antigen was used to identify TEX present in sera of patients with melanoma or head and neck squamous cell carcinoma (HNSCC) [25]. In contrast to plasma-derived sEV, TEX isolated from supernatants of cancer cell lines are putatively homogenous. These TEX derived from tumor cell lines are an excellent in vitro model for investigations of interactions of TEX with other cells. In fact, much of what is known about TEX signaling, uptake by responder cells, and reprogramming in TME is derived from in vitro and in vivo studies of TEX isolated from supernatants of tumor cell lines.

sEV have gained interest due to their essential role in "normal" intercellular signaling and communication, which impact the physiological balance and homeostasis as well as disease progression. [1,6,32–36]. Importantly, sEV can modulate the phenotype/functions of recipient cells, even those located in distant organs [2,3,35–38]. Moreover, the role of TEX in cancer progression has been reported for many cancer types, including ovarian, prostate, breast, lung, colorectal and gastric cancers, melanoma, and acute myeloid leukemia [26,37–44]. TEX are being intensively investigated because they play a key role in the reorganization of the TME, remodeling functions of the cells residing in the TME, and enhancing their contribution to tumorigenesis, metastasis, cancer immune escape, as well as resistance to cancer treatment [34,44–54]. The potential role of TEX in cancer biology is schematically illustrated in Figure 1. A better understanding of the mechanisms underlying TEX-mediated reprogramming of normal cells in TME is expected to be clinically significant, leading to improved cancer diagnosis/prognosis and treatment. In addition, TEX are considered to be an attractive source of cancer biomarkers.

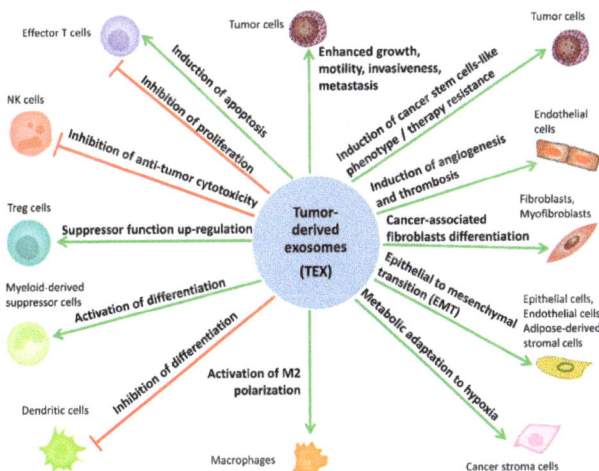

Figure 1. Role of tumor-derived small extracellular vesicles (sEV) (TEX) in cancer biology. Tumor-derived exosomes (TEX) are involved in intercellular signaling and communication between tumor cells and non-malignant cells residing in the tumor microenvironment. TEX reprogram these cells to acquire functions favoring tumor growth and metastasis. TEX-induced changes include enhancing cancer immune escape, remodeling of the tumor stroma, molecular and metabolic reprogramming, and promotion of angiogenesis. Green arrows indicate the processes stimulated by TEX. Red lines with blunt ends indicate processes inhibited by TEX.

3. General Features of Melanoma

Melanoma is the most aggressive skin cancer whose incidence has been increasing worldwide. Melanoma prognosis is generally poor, as it has a high potential for vascular invasion, metastasis, and recurrence [55–57]. Primary melanomas detected in an early stage and completely removed surgically show favorable outcome, with 5-year disease-specific survival rates of 99% [58]. However, melanoma cells tend to metastasize to distant sites, most often to lungs and brain, while evading the host immune system. Hence, the survival rate dramatically decreases when the cancer metastasizes, and 1-year survival rate drops to 35%–62% [57,59], while 5-year survival rate drops to 25% [58]. Currently, surgery is the treatment of choice for patients with cutaneous melanoma, and the adjuvant treatment scheme is usually tailored individually. Melanoma is sensitive to immune checkpoint inhibitors, such as anti-CTLA4 (anti-cytotoxic T-lymphocyte-associated protein 4 or anti-CD 152) and anti-PD1 (anti-programmed cell death protein 1 or anti-CD279) monoclonal antibodies (mAb), and to small-molecule targeted drugs, such as serine/threonine-protein kinase B-Raf (BRAF) or mitogen-activated protein kinase (MEK) inhibitors. Hence, different treatment schemes, including radiotherapy and/or adjuvant treatments with anti-BRAF/MEK inhibitors and anti-PD-1 mAb are currently used, depending on the patient's clinical situation [60]. Despite these novel combinatorial therapies, tumor escape from the immune control and development of primary or acquired therapy resistance that occurs in about half of melanoma patients remain the major therapeutic barrier [61–63]. Melanoma cells communicate with other cells present in the TME, including components of the immune system, via melanoma cell-derived exosomes (MTEX). Hence, in-depth knowledge of MTEX composition and function is expected to bring better understanding of the mechanisms determining the response of melanoma to treatments.

4. The Molecular Cargo of MTEX

4.1. The Proteome of MTEX

Recently, studies of proteomic profiles of cancer-derived sEV have been much intensified [64–67]. However, only limited data are available about the proteome of melanoma-derived TEX. A great part of the available literature focuses on in vitro studies with TEX isolated from supernatants of various melanoma cell lines [68–73]. Ex vivo studies performed with TEX isolated from the blood of melanoma patients are rare [74]. It is important to emphasize that only sEV derived from melanoma cell lines are "pure" MTEX, as those present in the plasma will be mixtures of sEV derived from many different cells. The available studies of MTEX have utilized different proteomic approaches. Most of them are based on shotgun LC-MS/MS strategies (i.e., tryptic digestion of proteins, followed by nano HPLC-MS/MS analysis of the resulting peptides), while others are based on LC-MS/MS analysis of proteins separated by 1D or 2D SDS-PAGE [75]. Currently available proteomic studies demonstrate differences in protein profiles of MTEX in comparison to melanocyte-derived sEV [68,69]. In addition, MTEX derived from melanoma cell lines with a different tumorigenic potential appeared to have distinct proteomic profiles [70]. Moreover, proteomic analysis of sEV present in the plasma of melanoma patients and healthy donors showed clear differences and revealed increased levels of TYRP2, VLA-4, and HSP70 in patients' samples [74]. However, the knowledge of the proteome in TEX produced by melanoma cells remains rather limited, and the available data are difficult to compare because they represent distinct experimental models. A summary of data on proteomics profiling of MTEX released by melanoma cell lines is presented in Table 1.

Table 1. Proteomics Profiling of Melanoma Cell-Derived Exosomes (MTEX) Released in Vitro by Melanoma Cell Lines.

Cell Line	Method of MTEX Purification and Characterization	MS Approach	Major Findings	Ref.
MeWo, SK-MEL-28 (human)	UC/TEM, WB, 1D/2D SDS-PAGE	MALDI-TOF MS/MS	A few proteins identified in MTEX for the first time: prostaglandin regulatory-like protein (PGRL), p120 catenin, syntaxin-binding proteins 1 and 2, septin 2 (Nedd5), ezrin, radixin, tryptophan/aspartic acid (WD) repeat-containing protein 1	[68]
A375 (human)	UC/TEM, NTA, WB	LC-MS/MS	Different sets of proteins present in MTEX and melanocyte-derived EV, including annexin A1, HAPLN1, GRP78, endoplasmin precursor (gp 96), TUBA1B, PYGB), ferritin, heavy polypeptide 1 (MTEX-upregulated), annexin A2, syntenin-1, MFGE8, OXCT (MTEX-downregulated)	[69]
MNT-1, G1, 501 mel, SKMEL28, Daju, A375M, 1205Lu (human)	UC+SEC/WB, TEM, NTA	nanoLC-MS/MS	Different sets of proteins present in MTEX from nontumorigenic, tumorigenic, and metastatic cell lines, including EGFR, PTK2/FAK1, EPHB2, SRC, LGALS1/LEG1, LGALS3/LEG3, NT5E/5NTD-CD73, NRAS, KIT, MCAM/MUC18, MET specific for metastatic cell lines	[70]
B16-F1 (murine)	UC+SEC/CEM, DLS, IA-FCM	uHPLC-MS	10 most abundant proteins: CD81, CD9, histones (H2A, H2B, H3.1, H4), heat shock proteins (HSPA5/GRP78, HSC71), syntetin-1	[71]
B16-F10 (murine)	UC+SEC, UF+SEC/TEM, NTA, WB	nanoLC-MS/MS	Different sets of proteins identified in low- and high-density MTEX, including ACTN4 and CCNY enriched in LD-MTEX and EPHA2 enriched in HD-MTEX	[72]
Mel501 (human)	UC+SEC/WB, CM	RPLC-MS/MS	Different sets of proteins identified in MTEX released in neutral and acidic environment (pH 6.7 and 6.0, respectively), including HRAS, NRAS, TIMP3, HSP90AB1, HSP90B1, HSPAIL, HSPA5, GANAB, gelsolin, and cofilin upregulated in acidic conditions.	[73]

Abbreviations: methods of EX purification: UC—ultracentrifugation, UF—ultrafiltration, SEC—size-exclusion chromatography; methods of EX characterization: NTA—nanoparticle tracking analysis, DLS—dynamic light scattering, TEM—transmission electron microscopy, CEM—cryo-electron microscopy, CM—confocal microscopy, WB—Western blotting.

4.2. Micro RNA Component of MTEX

Micro RNAs are small (19–25 nucleotides) non-coding RNAs that play an important role as regulators of cell differentiation, metabolism, proliferation, or innate and adaptive immunity [76–78]. Micro RNA profiles of TEX differ from miRNA profiles of their donor cancer cells as well as from profiles of sEV released by normal cells [78–81]. The majority of available works report miRNA signatures of pure MTEX released in vitro by melanoma cell lines [69,82–90]. Moreover, a few studies addressed miRNA composition of sEV derived from serum/plasma of melanoma patients [82,91–94]. Similar to proteomics data, few consistencies were observed among these studies due to different models applied. Nevertheless, there were 6 MTEX-upregulated miRNA species reported in more than one study: miR-494 [82,83], let-7c [69,84], miR-690 [84,85], miR-17 [84,91], and miR-494 [82,83], while miR-125b was reported to be downregulated in MTEX or sEV from plasma of melanoma patients [83,92]. Noteworthy, all the above mentioned miRs are known to be involved in cancer cell invasion, migration, and proliferation as well as in inflammatory processes linked to tumorigenesis and cancer progression [82–86,91,92].

Xiao et al. showed significant differences in miRNA content of exosomes isolated from normal melanocytes and malignant cell lines (HEMa-LP and A375), respectively [69]. In this study, 130 miRNAs were upregulated and 98 miRNAs downregulated in MTEX versus melanocyte-derived EX. The majority of differently expressed miRNAs were associated with tumor aggressiveness, including fifteen miRNAs known to be associated with melanoma metastasis: miR-138, miR-125b, miR-130a, miR-34a, miR-196a, miR-199a-3p, miR-25, miR-27a, miR-200b, miR-23b, miR-146a, miR-613, miR-205, miR-149, let-7c [69]. Another study reported enrichment of miRNA-494, which is known for its high metastatic potential, in MTEX released by A375 cells. A series of functional experiments performed by Li et al. demonstrated that intercellular transport of miR-494 in MTEX was responsible for melanoma metastasis [82]. Blocking of exosomal transfer of miR-494 by a knockdown (KO) of Rab27a induced cellular apoptosis and inhibited tumor growth and metastasis in vitro and in human xenografts [82].

Another analysis of the miRs upregulated in sEV of patients with metastatic melanoma (miR-17-5p, miR-19a-3p, miR-149-5p, miR-21, and miR-126-3p) focused on discovery of putative targets of these miRNAs [91]. Among their targets were genes associated with skin response to UV irradiation, genes coding the tumor protein p53 (TP53)/retinoblastoma protein (RB1) and genes related to the TGF-β/SMAD pathway. Upregulation of miRNAs controlling TP53/RB1 activation and the TGF-β/SMAD signaling pathway might play an important role in melanoma progression, as the TGFβ/SMAD pathway regulates the G1/S checkpoint in normal melanocytes [91]. Moreover, miR-17 was identified as a potential oncomiR not only in melanoma but also in other malignancies [93,94]. Association of miR-19a upregulation with increased melanoma invasiveness was confirmed by Levy et al. [95]. Upregulation of miR-21 and miR-19a is associated with increased proliferation, low apoptosis, invasiveness, and high metastatic potential, as reported for various human tumor cells [96,97], while KO of miR-21 in B16 melanoma cells reduced their metastatic potential [98,99]. The oncogenic properties of miR-21 may be a result of down-regulation of the tumor suppressors: PTEN, PDCD4 and the antiproliferative protein BTG2. In addition, miR-21 induced the IFN pathway with protumorigenic effects [98,99]. High abundance of another oncomiR—miR-1246 was detected in MTEX isolated from patient-derived melanoma cell lines, namely, DMBC9, -10, -11, and -12 [83,100]. Many other studies have confirmed its high concentration in sEV from the plasma of patients with various cancers, including melanoma [101,102]. The overexpression of miR-222 in MTEX and cells is also associated with tumor initiation, differentiation, increased cell motility, and invasion, as well as cancer progression [87]. MiR-222 inhibits anti-neoplastic functions of p27, CDKN1B, and c-Fos by down-modulation of their gene expression, reduces apoptosis, and allows proliferation by induction of the PI3K/AKT pathway [89]. Müller et al. showed the importance of let-7a in melanoma development [103]. Let-7a regulates the expression of integrin β-3, the promotor of melanoma progression. The loss of let-7a expression in MTEX derived from 8 different melanoma cell lines resulted in higher integrin β-3 levels in melanoma cells, enhancing their migratory and invasive potential [103]. Finally, let-7a was detected in serum EX as a factor differentiating stage I melanoma patients from non-melanoma subjects [104]. Altogether, the literature supports the key role played by miRs transferred by melanoma-associated TEX in oncogenesis and melanoma metastasis.

In addition to microRNA, MTEX contain mRNA transcripts of genes expressed in melanoma. Sets of mRNAs with different abundance in MTEX and in melanosome-derived exosomes were identified, including 945 transcripts associated with cancer and 364 associated with dermatological diseases [69]. Among upregulated transcripts there was DNA topoisomerase I (TOP1), which is known to be associated with aggressive, advanced tumors and poor prognosis in melanoma [69,105]. Among downregulated transcripts there were ATP-binding cassette, sub-family B, member 5 (ABCB5), which activates the NF-κB pathway enhancing p65 protein stability [106] and is also known to be closely co-regulated with melanoma tumor antigen p97 (tumor growth regulator—melanotransferrin, MTf) [107], and TYRP1 encoding tyrosinase-related protein 1, which is considered as an inhibitor of TYRP1-dependent miR-16 mediating tumor suppression [108,109].

5. Biological Activity of MTEX

The multi-level contribution of MTEX to tumorigenesis accounts for activation of biological processes enabling cancer immune evasion, as well as molecular and metabolic remodeling of tumor micro- and macro-environment, favoring cancer growth and metastasis. The in-depth knowledge of the pleiotropic role of MTEX in the natural history of melanoma has a great potential clinical application in the disease diagnosis, treatment design, and prognosis of patient's outcomes. MTEX are involved in a plethora of functions involved in initiation, progression, and metastasis of tumors, which is schematically depicted in Figure 2 (according to [26,37,73,74,83–150]). The most essential functions of MTEX are addressed more specifically in the following sub-chapters.

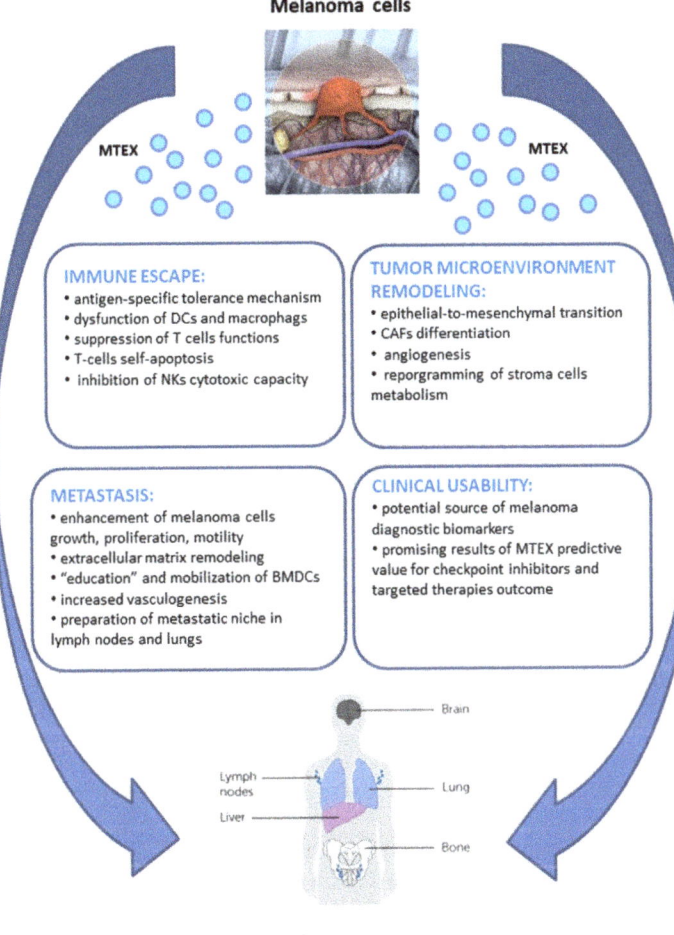

Figure 2. Pleiotropic effect of MTEX on melanoma biology.

5.1. MTEX Participate in the Reprogramming of Immune Cells

Growth and progression of cancer involve the escape from the immune surveillance as the sine qua non condition. Emerging evidence supports the idea that MTEX are involved in facilitating tumor escape from the host immune system [33,44,47,49,110–117]. However, in most of the studies reported in this context, melanoma cell lines were used as a source of MTEX. Düchler et al. showed that cancer-induced immunosuppression was mediated by MTEX, and involved an antigen-specific mechanism [118]. The authors provided evidence that MTEX transferred MHC class I receptor proteins from cancer cells to the surface of antigen-presenting cells (APC). At the same time, CD86 and CD40 (co-stimulatory molecules required for differentiation and proliferation of T cells) were down-regulated, while the production of immunosuppressive cytokine IL-6 was induced. Collaboration of TGF-β transported by

MTEX was also demonstrated in this process. The authors hypothesized that MTEX-mediated transfer of the combination of TAA-derived peptide-MHC complexes with immunosuppressive cytokines was a part of antigen-specific tolerance induction enabling melanoma immune escape [118]. The mechanism of melanoma immune escape is also related to the suppression of T cell functions. This can be attributed to an increased level of PD-L1 in MTEX. This immunosuppression is driven by the interaction between PD-L1 carried by MTEX and PD-1 receptors on $CD8^+$ T cells, leading to inhibition of T-cell functions [111,119]. MTEX are also enriched in Fas ligand (FasL) and APO2 ligand (APO2L)/TRAIL, both known as inducing factors of T cell-apoptosis [120]. Another possible mechanism for the suppression of T cell function by MTEX is through the upregulation of PTPN11 protein, which was found to negatively regulate interferon, IL-2, and T cell receptor signaling pathways [121]. Wu et al. confirmed that B16F0-derived MTEX are enriched with Ptpn11 mRNA and can increase PTPN11 dose-dependently in recipient cells. In addition to upregulating PTPN11 in lymphocytes, MTEX derived from B16F0 locally suppressed responses of cells to IL-12 (anti-tumor immunity enhancer) via inhibition of IL12RB2 expression in primary $CD8^+$ T cells. These inhibitory mechanisms of the immune cell response to IL-12 are complemented by B16F0 release of the Wnt-inducible signaling protein 1 (WISP1) that blocks T cell response to IL-12 [121,122]. Furthermore, the cargo of MTEX might alter mitochondrial respiration of cytotoxic T cells and up-regulate genes associated with the Notch signaling pathway [84]. Immunosuppressive activity of MTEX depends on their ligands that engage the T cell receptor (TCR) and IL-2 receptor (IL-2R). Recent studies showed that MTEX inhibited signaling and proliferation of activated primary $CD8^+$ T cells, inducing their apoptosis [25,32,90]. Furthermore, MTEX significantly promoted conversion of CD4(+) T cells to CD4(+)CD25(+)FOXP3(+) T regulatory cells (Treg) enhancing their suppressor functions [25]. Vignard et al. additionally confirmed decreased TCR signaling in T cells as a result of the enrichment in miRNAs regulating TCR signaling and TNF-α secretion (miR-3187-3p, miR-498, miR-122, miR149, miR-181a/b) in MTEX [90].

Accumulating evidence reveals that TNF is negatively regulated by miR-21. This may explain the effects of miR-21 on cell proliferation, migration, invasion, and transformation associated with excessive miR-21 levels in MTEX. Moreover, some results suggest that TNF can promote miR-21 biogenesis [123] as well as the turnover of PDCD4 in macrophages [124]. Yang et al. also showed that increased levels of miR-21 associated with a decreased level of TNF were consistent with elevated IL-10 protein expression and increased Arg1 macrophage expression, which could explain poor immune responses against cancer cells [98]. On the other hand, Fabri et al. reported that miR-21 which was found to be enriched in MTEX might also act as a ligand by binding to receptors of the Toll-like receptor (TLR) family members, murine TLR7, and human TLR8, in immune cells. Triggering the TLR-mediated prometastatic inflammatory response in responder cells might promote tumor growth and metastasis [125].

Stimulation of $TLR2^+$ DC by tumor-derived TLR2 ligands was reported to drive inhibitory signals leading to dysfunctional activity of DC in murine melanoma [126]. Modulation of immune response by MTEX was confirmed by Zhou et al. [85]. They observed that B16-derived MTEX induced apoptosis of $CD4^+$ T cells in vitro and promoted the growth of tumor cells implanted in mice. The opposite results were reported by blocking MTEX release (disrupting the expression of Rab27a), thus confirming the proposed mechanism. Further, they showed that B16-derived MTEX induced activation of caspase-3, caspase-7, and caspase-9, reducing the level of anti-apoptotic proteins, such as BCL-2, BCL-xL, and MCL-1 in $CD4^+$ T cells [85]. MTEX can also alter the functions of natural killer (NK) cells. They were found to modulate the tumor immune responses by inhibiting the cytotoxic activity of NKs and downregulating the expression of NKG2D, NKp30, NKP46, and NKG2C proteins on the surface of NK cells [26,42,127].

5.2. MTEX Participate in the Reprogramming of TME

TME plays a major role in cancer growth and evolution. Diverse cells such as fibroblasts, endothelial, epithelial, and mesenchymal cells or immune cells present in the TME might be reprogrammed by MTEX to favor tumor growth [45,56]. Accumulating data provide evidence that MTEX promote epithelial-to-mesenchymal transition (EMT), which promotes metastasis [46,48,55,57,128]. The mitogen-activated protein kinase (MAPK) signaling pathway is activated during the MTEX-mediated EMT, with the involvement of Let-7i, a miRNA modulator of EMT [104]. Furthermore, acquisition of the EMT-like phenotype is enforced by expression of other key regulators of EMT induction, including ZEB2 and Snail 2 [119,129]. Upregulation of ZEB2 and Snail 2 in primary melanocytes after co-culture with MTEX was confirmed by Xiao et al. This process was accompanied by decreased expression of E-cadherin and increased expression of vimentin [104]. The interplay between MTEX and myeloid stem cells (MSCs) induce the emergence of a tumor-like phenotype with PD-1 and mTOR overexpression in naïve MSCs in vitro and fast tumor progression in vivo [119]. Interaction networks build basing on genes overexpressed in recipient cells upon co-incubation with MTEX identified a variety of other exosomal molecules, apart from PD-1 and mTOR, which might affect tumor progressions, such as MET, Ras, RAF1, Mek, ERK1/2, MITF, BCL2, PI3K, Akt, KIT, JAK STAT3, or ETS1 [119].

MTEX transform fibroblasts into proangiogenic cancer-associated fibroblasts (CAF) in vitro and in vivo. CAF are known to support development of pre-cancerous micro- and macro-environments [86,130,131]. Zhao et al. discovered that incubation of MTEX with fibroblasts resulted in a significant increase of VCAM-1 expression, and this enhancement was even stronger when EX were derived from highly metastatic melanoma cells [131]. Overexpression of miR-155 in MTEX was found to be the trigger factor for the proangiogenic switch of fibroblasts into CAF [86]. MTEX-mediated delivery of miR-155 to fibroblasts suppressed expression of cytokine signaling 1 (SOCS1), that activates the JAK2/STAT3 signaling pathway which, in turn, regulates the expression of proangiogenic factors. Elevated expression of vascular endothelial growth factor A (VEGFa), fibroblast growth factor 2 (FGF2), and matrix metalloproteinase 9 (MMP9) in fibroblasts after incubation with MTEX was confirmed in this study [86]. Shu et al. also reported the presence of exosomal miR-155 and miR-210 across six melanoma cell lines [89] and showed that miRNA cargo of MTEX was capable of reprogramming the metabolism of human adult dermal fibroblasts (HADF). In this study, miR-155 upregulated glucose metabolism (i.e., increased glycolysis), while miR-210 decreased oxidative phosphorylation under non-hypoxic conditions. Exposure of HADF to MTEX resulted in upregulated aerobic glycolysis and downregulated oxidative phosphorylation in stromal fibroblasts, with consequently increasing extracellular acidification [89]. Furthermore, the acidic environment led to upregulation of over 50% of exosomal proteins involved in cancer progression in MTEX derived from the primary non-tumorigenic MEL501 cell line [73]. The upregulated proteins were associated with focal adhesion, actin cytoskeleton regulation, leukocyte trans-endothelial migration, regulation and modification of cell morphology, HSP family proteins, proteoglycans related to cancer, small GTPase mediated signal transduction, and epidermal growth factor receptor (EGFR) signaling pathways [73]. This shows that MTEX are important contributors to changes in the TME that are responsible for creating favorable conditions for the pre-metastatic niche. On the one hand accelerated aerobic glycolysis ensures more effective energy production, but on the other hand, the acidic microenvironment drives immune suppression and creates a pro-metastatic environment [73,89,132].

The pro-angiogenic effects of MTEX are well-documented. MTEX cargos are enriched in pro-angiogenic cytokines, including IL-1α, FGF, GCS-F, TNFα, leptin, TGFα, and VEGF [107]. MTEX also mediate the transfer of miR-9 from melanoma to endothelial cells (EC), which triggers the JAK-STAT pathway and enhances the migratory propensity of vascular cells as well as the formation of a tumor-supporting vascular net [133]. Additionally, it was reported that increased WNT5A signaling, which is known to promote melanoma metastasis, induced a Ca^{2+}-dependent release of exosomes containing the pro-angiogenic VEGF and MMP2 factors in melanoma cells [134].

5.3. MTEX Can Modulate Tumor Progression and Invasiveness

In general, TEX may induce tumor growth in vitro and in vivo [135,136]. It was reported that B16BL6-derived MTEX induced proliferation and inhibited apoptosis of murine melanoma B16BL6 cells, while inhibition of MTEX release by the N-Smase inhibitor suppressed melanoma growth. Noteworthy, the uptake of MTEX resulted in increased levels of cyclin D1, p-Akt (cell proliferation-related proteins), Bcl-2 (survival-related protein), and decreased level of Bax (apoptosis-related proteins) [137]. Peinado et al. reported that the oncoprotein MET selectively enriched in MTEX released by metastatic melanoma cells promoted the tumorigenic potential of melanoma [74]. Pre-conditioning of bone marrow (BM) with MTEX obtained from a highly metastatic melanoma B16-F10 cell line promoted mobilization of bone marrow-derived cells (BMDC), increasing tumor vasculogenesis, invasion, and metastasis. Comparative analysis of the protein content in MTEX from highly metastatic and poorly metastatic melanoma cells confirmed MET signaling as the principal mediator of BM progenitor cell "education". Pre-treatment of BM cells with B16-F10 MTEX resulted in HGF-induced S6 and ERK phosphorylation compared to non-treated controls. Effectors of MET-mediated BM progenitor cell mobilization, i.e., S6-kinase (mTOR pathway) and ERK (MAPK pathway), are known mediators of HGF/MET signaling. Further, the metastatic spread and organotropism of highly metastatic B16-F10 primary tumors were reduced by the BM of mice "educated" with the low-metastatic B16-F1 MTEX that lacked the MET receptor. These data suggested that non-metastatic MTEX might educate the BM and prevent metastatic disease, a finding that is worth further exploration. Finally, it was confirmed that MET expression was elevated in sEV circulating in the plasma of patients with metastatic melanoma [74]. Additionally, influence of metabotropic glutamate receptor 1 (GRM1) expressed on melanoma cells was tested for cell migration and invasiveness [138]. This neuronal receptor induces in vitro melanocytic transformation and spontaneous malignant melanoma development in vivo. Moreover, modulation (decrease) of GRM1 expression results in a decrease in both cell proliferation in vitro and tumor progression in vivo. Isola et al. verified a hypothesis that exosomes released by a GRM1-positive (metastatic) cell line made GRM1-negative (non-metastatic) cells acquire features characteristic for GRM1-positive cells, i.e., to migrate, invade, form colonies, and exhibit anchorage-independent cell growth. They found that acquiring these features was not connected with expression of this receptor on GRM1-negative cells. Another aspect of the potential role of MTEX in tumorigenesis is analysis of specific RAB genes involved in sEV secretion (RAB1A, RAB5B, RAB7, RAB27A) [74]. Rab27a is a regulator of protein trafficking and melanoma proliferation [139]. Reduced expression of Rab27a resulted in decreased sEV production, and in decreased release of pro-angiogenic factors (PlGF-2, osteopontin, and PDGF-AA) from tumor cells, interfering with BMDC mobilization and tumor invasiveness [74]. These results are in line with the latest findings of Guo and colleagues [140], who reported that the GTPase RAB27A was overexpressed in melanoma patients and correlated with poor patient survival. A loss of RAB27A expression in melanoma cell lines blocked invasion and cell motility in vitro, and spontaneous metastasis in vivo. Furthermore, RAB27A-expressing MTEX promoted the invasion phenotype of melanoma cells in contrast to MTEX without RAB27A [140]. All in all, these results suggest that RAB27A promotes the biogenesis of a distinct pro-invasive MTEX subpopulation [74,140].

MTEX are also involved in preparation of metastatic niche for melanoma in lymph nodes and lungs and in reprogramming of innate osteotropism of melanoma cells [74,141,142]. MTEX from a highly-metastatic B16-F10 cell line promoted lymph nodes (LN) metastasis in mice [142] and were detected after 24h in the interstitium of the lung, BM, liver, and spleen (organotropic sites for B16-F10 metastasis), but not in the circulatory system [74]. Several genes responsible for the recruitment of melanoma cells (stabilin 1, ephrin receptor β4, and αv integrin), extracellular matrix remodeling (Mapk14, uPA, laminin 5, Col 18α1, G-α13, p38), vascular growth (TNF-α, TNF-αip2, VEGF-B, HIF-1α, Thbs1) [142], and effectors of pre-metastatic niche formation such as S100A8, S100A9 [74] were upregulated by B16-F10 MTEX. The osteotropism of melanoma cells is related to the activation of the SDF-1/CXCR4/CXCR7 axis. MTEX were found to promote osteotropism of not-osteotropic melanoma cells (SK-Mel28, WM266) in vitro through membrane CXCR7 up-regulation. Thus, MTEX were found to contribute to bone metastasis in melanoma [141].

6. MTEX as Potential Clinical Biomarkers

MTEX present in body fluids of melanoma patients are a promising source of prognostic biomarkers as a new type of so-called liquid biopsy. Alegre et al. performed an analysis of the established melanoma biomarkers such as: MIA, S100B, and tyrosinase-related protein 2 (TYRP2) in sEV isolated from sera of stage IV melanoma patients, patients with no evidence of disease (NED), and healthy donors (HD) [37]. The levels of MIA and S100B were significantly higher in melanoma patients in comparison to HD and NED patients. Furthermore, patients with high EV concentration of MIA had shorter median survival compared to those with lower MIA levels (4 versus 11 months; $p < 0.05$). Hence, the data suggest the potential diagnostic and prognostic utility of MIA in plasma sEV [37]. Levels of MIA, along with growth/differentiation factor 15 precursor protein (GDF15) showed a significant increase in the whole secretome of uveal melanoma versus non-malignant cells [143], which was in line with the results of Alegre et al. [37]. Tenga et al. showed that miR-532-5p and miR-106b present in serum sEV could be used for classification of melanoma patients, including differentiation of patients with metastatic and non-metastatic disease and stage I-II patients from stage III-IV patients [144]. In addition, miR-17, miR-19a, miR-21, miR-126, and miR-149 were found to be expressed at significantly higher levels in patients with metastatic sporadic melanoma compared to familial melanoma patients or healthy controls [91]. On the other hand, levels of miR-125b in sEV were significantly lower in patients with advanced melanoma compared with disease-free patients with melanoma and healthy controls, while there was no statistical difference in the miR-125b levels between patients and controls when analyzing serum samples [92].

Melanoma is sensitive to immune checkpoint inhibitors (such as anti-CTLA4 and anti-PD1 monoclonal antibodies) and small-molecule targeted drugs (such as BRAF inhibitors and MEK inhibitors). However, many patients with melanoma fail to respond to these therapies, and the mechanisms of resistance to a therapy are not understood [61–63,145,146]. The accumulating data suggest the importance of MTEX in understanding these mechanisms and the role of MTEX as predictive biomarkers of response to immune therapies and outcome [55–57,147]. Higher levels of miR-497-5p in circulating sEV during MAPKi-based therapy of cutaneous metastatic melanoma patients (with BRAFV600 mutations) were significantly correlated with progression-free survival (hazard ratio of 0.27) [147]. Increased level of miR-497-5p was also associated with prolonged post-recurrence survival in resected metastases from patients with metastatic III (lymph nodes) and metastatic IV cutaneous malignant melanoma (CMM) [148]. Treatment with vemurafenib and dabrafenib induced miR-211-5p up-regulation in melanoma-derived EV, both in vitro and in vivo, thus promoting survival in parent melanoma cells despite a down-regulation of pERK1/2 by BRAF inhibitors [146]. What is more, transfection of miR-211 in low-expressing miR-211–5p melanoma cells resulted in enhanced proliferation of melanoma cells. What is more, 100-fold increase in miR-211–5p expression in vemurafenib-treated miR-211-5p-transfected cells was found with no reduction of cells proliferation upon BRAF inhibitor treatment. These findings suggest that miR-211-5p up-regulation upon vemurafenib treatment allows these cells to survive and grow into a population of cells that have reduced sensitivity to vemurafenib. Going further, inhibition of miR-211-5p in a vemurafenib resistant cell line decreased cell proliferation. The outcome of the study of Lunavat et al. leads to better understanding of possible mechanisms of acquiring by patients' resistance to the BRAF inhibitors treatment by showing that miR-211-5p can reduce the sensitivity to vemurafenib treatment in melanoma cells by regulating cellular proliferation. [146]. Another group of "new drugs" used in the treatment of melanoma are immune checkpoint inhibitors. Anti-PD-1 antibodies are frequently used in melanoma treatment to rejuvenate anti-tumor immunity, and in the majority of patients the response is durable, yet not all melanoma patients respond to this therapy [60,149]. Chen et al. reported positive correlation between exosomal-PD-L1 (Exo-PD-L1) level and IFN-γ, both in vitro using melanoma cell lines and in vivo in patients with metastatic melanoma [111]. Upregulation of PD-L1 by IFN-γ in metastatic melanoma leads to functional suppression of CD8+ T effector cells enabling melanoma growth and metastasis. In part, this explains low response rate to anti-PD-1 therapy (pembrolizumab). The level of circulating Exo-PD-L1 distinguished clinical responders from non-responders to pembrolizumab treatment. Since the level of exosomal PD-L1 was altered early during the anti-PD-1 therapy, the authors suggest that it might be an indicator of response to treatment [111]. A recent paper by Cordonnier et al. describes monitoring of circulating Exo-PD-L1 in melanoma patients treated with immune checkpoint inhibitors and BRAF/MEK inhibitors. This prospective clinical study confirmed a significantly higher level of Exo-PD-L1 in plasma of melanoma patients compared to soluble PD-L1 and demonstrated that the level of Exo-PD-L1 inversely correlated with patients' response to therapy [150]. The results of this clinical study provide a rationale for monitoring Exo-PD-L1 level as a potential predictor of the melanoma patients' response to treatment and outcome [150].

Clinical relevance of MTEX-based biomarkers is currently limited by the necessity of separation of MTEX from other fractions of sEV circulating in body fluids. Recently, however, the anti-CSPG4 mAb was used for the separation of MTEX and sEV produced by normal tissue from the plasma of melanoma patients [26–28]. CSPG4$^+$ MTEX captured from the plasma of melanoma patients are highly enriched in melanoma-associated antigens (MAA) in comparison to CSPG4(-) non-MTEX, including CSPG4, TYRP2, MelanA, Gp100, VLA4. Moreover, several immunostimulatory (CD40, CD40L, CD80, OX40, OX40L) and immunosuppressive (PDL-1, CD39, CD73, FasL, LAP-TGFβ, TRAIL, CTLA-4) proteins were enriched in MTEX compared to sEV purified from plasma of healthy donors [26,28]. Noteworthy, looking at individual differences among proteins in the cargo of MTEX and non-MTEX, significant correlations with disease activity were observed for both fractions of vesicles. For example, non-MTEX ability to induce apoptosis of T cells positively correlated with the disease stage [28]. The obtained data suggest that features of both MTEX and non-MTEX, as well as individual MTEX/total sEV ratios, might be useful for monitoring melanoma progression [26,28]. In addition to CSPG4, other melanoma-specific or enhanced proteins might also be considered as potential markers of MTEX. This includes several melanoma-associated antigens (MAA-4, MAA-B2, and melanoma antigen recognized by T-cells) found in MTEX released by 7 different melanoma cell lines with various phenotypic features (non-tumorigenic, tumorigenic, metastatic) [70]. Moreover, several other cancer-related proteins (NRAS, Src, c-Met, c-Kit, EGFR, MCAM, annexin A1, HAPLN1, LGALS1, GALS3, NT5E, and PMEL) were detected in MTEX originating from various melanoma cell lines [69,70]. Therefore, several candidates for MTEX-markers are known that could be used for the immune capture of MTEX circulating in the body fluids of melanoma patients. Hence, the emerging concept of MTEX-based biomarkers of melanoma will meet the necessary methodological support in the nearest future.

7. Future Directions

Although the number of publications reporting on sEV in melanoma is growing exponentially, the resulting knowledge remains limited. Most likely, this is due to several factors that impede research of sEV. First, no uniformly accepted nomenclature for EV has been established, creating havoc in the definition of investigated EV. Further, no standardized procedures for the isolation of different EV types exist, leading to differences in contamination levels and co-isolation of various vesicles. The criteria and methods of EV characterization are also not clear and seem to change as we progress in the understanding of the EV heterogeneity. Despite the recommendations updated yearly by the International Society of Extracellular Vesicles (ISEV), published papers often provide incomplete data creating further confusion. The emerging view of the complex biology of EV requires strict criteria for the definition of phenotypes, genotypes, and functions of participating EV. Specifically, in a large body of available data on melanoma-associated sEV in body fluids, their origin is often unclear. Until recently, melanoma cell lines had been the only reliable source of MTEX. However, research performed with vesicles produced by cell lines does not adequately reflect interactions taking place in body fluids or tissues. Separation of MTEX from plasma by immune capture allowed for a more relevant evaluation of their characteristics and functions in disease and comparisons of data between individual patients. While this represents considerable progress, ex vivo analysis of MTEX also provides only a limited view of their biological agenda in the TME and the periphery. In vivo studies of MTEX in murine models of melanoma are critical for the translation of signaling mediated by MTEX in vitro to cells, tissues, and organs in animals. Correlative studies of MTEX and clinical endpoints in melanoma progression, resistance, or response to therapies are growing in numbers and the concept of MTEX as a liquid tumor biopsy is slowly crystallizing. Understanding of multicellular MTEX-mediated signaling and their reprogramming activities in the TME opens a way for the use of MTEX-induced changes as yet another biomarker of disease activity. The next step is to develop and implement reliable means for the isolation and molecular characterization of MTEX from body fluids and tissues of patients with melanoma. At present, these methods are in the discovery stage, and the emerging results are promising not only due to successful subsetting of sEV into MTEX and non-MTEX, but also because of evidence that mechanistic and functional studies of MTEX can yield new and previously unsuspected information. For example, the ability of MTEX to simultaneously deliver to recipient cells multiple and often contradictory, i.e., suppressive vs. stimulatory signals have alerted us to the possibility of regulatory functions MTEX might exercise in vivo. Similarly, the realization that MTEX utilize surface proteins as well as miRs to transmit signals to recipient cells alerts us to ask why these two signaling pathways co-exist and how they impact the biology. As melanoma biomarkers, MTEX might provide a more reliable diagnostic, prognostic, or outcome data than total sEV isolated from body fluids. Future validation studies encompassing all aspects of MTEX isolation, characterization, and signaling will be necessary to move the field forward and translate current knowledge to clinically applicable strategies and methods. In this respect, antibody-based microarrays, multiparameter quantitative flow cytometry, and targeted proteomics are emerging as the tools applicable to serial monitoring of MTEX in body fluids of patients with melanoma. The future will likely see numerous such studies performed as part of clinical trials designed to validate the roles of MTEX in the biology of melanoma.

Author Contributions: All authors have read and agree to the published version of the manuscript. A.Z.—conception and drafting the article; P.W. and T.W.—critical revision of the article; M.P.—design and revision of the manuscript, funding and final approval of the version to be published.

Funding: This study was funded by the National Science Centre, Poland, Grant 2016/22/M/NZ5/00667 (to A.Z., M.P. and T.W.).

Conflicts of Interest: The authors declare no conflict of interest. The funders had no role in the design of the study; in the collection, analyses, or interpretation of data; in the writing of the manuscript, or in the decision to publish the results.

Abbreviations

AB	apoptotic bodies
APC	antigen presenting cells
BM	bone marrow
BMDC	bone marrow derived cells
CAF	cancer-associated fibroblasts
CEM	cryo-electron microscopy
CM	confocal microscopy
DC	differential centrifugation
DC	dendritic cells
DLS	dynamic light scattering
EC	endothelial cells
EMT	epithelial-to-mesenchymal transition
EV	extracellular vesicles
EX	exosomes
HADF	human adult dermal fibroblasts

IA-FCM	immune-affinity flow cytometry
KO	knockdown
MAA	melanoma associated antigens
mAb	monoclonal antibodies
MSC	myeloid stem cells
MTEX	melanoma cell-derived exosomes
MV	microvesicles
MVB	multivesicular bodies
NTA	nanoparticle tracking analysis
SEC	size-exclusion chromatography
SEM	scanning electron microscopy
sEV	small extracellular vesicles
TEM	transmission electron microscopy
TEX	tumor-derived exosomes
TME	tumor microenvironment
UC	ultracentrifugation
UF	ultrafiltration
WB	western blotting

References

1. Kalluri, R.; LeBleu, V.S. The biology, function, and biomedical applications of exosomes. *Science* **2020**, *367*, eaau6977. [CrossRef] [PubMed]
2. Willms, E.; Cabañas, C.; Mäger, I.; Wood, M.J.A.; Vader, P. Extracellular Vesicle Heterogeneity: Subpopulations, Isolation Techniques, and Diverse Functions in Cancer Progression. *Front. Immunol.* **2018**, *9*, 738. [CrossRef] [PubMed]
3. van Niel, G.; D'Angelo, G.; Raposo, G. Shedding light on the cell biology of extracellular vesicles. *Nat. Rev. Mol. Cell Biol.* **2018**, *19*, 213–228. [CrossRef]
4. Zaborowski, M.P.; Balaj, L.; Breakefield, X.O.; Lai, C.P. Extracellular Vesicles: Composition, Biological Relevance, and Methods of Study. *Bioscience* **2015**, *65*, 783–797. [CrossRef] [PubMed]
5. Yáñez-Mó, M.; Siljander, P.R.; Andreu, Z.; Zavec, A.B.; Borràs, F.E.; Buzas, E.I.; Buzas, K.; Casal, E.; Cappello, F.; Carvalho, J.; et al. Biological properties of extracellular vesicles and their physiological functions. *J. Extracell. Vesicles* **2015**, *4*, 27066. [CrossRef]
6. Minciacchi, V.R.; Freeman, M.R.; Di Vizio, D. Extracellular Vesicles in Cancer: Exosomes, Microvesicles and the Emerging Role of Large Oncosomes. *Semin. Cell Dev. Biol.* **2015**, *40*, 41–51. [CrossRef]
7. György, B.; Szabó, T.G.; Pásztói, M.; Pál, Z.; Misják, P.; Aradi, B.; László, V.; Pállinger, E.; Pap, E.; Kittel, A.; et al. Membrane vesicles, current state-of-the-art: Emerging role of extracellular vesicles. *Cell. Mol. Life Sci.* **2011**, *68*, 2667–2688. [CrossRef]
8. Théry, C.; Witwer, K.W.; Aikawa, E.; Alcaraz, M.J.; Anderson, J.D.; Andriansitohaina, R.; Antoniou, A.; Arab, T.; Archer, F.; Atkin-Smith, G.K.; et al. Minimal information for studies of extracellular vesicles 2018 (MISEV2018): A position statement of the International Society for Extracellular Vesicles and update of the MISEV2014 guidelines. *J. Extracell. Vesicles* **2019**, *8*, 1535750. [CrossRef]
9. Kowal, J.; Arras, G.; Colombo, M.; Jouve, M.; Morath, P.J.; Primdal-Bengtson, B.; Dingli, F.; Leow, D.; Tkach, M.; Théry, C. Proteomic comparison defines novel markers to characterize heterogeneous populations of extracellular vesicle subtypes. *Proc. Natl. Acad. Sci. USA* **2016**, *113*, 968–977. [CrossRef]
10. Abramowicz, A.; Widlak, P.; Pietrowska, M. Proteomic analysis of exosomal cargo: The challenge of high purity vesicle isolation. *Mol. Biosyst.* **2016**, *12*, 1407–1419. [CrossRef]
11. Gurunathan, S.; Kang, M.H.; Jeyaraj, M.; Qasim, M.; Kim, J.H. Review of the Isolation, Characterization, Biological Function, and Multifarious Therapeutic Approaches of Exosomes. *Cells* **2019**, *8*, 307. [CrossRef]
12. Zebrowska, A.; Skowronek, A.; Wojakowska, A.; Widlak, P.; Pietrowska, M. Metabolome of Exosomes: Focus on Vesicles Released by Cancer Cells and Present in Human Body Fluids. *Int. J. Mol. Sci.* **2019**, *20*, 3461. [CrossRef] [PubMed]
13. Théry, C.; Ostrowski, M.; Segura, E. Membrane vesicles as conveyors of immune responses. *Nat. Rev. Immunol.* **2009**, *9*, 581–593. [CrossRef]

14. Dixon, C.L.; Sheller-Miller, S.; Saade, G.R.; Fortunato, S.J.; Lai, A.; Palma, C.; Guanzon, D.; Salomon, C.; Menon, R. Amniotic Fluid Exosome Proteomic Profile Exhibits Unique Pathways of Term and Preterm Labor. *Endocrinology* **2018**, *159*, 2229–2240. [CrossRef]
15. Yu, J.; Lin, Y.; Xiong, X.; Li, K.; Yao, Z.; Dong, H.; Jiang, Z.; Yu, D.; Yeung, S.J.; Zhang, H. Detection of Exosomal PD-L1 RNA in Saliva of Patients With Periodontitis. *Front. Genet.* **2019**, *10*, 202. [CrossRef]
16. Grigor'eva, A.E.; Tamkovich, S.N.; Eremina, A.V.; Tupikin, A.E.; Kabilov, M.R.; Chernykh, V.V.; Vlassov, V.V.; Laktionov, P.P.; Ryabchikova, E.I. Exosomes in tears of healthy individuals: Isolation, identification, and characterization. *Biochem. Moscow Suppl. Ser. B* **2016**, *10*, 165. [CrossRef]
17. Wu, G.; Yang, G.; Zhang, R. Altered microRNA Expression Profiles of Extracellular Vesicles in Nasal Mucus From Patients With Allergic Rhinitis. *Allergy Asthma Immunol. Res.* **2015**, *7*, 449–457. [CrossRef]
18. Saunderson, S.C.; Dunn, A.C.; Crocker, P.R.; McLellan, A.D. CD169 mediates the capture of exosomes in spleen and lymph node. *Blood* **2014**, *123*, 208–216. [CrossRef] [PubMed]
19. Chiasserini, D.; van Weering, J.R.; Piersma, S.R.; Pham, T.V.; Malekzadeh, A.; Teunissen, C.E.; de Wit, H.; Jiménez, C.R. Proteomic analysis of cerebrospinal fluid extracellular vesicles: A comprehensive dataset. *J. Proteom.* **2014**, *106*, 191–204. [CrossRef]
20. Romancino, D.P.; Paterniti, G.; Campos, Y.; De Luca, A.; Di Felice, V.; d'Azzo, A.; Bongiovanni, A. Identification and characterization of the nano-sized vesicles released by muscle cells. *FEBS Lett.* **2013**, *587*, 1379–1384. [CrossRef]
21. Masyuk, A.I.; Huang, B.Q.; Ward, C.J.; Gradilone, S.A.; Banales, J.M.; Masyuk, T.V.; Radtke, B.; Splinter, P.L.; LaRusso, N.F. Biliary exosomes influence cholangiocyte regulatory mechanisms and proliferation through interaction with primary cilia. *Am. J. Physiol. Gastrointest. Liver Physiol.* **2010**, *299*, G990–G999. [CrossRef] [PubMed]
22. Runz, S.; Keller, S.; Rupp, C.; Stoeck, A.; Issa, Y.; Koensgen, D.; Mustea, A.; Sehouli, J.; Kristiansen, G.; Altevogt, P. Malignant ascites-derived exosomes of ovarian carcinoma patients contain CD24 and EpCAM. *Gynecol. Oncol.* **2007**, *107*, 563–571. [CrossRef] [PubMed]
23. Admyre, C.; Johansson, S.M.; Qazi, K.R.; Filén, J.J.; Lahesmaa, R.; Norman, M.; Neve, E.P.; Scheynius, A.; Gabrielsson, S. Exosomes with immune modulatory features are present in human breast milk. *J. Immunol.* **2007**, *179*, 1969–1978. [CrossRef]
24. Andreau, Z.; Yanez-Mo, M. Tetraspanins in extracellular vesicle formation and function. *Front. Immunol.* **2014**, *5*, 442. [CrossRef]
25. Wieckowski, E.U.; Visus, C.; Szajnik, M.; Szczepanski, M.J.; Storkus, W.J.; Whiteside, T.L. Tumor-Derived Microvesicles Promote Regulatory T Cell Expansion and Induce Apoptosis in Tumor-Reactive Activated CD8+ T Lymphocytes. *J. Immunol.* **2009**, *183*, 3720–3730. [CrossRef]
26. Sharma, P.; Diergaarde, B.; Ferrone, S.; Kirkwood, J.M.; Whietside, T.L. Melanoma cell-derived exosomes in plasma of melanoma patients suppress functions of immune effector cells. *Sci. Rep.* **2020**, *10*, 92. [CrossRef]
27. Ferrone, S.; Whiteside, T.L. Targeting CSPG4 for isolation of melanoma cell-derived exosomes from body fluids. *HNO* **2020**, *68*, 100–105. [CrossRef]
28. Sharma, P.; Ludwig, S.; Muller, L.; Hong, C.S.; Kirkwood, J.M.; Ferrone, S.; Whiteside, T.L. Immunoaffinity-based isolation of melanoma cell-derived exosomes from plasma of patients with melanoma. *J. Extracell. Vesicles* **2018**, *7*, 1435138. [CrossRef]
29. Melo, S.A.; Luecke, L.B.; Kahlert, C.; Fernandez, A.F.; Gammon, S.T.; Kaye, J.; LeBleu, V.S.; Mittendorf, E.A.; Weitz, J.; Rahbari, N.; et al. Glypican-1 identifies cancer exosomes and detects early pancreatic cancer. *Nature* **2015**, *523*, 177–182. [CrossRef]
30. Mizutani, K.; Terazawa, R.; Kameyama, K.; Kato, T.; Horie, K.; Tsuchiya, T.; Seike, K.; Ehara, H.; Fujita, Y.; Kawakami, K.; et al. Isolation of prostate cancer-related exosomes. *Anticancer Res.* **2014**, *34*, 3419–3423.
31. Hong, C.S.; Muller, L.; Boyiadzis, M.; Whiteside, T.L. Isolation and characterization of CD34+ blast-derived exosomes in acute myeloid leukemia. *PLoS ONE* **2014**, *9*, e103310. [CrossRef]
32. Raimondo, S.; Pucci, M.; Alessandro, R.; Fontana, S. Extracellular Vesicles and Tumor-Immune Escape: Biological Functions and Clinical Perspectives. *Int. J. Mol. Sci.* **2020**, *21*, 2286. [CrossRef] [PubMed]
33. Whiteside, T.L. Exosomes in Cancer: Another Mechanism of Tumor-Induced Immune Suppression. In *Tumor Immune Microenvironment in Cancer Progression and Cancer Therapy*; Kalinski, P., Ed.; Springer: Cham, Switzerland, 2017; Volume 1036, pp. 81–89. [CrossRef]

34. Whiteside, T.L. Tumor-Derived Exosomes and Their Role in Cancer Progression. *Adv. Clin. Chem.* **2016**, *74*, 103–141. [CrossRef] [PubMed]
35. Meldolesi, J. Exosomes and Ectosomes in Intercellular Communication. *Curr. Biol.* **2018**, *28*, R435–R444. [CrossRef]
36. Ludwig, A.K.; Giebel, B. Exosomes: Small vesicles participating in intercellular communication. *Int. J. Biochem. Cell Biol.* **2012**, *44*, 11–15. [CrossRef] [PubMed]
37. Alegre, E.; Zubiri, L.; Perez-Gracia, J.L.; González-Cao, M.; Soria, L.; Martín-Algarra, S.; González, A. Circulating melanoma exosomes as diagnostic and prognosis biomarkers. *Clin. Chim. Acta* **2016**, *454*, 28–32. [CrossRef] [PubMed]
38. Whiteside, T.L. The potential of tumor-derived exosomes for noninvasive cancer monitoring. *Expert Rev. Mol. Diagn.* **2015**, *15*, 1293–1310. [CrossRef] [PubMed]
39. Duijvesz, D.; Versluis, C.Y.; van der Fels, C.A.; Vredenbregt-van den Berg, M.S.; Leivo, J.; Peltola, M.T.; Bangma, C.H.; Pettersson, K.S.; Jenster, G. Immuno-based detection of extracellular vesicles in urine as diagnostic marker for prostate cancer. *Int. J. Cancer* **2015**, *137*, 2869–2878. [CrossRef]
40. Szajnik, M.; Derbis, M.; Lach, M.; Patalas, P.; Michalak, M.; Drzewiecka, H.; Szpurek, D.; Nowakowski, A.; Spaczynski, M.; Baranowski, W.; et al. Exosomes in Plasma of Patients with Ovarian Carcinoma: Potential Biomarkers of Tumor Progression and Response to Therapy. *Gynecol. Obstet.* **2013**, *4*, 003. [CrossRef]
41. Silva, J.; Garcia, V.; Rodriguez, M.; Compte, M.; Cisneros, E.; Veguillas, P.; Garcia, J.M.; Dominguez, G.; Campos-Martin, Y.; Cuevas, J.; et al. Analysis of exosome release and its prognostic value in human colorectal cancer. *Genes Chromosomes Cancer* **2012**, *51*, 409–418. [CrossRef]
42. Szczepanski, M.J.; Szajnik, M.; Welsh, A.; Whiteside, T.L.; Boyiadzis, M. Blast-derived microvesicles in sera from patients with acute myeloid leukemia suppress natural killer cell function via membrane-associated transforming growth factor-beta1. *Haematologica* **2011**, *96*, 1302–1309. [CrossRef] [PubMed]
43. Baran, J.; Baj-Krzyworzeka, M.; Weglarczyk, K.; Szatanek, R.; Zembala, M.; Barbasz, J.; Czupryna, A.; Szczepanik, A.; Zembala, M. Circulating tumour-derived microvesicles in plasma of gastric cancer patients. *Cancer Immunol. Immunother.* **2010**, *59*, 841–850. [CrossRef] [PubMed]
44. Zhang, L.; Yu, D. Exosomes in cancer development, metastasis, and immunity. *Biochim. Biophys. Acta Rev. Cancer* **2019**, *1871*, 455–468. [CrossRef] [PubMed]
45. Mashouri, L.; Yousefi, H.; Aref, A.R.; Ahadi, A.M.; Molaei, F.; Alahari, S.K. Exosomes: Composition, biogenesis, and mechanisms in cancer metastasis and drug resistance. *Mol. Cancer* **2019**, *18*, 75. [CrossRef]
46. Tung, K.H.; Ernstoff, M.S.; Allen, C.; Shu, S. A Review of Exosomes and their Role in The Tumor Microenvironment and Host-Tumor "Macroenvironment". *J. Immunol. Sci.* **2019**, *3*, 4–8. [CrossRef]
47. Wang, T.; Nasser, M.I.; Shen, J.; Qu, S.; He, Q.; Zhao, M. Functions of Exosomes in the Triangular Relationship between the Tumor, Inflammation, and Immunity in the Tumor Microenvironment. *J. Immunol. Res.* **2019**, *2019*, 4197829. [CrossRef]
48. Syn, N.; Wang, L.; Sethi, G.; Thiery, J.P.; Goh, B.C. Exosome-Mediated Metastasis: From Epithelial-Mesenchymal Transition to Escape from Immunosurveillance. *Trends Pharmacol. Sci.* **2016**, *37*, 606–617. [CrossRef]
49. Whiteside, T.L. Exosomes and tumor-mediated immune suppression. *J. Clin. Investig.* **2016**, *126*, 1216–1223. [CrossRef]
50. Whiteside, T.L. The role of tumor-derived exosomes in epithelial mesenchymal transition (EMT). *Transl. Cancer Res.* **2017**, *6*, S90–S92. [CrossRef]
51. Ludwig, N.; Yerneni, S.S.; Razzo, B.M.; Whiteside, T.L. Exosomes from HNSCC Promote Angiogenesis through Reprogramming of Endothelial Cells. *Mol. Cancer Res.* **2018**, *16*, 1798–1808. [CrossRef] [PubMed]
52. Barros, F.M.; Carneiro, F.; Machado, J.C.; Melo, S.A. Exosomes and Immune Response in Cancer: Friends or Foes? *Front. Immunol.* **2018**, *9*, 730. [CrossRef] [PubMed]
53. Czernek, L.; Düchler, M. Functions of Cancer-Derived Extracellular Vesicles in Immunosuppression. *Arch. Immunol. Ther. Exp.* **2017**, *65*, 311–323. [CrossRef] [PubMed]
54. Whiteside, T.L. Immune modulation of T-cell and NK (natural killer) cell activities by TEX (tumour-derived exosomes). *Biochem. Soc. Trans.* **2013**, *41*, 245–251. [CrossRef] [PubMed]
55. Tucci, M.; Mannavola, F.; Passarelli, A.; Stucci, L.S.; Cives, M.; Silvestris, F. Exosomes in melanoma: A role in tumor progression, metastasis and impaired immune system activity. *Oncotarget* **2018**, *9*, 20826–20837. [CrossRef]

56. Tucci, M.; Passarelli, A.; Mannavola, F.; Felici, C.; Stucci, L.S.; Cives, M.; Silvestris, F. Immune System Evasion as Hallmark of Melanoma Progression: The Role of Dendritic Cells. *Front. Oncol.* **2019**, *9*, 1148. [CrossRef]
57. Isola, A.L.; Eddy, K.; Chen, S. Biology, Therapy and Implications of Tumor Exosomes in the Progression of Melanoma. *Cancers* **2016**, *8*, 110. [CrossRef]
58. Siegel, R.L.; Miller, K.D.; Jemal, A. Cancer statistics, 2020. *CA Cancer J. Clin.* **2020**, *70*, 7–30. [CrossRef]
59. Osella-Abate, S.; Ribero, S.; Sanlorenzo, M.; Maule, M.M.; Richiardi, L.; Merletti, F.; Tomasini, C.; Marra, E.; Macripò, G.; Fierro, M.T.; et al. Risk factors related to late metastases in 1,372 melanoma patients disease free more than 10 years. *Int. J. Cancer* **2015**, *136*, 2453–2457. [CrossRef]
60. Rutkowski, P.; Wysocki, P.J.; Nasierowska-Guttmejer, A.; Jeziorski, A.; Wysocki, W.M.; Kalinka-Warzocha, E.; Świtaj, T.; Kozak, K.; Kamińska-Winciorek, G.; Czarnecka, A.M.; et al. Cutaneous melanomas. *Oncol. Clin. Pract.* **2019**, *15*, 1–19. [CrossRef]
61. Weiss, S.A.; Wolchok, J.D.; Sznol, M. Immunotherapy of Melanoma: Facts and Hopes. *Clin. Cancer Res.* **2019**, *25*, 5191–5201. [CrossRef]
62. Fujimura, T.; Fujisawa, Y.; Kambayashi, Y.; Aiba, S. Significance of BRAF Kinase Inhibitors for Melanoma Treatment: From Bench to Bedside. *Cancers* **2019**, *11*, 1342. [CrossRef] [PubMed]
63. Pasquali, S.; Hadjinicolaou, A.V.; Chiarion Sileni, V.; Rossi, C.R.; Mocellin, S. Systemic treatments for metastatic cutaneous melanoma. *Cochrane Database Syst. Rev.* **2018**, *2*, CD011123. [CrossRef] [PubMed]
64. Sun, Y.; Huo, C.; Qiao, Z.; Shang, Z.; Uzzaman, A.; Liu, S.; Jiang, X.; Fan, L.Y.; Ji, L.; Guan, X.; et al. Comparative Proteomic Analysis of Exosomes and Microvesicles in Human Saliva for Lung Cancer. *J. Proteome Res.* **2018**, *17*, 1101–1107. [CrossRef] [PubMed]
65. Luo, D.; Zhan, S.; Xia, W.; Huang, L.; Ge, W.; Wang, T. Proteomics study of serum exosomes from papillary thyroid cancer patients. *Endocr. Relat. Cancer* **2018**, *25*, 879–891. [CrossRef]
66. Gangoda, L.; Liem, M.; Ang, C.S.; Keerthikumar, S.; Adda, C.G.; Parker, B.S.; Mathivanan, S. Proteomic Profiling of Exosomes Secreted by Breast Cancer Cells with Varying Metastatic Potential. *Proteomics* **2017**, *17*, 23–24. [CrossRef]
67. Ludwig, S.; Marczak, L.; Sharma, P.; Abramowicz, A.; Gawin, M.; Widlak, P.; Whiteside, T.L.; Pietrowska, M. Proteomes of exosomes from HPV(+) or HPV(−) head and neck cancer cells: Differential enrichment in immunoregulatory proteins. *Oncoimmunology* **2019**, *8*, 1593808. [CrossRef]
68. Mears, R.; Craven, R.A.; Hanrahan, S.; Totty, N.; Upton, C.; Young, S.L.; Patel, P.; Selby, P.J.; Banks, R.E. Proteomic analysis of melanoma-derived exosomes by two-dimensional polyacrylamide gel electrophoresis and mass spectrometry. *Proteomics* **2004**, *4*, 4019–4031. [CrossRef] [PubMed]
69. Xiao, D.; Ohlendorf, J.; Chen, Y.; Taylor, D.D.; Rai, S.N.; Waigel, S.; Zacharias, W.; Hao, H.; McMasters, K.M. Identifying mRNA, microRNA and protein profiles of melanoma exosomes. *PLoS ONE* **2012**, *7*, e46874. [CrossRef]
70. Lazar, I.; Clement, E.; Ducoux-Petit, M.; Denat, L.; Soldan, V.; Dauvillier, S.; Balor, S.; Burlet-Schiltz, O.; Larue, L.; Muller, C.; et al. Proteome characterization of melanoma exosomes reveals a specific signature for metastatic cell lines. *Pigment Cell Melanoma Res.* **2015**, *28*, 464–475. [CrossRef]
71. Muhsin-Sharafaldine, M.R.; Saunderson, S.C.; Dunn, A.C.; Faed, J.M.; Kleffmann, T.; McLellan, A.D. Procoagulant and immunogenic properties of melanoma exosomes, microvesicles and apoptotic vesicles. *Oncotarget* **2016**, *7*, 56279–56294. [CrossRef]
72. Willms, E.; Johansson, H.J.; Mäger, I.; Lee, Y.; Blomberg, K.E.; Sadik, M.; Alaarg, A.; Smith, C.I.; Lehtiö, J.; El Andaloussi, S.; et al. Cells release subpopulations of exosomes with distinct molecular and biological properties. *Sci. Rep.* **2016**, *6*, 22519. [CrossRef] [PubMed]
73. Boussadia, Z.; Lamberti, J.; Mattei, F.; Pizzi, E.; Puglisi, R.; Zanetti, C.; Pasquini, L.; Fratini, F.; Fantozzi, L.; Felicetti, F.; et al. Acidic microenvironment plays a key role in human melanoma progression through a sustained exosome mediated transfer of clinically relevant metastatic molecules. *J. Exp. Clin. Cancer Res.* **2018**, *37*, 245. [CrossRef] [PubMed]
74. Peinado, H.; Alečković, M.; Lavotshkin, S.; Matei, I.; Costa-Silva, B.; Moreno-Bueno, G.; Hergueta-Redondo, M.; Williams, C.; García-Santos, G.; Ghajar, C.; et al. Melanoma exosomes educate bone marrow progenitor cells toward a pro-metastatic phenotype through MET. *Nat. Med.* **2012**, *18*, 883–891. [CrossRef] [PubMed]
75. Surman, M.; Stępień, E.; Przybyło, M. Melanoma-Derived Extracellular Vesicles: Focus on Their Proteome. *Proteomes* **2019**, *7*, 21. [CrossRef]
76. Kalluri, R. The biology and function of exosomes in cancer. *J. Clin. Investig.* **2016**, *126*, 1208–1215. [CrossRef]

77. Tsitsiou, E.; Lindsay, M.A. microRNAs and the immune response. *Trends Immunol.* **2008**, *29*, 343–351. [CrossRef]
78. Salehi, M.; Sharifi, M. Exosomal miRNAs as novel cancer biomarkers: Challenges and opportunities. *J. Cell. Physiol.* **2018**, *233*, 6370–6380. [CrossRef]
79. Sun, Z.; Shi, K.; Yang, S.; Liu, J.; Zhou, Q.; Wang, G.; Song, J.; Li, Z.; Zhang, Z.; Yuan, W. Effect of exosomal miRNA on cancer biology and clinical applications. *Mol. Cancer* **2018**, *17*, 147. [CrossRef]
80. Hessvik, N.P.; Phuyal, S.; Brech, A.; Sandvig, K.; Llorente, A. Profiling of microRNAs in exosomes released from PC-3 prostate cancer cells. *Biochim. Biophys. Acta* **2012**, *1819*, 1154–1163. [CrossRef]
81. Gajos-Michniewicz, A.; Duechler, M.; Czyz, M. MiRNA in melanoma-derived exosomes. *Cancer Lett.* **2014**, *347*, 29–37. [CrossRef]
82. Li, J.; Chen, J.; Wang, S.; Li, P.; Zheng, C.; Zhou, X.; Tao, Y.; Chen, X.; Sun, L.; Wang, A.; et al. Blockage of transferred exosome-shuttled miR-494 inhibits melanoma growth and metastasis. *J. Cell. Physiol.* **2019**, *234*, 15763–15774. [CrossRef] [PubMed]
83. Wozniak, M.; Peczek, L.; Czernek, L.; Düchler, M. Analysis of the miRNA Profiles of Melanoma Exosomes Derived Under Normoxic and Hypoxic Culture Conditions. *Anticancer Res.* **2017**, *37*, 6779–6789. [CrossRef] [PubMed]
84. Bland, C.L.; Byrne-Hoffman, C.N.; Fernandez, A.; Rellick, S.L.; Deng, W.; Klinke, D.J., 2nd. Exosomes derived from B16F0 melanoma cells alter the transcriptome of cytotoxic T cells that impacts mitochondrial respiration. *FEBS J.* **2018**, *285*, 1033–1050. [CrossRef] [PubMed]
85. Zhou, J.; Yang, Y.; Wang, W.; Zhang, Y.; Chen, Z.; Hao, C.; Zhang, J. Melanoma-released exosomes directly activate the mitochondrial apoptotic pathway of CD4+ T cells through their microRNA cargo. *Exp. Cell Res.* **2018**, *371*, 364–371. [CrossRef]
86. Zhou, X.; Yan, T.; Huang, C.; Xu, Z.; Wang, L.; Jiang, E.; Wang, H.; Chen, Y.; Liu, K.; Shao, Z.; et al. Melanoma cell-secreted exosomal miR-155-5p induce proangiogenic switch of cancer-associated fibroblasts via SOCS1/JAK2/STAT3 signaling pathway. *J. Exp. Clin. Cancer Res.* **2018**, *37*, 242. [CrossRef]
87. Felicetti, F.; De Feo, A.; Coscia, C.; Puglisi, R.; Pedini, F.; Pasquini, L.; Bellenghi, M.; Errico, M.C.; Pagani, E.; Carè, A. Exosome-mediated transfer of miR-222 is sufficient to increase tumor malignancy in melanoma. *J. Transl. Med.* **2016**, *1*, 56. [CrossRef]
88. Chen, L.; Karisma, V.W.; Liu, H.; Zhong, L. MicroRNA-300: A Transcellular Mediator in Exosome Regulates Melanoma Progression. *Front. Oncol.* **2019**, *9*, 1005. [CrossRef]
89. Shu, S.L.; Yang, Y.; Allen, C.L.; Maguire, O.; Minderman, H.; Sen, A.; Ciesielski, M.J.; Collins, K.A.; Bush, P.J.; Singh, P.; et al. Metabolic reprogramming of stromal fibroblasts by melanoma exosome microRNA favours a pre-metastatic microenvironment. *Sci. Rep.* **2018**, *8*, 12905. [CrossRef]
90. Vignard, V.; Labbé, M.; Marec, N.; André-Grégoire, G.; Jouand, N.; Fonteneau, J.F.; Labarrière, N.; Fradin, D. MicroRNAs in Tumor Exosomes Drive Immune Escape in Melanoma. *Cancer Immunol. Res.* **2020**, *8*, 255–267. [CrossRef]
91. Pfeffer, S.R.; Grossmann, K.F.; Cassidy, P.B.; Yang, C.H.; Fan, M.; Kopelovich, L.; Leachman, S.A.; Pfeffer, L.M. Detection of Exosomal miRNAs in the Plasma of Melanoma Patients. *J. Clin. Med.* **2015**, *4*, 2012–2027. [CrossRef]
92. Alegre, E.; Sanmamed, M.F.; Rodriguez, C.; Carranza, O.; Martín-Algarra, S.; González, A. Study of circulating microRNA-125b levels in serum exosomes in advanced melanoma. *Arch. Pathol. Lab. Med.* **2014**, *138*, 828–832. [CrossRef] [PubMed]
93. Greenberg, E.; Hershkovitz, L.; Itzhaki, O.; Hajdu, S.; Nemlich, Y.; Ortenberg, R.; Gefen, N.; Edry, L.; Modai, S.; Keisari, Y.; et al. Regulation of cancer aggressive features in melanoma cells by microRNAs. *PLoS ONE* **2011**, *6*, e18936. [CrossRef] [PubMed]
94. Rao, E.; Jiang, C.; Ji, M.; Huang, X.; Iqbal, J.; Lenz, G.; Wright, G.; Staudt, L.M.; Zhao, Y.; McKeithan, T.W.; et al. The miRNA-17 approximately 92 cluster mediates chemoresistance and enhances tumor growth in mantle cell lymphoma via pi3k/akt pathway activation. *Leukemia* **2012**, *26*, 1064–1072. [CrossRef] [PubMed]
95. Levy, C.; Khaled, M.; Iliopoulos, D.; Janas, M.M.; Schubert, S.; Pinner, S.; Chen, P.H.; Li, S.; Fletcher, A.L.; Yokoyama, S.; et al. Intronic miR-211 assumes the tumor suppressive function of its host gene in melanoma. *Mol. Cell* **2010**, *40*, 841–849. [CrossRef]
96. Si, M.L.; Zhu, S.; Wu, H.; Lu, Z.; Wu, F.; Mo, Y.Y. MiR-21-mediated tumor growth. *Oncogene* **2007**, *26*, 2799–2803. [CrossRef]

97. Zhu, S.; Wu, H.; Wu, F.; Nie, D.; Sheng, S.; Mo, Y.Y. MicroRNA-21 targets tumor suppressor genes in invasion and metastasis. *Cell Res.* **2008**, *18*, 350–359. [CrossRef]
98. Yang, C.H.; Yue, J.; Pfeffer, S.R.; Handorf, C.R.; Pfeffer, L.M. MicroRNA miR-21 regulates the metastatic behavior of b16 melanoma cells. *J. Biol. Chem.* **2011**, *286*, 39172–39178. [CrossRef] [PubMed]
99. Yang, C.H.; Yue, J.; Fan, M.; Pfeffer, L.M. IFN induces miR-21 through a signal transducer and activator of transcription 3-dependent pathway as a suppressive negative feedback on IFN-induced apoptosis. *Cancer Res.* **2010**, *70*, 8108–8116. [CrossRef] [PubMed]
100. Xu, Y.F.; Hannafon, B.N.; Khatri, U.; Gin, A.; Ding, W.Q. The origin of exosomal miR-1246 in human cancer cells. *RNA Biol.* **2019**, *16*, 770–784. [CrossRef]
101. Bhagirath, D.; Yang, T.L.; Bucay, N.; Sekhon, K.; Majid, S.; Shahryari, V.; Dahiya, R.; Tanaka, Y.; Saini, S. microRNA-1246 Is an Exosomal Biomarker for Aggressive Prostate Cancer. *Cancer Res.* **2018**, *78*, 1833–1844. [CrossRef]
102. Felicetti, F.; Errico, M.C.; Bottero, L.; Segnalini, P.; Stoppacciaro, A.; Biffoni, M.; Felli, N.; Mattia, G.; Petrini, M.; Colombo, M.P.; et al. The promyelocytic leukemia zinc finger-microRNA-221/-222 pathway controls melanoma progression through multiple oncogenic mechanisms. *Cancer Res.* **2008**, *68*, 2745–2754. [CrossRef]
103. Müller, D.; Bosserhoff, A. Integrin β3 expression is regulated by let-7a miRNA in malignant melanoma. *Oncogene* **2008**, *27*, 6698–6706. [CrossRef]
104. Xiao, D.; Barry, S.; Kmetz, D.; Egger, M.; Pan, J.; Rai, S.N.; Qu, J.; McMasters, K.M.; Hao, H. Melanoma cell-derived exosomes promote epithelial-mesenchymal transition in primary melanocytes through paracrine/autocrine signaling in the tumor microenvironment. *Cancer Lett.* **2016**, *376*, 318–327. [CrossRef] [PubMed]
105. Ryan, D.; Rafferty, M.; Hegarty, S.; O'Leary, P.; Faller, W.; Gremel, G.; Bergqvist, M.; Agnarsdottir, M.; Strömberg, S.; Kampf, C.; et al. Topoisomerase I amplification in melanoma is associated with more advanced tumours and poor prognosis. *Pigment Cell Melanoma Res.* **2010**, *23*, 542–553. [CrossRef] [PubMed]
106. Wang, S.; Tang, L.; Lin, J.; Shen, Z.; Yao, Y.; Wang, W.; Tao, S.; Gu, C.; Ma, J.; Xie, Y.; et al. ABCB5 promotes melanoma metastasis through enhancing NF-κB p65 protein stability. *Biochem. Biophys. Res. Commun.* **2017**, *492*, 18–26. [CrossRef] [PubMed]
107. Suryo Rahmanto, Y.; Dunn, L.; Richardson, D. The melanoma tumor antigen, melanotransferrin (p97): A 25-year hallmark—From iron metabolism to tumorigenesis. *Oncogene* **2007**, *26*, 6113–6124. [CrossRef] [PubMed]
108. Soengas, M.; Hernando, E. TYRP1 mRNA goes fishing for miRNAs in melanoma. *Nat. Cell Biol.* **2017**, *19*, 1311–1312. [CrossRef]
109. Gilot, D.; Migault, M.; Bachelot, L.; Journé, F.; Rogiers, A.; Donnou-Fournet, E.; Mogha, A.; Mouchet, N.; Pinel-Marie, M.L.; Mari, B.; et al. A non-coding function of TYRP1 mRNA promotes melanoma growth. *Nat. Cell Biol.* **2017**, *19*, 1348–1357. [CrossRef] [PubMed]
110. Li, X.; Wang, Y.; Wang, Q.; Liu, Y.; Bao, W.; Wu, S. Exosomes in cancer: Small transporters with big functions. *Cancer Lett.* **2018**, *435*, 55–65. [CrossRef]
111. Chen, G.; Huang, A.C.; Zhang, W.; Zhang, G.; Wu, M.; Xu, W.; Yu, Z.; Yang, J.; Wang, B.; Sun, H.; et al. Exosomal PD-L1 contributes to immunosuppression and is associated with anti-PD-1 response. *Nature* **2018**, *560*, 382–386. [CrossRef]
112. Kaiser, J. Malignant messengers. *Science* **2016**, *352*, 164–166. [CrossRef] [PubMed]
113. Chen, D.S.; Mellman, I. Elements of cancer immunity and the cancer-immune set point. *Nature* **2017**, *541*, 321–330. [CrossRef]
114. Muller, L.; Mitsuhashi, M.; Simms, P.; Gooding, W.E.; Whiteside, T.L. Tumor-derived exosomes regulate expression of immune function-related genes in human T cell subsets. *Sci. Rep.* **2016**, *6*, 20254. [CrossRef]
115. Bergmann, C.; Strauss, L.; Wang, Y.; Szczepanski, M.J.; Lang, S.; Johnson, J.T.; Whiteside, T.L. T regulatory Type 1 cells (Tr1) in squamous cell carcinoma of the head and neck: Mechanisms of suppression and expansion in advanced disease. *Clin. Cancer Res.* **2008**, *14*, 3706–3715. [CrossRef]
116. Clayton, A.; Al-Taei, S.; Webber, J.; Mason, M.D.; Tabi, Z. Cancer exosomes express CD39 and CD73, which suppress T cells through adenosine production. *J. Immunol.* **2011**, *187*, 676–683. [CrossRef] [PubMed]

117. Szajnik, M.; Czystowska, M.; Szczepanski, M.J.; Mandapathil, M.; Whiteside, T.L. Tumor-derived microvesicles induce, expand and up-regulate biological activities of human regulatory T cells (Treg). *PLoS ONE* **2010**, *5*, e11469. [CrossRef] [PubMed]
118. Düchler, M.; Czernek, L.; Peczek, L.; Cypryk, W.; Sztiller-Sikorska, M.; Czyz, M. Melanoma-Derived Extracellular Vesicles Bear the Potential for the Induction of Antigen-Specific Tolerance. *Cells* **2019**, *8*, 665. [CrossRef]
119. Gyukity-Sebestyén, E.; Harmati, M.; Dobra, G.; Németh, I.B.; Mihály, J.; Zvara, Á.; Hunyadi-Gulyás, É.; Katona, R.; Nagy, I.; Horváth, P.; et al. Melanoma-Derived Exosomes Induce PD-1 Overexpression and Tumor Progression via Mesenchymal Stem Cell Oncogenic Reprogramming. *Front. Immunol.* **2019**, *10*, 2459. [CrossRef]
120. Martínez-Lorenzo, M.J.; Anel, A.; Alava, M.A.; Piñeiro, A.; Naval, J.; Lasierra, P.; Larrad, L. The human melanoma cell line MelJuSo secretes bioactive FasL and APO2L/TRAIL on the surface of microvesicles. Possible contribution to tumor counterattack. *Exp. Cell Res.* **2004**, *295*, 315–329. [CrossRef]
121. Wu, Y.; Deng, W.; McGinley, E.C.; Klinke, D.J., 2nd. Melanoma exosomes deliver a complex biological payload that upregulates PTPN11 to suppress T lymphocyte function. *Pigment Cell Melanoma Res.* **2017**, *30*, 203–218. [CrossRef]
122. Kulkarni, Y.M.; Chambers, E.; McGray, A.J.R.; Ware, J.S.; Bramson, J.L.; Klinke, D.J. A quantitative systems approach to identify paracrine mechanisms that locally suppress immune response to Interleukin-12 in the B16 melanoma model. *Integr. Biol.* **2012**, *4*, 925–936. [CrossRef] [PubMed]
123. Cottonham, C.L.; Kaneko, S.; Xu, L. miR-21 and miR-31 converge on TIAM1 to regulate migration and invasion of colon carcinoma cells. *J. Biol. Chem.* **2010**, *285*, 35293–35302. [CrossRef]
124. Yasuda, M.; Schmid, T.; Rubsamen, D.; Colburn, N.H.; Irie, K.; Murakami, A. Downregulation of programmed cell death 4 by inflammatory conditions contributes to the generation of the tumor promoting microenvironment. *Mol. Carcinog.* **2010**, *49*, 837–848. [CrossRef] [PubMed]
125. Fabbri, M.; Paone, A.; Calore, F.; Galli, R.; Gaudio, E.; Santhanam, R.; Lovat, F.; Fadda, P.; Mao, C.; Nuovo, G.J.; et al. MicroRNAs bind to Toll-like receptors to induce prometastatic inflammatory response. *Proc. Natl. Acad. Sci. USA* **2012**, *109*, E2110–E2116. [CrossRef] [PubMed]
126. Tang, M.; Diao, J.; Gu, H.; Khatri, I.; Zhao, J.; Cattral, M.S. Toll-like Receptor 2 Activation Promotes Tumor Dendritic Cell Dysfunction by Regulating IL-6 and IL-10 Receptor Signaling. *Cell Rep.* **2015**, *13*, 2851–2864. [CrossRef]
127. Ashiru, O.; Boutet, P.; Fernández-Messina, L.; Agüera-González, S.; Skepper, J.N.; Valés-Gómez, M.; Reyburn, H.T. Natural killer cell cytotoxicity is suppressed by exposure to the human NKG2D ligand MICA*008 that is shed by tumor cells in exosomes. *Cancer Res.* **2010**, *70*, 481–489. [CrossRef] [PubMed]
128. Guo, Y.; Ji, X.; Liu, J.; Fan, D.; Zhou, Q.; Chen, C.; Wang, W.; Wang, G.; Wang, H.; Yuan, W.; et al. Effects of exosomes on pre-metastatic niche formation in tumors. *Mol. Cancer* **2019**, *18*, 39. [CrossRef]
129. Caramel, J.; Papadogeorgakis, E.; Hill, L.; Browne, G.J.; Richard, G.G.; Wierinckx, A.; Saldanha, G.; Osborne, J.; Hutchinson, P.; Tse, G.; et al. A switch in the expression of embryonic EMT-inducers drives the development of malignant melanoma. *Cancer Cell.* **2013**, *24*, 466–480. [CrossRef]
130. Hu, T.; Hu, J. Melanoma-derived exosomes induce reprogramming fibroblasts into cancer-associated fibroblasts via Gm26809 delivery. *Cell Cycle* **2019**, *18*, 3085–3094. [CrossRef]
131. Zhao, X.-P.; Wang, M.; Song, Y.; Song, K.; Yan, T.L.; Wang, L.; Li, K.; Shang, Z.J. Membrane microvesicles as mediators for melanoma-fibroblasts communication: Roles of the VCAM-1/VLA-4 axis and the ERK1/2 signal pathway. *Cancer Lett.* **2015**, *360*, 125–133. [CrossRef]
132. Hood, J.; Pan, H.; Lanza, G.; Wickline, S.A. Paracrine induction of endothelium by tumor exosomes. *Lab. Investig.* **2009**, *89*, 1317–1328. [CrossRef] [PubMed]
133. Zhuang, G.; Wu, X.; Jiang, Z.; Kasman, I.; Yao, J.; Guan, Y.; Oeh, J.; Modrusan, Z.; Bais, C.; Sampath, D.; et al. Tumour-secreted miR-9 promotes endothelial cell migration and angiogenesis by activating the JAK-STAT pathway. *EMBO J.* **2012**, *31*, 3513–3523. [CrossRef] [PubMed]
134. Ekström, E.J.; Bergenfelz, C.; von Bülow, V.; Serifler, F.; Carlemalm, E.; Jönsson, G.; Andersson, T.; Leandersson, K. WNT5A induces release of exosomes containing pro-angiogenic and immunosuppressive factors from malignant melanoma cells. *Mol. Cancer* **2014**, *13*, 88. [CrossRef] [PubMed]

135. Sento, S.; Sasabe, E.; Yamamoto, T. Application of a persistent heparin treatment inhibits the malignant potential of oral squamous carcinoma cells induced by tumor cell-derived exosomes. *PLoS ONE* **2016**, *11*, e0148454. [CrossRef]
136. Hazan-Halevy, I.; Rosenblum, D.; Weinstein, S.; Bairey, O.; Raanani, P.; Peer, D. Cell-specific uptake of mantle cell lymphoma-derived exosomes by malignant and non-malignant B-lymphocytes. *Cancer Lett.* **2015**, *364*, 59–69. [CrossRef] [PubMed]
137. Matsumoto, A.; Takahashi, Y.; Nishikawa, M.; Sano, K.; Morishita, M.; Charoenviriyakul, C.; Saji, H.; Takakura, Y. Accelerated growth of B16BL6 tumor in mice through efficient uptake of their own exosomes by B16BL6 cells. *Cancer Sci.* **2017**, *108*, 1803–1810. [CrossRef]
138. Isola, A.L.; Eddy, K.; Zembrzuski, K.; Goydos, J.S.; Chen, S. Exosomes released by metabotropic glutamate receptor 1 (GRM1) expressing melanoma cells increase cell migration and invasiveness. *Oncotarget* **2018**, *9*, 1187–1199. [CrossRef]
139. Ostrowski, M.; Carmo, N.B.; Krumeich, S.; Fanget, I.; Raposo, G.; Savina, A.; Moita, C.F.; Schauer, K.; Hume, A.N.; Freitas, R.P.; et al. Rab27a and Rab27b control different steps of the exosome secretion pathway. *Nat. Cell Biol.* **2009**, *12*, 19–30. [CrossRef] [PubMed]
140. Guo, D.; Lui, G.Y.L.; Lai, S.L.; Wilmott, J.S.; Tikoo, S.; Jackett, L.A.; Quek, C.; Brown, D.L.; Sharp, D.M.; Kwan, R.Y.Q.; et al. RAB27A promotes melanoma cell invasion and metastasis via regulation of pro-invasive exosomes. *Int. J. Cancer* **2019**, *144*, 3070–3085. [CrossRef]
141. Mannavola, F.; Tucci, M.; Felici, C.; Passarelli, A.; D'Oronzo, S.; Silvestris, F. Tumor-derived exosomes promote the in vitro osteotropism of melanoma cells by activating the SDF-1/CXCR4/CXCR7 axis. *J. Transl. Med.* **2019**, *17*, 230. [CrossRef] [PubMed]
142. Hood, J.L.; San, R.S.; Wickline, S.A. Exosomes released by melanoma cells prepare sentinel lymph nodes for tumor metastasis. *Cancer Res.* **2011**, *71*, 3792–3801. [CrossRef] [PubMed]
143. Angi, M.; Kalirai, H.; Prendergast, S.; Simpson, D.; Hammond, D.E.; Madigan, M.C.; Beynon, R.J.; Coupland, S.E. In-depth proteomic profiling of the uveal melanoma secretome. *Oncotarget* **2016**, *7*, 49623–49635. [CrossRef] [PubMed]
144. Tengda, L.; Shuping, L.; Mingli, G.; Jie, G.; Yun, L.; Weiwei, Z.; Anmei, D. Serum exosomal microRNAs as potent circulating biomarkers for melanoma. *Melanoma Res.* **2018**, *28*, 295–303. [CrossRef] [PubMed]
145. Larkin, J.; Ascierto, P.A.; Dréno, B.; Atkinson, V.; Liszkay, G.; Maio, M.; Mandalà, M.; Demidov, L.; Stroyakovskiy, D.; Thomas, L.; et al. Combined vemurafenib and cobimetinib in BRAF-mutated melanoma. *N. Engl. J. Med.* **2014**, *371*, 1867–1876. [CrossRef]
146. Lunavat, T.R.; Cheng, L.; Einarsdottir, B.O.; Olofsson Bagge, R.; Veppil Muralidharan, S.; Sharples, R.A.; Lässer, C.; Gho, Y.S.; Hill, A.F.; Nilsson, J.A.; et al. BRAFV600 inhibition alters the microRNA cargo in the vesicular secretome of malignant melanoma cells. *Proc. Natl. Acad. Sci. USA* **2017**, *114*, E5930–E5939. [CrossRef]
147. Svedman, F.C.; Lohcharoenkal, W.; Bottai, M.; Brage, S.E.; Sonkoly, E.; Hansson, J.; Pivarcsi, A.; Eriksson, H. Extracellular microvesicle microRNAs as predictive biomarkers for targeted therapy in metastastic cutaneous malignant melanoma. *PLoS ONE* **2018**, *13*, e0206942. [CrossRef]
148. Segura, M.F.; Belitskaya-Lévy, I.; Rose, A.E.; Zakrzewski, J.; Gaziel, A.; Hanniford, D.; Darvishian, F.; Berman, R.S.; Shapiro, R.L.; Pavlick, A.C.; et al. Melanoma MicroRNA signature predicts post-recurrence survival. *Clin. Cancer Res.* **2010**, *16*, 1577–1586. [CrossRef]
149. Ribas, A.; Hamid, O.; Daud, A.; Hodi, F.S.; Wolchok, J.D.; Kefford, R.; Joshua, A.M.; Patnaik, A.; Hwu, W.I.; Weber, J.S.; et al. Association of Pembrolizumab With Tumor Response and Survival Among Patients With Advanced Melanoma. *JAMA* **2016**, *315*, 1600–1609. [CrossRef]
150. Cordonnier, M.; Nardin, C.; Chanteloup, G.; Derangere, V.; Algros, M.P.; Arnould, L.; Garrido, C.; Aubin, F.; Gobbo, J. Tracking the evolution of circulating exosomal-PD-L1 to monitor melanoma patients. *J. Extracell. Vesicles* **2020**, *9*, 1. [CrossRef]

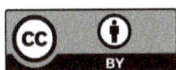

© 2020 by the authors. Licensee MDPI, Basel, Switzerland. This article is an open access article distributed under the terms and conditions of the Creative Commons Attribution (CC BY) license (http://creativecommons.org/licenses/by/4.0/).

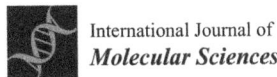

Article

Small Extracellular Vesicles Isolated from Serum May Serve as Signal-Enhancers for the Monitoring of CNS Tumors

Gabriella Dobra [1,2], Matyas Bukva [1,2], Zoltan Szabo [3], Bella Bruszel [3], Maria Harmati [1], Edina Gyukity-Sebestyen [1], Adrienn Jenei [4], Monika Szucs [5,6], Peter Horvath [1], Tamas Biro [7], Almos Klekner [4] and Krisztina Buzas [1,8,9],*

1. Laboratory of Microscopic Image Analysis and Machine Learning, Institute of Biochemistry, Biological Research Centre, H-6726 Szeged, Hungary; dobragab@yahoo.co.uk (G.D.); bukvamatyas@gmail.com (M.B.); harmatimarcsi@gmail.com (M.H.); e.gyukity.sebestyen@gmail.com (E.G.-S.); horvath.peter@brc.hu (P.H.)
2. Department of Medical Genetics, Doctoral School of Interdisciplinary Medicine, University of Szeged, H-6720 Szeged, Hungary
3. Department of Medical Chemistry, Faculty of Medicine, University of Szeged, H-6720 Szeged, Hungary; szabo.zoltan@med.u-szeged.hu (Z.S.); bruszel.bella@med.u-szeged.hu (B.B.)
4. Department of Neurosurgery, Clinical Centre, University of Debrecen, H-4032 Debrecen, Hungary; jenei.adrienn@med.unideb.hu (A.J.); aklekner@yahoo.com (A.K.)
5. Department of Medical Physics and Informatics, Faculty of Medicine, University of Szeged, H-6720 Szeged, Hungary; szucs.monika@med.u-szeged.hu
6. Department of Medical Physics and Informatics, Faculty of Science and Informatics, University of Szeged, H-6720 Szeged, Hungary
7. Department of Immunology, Faculty of Medicine, University of Debrecen, H-4032 Debrecen, Hungary; biro.lcmp@gmail.com
8. Department of Immunology, Faculty of Medicine, University of Szeged, H-6720 Szeged, Hungary
9. Department of Immunology, Faculty of Science and Informatics, University of Szeged, H-6720 Szeged, Hungary
* Correspondence: kr.buzas@gmail.com; Tel.: +36-62-432-340

Received: 26 June 2020; Accepted: 24 July 2020; Published: 28 July 2020

Abstract: Liquid biopsy-based methods to test biomarkers (e.g., serum proteins and extracellular vesicles) may help to monitor brain tumors. In this proteomics-based study, we aimed to identify a characteristic protein fingerprint associated with central nervous system (CNS) tumors. Overall, 96 human serum samples were obtained from four patient groups, namely glioblastoma multiforme (GBM), non-small-cell lung cancer brain metastasis (BM), meningioma (M) and lumbar disc hernia patients (CTRL). After the isolation and characterization of small extracellular vesicles (sEVs) by nanoparticle tracking analysis (NTA) and atomic force microscopy (AFM), liquid chromatography -mass spectrometry (LC-MS) was performed on two different sample types (whole serum and serum sEVs). Statistical analyses (ratio, Cohen's d, receiver operating characteristic; ROC) were carried out to compare patient groups. To recognize differences between the two sample types, pairwise comparisons (Welch's test) and ingenuity pathway analysis (IPA) were performed. According to our knowledge, this is the first study that compares the proteome of whole serum and serum-derived sEVs. From the 311 proteins identified, 10 whole serum proteins and 17 sEV proteins showed the highest intergroup differences. Sixty-five proteins were significantly enriched in sEV samples, while 129 proteins were significantly depleted compared to whole serum. Based on principal component analysis (PCA) analyses, sEVs are more suitable to discriminate between the patient groups. Our results support that sEVs have greater potential to monitor CNS tumors, than whole serum.

Keywords: extracellular vesicles; cancer biomarker; proteomics

1. Introduction

According to the World Health Organization (WHO), cancer is the second leading cause of death, accounting for an estimated 9.6 million cases in 2018. Globally, 1 in 6 deaths is due to cancer [1]. The cancer burden continues to grow worldwide, exerting tremendous physical, emotional and financial strain on individuals, families, communities and on health systems [2].

The diagnosis of central nervous system (CNS) tumors is based on CT and MRI scans, as well as on the histopathological analysis of samples obtained by biopsy or via surgical resection. However, these procedures are highly invasive, uncomfortable for the patient, bear a considerable risk of complications and provide limited information on tumor status. Therefore, biomarkers appropriate for monitoring disease progression and response to treatment are eagerly required. While repeated MRI scans serve as the standard method to follow patients, it has little prognostic value for long-term recurrence [3]. Thus, neuro-oncological research aims to identify novel biomarkers suitable for monitoring CNS tumors in clinical practice [4].

Liquid biopsy is in the spotlight of biomarker-focused research, as body fluids are easily accessible sources of biomarkers and are available with minimally invasive and low cost sampling procedures. Also, multiple sampling allows the monitoring of disease progression and therapeutic response [5]. Every cell, including neoplastic cells, release molecular markers into the circulation. Tumor-derived biomarkers include proteins, nucleic acids, circulating tumor cells, platelets and tumor-derived extracellular vesicles that accumulate in urine, cerebrospinal fluid, saliva and blood [6].

Blood is the most easily accessible source for biomarkers, thus it is frequently used to assess disease status in malignancies such as prostate, liver and ovarian cancers based on the serum concentrations of PSA, AFP and CA125, respectively. In neuro-oncology, blood-based biomarkers are mainly used to evaluate toxicity and safety of treatments to guide patient management. For example, myelosuppression is a common risk associated with temozolomide treatment and radiotherapy, thus standard practice dictates weekly tests of complete blood count, including whole blood cell differential and platelet counts during definitive chemoradiotherapy [7]. Finding biomarkers for blood-based CNS tumor monitoring is more challenging, as the blood-brain barrier (BBB) prevents the release of tumor-related biomarkers into peripheral blood. However, it would have outstanding benefits in clinical patient management, thus efforts to identify blood based biomarkers, including proteins, nucleic acids, circulating tumor cells and extracellular vesicles are currently in the forefront of neuro-oncological research [8].

Extracellular vesicles (EVs) are promising cancer biomarkers accessible via liquid biopsy, because they are cell-secreted, nano-sized and stably exist in all types of body fluids. EVs contain a sample of the cytosolic milieu, including an abundance of DNA, RNA, proteins and other analytes, while externally they also resemble their cell of origin [9]. EVs are small, lipid bilayer-enclosed vesicles released by both cancer and non-cancerous cells into the extracellular space [10].

EVs secreted by cancer cells communicate with neighboring stromal cells or even with cells at distant sites, inducing an alteration of the cell program [11,12]. Pre-metastatic niche formation has been shown in several tumors, for example, in pancreatic, lung, colorectal and ovarian cancers [13–16]. Also, EVs may be taken up by immune cells, leading to immunosuppression [17]. More recently, EVs have even gained a role in cancer diagnosis and therapy [18–20] as biomarker molecules that may be identified in different primary tumors with high sensitivity and specificity [21]. Regarding pancreatic cancer, Kalluri and colleagues found that glypican-1 (GPC1), a cell surface proteoglycan, is specifically enriched in circulating exosomes (30–200 nm endosome-derived EVs). GPC1 is suitable to differentiate early- and late-stage pancreatic cancer from benign diseases of the pancreas, with an accuracy of 100% [22]. The available evidence also supports that tumor-derived EVs can cross the BBB [23,24], however, currently no clinically relevant EV biomarkers are accepted for the monitoring of CNS tumors.

Several studies report on gene or protein expression analyses of CNS tumor tissue (specifically, glioblastoma), allowing to identify biomarkers that could be secreted into the blood and thus could be detected from serum samples. Recent studies have aimed to identify one and two specific biomarkers for the reliable evaluation of actual tumor status [25–27] but none of these proteins alone was found to be sufficiently specific and sensitive to serve as a monitoring marker.

Regarding that previous attempts to find surrogate serum markers for brain tumors have failed when based on a single or only few candidate factors, we made an attempt to identify a characteristic protein fingerprint of 10–20 candidate markers associated with CNS tumors.

For this purpose, 96 serum samples were collected from four patient groups according to the criteria of the National Ethical Committee and proteomics analysis was performed using liquid chromatography and mass spectrometry (LC-MS). The serum samples were obtained from patients diagnosed with the two most common types of brain tumors [28], namely malignant glioblastoma multiforme (GBM) and benign meningioma (M), as well as from patients with a prevalent brain metastasis [29] originating from non-small-cell lung cancer (BM). Patients with lumbar disc herniation served as controls (CTRL). Following a statistical selection, these four patient groups were compared with respect to the identified proteins. In parallel, small extracellular vesicles (sEVs) were isolated from the serum samples by differential centrifugation and proteomics and statistical analyses were also performed on these sEV samples, allowing to compare the suitability of these two different sample types. According to the best of our knowledge, this is the first study that compares the proteome of whole serum and serum-derived sEV samples. Results from the proteomics analysis indicate that using a protein fingerprint of serum-derived sEVs instead of analyzing whole serum increases the accuracy of distinguishing between the clinical samples, that is, between the patient groups. Our results support that sEVs have a greater potential for the proteomics-based monitoring of CNS tumors compared to whole serum analysis.

2. Results

2.1. EV Samples Show sEV Properties with Similar Concentration and Size Distribution in the Different Patient Groups

To verify the value of circulating extracellular vesicles as potential biomarkers for CNS tumors, EVs were isolated from the serum of patients with glioblastoma multiforme (GBM), single brain metastasis originating from non-small-cell lung cancer (BM) and meningioma (M), as well as from control patients with lumbar disc herniation (CTRL). Each group included 24 individuals of both genders with various ages. Extracellular vesicles were isolated from the sera by differential centrifugation and were characterized by atomic force microscopy (AFM) and nanoparticle tracking analysis (NTA). Pools of 6 samples were formed in all groups, allowing four parallel samples to be tested per group (see in Section 4.1). Western blot analyses were also performed to demonstrate the EV nature (Figure S1).

EVs were divided into subtypes based on their size range, separating small EVs (sEVs) and medium/large EVs (m/lEVs) [30]. AFM analysis revealed that the small EV subtype includes various structures. Mean and mode diameters of the particles, represented by an average of the 16 sample pools, were measured as 112 nm and 86 nm by NTA, respectively (Figure 1A).

The quantitative characterization of serum sEVs by NTA (Figure 1B) revealed no significant differences between the four patient groups regarding the size and concentration of circulating sEVs. However, within the groups high individual differences were observed in the measured parameters of the sEVs.

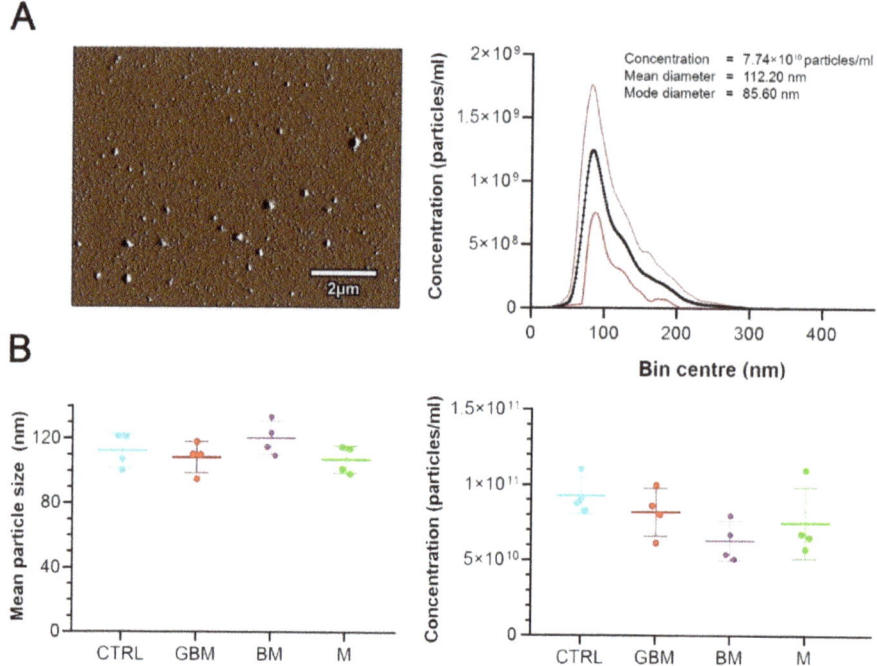

Figure 1. Characterization and quantitative properties of the small extracellular vesicle (sEV) samples. (**A**) Atomic force microscopy (AFM) image of sEV isolates displays vesicles with diameters within the range of 50–140 nm. The diagram shows the size distribution of the 96 sEV samples isolated from the serum, presenting the mean +/−95% CI values measured by nanoparticle tracking analysis (NTA). (**B**) Dot plots show the number and size distribution of small extracellular vesicles (sEVs) displayed in mean size (left) and concentration (right) values for each sample pools (4 samples/group).

2.2. Statistical Analysis of LC-MS Data Reveals Characteristic Proteomic Fingerprints for Each Patient Group and Informs on the Suitability of the Two Different Sample Types in Distinguishing CNS Tumors

We aimed to identify the differences between the four patient groups to reveal the characteristic protein profiles associated with the CNS tumors in point. Using an intensity ratio of >2 or <0.5 with Cohen's d effect size of 2 as a cut-off, we investigated which proteins show reliable intensity difference and which proteins can separate at least one group from the others based on a receiver operating characteristic (ROC) analysis. Moreover, utilizing principal component analysis (PCA) with k-means clustering, we were able to compare the suitability of the two different sample types to distinguish between the CNS tumors in point. Figure 2 shows the flowchart of LC-MS data processing and the results of the statistical analyses.

Proteomics analyses by LC-MS (Step 1) were performed on whole serum and sEV samples obtained from patients with GBM, BM, M and CTRL. Individual samples ($n = 24$) in each group were arranged into 4 pools (see in Section 4.1) to eliminate individual variances, reduce sample number, shorten the time of LC-MS measurements and reduce the need for materials. The Data independent acquisition (DIA) mode constructed spectral library revealed 311 proteins (see Table S1). Based on Pearson's correlation analyses (Step 2), one of the sEV control samples had to be excluded from further statistical analyses (Table S2). After excluding unreliable proteins, as well as proteins with missing values (Step 3), a total of 262 proteins remained for the final analysis.

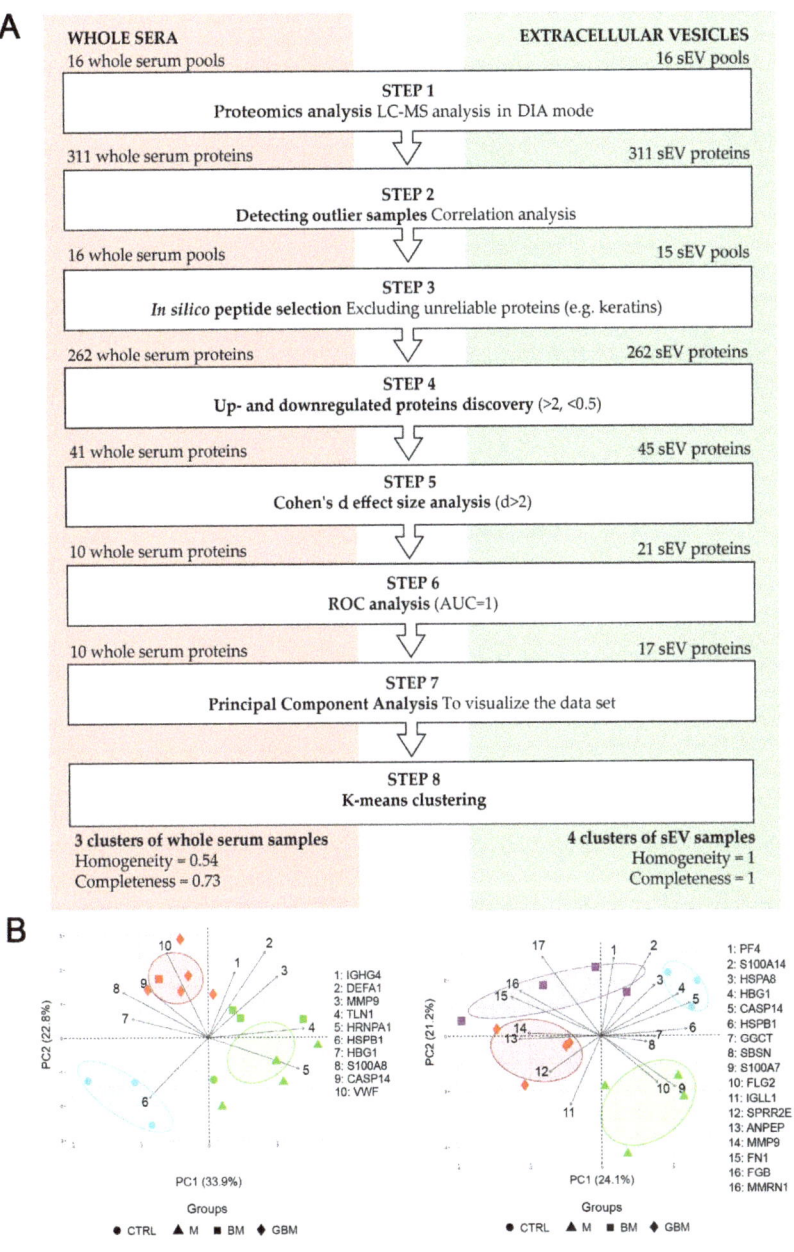

Figure 2. Statistical analysis of the proteome of whole serum (left) and sEV samples (right). (**A**) The flowchart shows the steps of selecting the proteins revealed by liquid chromatography and mass spectrometry (LC-MS) (**B**) The diagrams visualize the results of the principal component analysis (PCA) and k-means clustering. X and Y axes of PCA biplots show principal component 1 (PC1) and principal component 2 (PC2) with explained variances. Arrows represent the coefficients of each protein for PC1 versus the coefficients for PC2, showing the significance of each protein in influencing PCs. Different dots represent the 4 patient groups. Colors indicate the clusters formed by k-means clustering; ellipses indicating the 95% confidence interval were constructed around the barycenters of the clusters.

Following basic processing, up- and down-regulated protein discovery (Step 4) resulted in 41 whole serum proteins and 45 sEV proteins. In addition to comparing each CNS tumor group to CTRL, between-group differences among the CNS tumor groups were also assessed in the protein selection process. As clinically relevant incidence is an important consideration for selecting the proteins identified, Cohen's d effect size was adopted as an indicator of between-groups difference. The Cohen's d effect size analysis (Step 5) with a threshold of d > 2 yielded 10 and 21 proteins in the whole serum and sEV samples, respectively. In the ROC analyses (Step 6) 10 whole serum proteins (MMP9, HSPB1, CASP14, HBG1, IGHG4, DEFA1, VWF, HNRNPA1, S100A8, TLN1) and 17 sEV proteins (MMP9, HSPB1, CASP14, HBG1, FGB, GGCT, PF4, S100A7, FN1, ANPEP, FLG2, HSPA8, IGLL1, MMRN1, S100A14, SBSN, SPRR2E) were found to meet the AUC = 1 selection criteria. Table S3 includes the UniProt ID, Gene symbol, ratio of intensity means > 2 or < 0.5 and Cohen's d effect size > 2 parameters for the selected proteins. The two sample groups shared four significantly altered proteins (highlighted in Table S3), namely MMP9, CASP14, HBG1 and HSPB1.

Following protein selection, PCA (Step 7) was performed to visualize the dataset, where several potentially correlated proteins were projected into a smaller number of variables. K-means clustering (Step 8) on the whole serum PCA biplot resulted in 3 inhomogeneous or incomplete clusters. Calculated cluster homogeneity and completeness scores are 0.56 and 0.73, respectively. In contrast to whole serum samples, the clustering of sEV samples formed homogeneous and complete clusters, with homogeneity and completeness scores of 1. The results of the PCA analyses and k-means clustering indicate considerable differences between the whole serum and sEV samples (Figure 2B). We found that the accuracy of distinguishing between various CNS tumors can be increased using a protein panel from serum-derived sEVs, compared to analyzing whole serum samples.

2.3. Statistical Evaluation and IPA of LC-MS Data Revealed the Background of Suitability Differences between Whole Serum and sEV Samples

2.3.1. Quantitative Changes of the Proteome May Affect the Suitability of sEV Samples to Provide Biomarkers for CNS Tumor Status Monitoring

Statistical comparison of the proteome of sEV and whole serum samples was performed to reveal quantitative differences affecting the suitability of different sample types to provide biomarkers for CNS tumor status monitoring. Pairwise statistical comparison (Welch's test) was used to identify proteins significantly enriched or depleted in sEV samples compared to whole serum samples (Figure 3). Sixty-five proteins were found to be significantly enriched in sEV samples, while 129 proteins were significantly depleted ($p < 0.05$). Using our sEV purification protocol detailed in the Section 4, we obtained a uniform particle size range of sEVs but the magnitude of quantitative changes in the sEV versus whole serum proteome suggested the possible presence of lipoprotein and serum protein contaminations. The level of apolipoproteins was decreased in sEV enriched samples (sEV/serum mean ratio is 0.66), however this fraction could not be completely eliminated. Besides, well known high abundance serum proteins (e.g., ALB) dominated the protein content of sEV enriched samples too. However, the enrichment of non-tissue specific (ITGA2B, ITGB3, LGALS3BP), epithelial cell (CD5L) and platelet related (STOM, TSPAN9) EV marker proteins [31] confirms sEV enrichment (sEV/serum mean ratio is 26.58), while it also demonstrates the presence of sEVs produced during clotting.

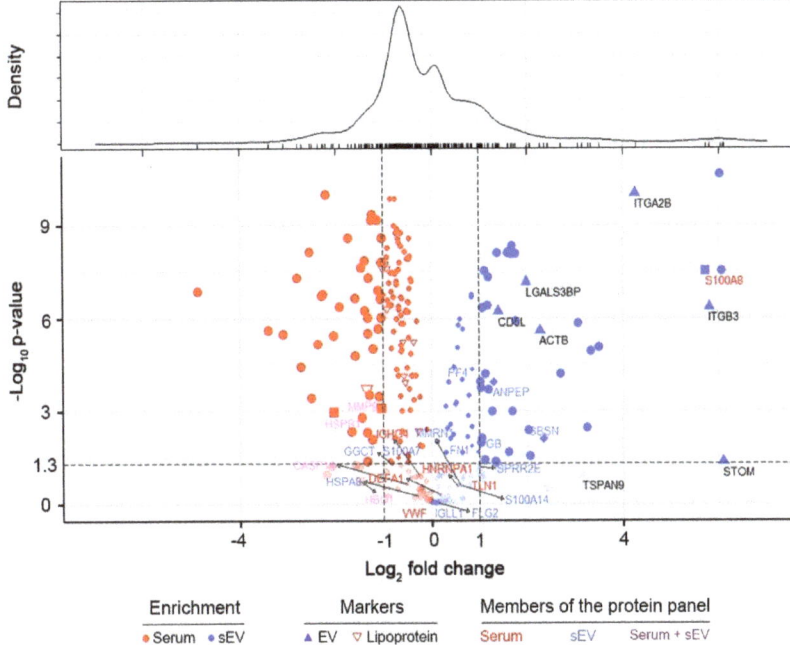

Figure 3. Quantitative comparison of the proteome of sEV and whole serum samples. Volcano plot represents the observed changes in average MS intensities in paired sEV vs. serum comparisons. Protein enrichment is marked with red and blue colored symbols in whole serum and sEVs, respectively. Lipoproteins (empty red upside-down triangles), elements of our whole serum protein panel (red letters, square symbols), sEV protein panel (blue letters, diamond symbols) and common members of the two protein panels (purple letters) are highlighted. Values of −log (p) were obtained from paired Welch's test in sEV/serum comparisons. Density estimation of log2 (fold change) values is shown on top.

Among the 17 proteins of the sEV marker panel described in Section 2.2 only 6 were significantly enriched in the sEV samples and 5 of the 10 proteins comprising the specific serum panel had higher abundance in whole serum (Figure 3). These findings suggest that the better suitability of sEV enriched samples to serve a biomarker source is not explained by a total increase in the abundance of specific proteins. (Detailed proteomics findings, protein annotation and sEV enrichment data are available in Table S1).

Additional sample processing (sEV isolation) may introduce higher technical variance in case of sEV samples, thus it may reduce the analytical suitability of this sample type. Our analysis revealed a similar level of variance for proteins quantified in each sample type (excluding contaminants)—median coefficients of variation within each patient group were in the ranges of 20.78–23.87% for sEV and 20.21–24.45% for serum samples (see Figure S2 for CV distributions).

2.3.2. Biological Background Might Be Responsible for the Increased Suitability of sEV Samples to Provide Biomarkers for CNS Tumor Status Monitoring

To gain insight into the biological background of the obtained proteomics data, IPA was applied. We performed 'Core Analyses' for whole serum and sEV data separately, yielding a list of significantly influenced 'Diseases and Functions' in each patient group ($p < 0.05$). Using 'Comparison Analysis,' we were able to develop heatmaps covering the relevant systemic and tumor-related functions, as well as the activated or inhibited immune functions (Figure 4A). Regarding whole serum samples, many of the significantly influenced functions identified are related to CNS involvement and active immune regulatory processes but the patient groups are not clearly distinguished on the heatmaps (Figure 4A, left panels). In contrast, on two of the three sEV proteome-based heatmaps M was evidently separated from the malignant tumor groups (Figure 4A, right panels), where tumor progression-related functions (e.g., angiogenesis, proliferation and migration of tumor cells) were detected to be highly activated and the activated immune functions (e.g., cell movement or activation of myeloid cells) predominate over inhibited immune functions (e.g., phagocytosis).

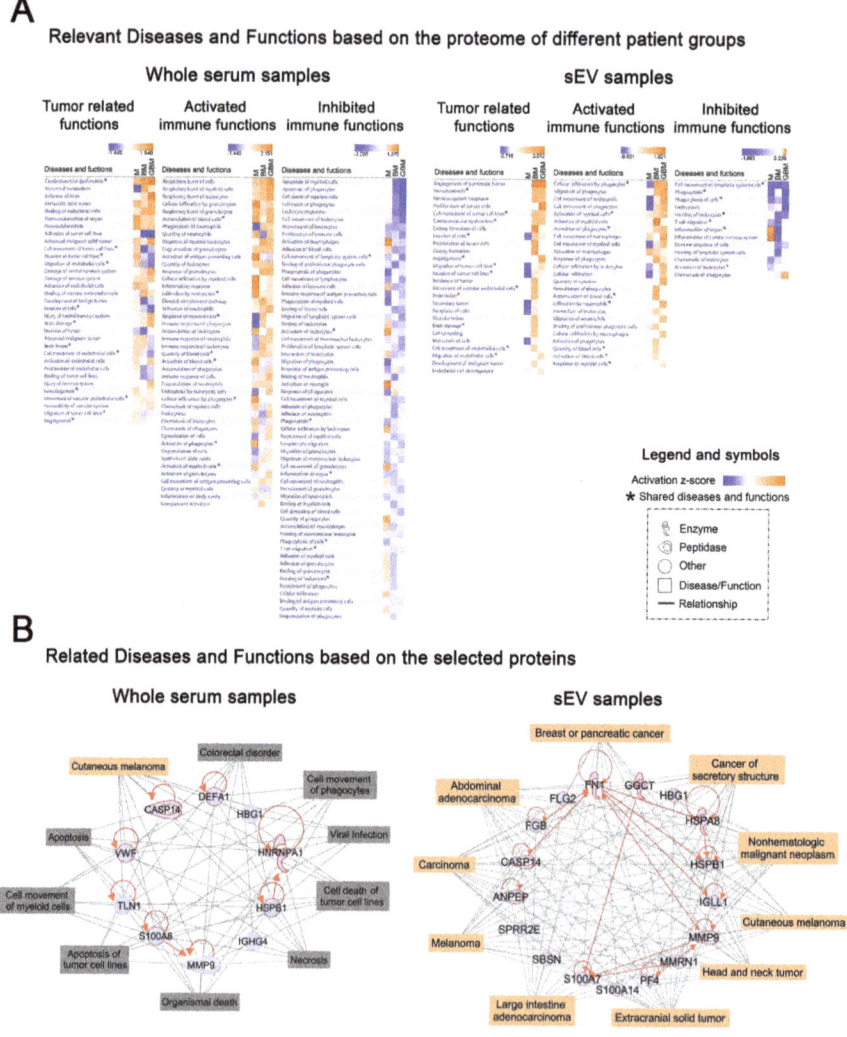

Figure 4. Ingenuity Pathway Analysis (IPA) analyses of whole serum (left) and sEV (right) data derived from the LC-MS analysis. (**A**) Heatmaps show relevant 'Diseases and Functions' in three separated panels related to systemic and tumor-related functions, as well as activated and inhibited immune functions. Z-score indicates activation or inhibition rates of the relevant 'Diseases and Functions' in the three tumorous patient groups compared to the control group. * symbol indicates the shared diseases and functions in whole serum and sEVs. (**B**) Networks display the selected 10 whole serum or 17 sEV proteins (blue symbols) and their relationships (red lines). Top ten related 'Diseases (highlighted in orange symbols) and Functions (highlighted in grey)' are connected by grey lines.

Next, we attempted to specify the common biological role of the characteristic protein profiles identified. Therefore, we elaborated two networks containing the selected 10 and 17 proteins identified based on whole serum and the sEV data, respectively (Figure 4B). Using the 'Grow tool,' the top ten influenced 'Diseases and Functions' were integrated into the networks. In case of the whole serum network (Figure 4B, left panel), nine different related 'Diseases and Functions' were identified, including viral infection, apoptosis, necrosis or cell movement of phagocytes and myeloid cells and only one was cancer-related. In contrast, the top ten influenced diseases identified on the sEV network based on the identified 17 proteins (Figure 4B, right panel) were all tumor-associated, suggesting their potential involvement in the pathophysiology of cancers.

3. Discussion

Non-invasive diagnostic tests are of outstanding clinical importance because of their minimal burden and risk to the patient, their repeatability, low cost, high information content and easy accessibility. In CNS tumors, a minimally invasive technique for describing the actual tumor status should be particularly important. Conventional MRI tests commonly used for the monitoring of CNS tumors are not absolutely appropriate for discriminating between various tumor types (e.g., cannot differentiate between glioblastomas and solitary metastases, CNS lymphomas or other glioma grades [32]) and cannot distinguish recurrence from pseudoprogression. Brain biopsies, as another option, are highly challenging and risky, especially when multiple sampling is required for long-term follow-up [33]. For several cancer types, blood-based tumor markers, such as PSA, AFP and CA125 have been introduced into clinical practice and research for the identification of further noninvasive biomarkers applicable for monitoring a wider scale of malignant diseases is ongoing [34]. However, regarding CNS tumors these studies have generally failed, presumably explained by several reasons, including (1) the barrier function of BBB (releasing less tumor 'information' into the systemic circulation), (2) the presence of molecules released into the blood from other sources and (3) possibly because of the complexity of tumor tissues (such as glioblastoma multiforme). These issues hamper attempts to use a single or only a few biomarkers to diagnose and monitor CNS tumors.

Based on these considerations, we aimed to detect the characteristic protein fingerprint of some common CNS tumors, trying to amplify the signal/information that brain tumors release into the circulation. For this purpose, the protein content of 96 clinical serum samples and related sEV samples isolated from the whole serum was measured by LC-MS. Serum samples were collected from three brain tumor groups considered as the most common malignant, benign and metastatic brain tumors (glioblastoma multiforme, meningioma [28] and brain metastasis of non-small-cell lung cancer [29]) and a control group (lumbar disc herniation).

To examine whether the proteomes of serum and sEV samples are suitable for differentiating between the CNS tumors in point, that is, whether they are applicable to diagnose and monitor the disease, the proteomes of these four patient groups were compared. The effectiveness of tumor type distinction may be increased if the analysis is restricted to proteins which exhibit significant between-group differences. Protein selection was carried out as described in literature [35] (using ratio of intensity means; Cohen's d effect size; ROC) but much stricter thresholds were applied (>2, <0.5; d > 2; AUC = 1, respectively). Statistical selection yielded a collection of proteins whose intensity showed significant between-group differences and thus these proteins could be reckoned as the most suitable molecules for distinguishing between the tumor types examined. Specifically, protein selection yielded a 10- and 17-membered protein panel for whole serum and sEV samples, respectively. While none of these proteins appeared to be able to distinguish between the patient groups individually, their combination was found to reliably discriminate between the different patient groups suggesting that instead of a few candidates, a specific protein panel is required for a perfect differentiation between various tumor types.

To evaluate group distinction efficiency, PCA with k-means clustering was carried out according to literature [36]. Homogeneity and completeness scores of the clusters were calculated to measure the performance of k-means clustering. Cluster homogeneity and completeness mean that each cluster contains only samples from the same group and all samples of a given group are assigned to the same cluster. Both scores are bounded below by 0 and above by 1. A score of 1 indicates perfect homogeneity or completeness. PCA revealed that sEV samples were more suitable for group distinction. Despite carefully selected and perfectly identical statistical analyses for the two sample types, the homogeneity and completeness scores for the whole serum analysis were 0.56 and 0.73, respectively, compared to scores 1 and 1 for the analysis of sEV samples. The explanation for these findings is illustrated on a PCA biplot (Figure 2). Regarding serum samples, the proteins that can separate two given groups by the appropriate ratio and effect size may have similar intensities in other groups as well. For example, DEFA1 is important in distinguishing the CTRL group from the BM and GBM groups, however, it shows similar intensities in the GBM and BM groups, hampering the separation of these groups (see DEFA1 arrow pointing between the BM and GBM groups in the whole serum PCA plot). Still, DEFA1 cannot be removed, because it plays a key role in separating the CTRL group from malignant tumors. In contrast, the majority of the proteins identified in the sEV samples were able to separate any given group from all the others.

To check whether the poorer performance of whole serum proteins in distinguishing between the patient groups is attributed to the number of the proteins considered, we performed another PCA analysis including only up- and down-regulated proteins selected from the whole identified panel (see Figure 2, Step 4), yielding a similar number of proteins for the two sample types. The PCA analysis of these 41 whole serum and 45 sEV proteins yielded similar results as the previous analysis of carefully selected proteins only and the sEV sample type proved to perform better again. Although the sEV sample was far from being perfect in this case (4 groups were recognized with a homogeneity score of 0.66 and a completeness score of 0.66), the results for the whole serum analysis indicated that not even the sample groups can be recognized based on these proteins only 2 groups were recognized, homogeneity—0.07, completeness: 0.40) (Figure S3). These findings support that sEVs have a better efficiency in distinguishing between various patient groups, irrespective of the order of magnitude of proteins analyzed for the comparison of sEV and whole serum samples.

To investigate the background of our observations, we performed a quantitative proteomics comparison of the two sample types. A quantitative evaluation of sEV purification protocols was suggested based on quantitative LC-MS based proteomics approach, using enrichment analysis of carefully selected sEV markers along with medium specific contamination marker proteins (e.g., lipoproteins and serum). To the best of our knowledge, we are the first group to quantitatively compare the proteome of serum derived small extracellular vesicles with that of the original whole serum samples. sEV enrichment may increase the relative abundance of proteins present in higher concentration within sEVs and the increased signal-to-noise ratio may be beneficial for the quantitative LC-MS analysis of such proteins. On the other hand, proteins in serum are originating from different sources of the human body. Any fractionation (e.g., enrichment of a specific sEV population) may decrease the suppressing effect of the uninformative protein fraction released from sources not specific for the target disease. No association was revealed between being a sEV marker and sEV enrichment, suggesting that it not the overall enrichment process that should be responsible for the increased suitability of sEV samples to provide biomarkers for CNS tumor monitoring. Instead, the removal of an uninformative protein fraction, providing a more specific sample, may explain why the sEV sample is more applicable for distinguishing between various CNS cancer patient groups. Compared to whole serum samples, EVs may be more suitable for investigating tumor related molecular patterns, as the characteristic fingerprint molecules are present in higher concentrations in sEV samples and are accompanied by less contaminating molecules that may bias the analytical findings.

To understand the biological background for our proteomics-based data, IPA was used for the separate analyses of whole serum and sEV data. 'Core Analyses' were performed, yielding a list of significantly influenced 'Diseases and Functions' comprising tumor-related functions as well as activated or inhibited immune functions in each patient group ($p < 0.05$). 'Comparison Analysis' was carried out to compare the affected 'Diseases and Functions' in the different patient groups. Regarding whole serum samples, many of the significantly influenced functions identified were associated with CNS involvement and active immune regulatory processes but the patient groups were not clearly distinguished on the heatmaps. In contrast, on the sEV proteome-based heatmaps the benign M was clearly separated from the malignant tumors, for which numerous tumor progression-related functions (e.g., angiogenesis, proliferation and migration of tumor cells) were found to be highly activated. The generated IPA heatmaps also revealed that the proteome of sEV samples may provide more specific information on the immune reactions characteristic to the patient groups. We assume that activated immune functions (e.g., cellular infiltration and migration of phagocytes) may play a crucial role in the development of an immune-suppressive microenvironment, while antitumoral immune responses (e.g., phagocytosis, inflammation) might be inhibited.

Serum is a dual source of biomolecular information on cancer, as it contains the molecules released by cancer cells, as well as those released during the immune system's tumor-specific responses [37]. Therefore, the differences observed in the serum vesicles isolated from different patient groups may not only mirror tumor-specific processes but also those related to the associated immune responses [38,39]. Samples enriched in sEVs can offer an amplified source of relevant information, representing not only the specific tumor tissue but also the associated immune responses. Thus, an appropriate protein panel, covering both sources, may have improved efficiency for CNS tumor classification and monitoring.

In addition, the networks developed based on the IPA 'Grow tool' demonstrated that the biological background of the sEV-based characteristic protein profile is more specifically associated with the tumor types compared with the whole serum based protein profile. The role of some of the proteins included in the sEV-based characteristic protein profile has already been described, for example in GBM biology, making these proteins promising targets for extracellular vesicle-based biomarker development [25].

In addition to the proteomics-based comparison of EV samples, we also examined the EV concentration of individual serum samples. Interestingly, no significant differences were detected between the four patient groups regarding the concentration of serum sEVs, with a mean size of 112.2 nm. Osti et al. observed higher EV plasma levels in GBM patients, brain metastases and extra-axial brain tumors compared to healthy controls. Other researchers also demonstrated higher EV concentration in tumorous patients, when unfractionated EV isolates [40] or a wider spectra of EVs were analyzed [41,42]. However, other non-neoplastic diseases of the central nervous system may also increase the number of small-sized circulating EVs, as it was demonstrated in acute ischemic stroke [43] or multiple sclerosis patients [44]. Our vesicle number measurement results, as well as the findings detailed above suggest that the elevated sEV concentration cannot be clearly attributed to the presence of the tumor as immune responses or other systemic responses also contribute to the circulating EV population. Our proteomics-based findings, coupled with the available literature data, suggest that circulating small-sized EVs show important qualitative but not quantitative differences between benign or malignant brain tumors and spinal disc herniation.

Liu and colleagues highlighted that serum is not the perfect choice for a representative sampling of circulating EVs [45], as a high fraction of EVs may be lost during coagulation and also blood components (e.g., platelets) may release microvesicles (MV) during clotting, altering the original MV content of blood samples. However, serum is still the preferred sample form for blood-based clinical diagnoses and it is a practical choice for future clinical developments. It should be noted that co-purification of proteins [46] and lipoprotein particles [47] in EV isolation methods is a common and well known challenge [31]. The presence of protein aggregates [48] and lipoproteins in sEV isolates may provide additional explanation for the lack of increase in the concentration of enriched sEV particles in cancer patients' serum, contrary to literature data on plasma [49] or serum samples [40]. Efforts to eliminate lipoproteins are described in numerous papers reporting on attempts to introduce more sophisticated methods (e.g., combination of ultracentrifugation and size-exclusion chromatography) [50]. In fact, these laborious and instrumentation demanding methods are of high importance in scientific research of the molecular contents of EVs but they may not be applicable in routine clinical practice. Our sEV isolation protocol has several advantages, as it does not require expensive equipment or highly trained professionals and the entire procedure (along with characterization) is performed within 4 h, therefore, this technique could be easily incorporated into clinical practice.

Our quantitative proteomics results demonstrate that even a simple sEV enrichment protocol can increase the diagnostic potential of serum samples for the identification and classification of patients with different CNS cancers. This finding also supports that even a low-efficacy sEV enrichment/purification method may be appropriate to enhance the analytical applicability of serum samples for CNS cancer monitoring, however, in such cases a quantitative description of enrichment efficiency is definitely required for the right interpretation of the analytical results [51].

In conclusion, our findings support that extracellular vesicles have a greater potential for the monitoring of CNS tumors compared to whole serum samples. Using EV samples is a possible way to amplify the signals released by brain tumors into the circulation. Given the easy-to-implement isolation and enrichment protocol established in this study, the introduction of EV analysis would be beneficial in clinical practice.

4. Materials and Methods

4.1. Patients

Blood samples of 96 patients treated between March 2015 and January 2018 in the Department of Neurosurgery, University of Debrecen were analyzed. Samples were obtained from patients with primary glioblastoma multiforme (GBM), meningioma (M) and single brain metastasis originating from non-small-cell lung cancer (BM). Control samples (CTRL) were collected from patients with spinal disc herniation without evidence of cancer. This non-tumor patient group served as control group in comparison to the patients having different intracranial tumor to distinguish the effects of tumorous processes from the CNS involvement on circulating sEVs. Each group contained 24 individuals with mixed ages and genders. As shown in the Table 1, six-sample-pools were created from the individuals, allowing four parallel samples to be tested per group. Blood samples were collected one day prior to neurosurgical procedure in each tumor case. None of the patients received radio- or chemotherapy before tumor resection. Blood samples were stored by the Neurosurgical Brain Tumor and Tissue Bank of Debrecen according to the criteria of the National Research Ethics Committee. An informed consent form was signed by each patient; the study was conducted in accordance with the Declaration of Helsinki. This study was carried out according to two ethical approvals, namely 51450-2/2015/EKU (0411/15), Medical Research Council, Scientific and Research Ethics Committee, Budapest, October 30, 2015 and 121/2019-SZTE, University of Szeged, Human Investigation Review Board, Albert Szent-Györgyi Clinical Centre, Szeged, 19 July 2019.

Table 1. Patient cohort [1].

♦ Glioblastoma Multiforme	GBM	GBM1	GBM2	GBM3	GBM4
Total No. of patients	$n = 24$	$n = 6$	$n = 6$	$n = 6$	$n = 6$
Age, Median (range)	67 (33–82)	64.5 (38–82)	69.5 (33–76)	67.5 (49–74)	66.5 (63–77)
Mean	64.9	62.7	63.8	64.7	68.5
Sex (%), Male	13 (54.2)	3 (50)	3 (50)	5 (83.3)	2 (33.3)
Female	11 (45.8)	3 (50)	3 (50)	1 (16.7)	4 (66.7)
■ Brain Metastasis	BM	BM1	BM2	BM3	BM4
Total No. of patients	$n = 24$	$n = 6$	$n = 6$	$n = 6$	$n = 6$
Age, Median (range)	64 (42–82)	66.5 (51–82)	68 (62–71)	63.5 (42–81)	59.5 (53–64)
Mean	64	67.7	67.5	59.7	59.5
Sex (%), Male	13 (54.2)	2 (33.3)	3 (50)	4 (66.7)	4 (66.7)
Female	11 (45.8)	4 (66.7)	3 (50)	2 (33.3)	2 (33.3)
▲ Meningioma	M	M1	M2	M3	M4

Table 1. Cont.

♦ Glioblastoma Multiforme	GBM	GBM1	GBM2	GBM3	GBM4
Total No. of patients	n = 24	n = 6	n = 6	n = 6	n = 6
Age, Median (range)	60 (30–79)	54.5 (39–69)	62 (30–66)	61.5 (44–75)	66.5 (52–79)
Mean	**58.0**	53.5	53	59.3	66
Sex (%), Male	**4 (16.7)**	0 (0)	0 (0)	1 (16.7)	3 (50)
Female	**20 (83.3)**	6 (100)	6 (100)	5 (83.3)	3 (50)
• Control	CTRL	CTRL1	CTRL2	CTRL3	CTRL4
Total No. of patients	n = 24	n = 6	n = 6	n = 6	n = 6
Age, Median (range)	50.5 (20–81)	46.5 (26–71)	47 (20–62)	70.5 (49–81)	52.5 (41–69)
Mean	**52.9**	46.5	45	67.2	53
Sex (%), Male	**9 (37.5)**	2 (33.3)	4 (66.7)	4 (66.7)	4 (66.7)
Female	**15 (62.5)**	4 (66.7)	2 (33.3)	2 (33.3)	2 (33.3)

[1] The table summarizes the main characteristics of the patient groups examined. Each group (average values highlighted in bald) included 24 individuals, converted into six-sample-pools to yield four samples per group for further analysis.

4.2. Preparation of Serum Samples, sEV Isolation and Characterization

Blood samples were collected into BD Vacutainer SST II Advance Tubes (Becton, Dickinson and Company, Franklin Lakes, NJ, USA), allowed to clot for at least 1 h at room temperature and centrifuged for 20 min at 3000× g, 10 °C to remove cells. Following the 3000× g centrifugation, the supernatant serum was transferred to new Eppendorf tubes and centrifuged for 30 min at 10,000× g, 4 °C to remove debris and large vesicles. One milliliter serum aliquot was diluted with DPBS (Ca^{2+}-free, Mg^{2+}-free, Lonza Group Ltd., Basel, Switzerland) to 8 mL and ultracentrifuged for 70 min, at 100,000× g, 4 °C (polycarbonate tubes, fixed angle T-1270 rotor, Thermo Fisher Scientific, Waltham, MA, USA). The pellet was resuspended in 100 uL DPBS and stored at −80 °C until further processing. This sEV isolation protocol served to reach intermediate recovery and intermediate specificity according to MISEV2018 [31].

SEVs were characterized by AFM (Oxford Instruments Asylum Research, Abingdon, UK), as described previously [52] and NTA using a NanoSight NS300 instrument (Malvern Panalytical Ltd., Malvern, UK) as it described below. Classical EV markers were presented by Western blot analyses using NuPAGE reagents and an XCell SureLock Mini-Cell System (Thermo Fisher Scientific, Waltham, MA, USA) according to manufacturer's protocols. For detection of the CD81 and Alix markers, we used rabbit anti-human CD81 (1:1000, Sigma-Aldrich, St. Louis, MO, USA) and rabbit anti-human Alix (1:1000, Sigma-Aldrich, St. Louis, MO, USA) primary antibody and HRP-conjugated anti-rabbit IgG (1:1000, R&D Systems, Minneapolis, MN, USA) secondary antibody.4.3. Quantitative analysis of sEVs by NTA.

As suggested by a recent study [53], sEVs were diluted in particle free DPBS and analyzed using a NanoSight NS300 instrument with 532 nm laser (Malvern Panalytical Ltd., Malvern, UK). The measurements were performed on the 16 sEV sample pools (described in 4.1). Six videos of 60 s were recorded for each sample under constant settings (Camera level: 15; Treshold: 4, 25 °C; 60–80 particles/frame) and analyzed to obtain data on size distribution and particle concentration.

4.3. Proteomic Analysis by LC-MS

4.3.1. 'In Solution' Digestion

Individual samples containing 20 µg protein were diluted to 10 µL with 0.1 M NH_4HCO_3 (pH = 8.0) buffer; 12 µL 0.1% RapiGest SF (Waters, Milford, MA, USA) and 2 µL 55 mM dithioeritritol solution was added and kept at 60 °C for 30 min to unfold and reduce proteins. A volume of 2 µL 200 mM iodo acetamide solution was added to alkylate the proteins which were kept for an additional 30 min in the dark at room temperature. The samples were digested overnight at 37 °C with trypsin (Thermo

Scientific, Waltham, MA, USA, enzyme/protein ratio: 0.4 to 1). The digestion was stopped by addition of 1 µL of concentrated formic acid.

4.3.2. LC-MS

The separation of the digested samples was carried out on a nanoAcquity UPLC, (Waters, Milford, MA, USA) using Waters ACQUITY UPLC M-Class Peptide C18 (130 Å, 1.78 µm, 75 µm × 250 mm) column with a nonlinear 90 min gradient. Eluents were water (A) and acetonitrile (B) containing 0.1 V/V% formic acid and the separation of the peptide mixture was performed at 45 °C with 0.35 µL/min flow rate using an optimized nonlinear LC gradient (3–40% B). The LC was coupled to a high-resolution Q Exactive Plus quadrupole-orbitrap hybrid mass spectrometer (Thermo Scientific, Waltham, MA, USA). The quantitative measurements of digested individual samples were performed in DIA mode. The survey scan for DIA method operated with 35,000 resolution. The full scan was performed between 380 to 1020 m/z. The AGC target was set to 5×10^6 or 120 ms maximum injection time. In the 400–1000 m/z region 22 m/z wide overlapping windows were acquired at 17,500 resolution (AGC target: 3×10^6 or 100 ms injection time, normalized collision energy: 27 for charge 2). The quantitative analysis was performed in Encyclopedia 0.81 [54] using default settings after deconvolution, peak picking and conversion of raw MS files to mzML format in Proteowizard [55]. A comprehensive spectral library [56] of 10,000 human proteins was used for peptide identification. Protein quantities calculated by the Encyclopedia software based on summed intensities of the automatically filtered peptides were used in further statistical evaluations.

4.4. Statistical Analysis

The collected data about the whole serum and extracellular vesicles were reduced and analyzed using statistical methods. Pearson's correlation analysis was used to investigate the outlier samples [57], contaminating proteins (cytokeratins) and proteins with missing values were excluded from the proteomic data [58]. Data were log-transformed to reduce skewness and increase linearity [59]. Cohen's d effect size was calculated to measure the difference between the protein intensity means, outcomes in two different groups [60,61]. Pairwise ROC analysis allowed us to find those proteins which can separate at least one group to the others [62]. The calculated ROC AUC (area under the ROC curve) values are accepted if it equals to 1. In order to transform several (potentially) correlated proteins into a (smaller) number of uncorrelated variables and visualize the dataset, PCA with k-means clustering was performed [63–66]. Homogeneity and completeness scores of the clusters were calculated to measure the performance of k-means clustering [67]. Two-tailed Welch's t-test was performed to identify the significantly enriched or depleted proteins in sEV samples. The statistical analyses were performed using R statistical program (version 3.6.3 with pROC, FactoMineR, factoextra and ggplot2 packages; Vienna, Austria), Python programming language (version 3.8, Scotts Valley, CA, USA) and Perseus (MaxQuant, Munich, Germany). Values of $p < 0.05$ were considered significant (see in Appendix A more detailed). GraphPad Prism 8 (San Diego, CA, USA) was used for further data visualization.

4.5. In Silico Analysis of LC-MS Data

Protein data derived from the LC-MS were analyzed by the IPA (Qiagen Bioinformatics, Hilden, Germany). Using fold change values, 'Core Analysis' were performed for whole serum and sEV data separately to identify 'Diseases and Functions,' which can be significantly influenced by the described proteomes ($p < 0.05$). After 'Comparison Analysis,' we created heatmaps of the relevant 'Diseases and Functions,' that is, tumor-related and immunological functions showing regulatory differences between the three CNS tumor groups. Activation z-score calculated by IPA indicates the extent and direction of the effect that given proteins have on function/disease.

The selected 10 whole serum proteins and 17 sEV proteins were introduced to custom pathways as well. Then, 'Connect tool' of IPA was used to reveal the relationships between these molecules and

'Grow tool' was applied to search the top ten 'Diseases and Functions' assigned to the 10 whole serum proteins or 17 sEV proteins. Results are displayed in two networks created by the IPA Path Designer.

Confidence level was set to 'Experimentally observed' for all IPA procedures, which enables literature data-based analysis but excludes unproven predictions.

4.6. Data Availability

All datasets generated during the current study are available from the corresponding author upon reasonable request.

We have submitted all relevant data of our experiments to the EV-TRACK [68] knowledgebase EV-TRACK ID: EV200080.

5. Conclusions

Our study aimed to detect the characteristic protein fingerprint of the most common CNS tumors. Intending to amplify the signal that brain tumors release into the circulation, in addition to the whole serum's, the protein content of the small extracellular vesicles isolated from the serum was also examined.

Comparative proteomic analysis suggests that sEVs may be more suitable for investigating tumor related molecular patterns, because these molecules are present in higher concentrations in sEV samples compared to whole serum samples and have less 'noise' that may bias the analytical findings. In silico analyses revealed that the biological background of the sEV-based characteristic protein profile of the samples is more specifically associated with the tumor types compared with the whole serum based protein profile. Samples enriched in sEVs can offer an amplified source of relevant information, representing not only the specific tumor tissue but also the associated immune responses.

These findings revealed that circulating small-sized extracellular vesicles were more suitable for separating different patient groups. The number of proteins applied for monitoring cannot be reduced to a few individual molecules, instead, a specific protein panel is required for perfect differentiation. To the best of our knowledge, we are the first group to quantitatively compare the proteome of serum derived small extracellular vesicles with that of the original whole serum samples.

In conclusion, our findings support that extracellular vesicles have a greater potential for monitoring CNS tumors, compared to whole serum samples. Considering that analyzing sEVs can be performed easily, incorporating our method into clinical practice would be of great benefit.

Supplementary Materials: Supplementary materials can be found at http://www.mdpi.com/1422-0067/21/15/5359/s1. Figure S1: Western blot analyses of classical EV markers, Figure S2: Intragroup Coefficients of variation (CV) distributions, Figure S3: PCA dotplot constructed after statistical selection based on the means of intensity ratio; Table S1: 311 membered protein table of DIA mode constructed spectral library; Table S2: Sample correlation matrix; Table S3: List of the selected proteins.

Author Contributions: Conceptualization, K.B.; methodology, G.D. and K.B.; validation, G.D., B.B. and A.J.; formal analysis G.D., M.B., Z.S., M.H., M.S.; investigation, G.D., M.B. and E.G.-S.; resources, A.K., P.H., T.B. and K.B.; writing—original draft preparation, G.D., M.B., Z.S. and M.H.; writing—review and editing, G.D. and K.B.; visualization, G.D, M.B., Z.S. and M.H.; supervision, A.K. and K.B.; project administration, G.D. and K.B.; funding acquisition, K.B. All authors have read and agreed to publish the final version of the manuscript.

Funding: This study was founded by the following research grants: GINOP-2.3.2-15-2016-00015 (K.B.); GINOP-2.2.1-15-2017-00052 (K.B.), 2017-1.2.1-NKP-2017-00002 "National Brain Research Program NAP 2.0" (A.K.), UNKP-19-4-SZTE-63 (K.B.), Janos Bolyai Research Scholarship of the Hungarian Academic of Sciences (K.B.).

Acknowledgments: The authors thank Lilla Pinter for her technical assistance and Zsolt Szegletes for taking the AFM images. The authors thank Dora Bokor, PharmD, for proofreading the manuscript.

Conflicts of Interest: The authors declare no conflict of interest. The funders had no role in the design of the study; in the collection, analyses, or interpretation of data; in the writing of the manuscript, or in the decision to publish the results.

Abbreviations

AFM	Atomic force microscopy
BBB	Blood brain barrier
BM	Brain metastasis originating from non-small-cell lung cancer
CNS	Central nervous system
CTRL	Controls – lumbar disc hernia patients
DIA	Data independent acquisition
EVs	Extracellular Vesicles
GBM	Primary glioblastoma multiforme
IPA	Ingenuity Pathway Analysis
LC-MS	Liquid chromatography - mass spectrometry
M	Meningioma
NTA	Nanoparticle tracking analysis
PCA	Principal component analysis
ROC	Receiver operating characteristic
sEVs	small extracellular vesicles

Appendix A. Detailed Description of the Statistical Analyses.

The collected data about the whole serum and extracellular vesicles were reduced and analyzed using statistical methods. Pearson's correlation analysis was used to investigate the outlier samples [57]. Contaminating proteins (cytokeratins) and proteins with missing values were excluded from the proteomic data [58]. Data were log-transformed to reduce skewness and increase linearity [59].

Cohen's d effect size was calculated to measure the difference between the protein intensity mean, outcomes in two different groups. The formula of the Cohen's d effect size

$$d = \frac{|\overline{X}_1 - \overline{X}_2|}{\sqrt{\frac{(n_1-1)SD_1^2 + (n_2-1)SD_2^2}{n_1+n_2-2}}}$$

where X is the mean protein intensity in a given group, SD is standard deviation and n is sample size [60]. In this study we say at least 2 effect size is necessary. It indicates that the mean of group 1 is at the 97.7 percentile of group 2, and the nonoverlapping area of the two distributions at least is 81.1% [61].

Pairwise ROC analysis allowed us to find those proteins which can separate at least one group to the others [62]. The ROC analysis use the true positive rate (sensitivity) and the true negative rate (specificity) at various threshold settings. Plotting the sensitivity against the 1-specificity we get the ROC curve, under the area under this curve measure the separability of the given variable (protein). AUC = 0.5 represents an unsuitable variable to the separate two groups. If AUC = 1, the separation using the actual variable is error-free. In our study the calculated AUC (area under the curve) values are accepted if it equals to 1.

In order to transform several (potentially) correlated proteins into a (smaller) number of uncorrelated variables, and visualize the dataset, principal component analysis (PCA) with k-means clustering was performed. The goal of PCA is to reduce a large number of correlated variables with a set of uncorrelated principal components. These components can be thought of as linear combinations of the original variables that are optimally weighted and derived from the correlation matrix of the data [63].

K-means clustering was performed on the obtained PCA score plots by Hartigan-Wong algorithm [64,65]. Optimal numbers of clusters were determined with Silhouette method and these recommended values were used for clustering [66].

Homogeneity and completeness scores of the clusters were calculated to measure the performance of k-means clustering Cluster homogeneity and completeness mean that each cluster contains only samples from the same group, and all samples of a given group are assigned to the same cluster. Both scores are bounded below by 0 and above by 1. A score of 1 indicates the perfect homogeneity or completeness. [67].

Two-tailed Welch's t-test was performed to identify significantly enriched or depleted proteins in sEV samples.

The statistical analyses were performed using R statistical program (version 3.6.3 with pROC, FactoMineR, factoextra and ggplot2 packages), Python programming language (version 3.8) and Perseus (MaxQuant). Values of $p < 0.05$ were considered significant. GraphPad Prism 8 was used for further data visualization.

References

1. World Health Organization. *WHO Guidelines for the Pharmacological and Radiotherapeutic Management of Cancer Pain in Adults and Adolescents*; World Health Organization, 2018; License: CC BY-NC-SA 3.0 IGO. Available online: https://apps.who.int/iris/handle/10665/279700 (accessed on 1 June 2020).
2. World Health Organization. *Guide to Cancer Early Diagnosis*; World Health Organization, 2017; License: CC BY-NC-SA 3.0 IGO. Available online: https://apps.who.int/iris/handle/10665/254500 (accessed on 1 June 2020).
3. Garden, G.A.; Campbell, B.M. Glial biomarkers in human central nervous system disease. *Glia* **2016**, *64*, 1755–1771. [CrossRef] [PubMed]
4. Staedtke, V.; Dzaye, O.; Holdhoff, M. Actionable molecular biomarkers in primary brain tumors. *Trends Cancer* **2016**, *2*, 338–349. [CrossRef] [PubMed]
5. Good, D.M.; Thongboonkerd, V.; Novak, J.; Bascands, J.L.; Schanstra, J.P.; Coon, J.J.; Dominiczak, A.; Mischak, H. Body fluid proteomics for biomarker discovery: Lessons from the past hold the key to success in the future. *J. Proteome Res.* **2007**, *6*, 4549–4555. [CrossRef] [PubMed]
6. Best, M.G.; Sol, N.; Zijl, S.; Reijneveld, J.C.; Wesseling, P.; Wurdinger, T. Liquid biopsies in patients with diffuse glioma. *Acta Neuropathol.* **2015**, *129*, 849–865. [CrossRef] [PubMed]
7. Gerber, D.E.; Grossman, S.A.; Zeltzman, M.; Parisi, M.A.; Kleinberg, L. The impact of thrombocytopenia from temozolomide and radiation in newly diagnosed adults with high-grade gliomas. *Neuro Oncol.* **2007**, *9*, 47–52. [CrossRef]
8. Cagney, D.N.; Sul, J.; Huang, R.Y.; Ligon, K.L.; Wen, P.Y.; Alexander, B.M. The FDA NIH Biomarkers, EndpointS and other Tools (BEST) resource in neuro-oncology. *Neuro Oncol.* **2018**, *20*, 1162–1172. [CrossRef]
9. Sheridan, C. Exosome cancer diagnostic reaches market. *Nat. Biotechnol.* **2016**, *34*, 359–360. [CrossRef]
10. Colombo, M.; Raposo, G.; Théry, C. Biogenesis, secretion and intercellular interactions of exosomes and other extracellular vesicles. *Annu. Rev. Cell Dev. Biol* **2014**, *30*, 255–289. [CrossRef] [PubMed]
11. Nogués, L.; Benito-Martin, A.; Hergueta-Redondo, M.; Peinado, H. The influence of tumour-derived extracellular vesicles on local and distal metastatic dissemination. *Mol. Asp. Med.* **2018**, *60*, 15–26. [CrossRef]
12. Hoshino, A.; Costa-Silva, B.; Shen, T.L.; Rodrigues, G.; Hashimoto, A.; Tesic Mark, M.; Molina, H.; Kohsaka, S.; Di Giannatale, A.; Ceder, S.; et al. Tumour exosome integrins determine organotropic metastasis. *Nature* **2015**, *527*, 329–335. [CrossRef] [PubMed]
13. Costa-Silva, B.; Aiello, N.M.; Ocean, A.J.; Singh, S.; Zhang, H.; Thakur, B.K.; Becker, A.; Hoshino, A.; Mark, M.T.; Molina, H.; et al. Pancreatic cancer exosomes initiate pre-metastatic niche formation in the liver. *Nat. Cell Biol.* **2015**, *17*, 816–826. [CrossRef] [PubMed]
14. Liu, Y.; Gu, Y.; Han, Y.; Zhang, Q.; Jiang, Z.; Zhang, X.; Huang, B.; Xu, X.; Zheng, J.; Cao, X. Tumor Exosomal RNAs Promote Lung Pre-metastatic Niche Formation by Activating Alveolar Epithelial TLR3 to Recruit Neutrophils. *Cancer Cell* **2016**, *30*, 243–256. [CrossRef] [PubMed]
15. Zeng, Z.; Li, Y.; Pan, Y.; Lan, X.; Song, F.; Sun, J.; Zhou, K.; Liu, X.; Ren, X.; Wang, F.; et al. Cancer-derived exosomal miR-25-3p promotes pre-metastatic niche formation by inducing vascular permeability and angiogenesis. *Nat. Commun.* **2018**, *9*, 5395. [CrossRef] [PubMed]
16. Feng, W.; Dean, D.C.; Hornicek, F.J.; Shi, H.; Duan, Z. Exosomes promote pre-metastatic niche formation in ovarian cancer. *Mol. Cancer* **2019**, *18*, 124. [CrossRef] [PubMed]
17. Chen, G.; Huang, A.C.; Zhang, W.; Zhang, G.; Wu, M.; Xu, W.; Yu, Z.; Yang, J.; Wang, B.; Sun, H.; et al. Exosomal PD-L1 contributes to immunosuppression and is associated with anti-PD-1 response. *Nature* **2018**, *560*, 382–386. [CrossRef] [PubMed]

18. Scavo, M.P.; Depalo, N.; Tutino, V.; De Nunzio, V.; Ingrosso, C.; Rizzi, F.; Notarnicola, M.; Curri, M.L.; Giannelli, G. Exosomes for Diagnosis and Therapy in Gastrointestinal Cancers. *Int. J. Mol. Sci.* **2020**, *21*, 367. [CrossRef] [PubMed]
19. Basu, B.; Ghosh, M.K. Extracellular Vesicles in Glioma: From Diagnosis to Therapy. *Bioessays* **2019**, *41*, e1800245. [CrossRef]
20. Kosaka, N.; Kogure, A.; Yamamoto, T.; Urabe, F.; Usuba, W.; Prieto-Vila, M.; Ochiya, T. Exploiting the message from cancer: The diagnostic value of extracellular vesicles for clinical applications. *Exp. Mol. Med.* **2019**, *51*, 31. [CrossRef]
21. Möhrmann, L.; Huang, H.J.; Hong, D.S.; Tsimberidou, A.M.; Fu, S.; Piha-Paul, S.A.; Subbiah, V.; Karp, D.D.; Naing, A.; Krug, A. Liquid biopsies using plasma exosomal nucleic acids and plasma cell-free DNA compared with clinical outcomes of patients with advanced cancers. *Clin. Cancer Res.* **2018**, *24*, 181–188. [CrossRef]
22. Melo, S.A.; Luecke, L.B.; Kahlert, C.; Fernandez, A.F.; Gammon, S.T.; Kaye, J.; LeBleu, V.S.; Mittendorf, E.A.; Weitz, J.; Rahbari, N.; et al. Glypican-1 identifies cancer exosomes and detects early pancreatic cancer. *Nature* **2015**, *523*, 177–182. [CrossRef]
23. Choy, C.; Jandial, R. Breast Cancer Exosomes Breach the Blood-Brain Barrier. *Neurosurgery* **2016**, *78*, N10-1. [CrossRef] [PubMed]
24. García-Romero, N.; Carrión-Navarro, J.; Esteban-Rubio, S.; Lázaro-Ibáñez, E.; Peris-Celda, M.; Alonso, M.M.; Guzmán-De-Villoria, J.; Fernández-Carballal, C.; de Mendivil, A.O.; García-Duque, S.; et al. DNA sequences within glioma-derived extracellular vesicles can cross the intact blood-brain barrier and be detected in peripheral blood of patients. *Oncotarget* **2017**, *8*, 1416–1428. [CrossRef] [PubMed]
25. Gollapalli, K.; Ray, S.; Srivastava, R.; Renu, D.; Singh, P.; Dhali, S.; Bajpai Dikshit, J.; Srikanth, R.; Moiyadi, A.; Srivastava, S. Investigation of serum proteome alterations in human glioblastoma multiforme. *Proteomics* **2012**, *12*, 2378–2390. [CrossRef] [PubMed]
26. Gállego Pérez-Larraya, J.; Paris, S.; Idbaih, A.; Dehais, C.; Laigle-Donadey, F.; Navarro, S.; Capelle, L.; Mokhtari, K.; Marie, Y.; Sanson, M.; et al. Diagnostic and prognostic value of preoperative combined GFAP, IGFBP-2 and YKL-40 plasma levels in patients with glioblastoma. *Cancer* **2014**, *120*, 3972–3980. [CrossRef] [PubMed]
27. Figueroa, J.M.; Carter, B.S. Detection of glioblastoma in biofluids. *J. Neurosurg.* **2018**, *129*, 334–340. [CrossRef] [PubMed]
28. Ostrom, Q.T.; Gittleman, H.; Truitt, G.; Boscia, A.; Kruchko, C.; Barnholtz-Sloan, J.S. CBTRUS Statistical Report: Primary Brain and Other Central Nervous System Tumors Diagnosed in the United States in 2011-2015. *Neuro Oncol.* **2018**, *20*, iv1–iv86. [CrossRef]
29. Fox, B.D.; Cheung, V.J.; Patel, A.J.; Suki, D.; Rao, G. Epidemiology of Metastatic Brain Tumors. *Neurosurg. Clin. N. Am.* **2011**, *22*, 1–6. [CrossRef]
30. Théry, C.; Witwer, K.W.; Aikawa, E.; Alcaraz, M.J.; Anderson, J.D.; Andriantsitohaina, R.; Antoniou, A.; Arab, T.; Archer, F.; Atkin-Smith, G.K.; et al. Minimal information for studies of extracellular vesicles 2018 (MISEV2018): A position statement of the International Society for Extracellular Vesicles and update of the MISEV2014 guidelines. *J. Extracell. Vesicles* **2018**, *7*, 1535750. [CrossRef]
31. de Menezes-Neto, A.; Sáez, M.J.; Lozano-Ramos, I.; Segui-Barber, J.; Martin-Jaular, L.; Ullate, J.M.; Fernandez-Becerra, C.; Borrás, F.E.; Del Portillo, H.A. Size-exclusion chromatography as a stand-alone methodology identifies novel markers in mass spectrometry analyses of plasma-derived vesicles from healthy individuals. *J. Extracell. Vesicles* **2015**, *4*, 27358. [CrossRef]
32. Weber, M.A.; Zoubaa, S.; Schlieter, M.; Jüttler, E.; Huttner, H.B.; Geletneky, K.; Ittrich, C.; Lichy, M.P.; Kroll, A.; Debus, J.; et al. Essig Diagnostic performance of spectroscopic and perfusion MRI for distinction of brain tumors. *Neurology* **2006**, *66*, 1899–1906. [CrossRef]
33. Shankar, G.M.; Balaj, L.; Stott, S.L.; Nahed, B.; Carter, B.S. Liquid biopsy for brain tumors. *Expert Rev. Mol. Diagn.* **2017**, *17*, 943–947. [CrossRef] [PubMed]
34. Marrugo-Ramírez, J.; Mir, M.; Samitier, J. Blood-Based Cancer Biomarkers in Liquid Biopsy: A Promising Non-Invasive Alternative to Tissue Biopsy. *Int. J. Mol. Sci.* **2018**, *21*, 2877. [CrossRef] [PubMed]
35. Miyauchi, E.; Furuta, T.; Ohtsuki, S.; Tachikawa, M.; Uchida, Y.; Sabit, H.; Obuchi, W.; Baba, T.; Watanabe, M.; Terasaki, T.; et al. Identification of blood biomarkers in glioblastoma by SWATH mass spectrometry and quantitative targeted absolute proteomics. *PLoS ONE* **2018**, *13*, e0193799. [CrossRef] [PubMed]

36. Rhie, S.K.; Perez, A.A.; Lay, F.D.; Schreiner, S.; Shi, J.; Polin, J.; Farnham, P.J. A high-resolution 3D epigenomic map reveals insights into the creation of the prostate cancer transcriptome. *Nat. Commun.* **2019**, *10*, 4154. [CrossRef] [PubMed]
37. Anderson, K.S.; LaBaer, J. The sentinel within: Exploiting the immune system for cancer biomarkers. *J. Proteome Res.* **2005**, *4*, 1123–1133. [CrossRef] [PubMed]
38. Wen, C.; Seeger, R.C.; Fabbri, M.; Wang, L.; Wayne, A.S.; Jong, A.Y. Biological roles and potential applications of immune cell-derived extracellular vesicles. *J. Extracell. Vesicles* **2017**, *6*, 1400370. [CrossRef] [PubMed]
39. Veerman, R.E.; Güçlüler Akpinar, G.; Eldh, M.; Gabrielsson, S. Immune Cell-Derived Extracellular Vesicles –Functions and Therapeutic Applications. *Trends Mol. Med.* **2019**, *25*, 382–394. [CrossRef]
40. Gercel-Taylor, C.; Atay, S.; Tullis, R.H.; Kesimer, M.; Taylor, D.D. Nanoparticle analysis of circulating cell-derived vesicles in ovarian cancer patients. *Anal. Biochem.* **2012**, *428*, 44–53. [CrossRef]
41. Lázaro-Ibáñez, E.; Sanz-Garcia, A.; Visakorpi, T.; Escobedo-Lucea, C.; Siljander, P.; Ayuso-Sacido, A.; Yliperttula, M. Different gDNA content in the subpopulations of prostate cancer extracellular vesicles: Apoptotic bodies, microvesicles and exosomes. *Prostate* **2014**, *74*, 1379–1390. [CrossRef]
42. König, L.; Kasimir-Bauer, S.; Bittner, A.K.; Hoffmann, O.; Wagner, B.; Santos Manvailer, L.F.; Kimmig, R.; Horn, P.A.; Rebmann, V. Elevated levels of extracellular vesicles are associated with therapy failure and disease progression in breast cancer patients undergoing neoadjuvant chemotherapy. *Oncoimmunology* **2017**, *27*, e1376153. [CrossRef]
43. Ji, Q.; Ji, Y.; Peng, J.; Zhou, X.; Chen, X.; Zhao, H.; Xu, T.; Chen, L.; Xu, Y. Increased Brain-Specific MiR-9 and MiR-124 in the Serum Exosomes of Acute Ischemic Stroke Patients. *PLoS ONE* **2016**, *11*, e0163645. [CrossRef] [PubMed]
44. Galazka, G.; Mycko, M.P.; Selmaj, I.; Raine, C.S.; Selmaj, K.W. Multiple sclerosis: Serum-derived exosomes express myelin proteins. *Mult. Scler.* **2018**, *24*, 449–458. [CrossRef] [PubMed]
45. Liu, M.-L.; Werth, V.P.; Williams, K.J. Blood plasma versus serum: Which is right for sampling circulating membrane microvesicles in human subjects? *Ann. Rheum. Dis.* **2020**, *79*, e73. [CrossRef] [PubMed]
46. Smolarz, M.; Pietrowska, M.; Matysiak, N.; Mielańczyk, Ł.; Widłak, P. Proteome Profiling of Exosomes Purified from a Small Amount of Human Serum: The Problem of Co-Purified Serum Components. *Proteomes* **2019**, *7*, 18. [CrossRef]
47. Sódar, B.W.; Kittel, Á.; Pálóczi, K.; Vukman, K.V.; Osteikoetxea, X.; Szabó-Taylor, K.; Németh, A.; Sperlágh, B.; Baranyai, T.; Giricz, Z.; et al. Low-density lipoprotein mimics blood plasma-derived exosomes and microvesicles during isolation and detection. *Sci. Rep.* **2016**, *6*, 24316. [CrossRef] [PubMed]
48. Filipe, V.; Hawe, A.; Jiskoot, W. Critical evaluation of Nanoparticle Tracking Analysis (NTA) by NanoSight for the measurement of nanoparticles and protein aggregates. *Pharm. Res.* **2010**, *27*, 796–810. [CrossRef] [PubMed]
49. Osti, D.; Del Bene, M.; Rappa, G.; Santos, M.; Matafora, V.; Richichi, C.; Faletti, S.; Beznoussenko, G.V.; Mironov, A.; Bachi, A.; et al. Clinical Significance of Extracellular Vesicles in Plasma from Glioblastoma Patients. *Clin. Cancer Res.* **2019**, *25*, 266–276. [CrossRef]
50. Karimi, N.; Cvjetkovic, A.; Jang, S.C.; Crescitelli, R.; Hosseinpour Feizi, M.A.; Nieuwland, R.; Lötvall, J.; Lässer, C. Detailed analysis of the plasma extracellular vesicle proteome after separation from lipoproteins. *Cell Mol. Life Sci.* **2018**, *75*, 2873–2886. [CrossRef]
51. Xu, R.; Greening, D.W.; Zhu, H.J.; Takahashi, N.; Simpson, R.J. Extracellular vesicle isolation and characterization: Toward clinical application. *J. Clin. Investig.* **2016**, *126*, 1152–1162. [CrossRef]
52. Harmati, M.; Tarnai, Z.; Decsi, G.; Kormondi, S.; Szegletes, Z.; Janovak, L.; Dekany, I.; Saydam, O.; Gyukity-Sebestyen, E.; Dobra, G.; et al. Stressors alter intercellular communication and exosome profile of nasopharyngeal carcinoma cells. *J. Oral Pathol. Med.* **2017**, *46*, 259–266. [CrossRef]
53. Parsons, M.E.M.; McParland, D.; Szklanna, P.B.; Guang, M.H.Z.; O'Connell, K.; O'Connor, H.D.; McGuigan, C.; Ní Áinle, F.; McCann, A.; Maguire, P.B. A Protocol for Improved Precision and Increased Confidence in Nanoparticle Tracking Analysis Concentration Measurements between 50 and 120 nm in Biological Fluids. *Front. Cardiovasc. Med.* **2017**, *4*, 68. [CrossRef] [PubMed]
54. Searle, B.C.; Pino, L.K.; Egertson, J.D.; Ting, Y.S.; Lawrence, R.T.; MacLean, B.X.; Villén, J.; MacCoss, M.J. Chromatogram libraries improve peptide detection and quantification by data independent acquisition mass spectrometry. *Nat. Commun.* **2018**, *9*, 5128. [CrossRef] [PubMed]

55. Chambers, M.; Maclean, B.; Burke, R.; Amodei, D.; Ruderman, D.L.; Neumann, S.; Gatto, L.; Fischer, B.; Pratt, B.; Egertson, J.; et al. A cross-platform toolkit for mass spectrometry and proteomics. *Nat. Biotechnol.* **2012**, *30*, 918–920. [CrossRef] [PubMed]
56. Rosenberger, G.; Koh, C.C.; Guo, T.; Röst, H.L.; Kouvonen, P.; Collins, B.C.; Heusel, M.; Liu, Y.; Caron, E.; Vichalkovski, A.; et al. A repository of assays to quantify 10,000 human proteins by SWATH-MS. *Sci. Data* **2014**, *1*, 140031. [CrossRef] [PubMed]
57. Metz, T.O.; Qian, W.J.; Jacobs, J.M.; Gritsenko, M.A.; Moore, R.J.; Polpitiya, A.D.; Monroe, M.E.; Camp, D.G., 2nd; Mueller, P.W.; Smith, R.D. Application of proteomics in the discovery of candidate protein biomarkers in a diabetes autoantibody standardization program sample subset. *J. Proteome Res.* **2008**, *7*, 698–707. [CrossRef] [PubMed]
58. Hodge, K.; Have, S.T.; Hutton, L.; Lamond, A.I. Cleaning up the masses: Exclusion lists to reduce contamination with HPLC-MS/MS. *J. Proteom.* **2013**, *88*, 92–103. [CrossRef] [PubMed]
59. Curran-Everett, D. Explorations in statistics: The log transformation. *Adv. Physiol. Educ.* **2018**, *42*, 343–347. [CrossRef]
60. Lakens, D. Calculating and reporting effect sizes to facilitate cumulative science: A practical primer for t-tests and ANOVAs. *Front. Psychol.* **2013**, *4*, 863. [CrossRef]
61. Cohen, J. *Statistical Power Analysis for the Behavioral Sciences*, 2nd ed.; Routledge: New York, NY, USA, 1988. [CrossRef]
62. Fawcett, T. An introduction to ROC analysis. *Pattern Recognit. Lett.* **2006**, *27*, 861–874. [CrossRef]
63. Husson, F.; Le, S.; Pagès, J. *Exploratory Multivariate Analysis by Example Using R*, 2nd ed.; Chapman and Hall/CRC: New York, NY, USA, 2017. [CrossRef]
64. Hartigan, J.A.; Wong, M.A. Algorithm AS 136: A K-Means Clustering Algorithm. *J. Appl. Stat.* **1979**, *28*, 100. [CrossRef]
65. Ding, C.; He, X. K-means clustering via principal component analysis. In Proceedings of the Twenty-First International Conference on Machine Learning, Banff, AB, Canada, 4–8 July 2004; Association for Computing Machinery: New York, NY, USA, 2004. [CrossRef]
66. Rousseeuw, P.J. Silhouettes: A graphical aid to the interpretation and validation of cluster analysis. *J. Comput. Appl. Math.* **1987**, *20*, 53–65. [CrossRef]
67. Pedregosa, F.; Varoquaux, G.; Gramfort, A.; Michel, V.; Thirion, B.; Grisel, O.; Blondel, M.; Prettenhofer, P.; Weiss, R.; Dubourg, V.; et al. Scikit-learn: Machine Learning in Python. *J. Mach. Learn. Res.* **2012**, *12*, 2825–2830.
68. Van Deun, J.; Mestdagh, P.; Agostinis, P.; Akay, Ö.; Anand, S.; Anckaert, J.; Martinez, Z.A.; Baetens, T.; Beghein, E.; Bertier, L.; et al. EV-TRACK: Transparent reporting and centralizing knowledge in extracellular vesicle research. *Nat. Methods* **2017**, *14*, 228–232. [CrossRef] [PubMed]

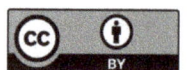

© 2020 by the authors. Licensee MDPI, Basel, Switzerland. This article is an open access article distributed under the terms and conditions of the Creative Commons Attribution (CC BY) license (http://creativecommons.org/licenses/by/4.0/).

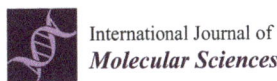

Article

Analysis of Serum miRNA in Glioblastoma Patients: CD44-Based Enrichment of Extracellular Vesicles Enhances Specificity for the Prognostic Signature

Theophilos Tzaridis [1,2,3,†], Katrin S Reiners [1,*,†], Johannes Weller [2], Daniel Bachurski [4], Niklas Schäfer [2], Christina Schaub [2], Michael Hallek [4], Björn Scheffler [5], Martin Glas [6], Ulrich Herrlinger [2], Stefan Wild [7], Christoph Coch [1,7,†] and Gunther Hartmann [1,†]

1. Institute of Clinical Chemistry and Clinical Pharmacology, University of Bonn, 53127 Bonn, Germany; theophilos.tzaridis@ukbonn.de (T.T.); ccoch@uni-bonn.de (C.C.); Gunther.Hartmann@uni-bonn.de (G.H.)
2. Division of Clinical Neurooncology, Department of Neurology, Center of Integrated Oncology Aachen-Bonn-Cologne-Düsseldorf, Partner Site Bonn, University Hospital Bonn, 53127 Bonn, Germany; Johannes.weller@ukbonn.de (J.W.); Niklas.Schaefer@ukbonn.de (N.S.); Christina.Schaub@ukbonn.de (C.S.); Ulrich.Herrlinger@ukbonn.de (U.H.)
3. Tumor Initiation & Maintenance Program, NCI-Designated Cancer Center, Sanford Burnham Prebys Medical Discovery Institute, La Jolla, CA 92037, USA
4. Department I of Internal Medicine, Center for Integrated Oncology Aachen-Bonn-Cologne-Düsseldorf, Partner Site Cologne, CECAD Center of Excellence on "Cellular Stress Responses in Aging-Associated Diseases", Center for Molecular Medicine Cologne, University of Cologne, 50937 Cologne, Germany; Daniel.Bachurski@uk-koeln.de (D.B.); Michael.hallek@uk-koeln.de (M.H.)
5. DKFZ-Division Translational Neurooncology at the West German Cancer Center (WTZ), German Cancer Consortium (DKTK), DKFZ Heidelberg & Partner Site Univ Hospital Essen, 45147 Essen, Germany; b.scheffler@dkfz-heidelberg.de
6. Division of Clinical Neurooncology, Department of Neurology and West German Cancer Center (WTZ), German Cancer Consortium, University Hospital Essen, 45147 Essen, Germany; martin.glas@uk-essen.de
7. Miltenyi Biotec & Biomedicine GmbH, 51429 Bergisch Gladbach, Germany; StefanW@Miltenyi.com
* Correspondence: kreiners@uni-bonn.de
† These authors contributed equally to this work.

Received: 18 August 2020; Accepted: 28 September 2020; Published: 29 September 2020

Abstract: Glioblastoma is a devastating disease, for which biomarkers allowing a prediction of prognosis are urgently needed. microRNAs have been described as potentially valuable biomarkers in cancer. Here, we studied a panel of microRNAs in extracellular vesicles (EVs) from the serum of glioblastoma patients and evaluated their correlation with the prognosis of these patients. The levels of 15 microRNAs in EVs that were separated by size-exclusion chromatography were studied by quantitative real-time PCR, followed by CD44 immunoprecipitation (SEC + CD44), and compared with those from the total serum of glioblastoma patients ($n = 55$) and healthy volunteers ($n = 10$). Compared to total serum, we found evidence for the enrichment of miR-21-3p and miR-106a-5p and, conversely, lower levels of miR-15b-3p, in SEC + CD44 EVs. miR-15b-3p and miR-21-3p were upregulated in glioblastoma patients compared to healthy subjects. A significant correlation with survival of the patients was found for levels of miR-15b-3p in total serum and miR-15b-3p, miR-21-3p, miR-106a-5p, and miR-328-3p in SEC + CD44 EVs. Combining miR-15b-3p in serum or miR-106a-5p in SEC + CD44 EVs with any one of the other three microRNAs in SEC + CD44 EVs allowed for a prognostic stratification of glioblastoma patients. We have thus identified four microRNAs in glioblastoma patients whose levels, in combination, can predict the prognosis for these patients.

Keywords: biomarkers; glioblastoma; extracellular vesicles; microRNA; immunoprecipitation; CD44

1. Introduction

Glioblastomas lacking isocitrate-dehydrogenase (*IDH*) 1 or 2 mutations (IDH-wildtype glioblastomas) are the most aggressive primary brain tumors, mainly occurring in adults, and exhibit a dismal prognosis [1]. First-line treatment includes surgical resection if feasible, followed by radiochemotherapy with temozolomide (TMZ) [2]. Despite a large number of studies on biomarkers for glioblastoma, only one has regularly been applied for prognostic stratification in routine clinical use: Promoter methylation of the *O-6-methylguanine-DNA methyltransferase* (*MGMT*) gene in tumor tissue. Promoter methylation of the *MGMT* gene leads to impaired DNA-repair mechanisms and not only correlates with superior survival, but also leads to a better response to TMZ treatment [3]. Based on this observation, novel data show an enhanced response of combination therapy with TMZ and lomustine (CCNU) for patients with tumors harboring *MGMT*-promoter methylation, and this intensified treatment does not compromise the patients' quality-of-life [4,5]. Due to the limited number of treatment options for recurrent disease [6], biomarkers capable of stratifying patients are crucial.

MicroRNAs (miRNAs) are non-coding single-stranded RNA molecules with a length of 21–25 nucleotides [7]. After initial processing in the nucleus by RNA polymerases II and III [8], the precursor miRNA (pre-miRNA) is transported into the cytoplasm and then processed by the cytoplasmic RNase III protein Dicer, thereby creating mature miRNA [7–9]. The purpose of the mature microRNAs is complex, and not yet fully understood, but usually involves the regulation (mostly repression) of gene expression by binding to either the 3′- or the 5′-untranslated region (UTR) of mRNAs [8,10,11]. microRNAs are loaded into an Argonaute protein (Ago) as part of the RNA-induced silencing complex (RISC) and are thereby protected from cytoplasmic nucleases [7].

The role of microRNAs in glioblastoma has already been extensively examined. They have been shown to be involved in invasiveness and proliferation (e.g., hsa-miR-21 or hsa-miR-15b) [12], to induce angiogenesis [13], and to modulate the innate immune system by polarizing it towards M2 macrophages and thereby inducing an immunosuppressive environment (hsa-miR-21 and hsa-miR-451) [13]. Interestingly, many of these functions require the trafficking of miRNA between cells, which occurs through either gap junctions or the exchange of extracellular vesicles (EVs) [13,14]. While some miRNAs are mainly found in miRNA-binding protein complexes, such as Ago-2, or high-density lipoproteins (HDL), other types of miRNAs are uniquely packaged into EVs [15], which makes them a potentially interesting biomarker in tumor diagnostics [16].

EVs are small particles formed by either direct budding of the plasma membrane (typically "large EVs") or by the fusion of a multivesicular endosome with the plasma membrane (typically "small EVs"), thus releasing the EVs into the extracellular space [17]. In a recent study, we identified relevant protein markers that are highly elevated in EVs from the serum of patients with glioblastoma, compared to those from healthy volunteers (HV), and these proteins are capable of detecting tumor progression [18]. Many studies have identified microRNAs in the biofluids (e.g., cerebrospinal fluid (CSF), serum and plasma) of patients with glioblastoma, which can be EV-independent [19] or contained in EVs [20]. While some reports have demonstrated the upregulation of microRNAs in patients with high-grade glioma compared to low-grade glioma [21], no report has thus far shown the potential of microRNAs in biofluids to stratify patients into different prognostic groups at critical time-points during treatment. Moreover, it is unknown whether the detection of any relevant microRNAs in the serum of glioma patients can be enhanced through specifically capturing tumor-derived EVs.

In this study, we evaluated suitable methods for the separation of EVs that could enrich the potentially glioblastoma-relevant microRNAs within the samples. In addition, we tested whether these microRNAs could serve as biomarkers to determine patient prognosis when purified from serum EVs (EV microRNAs) or as microRNAs directly from total serum (total serum microRNAs).

2. Results

2.1. Enrichment of Disease-Relevant microRNAs in Serum EV Samples Using Size-Exclusion Chromatography (SEC) Followed by CD44-Based Immunoprecipitation

Our study included 55 patients in total, 26 (47.3%) of which were treated within the multicenter Phase III CeTeG/NOA-09 trial [4] and 29 (52.7%) in the Division of Clinical Neurooncology of the University Hospital of Bonn. The median age at diagnosis was 56 years (range: 19–77 years) and the median overall survival was 2.35 years (range: 0.39–5.17 years). The vast majority of patients (53/55, i.e., 96.4%) had *IDH*-wildtype tumors and *MGMT* promoter methylation was observed in 33 (60%) cases (Table S1). Sampling was performed at the Q3 time point (i.e., the third quarter of the first year after diagnosis, 6–9 months after the initiation of primary radiotherapy and chemotherapy) for 54/55 patients and in the fifth month for one patient. Consistent with previous results [21], serum from glioblastoma patients showed a much higher concentration of small EVs (size range: 87–166 nm) compared to HV when they were isolated by using size-exclusion chromatography (SEC, Figure 1A). In order to specifically isolate relevant glioblastoma-associated EVs, we subsequently performed immunoprecipitation using CD44 (SEC + CD44), which we had previously identified in a screen of serum EV proteins as being important in tumor progression [18]. Using this technique, we were able to capture a distinct EV subpopulation, as shown in Figure 1. Immunodetection was used to determine the presence of EV marker proteins flotillin-1 and CD9. Calnexin, which is a protein associated with the endoplasmic reticulum, serum protein albumin and apolipoprotein-A1 were absent or strongly reduced after EV isolation via SEC + CD44 (Figure 1C). Transmission electron microscopy (TEM) analysis showed that the CD44-enriched fraction mainly contained EVs with a size and shape typical of small EVs (Figure 1B). The TEM images show that lipoprotein contamination present after SEC (Figure 1B, left lane) is diminished after additional immunoprecipitation with CD44 beads (Figure 1B, middle lane). To allow the quantification of SEC + CD44 EVs, they were effectively diluted from capture-beads (visible as small black dots in middle lane pictures), as shown in Figure 1B, in the right lane.

Based on extensive screening of the literature, we selected 15 microRNAs that have been described to be present and relevant in the serum and plasma of glioblastoma patients (Table S2). Out of these 15 pre-screened microRNAs, we identified eight that consistently had Ct values lower than 36 in our glioblastoma patients. To determine if these miRNAs are more abundant in CD44-enriched EVs (SEC + CD44 EVs) compared to miRNAs isolated from total serum, we studied the levels of these microRNAs in the serum of glioblastoma patients ($n = 55$) at the Q3 time point. In total, we detected an enrichment of five out of the eight microRNAs tested in SEC + CD44-purified EVs compared to total serum (miR-21-3p, miR-106a-5p, miR-155-5p, and let-7a-5p with significantly higher levels and miR-486-5p with a non-significant trend toward a higher level, Figure 2A–H). Two out of eight miRNAs showed significantly higher levels in total serum compared to the purified EVs (miR-15b-3p and miR-23a-3p, Figure 2), indicating that these miRNAs are not enriched in SEC + CD44 EVs.

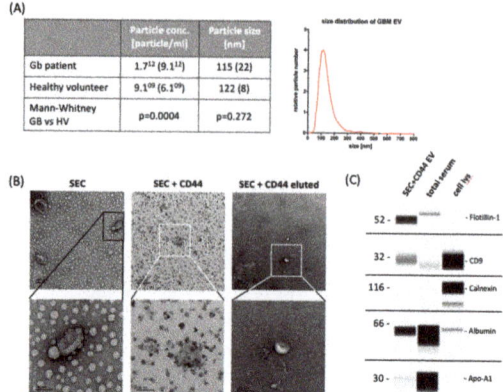

Figure 1. Yield and characteristics of serum-derived extracellular vesicles. (**A**) NTA of extracellular vesicles (EVs) isolated from 500 μL serum by size-exclusion chromatography (SEC) to determine the yield and particle size. The table states the mean particle concentration and mean modal size of 55 glioblastoma patients and 5 healthy volunteers (HV). Standard deviation is given in parentheses; histograms: exemplary size distribution of glioblastoma-EVs measured by NTA. (**B**) Transmission electron microscopy images showing the typical EV morphology. Scale bar represents, in all images, 200 nm in the upper row (30k × magnification) and 100 nm in the lower row (110k × magnification). Images in the left lane show EVs after SEC, middle lane images show CD44-captured SEC-EVs, and right lane images represent EVs that were diluted from CD44-beads. (**C**) Wes ProteinSimple immunodetection confirming the presence of the EV-markers flotillin-1 and CD9 and the absence of non-EV protein calnexin in SEC + CD44 EV preparations. Cell and total serum lysates were used as positive controls for the non-EV marker calnexin, apolipoprotein A1, and serum albumin, respectively. NTA = nanoparticle tracking analysis; cell lys = cell lysate of PBMCs (1:10) or glioblastoma cell line Gli36 (1:100); Apo-A1 = apolipoprotein A1.

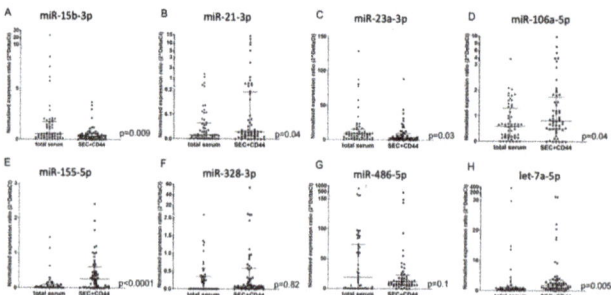

Figure 2. Comparison of microRNA detection in glioblastoma serum, depending on the source. (**A**) miR-15b-3p, (**B**) miR21-3p, (**C**) miR-23a-3p, (**D**) miR-106-5p, (**E**) miR-155-5p, (**F**) miR-328-3p, (**G**) miR-486-5p, (**H**) let-7a-5p. Depicted is the normalized expression ratio ($2^{\wedge}$deltaCt) of eight microRNAs (**A**–**H**) in total serum and in SEC + CD44-purified EVs from the serum of glioblastoma patients ($n = 55$). Expression levels were compared using a Wilcoxon rank sum test. Note that miR-15b-3p shows higher levels in total serum, as opposed to miR-21-3p and miR-106a-5p, which are upregulated in SEC + CD44 EVs. For miR-328-3p, no consistent up- or downregulation was observed between the two samples, which was partially because only 26/55 (47%) total serum samples were above the limit of detection. Bars depict the median value and the interquartile range.

When comparing SEC + CD44-purified EV microRNA from the serum of glioblastoma patients to HV, we saw significantly higher levels of miR-15b-3p, miR-21-3p, miR-155-5p, and let-7a-5p in glioblastoma patients ($p = 0.01$, $p = 0.001$, $p = 0.01$, and $p = 0.008$, respectively) and a non-significant trend for miR-23a-3p and miR-106a-5p ($p = 0.18$ and $p = 0.07$, respectively), while no significant difference was detected for miR-23a-3p, miR-328-3p, and miR-486-5p ($p = 0.45$ and $p = 0.48$ respectively, Figure 3A–H).

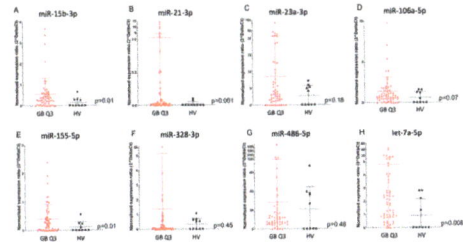

Figure 3. MicroRNA expression in SEC + CD44 EV. Normalized expression ratio (2^deltaCt) of eight microRNAs (**A–H**) in SEC + CD44 EV from glioblastoma patients ($n = 55$) versus HV ($n = 10$, average of two time points). (**A**) miR-15b-3p, (**B**) miR21-3p, (**C**) miR-23a-3p, (**D**) miR-106-5p, (**E**) miR-155-5p, (**F**) miR-328-3p, (**G**) miR-486-5p, (**H**) let-7a-5p. Expression levels were compared using the Mann–Whitney U test. Bars depict the median value and the interquartile range.

2.2. Four SEC+CD44-EV miRNAs and Total Serum miR-15b-3p Correlate with Survival in Glioblastoma Patients

To evaluate the prognostic potential of different microRNAs, we correlated the normalized expression ratio with the overall survival of glioblastoma patients ($n = 55$). miR-15b-3p, miR-21-3p, miR-106a-5p, and miR-328-3p in SEC + CD44 EVs showed a significant correlation with survival, with miR-15b-3p, miR-21-3p, and miR-328-3p exhibiting a negative correlation (high levels were associated with an inferior prognosis) and miR-106a-5p a positive correlation (high levels were associated with a better prognosis; Table 1A). While miR-15b-3p showed a weak correlation (Spearman r = −0.27), miR-21-3p, miR-106a-5p, and miR-328-3p showed intermediate correlation values (absolute Spearman r > 0.34). Interestingly, when considering total serum microRNAs, only miR-15b-3p correlated with inferior survival (Spearman r = 0.4) and miR-328-3p was not measurable in 29/55 (53%) patients (Table 1B). For all of the other microRNAs analyzed, no correlation with survival was found in either SEC + CD44 EVs or total serum (data not shown).

Interestingly, we found distinct differences of miR levels in SEC + CD44 EVs, depending on the MGMT promoter methylation status, with miR-15b-3p, miR-21-3p, and miR328-3p being enriched in MGMT-non-methylated and miR-106a-5p in MGMT-methylated patient samples (Figure S1). For total serum, we saw higher levels of miR-15b-3p in MGMT-non-methylated compared to MGMT-methylated patient samples (Figure S2). When only assessing the prognostic potential of the above-mentioned markers for MGMT-methylated patients, we observed a non-significant correlation with overall survival for miR-21-3p and miR-328-3p in SEC + CD44 EVs (data not shown).

The four microRNAs that were identified as putative prognostic markers were selected for dichotomous assessment based on the median of the normalized expression ratios and using Kaplan–Meier curves for data visualization. To define the subgroups, we calculated the median value of the normalized expression for each microRNA and split the patients into two groups, with one group including patients with expression values lower than the median and the other group with values equal to or higher than the median. In an analysis of single SEC + CD44 EV microRNAs, we saw a curve separation for all four miRNAs, which was less pronounced for miR-15b-3p and miR-328-3p (Figure 4A–D). Consistent with our correlation data, the subgroup of patients with levels of miR-106a-5p higher than the median had a clear survival benefit compared to those with lower levels, as opposed to miR-21-3p, where high levels of the miRNA defined a prognostically inferior group (Figure 4B,C).

Table 1. Correlation of the survival of 55 patients with microRNA levels from SEC + CD44 EV (**A**) or total serum (**B**) using the Spearman's rank correlation coefficient, r. Depicted are the Spearman r values showing either a positive or negative correlation, the p value, and the degree of significance (* $p < 0.05$, ** $p < 0.01$, *** $p < 0.001$, n.s. = not significant). For miR-328-3p in total serum, no correlation with survival was calculated because 53% of the values were non-measurable.

(A)				
SEC + CD44	miR15b-3p	miR-21-3p	miR-328-3p	miR-106-5p
Spearman R	−0.2746	−0.4372	−0.3407	0.3501
p (two-tailed)	0.043	0.00008	0.011	0.009
p value	*	***	*	**
(B)				
Total serum	miR15b-3p	miR-21-3p	miR-328-3p	miR-106-5p
Spearman R	−0.3947	0.0225	-	0.06753
p (two-tailed)	0.003	0.78	-	0.62
p value	**	n.s.	-	n.s.

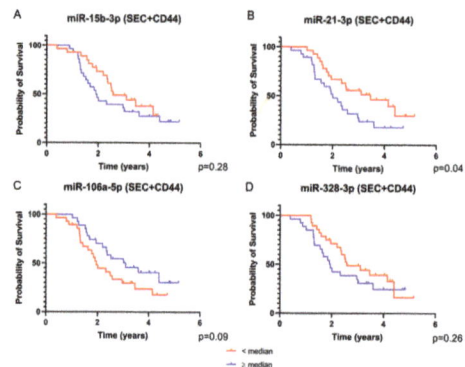

Figure 4. Survival analysis based on the expression of SEC + CD44 EV microRNA. Depicted are survival curves using a dichotomous assessment based on microRNA levels of SEC + CD44 EVs. ((**A**) miR-15b-3p, (**B**) miR-21-3p, (**C**) miR-106a-5p, (**D**) miR-328-3p) from glioblastoma patient serum ($n = 55$). Red color indicates patients with values equal to or higher than the median and blue color represents values lower than the median normalized expression ratio. Note that all four microRNAs were able to stratify the patients into different prognostic subgroups, albeit not reaching statistical significance. The p value for miR-21-3p is above the critical Benjamini–Hochberg value (0.03, Tables S3 and S4). Also note that for miR-106a-5p, higher values correlate with a better prognosis.

In analyses of single total serum microRNAs, we observed a clear curve separation for miR-15b-3p, as opposed to miR-21-3p and miR-106a-5p (Figure 5A–C). For miR-328-3p, no Kaplan–Meier curve was generated, because more than 50% of the values were below the detection limit.

2.3. Combination of SEC + CD44-EV- and Total Serum-microRNAs Allows Patient Stratification into Prognostically Relevant Subgroups

We next sought to determine whether a combination of different microRNAs results allows a more precise survival prediction compared to single microRNA analysis. Indeed, when we combined the analysis of miR-15b-3p in total serum with each of the other three EV-contained microRNAs, the prediction of prognosis was improved (based on the *p*-value determined) compared to the single microRNA analyses (Figure 6A–C).

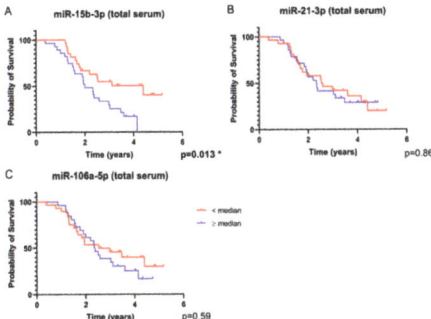

Figure 5. Survival analysis based on total serum microRNA expression. Depicted are survival curves using a dichotomous assessment based on microRNA levels ((**A**) miR-15b-3p, (**B**) miR-21-3p, (**C**) miR-106a-5p) from total serum of glioblastoma patients ($n = 55$). Red color indicates patients with values equal to or higher than the median and blue color represents values lower than the median normalized expression ratio. For miR-328-3p, no graph was generated because more than 50% of the values were non-measurable. Note that the separation of the curves based on miR-15b-3p is significant after Benjamini–Hochberg correction for multiple testing (Tables S3 and S4).

When combining markers tested only in SEC + CD44 EVs, three of these combinations, always including miR-106a-5p as one of the two microRNAs, yielded prognostically significant subgroups (Figure 7A–C). Because comparing multiple variables can give a bias and lead to a high risk of false significant results (type I error), we applied Benjamini–Hochberg correction [22]. Importantly, the combinations of microRNAs in Figures 6 and 7, as well as miR-15b-3p in total serum (Figure 5A), remained significant after this correction, as opposed to a single analysis of miR-21-3p (Figure 4B).

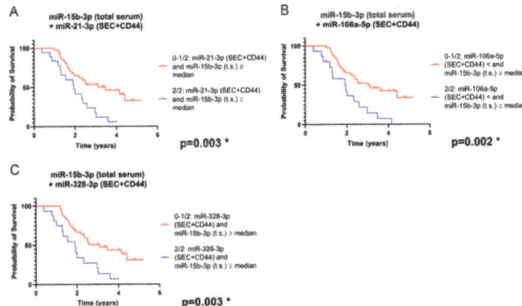

Figure 6. Survival analysis based on a combination of microRNA levels in total serum (t.s.) and/or SEC + CD44 EVs (combinations: miR-15b-3p in t.s. plus (**A**): miR-21-3p in SEC + CD44 EVs; (**B**): miR-106a-5p in SEC + CD44 EVs; (**C**): miR-328-3p in SEC + CD44 EVs). Depicted are survival curves using a dichotomous assessment from glioblastoma patients ($n = 55$) in both SEC + CD44 separated serum EVs and total serum. Blue color indicates patients whose microRNA profile fulfils both conditions, while red color indicates patients whose profile fulfils at most one out of two conditions. Note that the combination of miR-15b-3p in serum with each of these four microRNAs in SEC + CD44 EVs allowed for a prognostic stratification of this patient population, even after Benjamini–Hochberg correction (Table S1).

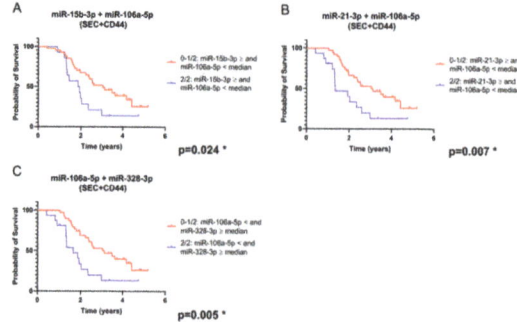

Figure 7. Survival analysis based on the expression of a combination of microRNAs isolated from SEC + CD44 EV (combinations: miR-106a-5p plus (**A**): miR-15b-3p; (**B**): miR-21-3p in SEC + CD44 EVs; (**C**): miR-328-3p). Depicted are survival curves using a dichotomous assessment based on a combination of microRNA levels from glioblastoma patients ($n = 55$) in SEC + CD44 separated serum EVs. Blue color indicates patients whose microRNA profile fulfils both conditions, while red color indicates patients whose profile fulfils at most one out of two conditions. Note that the combination of miR-106a-5p with each of the other three microRNAs allowed for a prognostic stratification of this patient population, even after Benjamini–Hochberg correction for multiple testing (Tables S3 and S4).

3. Discussion

In this study, we report on a new method for EV separation using the already established method of size-exclusion chromatography (by using qEV columns from IZON®), followed by immunoprecipitation with CD44-conjugated beads, thereby allowing specific enrichment of glioblastoma-associated EVs from patient serum. Using this novel method for EV separation, as well as total serum analyses, we identified a panel of four miRNAs suitable as biomarkers (alone or in combination) that allow for the prognostic stratification of glioblastoma patients at a relevant time point of the disease course.

Glioblastoma is a devastating disease which is currently lacking established biomarkers to aid in the prediction of prognosis and treatment decisions. Although progression-free survival (PFS) has been discussed as a surrogate parameter for overall survival in clinical trials of glioblastoma [23], it is mainly based on radiological findings [24,25], which are known to yield equivocal results [26]. Therefore, identifying biomarkers which would predict prognosis at an early time point during treatment is crucial. The median PFS is heterogeneous, and frequently ranges from 6 to 8 months [27,28]. In this study, we therefore chose the third quartile (6–9 months after the start of the adjuvant treatment) as a time for measuring microRNAs in serum and serum-derived EVs. Robust and feasible prognostic biomarkers at this critical time-point could therefore be highly relevant for the course of disease and help both patients and physicians in developing treatment strategies.

We have previously identified a key role for CD44, found on the surface of serum-EVs from glioblastoma patients, in the detection of tumor progression [18]. Due to a high upregulation of CD44 in glioblastoma patients compared to HV, we hypothesized that the immunoprecipitation of EVs with CD44 would lead to an enrichment of glioblastoma-specific EVs. The rationale for first separating the EVs using SEC was to ensure a purer sample of CD44-carrying EVs and minimize the risk of capturing EV-independent CD44, which is known to be present on various cell types, including T-cells and macrophages [29]. Furthermore, we intended to reduce the amount of soluble CD44 in the sample, which is shed by matrix-metalloproteases from the surface of tumor and non-tumor cells [30]. CD44 can also be found on EVs from different non-malignant cells, such as B- or T-cells [31,32], thus, we cannot exclude the possibility that some non-glioblastoma EVs are found in our SEC + CD44 EV fractions. However, the analysis of SEC-enriched serum-derived EVs from HV showed significantly lower CD44 levels compared to EVs from the serum of glioblastoma patients, indicating that CD44-positive EVs are enriched and highly relevant in glioblastoma patients [18]. This is in line with the intriguing hypothesis that glioblastoma is actually a systemic disease, as glioblastoma cells are known to affect non-tumor cells [33], suggesting that the EV-composition of glioblastoma patients differs from that of HV and thus could serve as a biomarker, irrespective of their origin.

The microRNAs selected for this project have all previously been studied in glioblastoma, either in total serum or EVs [19,20,34–36]. While some of these papers report that the majority of extracellular microRNAs are found bound to Ago [14], other studies claim that the majority of extracellular microRNAs are found inside small or large EVs [15,37,38]. Either way, it is clear that EV-associated microRNAs play a central role in intercellular communication and are capable of regulating key oncogenic processes, such as metastasis formation [16,39]. Ebrahimkhani et al. performed deep sequencing of exosomal microRNAs and discovered a panel of microRNAs that were not only upregulated in EVs from glioma patients, but were also capable of discriminating between *IDH*-mutated glioma and *IDH*-wildtype glioblastoma [34]. To account for differences between microRNAs found in total serum and glioblastoma-associated EVs, we examined the microRNA levels in both states and found a significant upregulation in four out of eight microRNAs, thus supporting our rationale for an enrichment of the relevant microRNAs through this isolation technique. Intriguingly, miR-328-3p, which was one of the microRNAs implicated in Ebrahimkhani et al. [34], did not show an increased concentration in EVs, yet its levels correlated with survival in our glioblastoma cohort. This finding underlines the importance of biological relevance rather than absolute quantitative changes in biomarker concentrations. miR-23, albeit having no prognostic significance in our study, might exude biological relevance based on its relatively strong increase in glioblastoma EVs. On the other hand, miR-15b-3p was found at higher levels in total serum and possessed the highest prognostic relevance using single microRNA analysis, while allowing for an even better stratification when combined with other microRNAs in SEC + CD44 EVs. Therefore, our data suggest that both targeted EV and total serum microRNAs should be studied for assessing the prognosis of glioblastoma patients. Notably, this is, to the best of our knowledge, the first study highlighting the prognostic potential of these biomarkers for glioblastoma patients.

The assessment of microRNA levels based on the MGMT methylation status showed that microRNAs indicating a non-favorable outcome (miR-15b-3p, miR-21-3p, and miR328-3p) were elevated in MGMT-non-methylated patient samples, while miR106a-5p showed lower levels compared to MGMT-methylated samples, thereby possibly highlighting a correlation of microRNAs with biologically aggressive tumors. While we only saw non-significant trends towards inferior survival for MGMT-methylated patients showing higher levels of miR-21-3p and miR-328-3p (data not shown), caution is warranted due to the low patient numbers.

All of the microRNAs from our prognostic panel have also been shown to carry important biological functions in glioblastoma, although their up- or downregulation in glioblastoma has not been conclusively resolved. miR-21-3p in EVs secreted by glioblastoma cells is known to promote oncogenesis, angiogenesis, and microglia activation [13] and has unanimously been described to be upregulated in the plasma of glioma patients [40], which is consistent with our data showing higher levels of miR-21-3p in glioblastoma-EVs compared to HV, as well as prognostic significance in SEC + CD44-purified EVs. The levels of miR-15b have also been shown to correlate with a high proliferation of glioma cells in vitro [12], but the levels in the serum of glioma patients were lower compared to HV [41]. Nevertheless, higher serum levels of miR-15b correlated with a higher WHO grade, thereby indicating that more aggressive tumors exhibit higher ratios of this microRNA compared to less proliferative tumors, which corresponds to the survival data in our study. Contradictory data have been published regarding the roles of miR-106a and miR-328 in glioma. High levels of miR-106a in glioma cells have been associated with reduced proliferation and increased apoptosis [12], but in other publications, have been associated with invasiveness [42]. Zhi and colleagues identified Fas-activated serine/threonine kinase (FASTK) as a direct target of miR-106a-5p and showed that a reduced expression of miR-106a-5p or increased expression of FASTK is significantly associated with poor survival in human astrocytoma patients [43], which is compatible with our data. While miR-328 has been shown to mediate the invasiveness of glioma cells via the downregulation of *Secreted Frizzled-related protein 1* (*SFRP1*) [44], Ebrahimkhani et al. reported that serum EVs from glioblastoma patients exhibited lower levels of miR-328 compared to HV [34]. Notably, the EVs used in this study were non-specifically purified from whole serum. Therefore, it would be tempting to speculate that a more specific separation of EVs using CD44 as a target antigen, and thereby enriching the population for glioblastoma EVs, would lead to a correlation of high miR-328 levels with a lower prognosis, as was the case in our study and as reported by Delic et al. [44].

In this study, we used serum as the biofluid source for miRNAs. While plasma used to be the preferred biomaterial for conducting EV studies, because coagulation activates platelets, resulting in an increased release of platelet-derived EVs [45], EVs and microRNAs are now increasingly being evaluated from the serum of glioblastoma patients [19,34]. Intriguingly, large-scale studies of different RNA subclasses, including microRNAs, in biofluids revealed only minor differences in the concentrations between serum and plasma [46,47]. These differences increased substantially if different RNA-extraction and EV-separation methods were applied, implying that both biofluids could yield similar results when established and validated protocols are used for purification. In our study, we used the miRNeasy kit by Qiagen for RNA extraction, as this method was identified as a suitable extraction method for high-yield and high-quality exosomal RNA [47]. There is still debate over what is the most suitable reference microRNA for calculating deltaCt. While some studies have used raw Ct values or exogenous non-human microRNAs as a reference, newer studies have discouraged the use of these conventions and instead recommend the use of at least one, and ideally two, microRNAs as a reference [48]. Based on these findings, we had previously performed screening for suitable reference microRNAs and identified miR-103 and miR-484 as two reliable housekeeper miRNAs (data not shown).

This is, to the best of our knowledge, the first study defining a microRNA signature (in EVs and cell-depleted serum) that shows a direct correlation with the survival of glioblastoma patients, thereby allowing prognostic stratification. Moreover, we introduce a novel approach for separating and enriching glioblastoma-specific EVs by combining size-exclusion chromatography and immunoprecipitation with CD44 as a unique target antigen. This optimized enrichment of glioblastoma-specific EVs leads to a more precise and sensitive prediction of prognosis compared to an unspecific serum-derived microRNA analysis. These encouraging data remain to be confirmed in larger prospective clinical trials, which could then pave the way for the introduction of an miRNA biomarker signature for clinicians, using methods that are feasible and time-efficient for routine diagnostic laboratories.

4. Materials and Methods

4.1. Ethical Approval

Studies on two cohorts of glioblastoma patients were separately approved by the Ethical Committee of the University of Bonn (protocol number for patients treated in Bonn: 182/08 and in the CeTeG/NOA-09 trial: 093/10) and on HV (Protocol number: 007/17).

4.2. Sample Collection

Serum was collected in 9 mL serum (S-Monovette, Sarstedt, Nuembrecht, Germany) tubes from HV and glioblastoma patients. For glioblastoma patients, blood was drawn at the time of an MRI visit in the third quartile period of their adjuvant treatment (i.e., 6–9 months after the initial diagnosis). For HV, blood was drawn at two different time-points with a time interval of three months. After a resting period of 30 min at room temperature (RT), the samples were centrifuged for 15 min at $2000\times g$ at RT, followed by a further centrifugation step for 20 min at $3000\times g$ at 6 °C. After filtration with a 0.45 µm filter, the serum was stored in aliquots at −80 °C.

4.3. EV Separation

EVs from serum samples were separated by size-exclusion chromatography (SEC) using the sepharose-based qEV columns (iZON Science, Christchurch, New Zealand), according to the manufacturer's recommendations. In short, 0.5 mL of serum was applied to the column and the EVs were eluted with Hank's balanced salt solution (HBSS). Next, 500 µL fractions were collected, fractions 8 to 10 were pooled, and a protease inhibitor (cOmplete, EDTA-free Protease Inhibitor Cocktail, Roche, Mannheim, Germany) was added to a final one-fold dilution. Subsequently, the combined fractions 8–10 (in total, 1.5 mL) were used for immunoprecipitation with 50 µL CD44-conjugated MicroBeads (CD44: Clone DB105) that were specifically designed for EV isolation and produced for this study. Separation of the EV-bound MicroBeads was performed with µColumns using the µMACS separator, according to the manufacturer's protocol (all Miltenyi Biotec, Bergisch Gladbach, Germany). EVs were eluted in 110 µL HBSS (ThermoFisher Scientific, Waltham, MA, USA) with protease inhibitor (Roche, Mannheim, Germany).

4.4. Nanoparticle Tracking Analysis (NTA)

As previously described, ZetaView Nanoparticle Tracking (Particle Metrix, Meerbusch, Germany) was used for NTA, according to the manufacturer's guidelines [49].

4.5. Transmission Electron Microscopy (TEM)

TEM was conducted based on the protocol previously described by Bachurski et al. [49]. Briefly, after loading 5 µL of an EV sample onto formvar-coated copper grids (Science Services, Munich, Germany), the EVs were fixed with 2% paraformaldehyde for 5 min, washed with PBS, fixed again for 5 min with 1% glutaraldehyde, washed with ddH$_2$O, and incubated with contrast dye (1.5% uranyl acetate) for 4 min. Images were captured with a Gatan OneView 4K camera (Gatan, Pleasanton, CA, USA) on a Jem-2100Plus microscope (JEOL) operating at 200 kV.

4.6. Wes^{TM} Simple Immunodetection

The presence of the EV markers CD9 and flotillin-1 and the absence of the endoplasmic-reticulum protein calnexin in the purified EV samples were confirmed using Wes^{TM} Simple Western technology with the Wes instrument (ProteinSimple, San Jose, CA, USA). In this study, 3 µL EVs were combined with 1 µL 0.1 × sample buffer and 1 µL 5 × fluorescent master mix for each lane. Analyses for flotillin-1 (clone 18/flotillin-1; BD Biosciences, Dilution: 1:100), calnexin (clone: C5C9; Cell Signaling Technology, Dilution: 1:80), apolipoprotein A1 (polylonal, R&D Systems, Concentration: 5 µg/mL), and human serum albumin polylonal (R&D Systems, Concentration: 5 µg/mL) were conducted under reducing (DTT-based buffer) conditions, while CD9 (clone D801A, Cell Signaling Technology, Dilution: 1:80) analysis was run under non-reducing conditions and using the 12–230 kDa Wes Separation Module. Anti-rabbit, anti-mouse, and anti-goat antibody detection modules (all from ProteinSimple) were used, according to the manufacturer's instructions. The default run conditions were changed to stocking-gel uptake: 22 s; sample uptake: 15 s; primary-antibody: 90 min; and secondary-antibody: 40 min incubation. Data analysis was performed with Compass software (ProteinSimple).

4.7. RNA Extraction and Quantitative Real-Time Polymerase Chain Reaction (qRT-PCR)

RNA extraction was performed using the Qiagen Micro-RNeasy kit, according to the manufacturer's protocol (Qiagen, Hilden, Germany). Following RNA extraction, equal volumes of the RNA samples were used for cDNA synthesis using a TaqMan Advanced miRNA cDNA Synthesis Kit, according to the manufacturer's protocol (ThermoFisher Scientific, Waltham, MA, USA). qRT-PCR was performed by using a QuantStudio 7 with TaqMan Advanced Control miRNA Assay (Table S2, both ThermoFisher Scientific, Waltham, MA, USA). miR-103a-3p and miR-484 were used as reference miRNAs (Table S2). The QuantStudio 7 PCR protocol included (1) enzyme activation at 95 °C for 20 s and (2) 40 cycles of denaturation (1 s at 95 °C) and annealing/extension (20 s at 60 °C).

4.8. Data Deposition

We have submitted all relevant data from our experiments to the EV-TRACK knowledgebase (EV-TRACK ID: 200051) [50].

4.9. Statistical Analysis

Statistical analysis was performed using GraphPad Prism software (Version 8.2.1, La Jolla, CA, USA). A Mann–Whitney U test was used to detect differences in the EV concentration, as well as differences in microRNAs between glioblastoma patients and HV. To compare levels of microRNAs isolated from total serum and SEC + CD44 EVs, a Wilcoxon signed-rank test was applied. Survival curves were generated using Kaplan–Meier plots and groups were evaluated using a log-rank test. The correlation of microRNA levels with survival was investigated using a nonparametric Spearman's rank correlation coefficient.

Since multiple microRNAs were tested, we corrected for multiple testing using the Benjamini–Hochberg procedure [22]. Out of the measured microRNAs used for dichotomous survival analysis, four out of four were measurable in SEC + CD44, but only three out of four in cell-depleted serum (miR-15b-3p, miR-21-3p, and miR-106a-5p, but not miR-328-3p). Therefore, we included seven groups in the single analysis and 21 in the two-fold combination analysis (Tables S3 and S4), leading to a total of m = 28 groups. After ranking the p-values (value i, range 1–28) and defining a false discovery rate (FDR = q) of 10%, we calculated the Benjamini–Hochberg critical value q*(i/m). If the log-rank p value was below the Benjamini–Hochberg critical value, the p values were considered statistically significant (*).

5. Conclusions

A panel of four microRNAs (miR-15b-3p, miR-21-3p, miR-106a-5p, and miR-328-3p) isolated from extracellular vesicles that were purified using size-exclusion chromatography and CD44-based immunoprecipitation in combination with total serum analysis allowed us to predict the prognosis of glioblastoma patients. Further analyses in larger prospective clinical trials are still warranted before these novel biomarkers become established in routine clinical practice.

Supplementary Materials: The following are available online at http://www.mdpi.com/1422-0067/21/19/7211/s1.

Author Contributions: Conceptualization, T.T., G.H., S.W., C.C. and K.S.R.; methodology, T.T., S.W., C.C. and K.S.R.; visualization, T.T. and K.S.R.; validation, K.S.R.; formal analysis, T.T., J.W. and K.S.R.; investigation, T.T., G.H., U.H., C.C. and K.S.R.; resources, D.B., N.S., C.S., M.H., B.S., M.G., G.H. and S.W.; data curation, T.T., C.C. and K.S.R.; writing—original draft preparation, T.T. and K.S.R.; writing—review and editing, T.T., J.W., D.B., N.S., C.S., M.H., B.S., M.G., G.H., U.H., S.W., C.C. and K.S.R.; supervision, G.H., U.H., C.C. and K.S.R.; project administration, G.H.; funding acquisition, T.T. and G.H. All authors have read and agreed to the published version of the manuscript.

Funding: This research was funded by the University of Bonn (BONFOR scholarship awarded to T.T., grant number O-129.0106) and by the Deutsche Forschungsgemeinschaft (DFG, German Research Foundation) under Germany's Excellence Strategy—EXC2151–390873048, of which G.H. is a member.

Acknowledgments: We thank Dagmar Christoph for excellent technical assistance and Meghan Campbell for her valuable input on the manuscript. We acknowledge Christiane Landwehr for her excellent trial and project management.

Conflicts of Interest: U.H. reports grants and personal fees from Roche; personal fees and non-financial support from Medac and Bristol-Myers Squibb; and personal fees from Novocure, Novartis, Daichii-Sankyo, Riemser, and Noxxon. N.S. reports personal fees and other support from Roche and received honoraria for advisory board from Bayer. M.G. reports grants, personal fees, and other support from Novocure and Medac, and personal fees from Merck. C.S. reports personal fees from Roche. S.W. and C.C. are employed by Miltenyi Biomedicine. All other authors declare no conflicts of interest.

Abbreviations

MDPI   Multidisciplinary Digital Publishing Institute
LD   linear dichroism
EV   extracellular vesicles
HV   healthy volunteers
SEC   size-exclusion chromatography

References

1. Taylor, O.G.; Brzozowski, J.S.; A Skelding, K. Glioblastoma multiforme: An overview of emerging therapeutic targets. *Front. Oncol.* **2019**, *9*, 963. [CrossRef]
2. Stupp, R.; Mason, W.P.; Van Den Bent, M.J.; Weller, M.; Fisher, B.; Taphoorn, M.J.; Belanger, K.; Brandes, A.A.; Marosi, C.; Bogdahn, U.; et al. Radiotherapy plus concomitant and adjuvant temozolomide for glioblastoma. *N. Engl. J. Med.* **2005**, *352*, 987–996. [CrossRef]
3. Hegi, M.E.; Diserens, A.C.; Gorlia, T.; Hamou, M.F.; De Tribolet, N.; Weller, M.; Kros, J.M.; Hainfellner, J.A.; Mason, W.; Mariani, L.; et al. MGMT gene silencing and benefit from temozolomide in glioblastoma. *N. Engl. J. Med.* **2005**, *352*, 997–1003. [CrossRef]
4. Herrlinger, U.; Tzaridis, T.; Mack, F.; Steinbach, J.P.; Schlegel, U.; Sabel, M.; Hau, P.; Kortmann, R.-D.; Krex, D.; Grauer, O.; et al. Lomustine-temozolomide combination therapy versus standard temozolomide therapy in patients with newly diagnosed glioblastoma with methylated MGMT promoter (CeTeG/NOA–09): A randomised, open-label, phase 3 trial. *Lancet* **2019**, *393*, 678–688. [CrossRef]
5. Weller, J.; Tzaridis, T.; Mack, F.; Steinbach, J.P.; Schlegel, U.; Hau, P.; Krex, D.; Grauer, O.; Goldbrunner, R.; Bähr, O.; et al. Health-related quality of life and neurocognitive functioning with lomustine–temozolomide versus temozolomide in patients with newly diagnosed, MGMT-methylated glioblastoma (CeTeG/NOA-09): A randomised, multicentre, open-label, phase 3 trial. *Lancet Oncol.* **2019**, *20*, 1444–1453. [CrossRef]
6. Wick, W.; Osswald, M.; Wick, A.; Winkler, F. Treatment of glioblastoma in adults. *Ther. Adv. Neurol. Disord.* **2018**, *11*, 1756286418790452. [CrossRef]
7. Wahid, F.; Shehzad, A.; Khan, T.; Kim, Y.Y. MicroRNAs: Synthesis, mechanism, function, and recent clinical trials. *Biochim. Biophys. Acta* **2010**, *1803*, 1231–1243. [CrossRef]
8. O'Brien, J.; Hayder, H.; Zayed, Y.; Peng, C. Overview of MicroRNA Biogenesis, Mechanisms of Actions, and Circulation. *Front. Endocrinol. (Lausanne)* **2018**, *9*, 402. [CrossRef]
9. Knight, S.W.; Bass, B.L. A Role for the RNase III Enzyme DCR-1 in RNA Interference and Germ Line Development in Caenorhabditis elegans. *Science* **2001**, *293*, 2269–2271. [CrossRef]
10. Zhang, J.; Zhou, W.; Liu, Y.; Liu, T.; Li, C.; Wang, L. Oncogenic role of microRNA-532-5p in human colorectal cancer via targeting of the 5′UTR of RUNX3. *Oncol. Lett.* **2018**, *15*, 7215–7220. [CrossRef]
11. Huntzinger, E.; Izaurralde, E. Gene silencing by microRNAs: Contributions of translational repression and mRNA decay. *Nat. Rev. Genet.* **2011**, *12*, 99–110. [CrossRef] [PubMed]
12. Møller, H.G.; Rasmussen, A.P.; Andersen, H.H.; Johnsen, K.B.; Henriksen, M.; Duroux, M. A Systematic Review of MicroRNA in Glioblastoma Multiforme: Micro-modulators in the Mesenchymal Mode of Migration and Invasion. *Mol. Neurobiol.* **2013**, *47*, 131–144. [CrossRef]
13. Buruiană, A.; Florian, Ș.I.; Florian, I.A.; Timiș, T.L.; Mihu, C.M.; Miclăuș, M.; Oșan, S.; Hrapșa, I.; Cataniciu, R.C.; Farcaș, M.; et al. The Roles of miRNA in Glioblastoma Tumor Cell Communication: Diplomatic and Aggressive Negotiations. *Int. J. Mol. Sci.* **2020**, *21*, 1950. [CrossRef] [PubMed]
14. Arroyo, J.D.; Chevillet, J.R.; Kroh, E.M.; Ruf, I.K.; Pritchard, C.C.; Gibson, D.F.; Mitchell, P.S.; Bennett, C.F.; Pogosova-Agadjanyan, E.L.; Stirewalt, D.L.; et al. Argonaute2 complexes carry a population of circulating microRNAs independent of vesicles in human plasma. *Proc. Natl. Acad. Sci. USA* **2011**, *108*, 5003–5008. [CrossRef]
15. Bayraktar, R.; Van Roosbroeck, K.; Calin, G.A. Cell-to-cell communication: microRNAs as hormones. *Mol. Oncol.* **2017**, *11*, 1673–1686. [CrossRef]
16. Valadi, H.; Ekstrom, K.; Bossios, A.; Sjöstrand, M.; Lee, J.J.; Lötvall, J. Exosome-mediated transfer of mRNAs and microRNAs is a novel mechanism of genetic exchange between cells. *Nat. Cell Biol.* **2007**, *9*, 654–659. [CrossRef]

17. Théry, C.; Ostrowski, M.; Segura, E. Membrane vesicles as conveyors of immune responses. *Nat. Rev. Immunol.* **2009**, *9*, 581–593. [CrossRef]
18. Tzaridis, T.; Reiners, K.; Herrlinger, U.; Gunther, H.; Scheffler, B.; Glas, M.; Coch, C. CBMT-17. Novel Approach of Utilising Serum/Plasma ev and Cell-Free RNA for Treatment Monitoring in Glioblastoma Patients. *Neuro Oncol.* **2018**, *20*, vi35–vi36. [CrossRef]
19. Kros, J.M.; Mustafa, D.M.; Dekker, L.J.; Smitt, P.A.S.; Luider, T.M.; Zheng, P.-P. Circulating glioma biomarkers. *Neuro Oncol.* **2015**, *17*, 343–360. [CrossRef]
20. Santangelo, A.; Imbrucè, P.; Gardenghi, B.; Belli, L.; Agushi, R.; Tamanini, A.; Munari, S.; Bossi, A.M.; Scambi, I.; Benati, N.; et al. A microRNA signature from serum exosomes of patients with glioma as complementary diagnostic biomarker. *J. Neuro Oncol.* **2018**, *136*, 51–62. [CrossRef]
21. Wang, H.; Jiang, D.; Li, W.; Xiang, X.; Zhao, J.; Yu, B.; Wang, C.; He, Z.; Zhu, L.; Yang, Y. Evaluation of serum extracellular vesicles as noninvasive diagnostic markers of glioma. *Theranostics* **2019**, *9*, 5347–5358. [CrossRef]
22. Benjamini, Y.; Hochberg, Y. Controlling the False Discovery Rate: A Practical and Powerful Approach to Multiple Testing. *J. R. Stat. Soc.* **1995**, *57*, 289–300. [CrossRef]
23. Han, K.; Ren, M.; Wick, W.; Abrey, L.; Das, A.; Jin, J.; Reardon, D.A. Progression-free survival as a surrogate endpoint for overall survival in glioblastoma: A literature-based meta-analysis from 91 trials. *Neuro Oncol.* **2014**, *16*, 696–706. [CrossRef]
24. Chukwueke, U.N.; Wen, P.Y. Use of the Response Assessment in Neuro-Oncology (RANO) criteria in clinical trials and clinical practice. *CNS Oncol.* **2019**, *8*, CNS28. [CrossRef]
25. Ellingson, B.M.; Wen, P.Y.; Cloughesy, T.F. Modified Criteria for Radiographic Response Assessment in Glioblastoma Clinical Trials. *Neurotherapeutics* **2017**, *14*, 307–320. [CrossRef]
26. Galldiks, N.; Kocher, M.; Langen, K.-J. Pseudoprogression after glioma therapy: An update. *Expert Rev. Neurother.* **2017**, *17*, 1109–1115. [CrossRef]
27. Kelly, C.; Majewska, P.; Ioannidis, S.; Raza, M.H.; Williams, M. Estimating progression-free survival in patients with glioblastoma using routinely collected data. *J. Neuro Oncol.* **2017**, *135*, 621–627. [CrossRef]
28. Majewska, P.; Ioannidis, S.; Raza, M.H.; Tanna, N.; Bulbeck, H.; Williams, M. Postprogression survival in patients with glioblastoma treated with concurrent chemoradiotherapy: A routine care cohort study. *CNS Oncol.* **2017**, *6*, 307–313. [CrossRef]
29. Senbanjo, L.T.; Chellaiah, M.A. CD44: A Multifunctional Cell Surface Adhesion Receptor Is a Regulator of Progression and Metastasis of Cancer Cells. *Front. Cell Dev. Biol.* **2017**, *5*, 18. [CrossRef]
30. Stamenkovic, I.; Yu, Q. Shedding Light on Proteolytic Cleavage of CD44: The Responsible Sheddase and Functional Significance of Shedding. *J. Investig. Dermatol.* **2009**, *129*, 1321–1324. [CrossRef]
31. Buschow, S.I.; Van Balkom, B.W.M.; Aalberts, M.; Heck, A.J.R.; Wauben, M.; Stoorvogel, W. MHC class II-associated proteins in B-cell exosomes and potential functional implications for exosome biogenesis. *Immunol. Cell Biol.* **2010**, *88*, 851–856. [CrossRef] [PubMed]
32. Perez-Hernandez, D.; Gutiérrez-Vázquez, C.; Jorge, I.; López-Martín, S.; Ursa, A.; Sánchez-Madrid, F.; Vázquez, J.; Yáñez-Mó, M. The Intracellular Interactome of Tetraspanin-enriched Microdomains Reveals Their Function as Sorting Machineries toward Exosomes. *J. Biol. Chem.* **2013**, *288*, 11649–11661. [CrossRef] [PubMed]
33. Rak, J.; Milsom, C.; Yu, J. Vascular determinants of cancer stem cell dormancy-do age and coagulation system play a role? *APMIS* **2008**, *116*, 660–676. [CrossRef]
34. Ebrahimkhani, S.; Vafaee, F.; Hallal, S.; Wei, H.; Lee, M.Y.T.; Young, P.E.; Satgunaseelan, L.; Beadnall, H.; Barnett, M.H.; Shivalingam, B.; et al. Deep sequencing of circulating exosomal microRNA allows non-invasive glioblastoma diagnosis. *NPJ Precis. Oncol.* **2018**, *2*, 28. [CrossRef]
35. Niyazi, M.; Pitea, A.; Mittelbronn, M.; Steinbach, J.; Sticht, C.; Zehentmayr, F.; Piehlmaier, D.; Zitzelsberger, H.; Ganswindt, U.; Rödel, C.; et al. A 4-miRNA signature predicts the therapeutic outcome of glioblastoma. *Oncotarget* **2016**, *7*, 45764–45775. [CrossRef]
36. Wei, Z.; Batagov, A.O.; Schinelli, S.; Wang, J.; Wang, Y.; El Fatimy, R.; Rabinovsky, R.; Balaj, L.; Chen, C.C.; Hochberg, F.; et al. Coding and noncoding landscape of extracellular RNA released by human glioma stem cells. *Nat. Commun.* **2017**, *8*, 1145. [CrossRef]
37. Gallo, A.; Tandon, M.; Alevizos, I.; Illei, G.G. The Majority of MicroRNAs Detectable in Serum and Saliva Is Concentrated in Exosomes. *PLoS ONE* **2012**, *7*, e30679. [CrossRef]

38. Hunter, M.P.; Ismail, N.; Zhang, X.; Aguda, B.D.; Lee, E.J.; Yu, L.; Xiao, T.; Schafer, J.; Lee, M.-L.T.; Schmittgen, T.D.; et al. Detection of microRNA Expression in Human Peripheral Blood Microvesicles. *PLoS ONE* **2008**, *3*, e3694. [CrossRef]
39. Kosaka, N.; Iguchi, H.; Hagiwara, K.; Yoshioka, Y.; Takeshita, F.; Ochiya, T. Neutral Sphingomyelinase 2 (nSMase2)-dependent Exosomal Transfer of Angiogenic MicroRNAs Regulate Cancer Cell Metastasis. *J. Biol. Chem.* **2013**, *288*, 10849–10859. [CrossRef]
40. Ilhan-Mutlu, A.; Wagner, L.; Woehrer, A.; Furtner, J.; Widhalm, G.; Marosi, C.; Preusser, M. Plasma MicroRNA-21 Concentration May Be a Useful Biomarker in Glioblastoma Patients. *Cancer Investig.* **2012**, *30*, 615–621. [CrossRef]
41. Yang, C.; Wang, C.; Chen, X.; Chen, S.; Zhang, Y.; Zhi, F.; Wang, J.; Li, L.; Zhou, X.; Li, N.; et al. Identification of seven serum microRNAs from a genome-wide serum microRNA expression profile as potential noninvasive biomarkers for malignant astrocytomas. *Int. J. Cancer* **2013**, *132*, 116–127. [CrossRef] [PubMed]
42. Lavon, I.; Zrihan, D.; Granit, A.; Einstein, O.; Fainstein, N.; Cohen, M.A.; Cohen, M.A.; Zelikovitch, B.; Shoshan, Y.; Spektor, S.; et al. Gliomas display a microRNA expression profile reminiscent of neural precursor cells. *Neuro Oncol.* **2010**, *12*, 422–433. [CrossRef] [PubMed]
43. Zhi, F.; Zhou, G.; Shao, N.; Xia, X.; Shi, Y.; Wang, Q.; Zhang, Y.; Wang, R.; Xue, L.; Wang, S.; et al. miR-106a-5p Inhibits the Proliferation and Migration of Astrocytoma Cells and Promotes Apoptosis by Targeting FASTK. *PLoS ONE* **2013**, *8*, e72390. [CrossRef]
44. Delic, S.; Lottmann, N.; Stelzl, A.; Liesenberg, F.; Wolter, M.; Götze, S.; Zapatka, M.; Shiio, Y.; Sabel, M.C.; Felsberg, J.; et al. MiR-328 promotes glioma cell invasion via SFRP1-dependent Wnt-signaling activation. *Neuro Oncol.* **2014**, *16*, 179–190. [CrossRef] [PubMed]
45. Ambrose, A.; Alsahli, M.A.; Kurmani, S.A.; Goodall, A.H. Comparison of the release of microRNAs and extracellular vesicles from platelets in response to different agonists. *Platelets* **2018**, *29*, 446–454. [CrossRef]
46. Murillo, O.D.; Thistlethwaite, W.; Rozowsky, J.; Subramanian, S.L.; Lucero, R.; Shah, N.; Jackson, A.R.; Srinivasan, S.; Chung, A.; Laurent, C.D.; et al. exRNA Atlas Analysis Reveals Distinct Extracellular RNA Cargo Types and Their Carriers Present across Human Biofluids. *Cell* **2019**, *177*, 463–477.e15. [CrossRef]
47. Srinivasan, S.; Yeri, A.; Cheah, P.S.; Chung, A.; Danielson, K.M.; De Hoff, P.; Filant, J.; Laurent, C.D.; Laurent, L.D.; Magee, R.; et al. Small RNA Sequencing across Diverse Biofluids Identifies Optimal Methods for exRNA Isolation. *Cell* **2019**, *177*, 446–462.e16. [CrossRef]
48. Occhipinti, G.; Giulietti, M.; Principato, G.; Piva, F. The choice of endogenous controls in exosomal microRNA assessments from biofluids. *Tumor Biol.* **2016**, *37*, 11657–11665. [CrossRef]
49. Bachurski, D.; Schuldner, M.; Nguyen, P.-H.; Malz, A.; Reiners, K.S.; Grenzi, P.C.; Babatz, F.; Schauss, A.C.; Hansen, H.P.; Hallek, M.; et al. Extracellular vesicle measurements with nanoparticle tracking analysis—An accuracy and repeatability comparison between NanoSight NS300 and ZetaView. *J. Extracell. Vesicles* **2019**, *8*, 1596016. [CrossRef]
50. Van Deun, J.; EV-TRACK Consortium; Mestdagh, P.; Agostinis, P.; Akay, Ö.; Anand, S.; Anckaert, J.; Martinez, Z.A.; Baetens, T.; Beghein, E.; et al. EV-TRACK: Transparent reporting and centralizing knowledge in extracellular vesicle research. *Nat. Methods* **2017**, *14*, 228–232. [CrossRef]

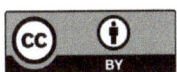

© 2020 by the authors. Licensee MDPI, Basel, Switzerland. This article is an open access article distributed under the terms and conditions of the Creative Commons Attribution (CC BY) license (http://creativecommons.org/licenses/by/4.0/).

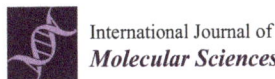

Article

Suppression of Ovarian Cancer Cell Growth by AT-MSC Microvesicles

Agnieszka Szyposzynska, Aleksandra Bielawska-Pohl, Agnieszka Krawczenko, Olga Doszyn, Maria Paprocka and Aleksandra Klimczak *

Laboratory of Biology of Stem and Neoplastic Cells, Hirszfeld Institute of Immunology and Experimental Therapy, Polish Academy of Sciences, R. Weigla 12, 53-114 Wroclaw, Poland; agnieszka.szyposzynska@hirszfeld.pl (A.S.); aleksandra.bielawska-pohl@hirszfeld.pl (A.B.-P.); agnieszka.krawczenko@hirszfeld.pl (A.K.); olga.doszyn@hirszfeld.pl (O.D.); maria.paprocka@hirszfeld.pl (M.P.)
* Correspondence: aleksandra.klimczak@hirszfeld.pl; Tel.: +48-71-3371-172 (ext. 118)

Received: 20 November 2020; Accepted: 27 November 2020; Published: 30 November 2020

Abstract: Transport of bioactive cargo of microvesicles (MVs) into target cells can affect their fate and behavior and change their microenvironment. We assessed the effect of MVs derived from human immortalized mesenchymal stem cells of adipose tissue-origin (HATMSC2-MVs) on the biological activity of the ovarian cancer cell lines ES-2 (clear cell carcinoma) and OAW-42 (cystadenocarcinoma). The HATMSC2-MVs were characterized using dynamic light scattering (DLS), transmission electron microscopy, and flow cytometry. The anti-tumor properties of HATMSC2-MVs were assessed using MTT for metabolic activity and flow cytometry for cell survival, cell cycle progression, and phenotype. The secretion profile of ovarian cancer cells was evaluated with a protein antibody array. Both cell lines internalized HATMSC2-MVs, which was associated with a decreased metabolic activity of cancer cells. HATMSC2-MVs exerted a pro-apoptotic and/or necrotic effect on ES-2 and OAW-42 cells and increased the expression of anti-tumor factors in both cell lines compared to control. In conclusion, we confirmed an effective transfer of HATMSC2-MVs into ovarian cancer cells that resulted in the inhibition of cell proliferation via different pathways, apoptosis and/or necrosis, which, with high likelihood, is related to the presence of different anti-tumor factors secreted by the ES-2 and OAW-42 cells.

Keywords: ovarian cancer cells; ES-2; OAW-42; microvesicles; adipose tissue origin mesenchymal stem cells

1. Introduction

Today, ovarian cancer is one of the most dangerous types of cancer in women. This is associated with a lack of screening tests and late diagnosis. Moreover, the disease has no symptoms in the early stages. Currently, various ovarian cancer therapies are used depending on the histological type of ovarian cancer, its stage, and the patient's predisposition. Standard treatment is a surgery combined with platinum-based chemotherapy [1]. Clinical trials focus primarily on an anti-angiogenic strategy [Vascular endothelial growth factor (VEGF) inhibition] or on modulating the immune system [2]. An extremely important field in oncology is research focused on cancer stem cells (CSCs). Cancer stem cells constitute a small population of tumor cells and play an important role in metastasis. Moreover, these cells are resistant to widely used drugs, which often leads to tumor recurrence [3]. Thus, a search for effective factors is needed that inhibit the biological activity of CSCs.

Mesenchymal stem/stromal cells (MSCs) are multipotent cells that reside in the majority of human tissues and organs, and in steady-state conditions, are responsible for the maintenance of tissue homeostasis [4,5]. Cells with MSC characteristics can be isolated from various source tissues, such as bone marrow, adipose tissue, dental pulp, skin, skeletal muscle, or perinatal tissues, including the umbilical cord, cord blood, Warton's jelly, and amniotic fluid. The tissue source of MSCs affects their cellular phenotype and biological properties [6]. MSCs and their derivates are a promising tool in clinical applications thanks to their high proliferative potential, longevity, and immunomodulatory properties [7,8].

Extracellular vesicles (EVs), such as exosomes and microvesicles (MVs), play an important role as mediators of cell-to-cell communication [9]. EVs are released by all normal, apoptotic, and neoplastic cells [10]. The transport of bioactive cargo, such as proteins, lipids, or nucleic acids, into the recipient cells may affect their phenotype and biological activity [11].

The tumor microenvironment consist not only of tumor cells, but also fibroblasts, smooth muscle cells, immune cells, endothelial cells, and mesenchymal stem cells [12]. Cell-to-cell communication in tumor niches takes place through direct contact between the surrounding cells and gap junctions or through the paracrine activity of the cells (e.g., the release of soluble factors or EVs).

The effect of EVs derived from MSCs of different tissue origin on cancer cells is not well understood. Different studies have confirmed the pro-tumorigenic [13] or anti-tumorigenic activity [14] of EVs derived from MSCs on ovarian cancer cells. This effect depends on the origin of the MSCs, methods of EV isolation, and tumor type [15].

The aim of this study was to examine the effect of MVs derived from immortalized human MSCs of adipose tissue origin (HATMSC2-MVs) on the biological activity of two ovarian cancer cell lines: ES-2, representing poorly differentiated ovarian clear cell carcinoma, and OAW-42, representing ovarian cystadenocarcinoma, with different genetic backgrounds and therapeutic responses. These two cell lines were characterized according to their phenotype and the secretion profile of cytokines and trophic factors released in response to MV treatment. Moreover, we investigated the proliferation and cell death processes/pathways (apoptosis and necrosis) of ovarian cancer cells in the presence of different ratios of HATMSC2-MVs and target cells.

2. Results

2.1. Characterization of HATMSC2-Derived MVs

Size distribution of MVs was analyzed using dynamic light scattering (DLS). In the histogram, a single distinct peak characteristic for MVs was observed, confirming the presence of a homogenous population of MVs. The average size of MVs, assessed using DLS, was 456 nm (Figure 1a). The size of individual MVs was confirmed using transmission electron microscopy (TEM) imaging (Figure 1b).

Isolation efficiency, using the flow cytometry method, revealed that the average number of MVs was 172×10^6 MVs/mL (Figure 1c). A Bradford assay was performed to estimate the protein concentration within the MVs, and the average protein concentration was assessed at 169.8 µg/mL.

2.2. Surface Marker Analysis of HATMSC2 Cells and HATMSC2-MVs

The HATMSC2 cells and HATMSC2-MVs were tested for the presence of MSC markers CD73, CD90, CD105, the HLA ABC and HLA DR antigens, and the leukocyte marker CD45. The analysis confirmed the presence of CD73, CD90, and CD105 on the surface of HATMSC2 cells. The cells were also positive for the HLA ABC antigen and negative for the HLA DR antigen and for the pan-leukocyte antigen CD45 [16]. Importantly, HATMSC2-MVs expressed surface markers typical for MSCs, including CD73 (50.50 ± 2.18% of the population), CD90 (90.67 ± 5.36% of the population), CD105 (45.32 ± 3.24% of the population), and HLA ABC (88.20 ± 4.61% of the population). HATMSC2-MVs did not express HLA DR or CD45 (Figure 2).

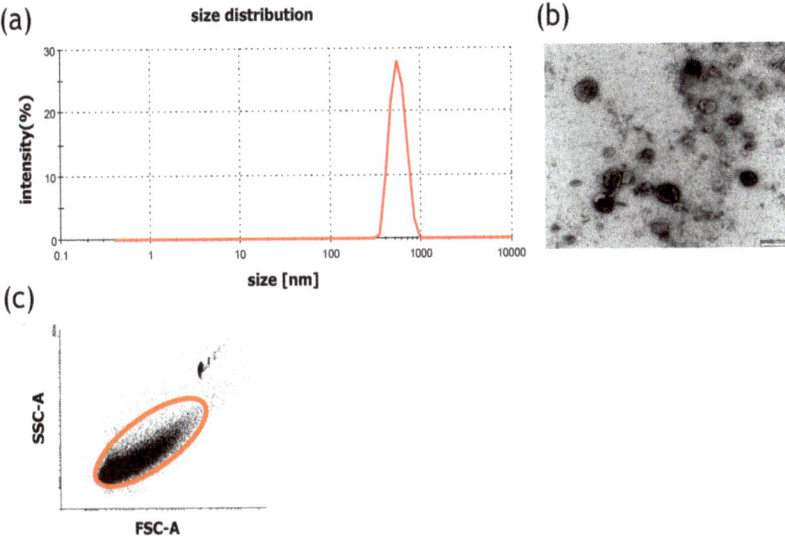

Figure 1. Characteristics of HATMSC2-MVs (**a**) Representative HATMSC2-MV size distribution histogram obtained using dynamic light scattering analysis. (**b**) Representative transmission electron microscopy image of HATMSC2-MVs, bars represent 500 nm. (**c**) Representative dot plot showing forward scatter (FSC) vs. side scatter (SSC). Gate R-1 shows the population of HATMSC2-MVs, and gate R-2 represents the counting beads. HATMSC2-MVs—microvesicles derived from immortalized human mesenchymal stem cells of adipose tissue origin.

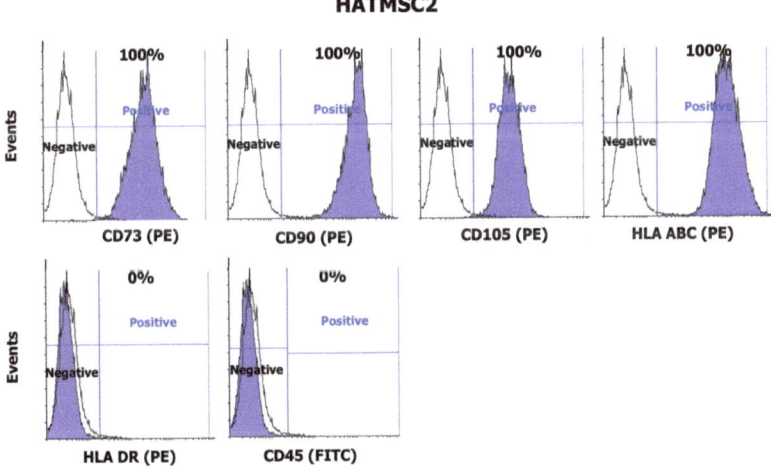

Figure 2. *Cont.*

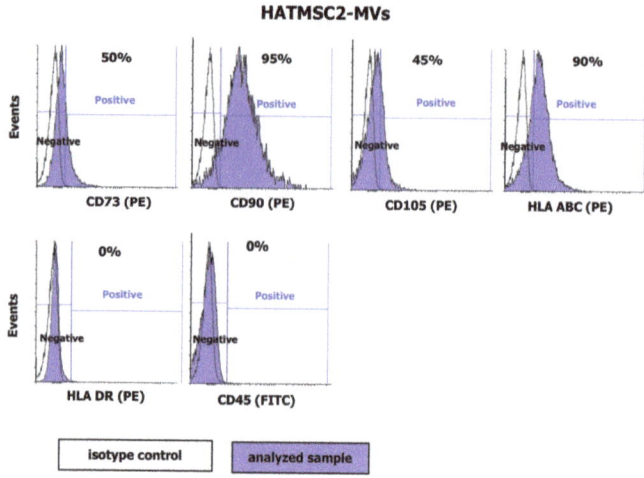

Figure 2. Representative flow cytometry histograms of flow cytometry analysis of mesenchymal stem cells markers (CD73, CD90, CD105, HLA ABC, HLA DR, and CD45) on HATMSC2 cells and HATMSC2-MVs from three independent experiments. Cells and MVs were stained with selected antibodies conjugated with fluorochromes. Blue filled histograms correspond to HATMSC2 cells and HATMSC2-MVs labeled with defined antibodies, and empty histograms represent the isotype controls. HATMSC2-MVs—microvesicles derived from immortalized human mesenchymal stem cells of adipose tissue origin.

2.3. Internalization of HATMSC2-MVs into Ovarian Cancer Cells

The internalization of fluorescently-labeled HATMSC2-MVs into ovarian cancer cell lines was analyzed using three-dimensional microscopic imaging. HATMSC2-MV co-culture with target cells (ES-2 and OAW-42 cell lines) for 24 h resulted in the incorporation of the MVs into ES-2 and OAW-42 cells, as shown by green fluorescence (DiO) expression in the cytoplasm of the target cells across the Z-stack slices (Figure 3a).

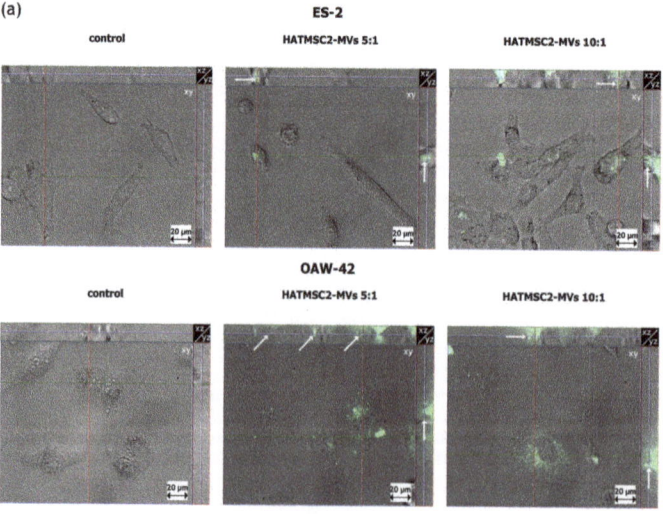

Figure 3. *Cont.*

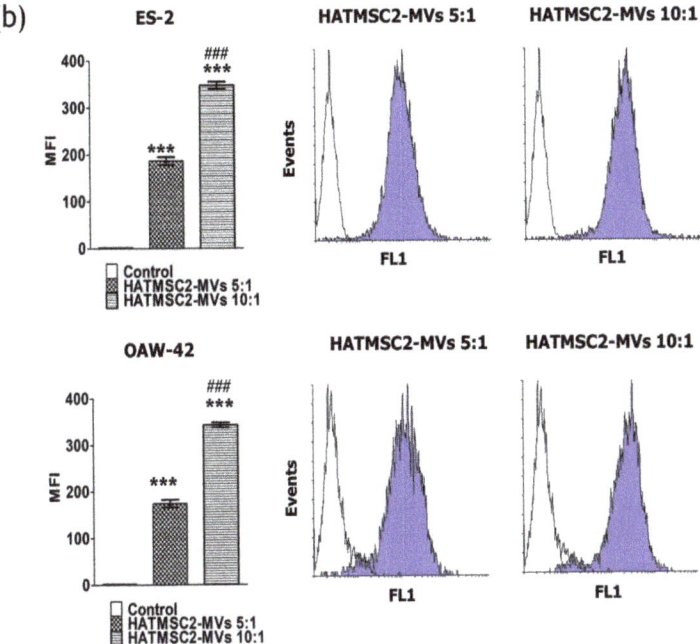

Figure 3. Internalization of HATMSC2-MVs into ovarian cancer cells. (**a**) Images from three-dimensional microscopic analysis of HATMSC2-MV internalization into ES-2 and OAW-42 cells at different ratios. The images were taken using an inverted microscope after 24 h of incubation with fluorescently-labeled HATMSC2-MVs (scale bar: 20 μm). A set of representative orthogonal slices is shown. Each image in a group consists of a large middle segment that represents the midpoint of the Z-stack in the *xy* plane; a narrow top segment that represents the *xz* plane; and a narrow segment on the right that represents the *yz* plane. The arrows point to MVs that have been taken up into the cell. (**b**) Bottom left panel, the bar graph represents the mean fluorescence intensity (MFI) of ES-2 cells treated with fluorescently labeled HATMSC2-MVs at different ratios. Untreated cells without MVs served as a control. Right panel, flow cytometry analysis of HATMSC2-MV internalization. Empty histograms represent the control for untreated cells, and blue filled histograms show the green fluorescence of ovarian cancer cells ES-2 and OAW-42 after HATMSC2-MV internalization at different ratios. The data represent mean ± SEM values from three independent experiments performed in duplicate. *** $p < 0.001$ calculated vs. control, ### $p < 0.001$ calculated vs. The HATMSC2-MVs 5:1 treatment. HATMSC2-MVs—microvesicles derived from immortalized human mesenchymal stem cells of adipose tissue origin.

Furthermore, the uptake of HATMSC2-MVs by ovarian cancer cells was confirmed by an increase in mean fluorescence intensity (MFI), as analyzed using flow cytometry. The results showed a significant increase in MFI in the ES-2 and OAW-42 cell lines treated with HATMSC2-MVs for both the ratios of 5:1 and 10:1 (the number of MVs to one target cell) compared to the control groups ($p < 0.001$). Moreover, this effect was dose-dependent, and significant differences between the ratios 5:1 and 10:1 ($p < 0.001$) were observed (Figure 3b).

2.4. Anti-Proliferative Activity of HATMSC2-MVs

The anti-proliferative activity of HATMSC2-MVs was analyzed using the MTT assay. ES-2 and OAW-42 cells were treated with MVs at four different ratios: 1:1, 5:1, 10:1, and 100:1. The HATMSC-MV treatment caused a significant decrease in OAW-42 cell proliferation on day 3 ($p < 0.01$) at a ratio of 100:1 (Figure 4a). The anti-proliferative activity of the MVs used at a ratio of 100:1 in OAW-42 cells on day 3 was also shown on a microscopic images of calcein-stained ovarian cancer cells (Figure 4b).

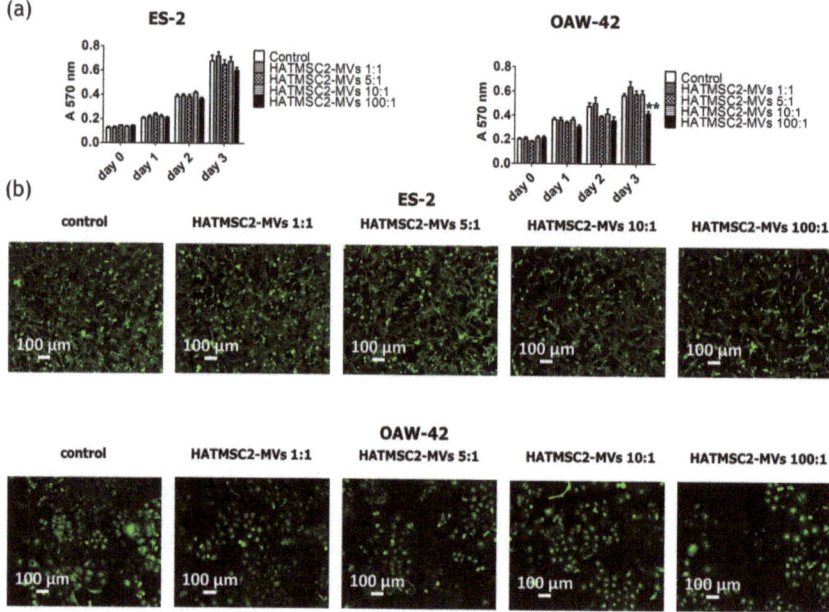

Figure 4. Effect of HATMSC2-MVs on the proliferation activity of ovarian cancer cells. (**a**) Proliferation activity of ES-2 and OAW-42 cells cultured in standard conditions was measured using an MTT assay on day 0, 1, 2, and 3 following treatment with HATMSC2-MVs at different ratios. Untreated cells without MVs served as a control. The data represent mean ± SEM values from four independent experiments performed in triplicate. ** $p < 0.01$ calculated vs. control on a given day. (**b**) Representative images from microscopic analysis of the morphology of ovarian cancer cells treated with HATMSC2-MVs at different ratios. ES-2 and OAW-42 cells were co-incubated with HATMSC2-MVs for 72 h. Afterwards, the cells were stained with Calcein AM and images were taken using an inverted microscope (scale bar: 100 µm). HATMSC2-MVs—microvesicles derived from immortalized human mesenchymal stem cells of adipose tissue origin.

2.5. Effect of HATMSC2-MVs on Cell Cycle Progression

The effect of HATMSC2-MVs on cell cycle progression was tested using flow cytometry analysis of ES-2 and OAW-42 cells stained with propidium iodide. We observed an increase in the percentage of cells in the sub-G1 phase (dead cells) in the samples treated with the MV ratio of 100:1 in ES-2 cells, compared to the control group (mean 2.57 ± 0.54% vs. 0.79 ± 0.05%; $p < 0.01$). Similarly, in OAW-42 cells treated with the MVs ratio of 100:1, the percentage of cells in the sub-G1 phase increased to 15.66 ± 2.86% compared to 2.74 ± 0.48% in control group ($p < 0.001$). Moreover, in OAW-42 cells treated with an MVs ratio of 100:1, the percentage of cells in the G0/G1 phase decreased from 63.06 ± 1.49% in the control group to 55.87 ± 1.37% in the test group ($p < 0.01$), (Figure 5).

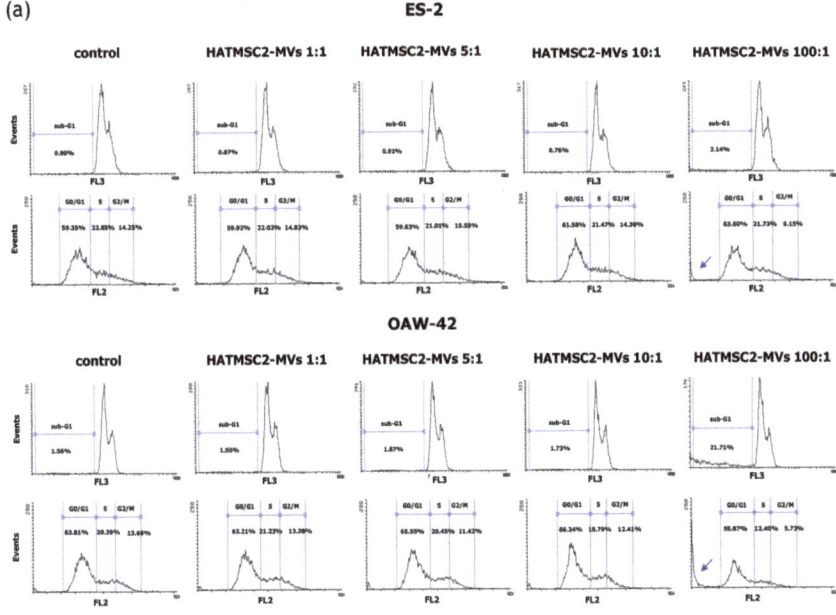

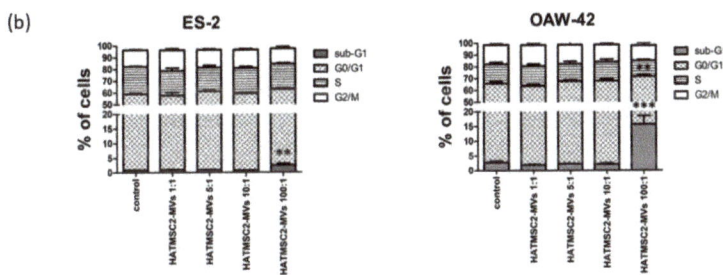

Figure 5. Effect of HATMSC2-MVs on the cell cycle progression of ovarian cancer cells. (**a**) Representative flow cytometry histograms showing cell cycle progression in ES-2 and OAW-42 cells treated with HATMSC2-MVs at different ratios. Untreated cells without MVs served as a control. Arrows represent the increased peaks in the sub-G1 phase of the cell cycle. (**b**) Percentages of cells in the sub-G1, G0/G1, S, and G2/M phases were determined using Flowing Software 2. The data represent mean ± SEM values from three independent experiments performed in duplicate. *** $p < 0.001$, ** $p < 0.01$ calculated vs. control. HATMSC2-MVs—microvesicles derived from immortalized human mesenchymal stem cells of adipose tissue origin

2.6. Proapoptotic Activity of HATMSC2-MVs

We examined the impact of HATMSC2-MVs on ovarian cancer cell survival. Cell death processes, such as apoptosis and necrosis, were assessed using flow cytometry after 72 h of co-culture of HATMSC2-MVs with ES-2 and OAW-42 cells at the ratios of 1:1, 5:1, 10:1, and 100:1. Untreated cells served as a control. The obtained results revealed that the HATMSC2-MVs treatment affected cell viability depending on the ratio of HATMSC2-MVs and cancer cells. The ratio of MVs 100:1 had the greatest impact on cell viability, both in the ES-2 and OAW-42 cells (Figure 6).

In ES-2 cells, the percentage of live cells treated with HATMSC2-MVs decreased to 61.23 ± 7.71% for the ratio of 100:1 vs. control (89.65 ± 0.99%; $p < 0.001$). The average percentage of early apoptotic cells increased to 8.22 ± 1.32% vs. control 1.95 ± 0.41%, ($p < 0.001$), whereas the average percentage of late apoptotic cells increased to 11.75 ± 3.22% vs. control 2.79 ± 0.32%, ($p < 0.01$). The average percentage of ES-2 necrotic cells increased to 18.81 ± 4.79% vs. control 5.72 ± 0.81%, ($p < 0.01$).

In OAW-42 cells, the percentage of live cells treated with HATMSC2-MVs decreased to 47.78 ± 10.11% for the ratio of 100:1 vs. control (86.17 ± 2.12%, $p < 0.001$). The average percentage of late apoptotic cells increased to 18.53 ± 5.17% vs. control 1.57 ± 0.34%, ($p < 0.001$). The average percentage of OAW-42 necrotic cells increased to 27.51 ± 5.04% vs. control 10.70 ± 2.02%, ($p < 0.001$).

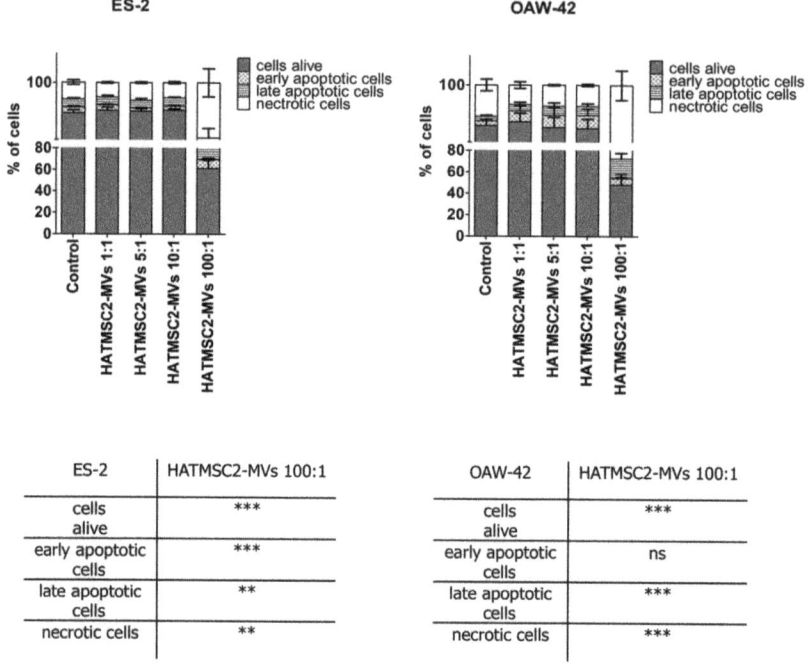

ES-2	HATMSC2-MVs 100:1	OAW-42	HATMSC2-MVs 100:1
cells alive	***	cells alive	***
early apoptotic cells	***	early apoptotic cells	ns
late apoptotic cells	**	late apoptotic cells	***
necrotic cells	**	necrotic cells	***

Figure 6. Quantification of cell viability after treatment with HATMSC2-MVs for 72 h at different ratios, determined using flow cytometric analysis of the apoptotic and necrotic cells via the double-staining of ES-2 and OAW-42 cells with propidium iodide and Annexin V. The percentages of alive, early apoptotic, late apoptotic, and necrotic cells were determined using Flowing Software 2. The data represent mean ± SEM values from five independent experiments performed in duplicate. *** $p < 0.001$, ** $p < 0.01$ calculated vs. control, ns: non-significant results. HATMSC2-MVs—microvesicles derived from immortalized human mesenchymal stem cells of adipose tissue origin.

2.7. Effect of HATMSC2-MVs on the Phenotype of Ovarian Cancer Cell Lines

To determine the effect of HATMSC2 -MVs on the phenotype of ovarian cancer cell lines treated at the ratios of 10:1 and 100:1, we tested the presence of the CD34, CD44, CD133, SSEA4, CD73, CD90, and CD105 markers using flow cytometry. The results showed that both cell lines, ES-2 and OAW-42, were positive for the adhesion molecule CD44 (Figure 7). However, the expression of the CD44 marker was higher (97.80% ± 2.20% of the population) for the ES-2 cells compared to OAW-42 cells (78.36% ± 3.20% of the population). Both ES-2 and OAW-42 cell lines were negative for CD34 and CD133 and for the pluripotency-related marker SSEA4. An analysis of the expression of MSC markers showed that both ES-2 and OAW-42 were positive for CD73 and CD90, whereas the CD105 marker was detected in ES-2 cells (98.20% ± 1.79% of the population), but not in OAW-42 cells (Figure 7a). The HATMSC2-MVs treatment did not affect the phenotype of ES-2 and OAW-42 cells (Figure 7b).

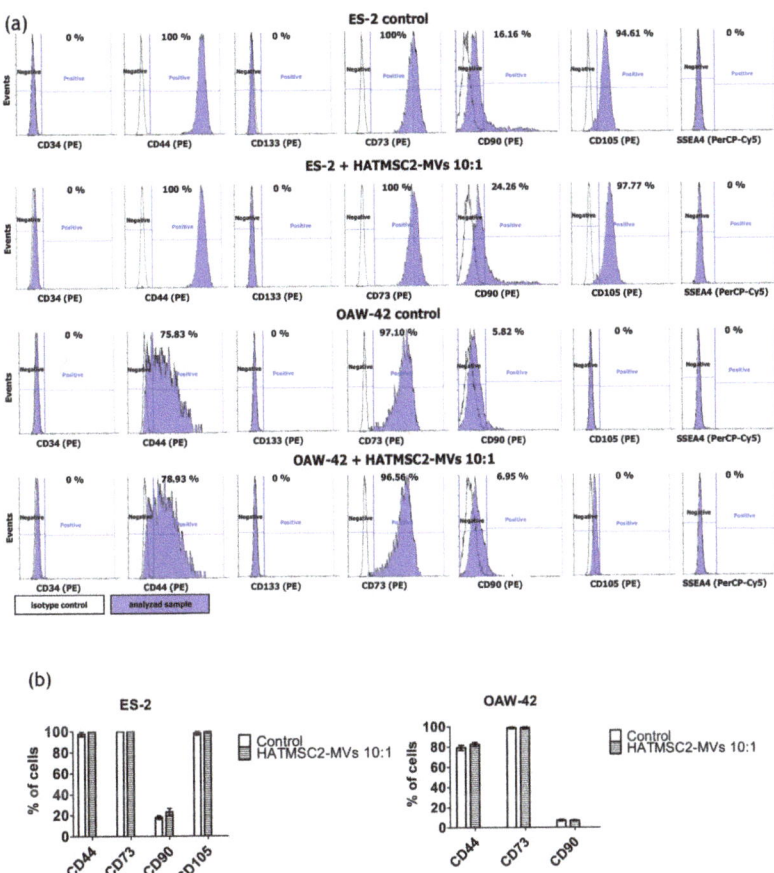

Figure 7. Characteristics of human ovarian cancer cell lines before and after HATMSC2-MV treatment at different ratios. (a) Representative histograms of flow cytometry analysis for surface markers (CD34, CD44, CD133, SSEA4, CD73, CD90, and CD105) on the ES-2 and OAW-42 cell lines. The cells were stained with selected antibodies conjugated with fluorochromes. Blue filled histograms correspond to ES-2 and OAW-42 cells, labeled with defined antibodies, and empty histograms represent the isotype controls. (b) The percentages of cells positive for selected markers were determined using Flowing Software 2. The data represent mean ± SEM values from three independent experiments. HATMSC2-MVs—microvesicles derived from immortalized human mesenchymal stem cells of adipose tissue origin.

2.8. Effect of HATMSC2-MVs on the Secretion Profile of Ovarian Cancer Cell Lines

The effect of HATMSC2-MVs on the biological properties of ovarian cancer cells was determined in all experiments at different ratios of MVs to cancer cells (1:1, 5:1, 10:1 and 100:1). However, the best effect was seen when a ratio of 100:1 was used. Therefore, to determine the effect of HATMSC2-MVs on the secretion profile of the ES-2 and OAW-42 cell lines, only the ratio of 100:1 was used. The secretion profile was evaluated using a human cytokine antibody array (Figure 8a). Most of the 120 cytokines and trophic factors identified in this analysis affect cancer cells either by promoting cancer growth or through their anti-tumor properties. For the ES-2 cells treated with HATMSC2-MVs, among cancer-promoting cytokines and trophic factors, a decrease was observed for angiogenesis-related cytokines, such as growth related oncogene-alpha (GRO-alpha) (by 53%), angiopoietin 2 (by 10%), VEGF (by 44%), and VEGFD (by 8%), and for the pro-angiogenic and pro-inflammatory cytokines IL-6 (by 15%), IL-8 (by 36%), MIP-1α (by 7%), and MIP-1β (by 8%). The levels of apoptosis-related TRAIL-R3 and TRAIL-R4 also decreased (by 10% and 14%, respectively). However, an increase was observed in the levels of the pro-inflammatory cytokines IL-1α (by 18%), IL-1β (by 21%), MCP-1 (by 43%), MIG (by 28%), TNFα (by 13%), IL-13 (by 6%), eotaxin (by 16%), and eotaxin-2 (by 21%), and growth factors bFGF (by 9%), EGF (by 33%), and HGF (by 21%). On the other hand, we observed an increase in the levels of several anti-cancer cytokines, such as IL-1 receptor antagonist (IL-1ra) (by 42%), IL-2 by (21%), IL-2 receptor alpha chain (IL-2Ra) (by 13%), IL-12 (by 6% and 10% for the p40 and p70 subunits, respectively), IL-15 (by 34%), and IFN-γ (by 43%). Nevertheless, the overall number of expressed cytokines in the ES-2 cells was 92; however, the expression of a majority of these cells differed before and after the HATMSC2-MV treatment (Figure 8b).

For the OAW-42 cells, the overall number of expressed cytokines increased from 58 in the control group to 87 after the MV treatment. However, most of these cytokines did not show a major difference in expression between the control and test groups. Among the tumor-promoting cytokines, we observed a decrease in the levels of the pro-angiogenic and pro-inflammatory cytokines GRO-alpha (by 192%), VEGF (by 34%), IL-6 (by 176%), IL-8 (by 204%), and RANTES (by 16%), and an increase in other cytokines, such as eotaxin-2 (by 8%), eotaxin-3 (by 6%), IL-1β (by 24%), MIG (by 18%), TNFα (by 36%), TGF-beta1 (by 21%), and -beta3 (by 34%), bFGF (by 15%), TRAIL-R3 (by 11%), and TRAIL-R4 (by 15%). An increase in the levels of anti-cancer cytokines was similar as observed for the ES-2 cells. All data were presented as a heat map (Figure 8b); selected cytokines which exhibited the largest differences between the treated cells and the control group were additionally shown on a column graph (Figure 8c).

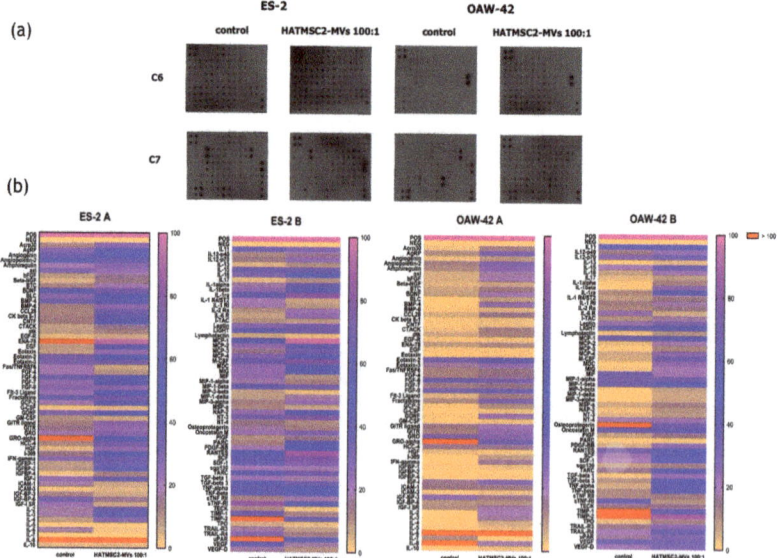

Figure 8. *Cont.*

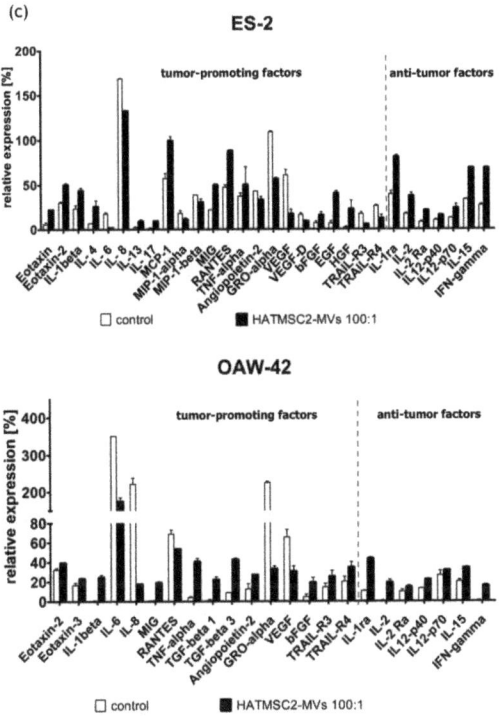

Figure 8. Effect of HATMSC2-MVs on the secretion profiles of ovarian cancer cell lines. (**a**) Scans of representative antibody arrays for ES-2 and OAW-42 supernatants. Untreated cells served as a control. The signal intensity for each antibody spot is proportional to the relative concentration of the antigen in the sample. (**b**) Heat map of cytokine levels for the ES-2 and OAW-42 supernatants; magenta and yellow indicate higher and lower expression limits, respectively. Outstanding values (above 100% of positive control) are depicted in red. Data are normalized to the internal positive control spots, which are consistent between the arrays and represent 100%. The data represent the mean from a duplicate assessment. (**c**) Column graph representing selected proteins (equal to or above 10% of the positive control). The data are presented as mean ± SEM values from a duplicate assessment. HATMSC2-MVs—microvesicles derived from immortalized human mesenchymal stem cells of adipose tissue origin.

3. Discussion

The paracrine activity of cells via EVs is an important link in cell-to-cell communication. Recent research has shown that EVs derived from MSCs play an important role in tumor microenvironment. Tumor cells secrete EVs to reprogram the mesenchymal stem cells present in the tumor microenvironment. The reprogrammed MSCs release exosomes that affect other cells in the tumor niche, such as fibroblasts, endothelial cells, and immune cells, inducing their pro-tumorigenic activity [17]. However, the effect of MVs derived from outside the tumor microenvironment, e.g., from the MSCs of adipose tissue origin, on cancer cells is not well understood and still debatable. The purpose of this study was to analyze the biological behavior of two histologically different ovarian cancer cell lines, ES-2 and OAW-42, in response to HATMSC2-MV treatment. In this study, we investigated whether MVs derived from human immortalized MSCs of adipose tissue origin may represent a new form of supportive therapy in ovarian cancer treatment. Flow cytometry and microscopic analysis confirmed the internalization of HATMSC2-MVs into target cells. Moreover, in all functional experiments, we used untouched MVs, but not the MVs lysate tested by different research groups [14]. We showed that treatment with HATMSC2-MVs gradually decreased the proliferation of ES-2 and OAW-42 cells, depending on the dose; however, a significant effect was observed on day 3, only for the OAW-42 cell line, when the highest ratio of HATMSC2-MVs of 100:1 (100 MVs per cell) was used. Similar results were obtained by Reza et al. [14], who reported an anti-proliferative and pro-apoptotic effect of ATMSC exosomes on ovarian cancer cells. The main mechanism involved in the action of the exosomes was the transfer of different miRNAs into the recipient cells. However, Reza et al. used protease or RNase-digested exosomes. The anti-proliferative activity of MVs derived from BM-MSCs was also confirmed in vitro on the SKOV3 cell line and in vivo through an intra-tumor injection of MVs into an established tumor generated by a subcutaneous injection of these cells into SCID mice [18]. On the other hand, Dong et al. [19] showed that EVs derived from MSCs isolated from the umbilical cord increased the proliferation of lung adenocarcinoma cells by transporting miR-410 to target cells.

Further experiments involving an analysis of cell cycle progression and cell death processes, such as apoptosis and necrosis, confirmed that HATMSC2-MV treatment affected cancer cell viability. The cell cycle analysis showed that treatment with HATMSC2-MVs, at the ratio of 100:1, significantly increased the percentage of cells of both cell lines in the sub-G1 phase compared to control; however, the increase of OAW-42 cells in the sub-G1 phase was significantly higher compared to the ES-2 cell line. The increased number of cells in the sub-G1 phase suggests that both ovarian cancer cell lines underwent cell death via apoptosis. A similar pro-apoptotic effect of the bioactive factors derived from MSCs isolated from human Wharton's jelly and applied in the form of a conditioned medium or Wharton's jelly-MSCs lysate was observed in a study on the OVCAR3 and SCOV3 ovarian cancer cell lines, confirming the anti-cancer properties of the MSC secretome [20]. The pro-apoptotic effect of HATMSC2-MVs on the examined ovarian cancer cell lines was also confirmed through flow cytometry analysis of cell death processes, distinguishing between apoptosis and necrosis. When HATMSC2-MVs were cultured with ovarian cancer cell lines at the ratio of 100:1, we observed a significant increase in the percentage of early and late apoptotic cells for the ES-2 cells, whereas in the OAW-42 cells, a substantial increase was observed for late apoptotic cells. Moreover, in both cells lines, HATMSC2-MVs significantly increased the percentage of necrotic cells. These results suggest that HATMSC2-MVs at a ratio of 100:1 induce mechanisms governing ovarian cancer cell death via both apoptosis and necrosis. Studies on the anti-cancer properties of the MSC secretome report that co-culture of MSCs of different tissue origin with ovarian cancer cell lines increases apoptosis with varying effects [21]. Interestingly, the percentage of apoptotic cells was higher when the supernatant derived from AT-MSCs was applied compared to the supernatants derived from BM-MSCs and UC-MSCs [21].

Additionally, we assessed the secretion profile of ovarian cancer cell lines and the effect of HATMSC2-MVs on the presence of the produced cytokines and trophic factors with different functions; one set of bioactive factors is known to promote cancer cells growth and metastasis, and the second set of cytokines is associated with anti-tumor properties. The differences in the secretion profiles of the examined ovarian cancer cell lines correlated with the histological type of the tumor. ES-2 cells were derived from clear cell carcinoma, with a good prognosis for the patient when diagnosed at an early stage of the disease and poor survival when diagnosed at an advanced stage, because this type of ovarian cancer is often more resistant to chemotherapy than serous cystadenocarcinoma, represented by the OAW-42 cell line [22]. The presence of cancer-promoting cytokines and chemokines, such as IL-6, IL-8, GRO-alpha, MIP-1α, MIP-1β, angiopoetin-2, and VEGF, which are associated with tumor growth, metastatic properties, and a poor prognosis, was detected in the supernatants collected from both ES-2 cells and OAW-42 cells. The application of HATMSC2-MVs resulted in a substantial decrease in IL-6, IL-8, GRO-alpha, and VEGF secretion in both cell lines. IL-8 is a pleiotropic chemokine with a dual function, which acts as a chemoattractant for neutrophils, inducing innate immune responses, whereas in the ovarian cancer environment, it contributes to the pro-survival activity of tumor cells and resistance to chemotherapy. A high production of IL-8 correlates with faster proliferation and increases the potential of angiogenesis, adhesion, and invasion of platinum sensitive (PEA1 and PEO14) and platinum resistant (PEA2 and PEO23) cell lines [23]. Browne et al. demonstrated a significant increase in the expression of IL-8 in specimens of the serous type of ovarian cancer compared to clear cancer ovarian carcinoma tissue [24]. The HATMSC2-MVs markedly inhibit IL-8 production in both examined cell lines in vitro. This effect can be used as a potential supportive therapy for ovarian cancer treatment. IL-6 was present in the OAW-42 culture supernatant at a very high level, in contrast to the ES-2 cells. It is well known that IL-6 plays a crucial role in the stimulation of inflammatory cytokine production, tumor angiogenesis, cell proliferation, and tumor macrophage infiltration [25]. A high production of IL-6 by ovarian cancer cells contributes to tumor progression and correlates with a poor prognosis [26]. The HATMSC2-MVs inhibit the activity of IL-6, and in conjunction with a decreased level of IL-8, may exert suppressive effects on the ovarian cancer cell line. GRO-alpha and VEGF were produced by ES-2 and OAW-42 cells; however, the GRO-alpha level markedly exceeded the VEGF level. Both growth factors, GRO-alpha and VEGF, are important for tumor growth and metastasis, especially in terms of supporting cancer angiogenesis. The diverse production of cytokines and growth factors by ovarian cancer cells is associated with the biological activity of cancer cells and may affect tumor progression, as reported in a study performed simultaneously on a set of 120 cytokines in ovarian cancer ascites [25]. Our study determined that HATMSC2-MVs substantially reduced the secretion of GRO-alpha and VEGF in both cell lines. Numerous growth factors and cytokines, including those assessed in our study, such as IL-6, IL-8, MCP-1, RANTES, GRO-alpha, and VEGF, are involved in promoting tumor growth and ovarian cancer cell aggressiveness. Therefore, characterizing cytokine secretion may provide information on the functional profile of cancer cells. This may help to create targeted therapy for ovarian cancer, in which angiogenesis is inhibited by a blockage of NF-κB, suppressing VEGF and IL-8 activity [27], or by targeting CXCR2, the key receptor for the GRO-alpha and IL-8 chemokine activity [28]. RANTES (CCL5) level decreased only in OAW-42 cells after the HATMSC2-MVs treatment. RANTES is involved in trafficking immune cells into the inflammation site and acts as a co-activator of T cells promoting the polarization of the immune response towards the Th1 profile. In the ovarian cancer microenvironment, RANTES acts through paracrine or autocrine signaling to promote tumor cell migration, invasion, and metastasis [29]. In contrast, MCP-1 was detected in supernatants collected from ES-2 cells, and its level increased after the HATMSC2-MV treatment. The main function of MCP-1 in the tumor microenvironment is to attract tumor-associated monocytes (TAMs) [30]. Research performed by Furukawa et al. [30] demonstrated that the MCP-1 chemokine promoted the invasion and adhesion of the ovarian cancer cell line SKOV3, contributing to the progression of tumors. Tumor necrosis factor-related apoptosis-inducing ligand (TRAIL)-R3 and –R4 are known as the negative regulators of TRAIL-mediated apoptosis in cancer cells [31–33]. The internalization of HATMSC2-MVs by the examined cell lines exerts a different effect on ovarian cancer cells, and decrease the level of TRAIL-R3 and TRAIL-R4 in ES-2 cells and increase their level in OAW-42 cell lines. The downregulation of TRAIL-R3 and TRAIL-R4 is associated with an increased level of early apoptotic cells in the ES-2 cell line treated with the 100:1 ratio. A very recent study, performed on a murine xenograft model, documented that the EVs isolated from the TRAIL expressing cell line 293T in combination with cyclin-dependent kinase inhibitor (dinaciclib) successfully inhibited the growth of human lung cancer cell lines NCI-H727 and A549 and the human breast adenocarcinoma cell line MDAMB231 by inducing apoptosis [34].

The HATMSC2-MVs used in this study affect both histologically different cell lines, the ES-2 cells and the OAW-42 cells, by increasing the production of tumor-suppressive cytokines, such as IL-1ra, IL-2, IL-2Ra, IL-12-p40, IL12-p70, IL-15, and IFN-γ. Studies that used bioactive factors released to the culture medium from Wharton's jelly MSCs led to a similar inhibition of the proliferation of the ovarian cancer cell line OVCAR3 through a decreased expression of oncogenic cytokines and growth factors and an increased expression of anti-tumor related cytokines [35]. The anti-inflammatory properties of IL-1ra, a naturally occurring inhibitor to IL-1, contribute to tumor growth inhibition by competitive binding to IL-1 receptors blocking cancer-promoting activity of IL-1 [36]. The anti-proliferative effect of ovarian cancer cell lines can be also supported by an increased production of IFN-γ following the exposure of cells to HATMSC2-MVs, as documented in both examined cell lines. It has been reported that IFN-α and IFN-γ, applied in combination with IL-4 fused to Pseudomonas exotoxin, inhibit tumor growth in an experimental mouse model of human ovarian cancer. The anti-tumor effect was accomplished by the activation of the IFN signaling pathways and the subsequent activation of molecules inducing apoptotic cell death [37]. Characterization of a wide range of tumor-promoting factors and anti-tumor cytokines after ovarian cancer cell expose to HATMSC2-MVs provides information on how they affect the production of functional cytokines and shed light on the mechanism altering the behavior of ovarian cancer cells in response to MV treatment.

Consequently, we characterized the ovarian cancer cell lines ES-2 and OAW-42 for the presence of CSC and MSC markers. The results showed that the ES-2 and OAW-42 cells were positive for CD44 and negative for CD133, and that the application of HATMSC2-MVs had no effect on the expression of these markers. Similar results were reported by Tudrej et al., who showed that CD44 expression was higher for ES-2 cells compared to OAW-42 cell lines [38]. They found a small subpopulation of ES-2 cells positive for the CD133 marker expression (around 0.2%). However, we did not observe any CD133 positive cells in our study. To our best knowledge, the expression of specific MSC markers on ovarian cancer cell lines has been studied in the form of a single MSC marker as a potential therapeutic target [39–42], whereas a complete analysis of MSC markers has been performed in a limited number of studies concerning the biological activity of ovarian cancer cell lines [21]. Our results revealed that both ES-2 and OAW-42 cells were strongly positive for CD73, and that HATMSC2-MVs had no impact on CD73 expression. CD73, also known as cell surface nucleotidase, is an immunosuppressive enzyme involved in tumor progression and metastasis, and its expression is associated with a poor prognosis for high-grade serous ovarian cancer [42]. The functional inhibition of CD73 via either a chemical compound or a neutralizing antibody reduced the tumorigenesis of primary high-grade serous epithelial ovarian cancer cells [41]. In contrast, CD90 was present on a limited population of both examined cell lines, and co-culture of ES-2 and OAW-42 cells with HATMSC2-MVs at a ratio of 1:10 did not increase the expression of this marker. It was reported previously that the overexpression of CD90 inhibited the sphere-forming ability of SKOV3 cell lines and increased cell apoptosis. These studies also suggest that CD90 may decrease cell growth through a downregulation of the expression of other CSC markers, including CD133 and CD24 [40]. Interestingly, the CD105 molecule was detected only on poorly-differentiated ES-2 cells, but not on the better-differentiated OAW-42 cells. This finding confirmed the mesenchymal phenotype of ES-2 cells, which is associated with increased aggressiveness and metastatic potential. The HATMSC2-MVs have no marked impact on CD105 expression in either of the cell lines. Studies on the biological role of CD105 in ovarian cancer revealed that high CD105, CD44, or CD106 expression was associated with drug resistance, an advanced stage of the disease, poor differentiation, and high rate of cancer relapse [43]. The downregulation of CD105 expression with a clinically relevant CD105-neutralizing mAb (TRC105) inhibited high-grade serous cancer metastasis, reduced ascites, and hampered the growth of abdominal tumor nodules in animal models of ovarian cancer [39].

A systematic review, introducing the impact of experimental anti-tumor cellular therapies involving MSCs of different human tissue origin, also highlights the possibility to use MSC secretome, in the form of a conditioned medium or EVs, as a cell-free therapy to inhibit cancer growth [44]. Thus, MVs may serve as a carrier for the delivery of therapeutic agents to target cells. A modification of primary MSCs for the secretion of inhibitory growth factors and pro-apoptotic factors may be employed to prepare the MVs carrying the pro-apoptotic signal and transport them to target ovarian cancer cells. Thus, MVs may be applied as a supportive therapy to enhance the therapeutic effect of chemotherapy, especially for multidrug resistant cancers.

In conclusion, we confirmed an effective transfer of HATMSC2-MVs into target ovarian cancer cells, which affected the biological behavior of these cells. Our results revealed that HATMSC2-MVs inhibit tumor cell proliferation in the two histologically distinct ovarian cancer cell lines via different pathways, apoptosis and/or necrosis. This phenomenon, with high likelihood, is related to the secretion of the different anti-tumor factors by the ES-2 (representing poorly differentiated ovarian clear cell carcinoma), and OAW-42 (representing ovarian cystadenocarcinoma) cell lines treated with HATMSC2-MVs. However, further studies are needed to determine the possible mechanisms involved in HATMSC2-MV-mediated effect on target cells, as well as to validate their anti-tumorigenic potential with respect to cancer cells isolated from human tissues. Therefore, understanding the mechanisms involved in the bilateral interaction between the MVs and ovarian cancer cells may be help to design new treatment modalities for an effective anti-tumor cell-free therapy.

4. Materials and Methods

4.1. Cell Culture

The ES-2 cell line was purchased from ATCC (American Type Culture Collection, Manassas, VA, USA) (catalog number: CRL-1978™). The cells were cultured in the DMEM and OptiMEM GlutaMax media, mixed in equal proportions. The DMEM medium was supplemented with 10% FBS (Gibco, Thermo Scientific, Carlsbad, CA, USA), a 1% penicillin/streptomycin solution (Gibco, Thermo Scientific, Carlsbad, CA, USA) and L-glutamine (Gibco, Thermo Scientific, Carlsbad, CA, USA). The OptiMEM GlutaMax medium was supplemented with 3% FBS (Gibco, Thermo Scientific, Carlsbad, CA, USA) and a 1% penicillin/streptomycin solution (Gibco, Thermo Scientific, Carlsbad, CA, USA).

The OAW-42 cell line was purchased from ECACC (European Collection of Authenticated Cell Cultures, Salisbury, United Kingdom) (catalog number: 85073102). The cells were cultured in the same media conditions, mixed in equal proportions, and additionally supplemented with a 10 µg/mL insulin solution (Sigma-Aldrich, St. Louis, MO, USA).

All cells were cultured in standard conditions (21% O_2, 5% CO_2, 95% humidity, 37 °C temperature). Upon reaching 70–80% confluence, the cells were harvested with a 0.05% trypsin/0.02% EDTA (*w/v*) solution (IIET, Wroclaw, Poland) and seeded onto new culture flasks.

The human mesenchymal stem cell line HATMSC2 was established in our laboratory using the hTERT and pSV402 plasmids, as described in a previous study [16].

4.2. MV Isolation Using Sequential Centrifugation

MVs were isolated according to the well-established protocol developed in our laboratory [45] based on the procedure introduced in the previous study [46]. HATMSC2 cells were cultured in multi-layer cell culture flasks (Nunc TripleFlasks, Thermo Scientific, Carlsbad, CA, USA) using DMEM + 10% FBS until they reached 75% confluence. Next, the cells were cultured in serum-free media in hypoxic conditions (1% O_2) for 48 h to enhance the release of MVs. The conditioned media collected from the HATMSC2 cultures were mixed to obtain a homogenous starting material before the isolation of MVs. In the next step, the conditioned media were centrifuged at 300× *g* for 10 min at 4 °C, and at 2000× *g* for 10 min at 4 °C, in order to remove cellular debris and apoptotic bodies. Subsequently, the supernatants were subjected to double centrifugation at 12,000× *g* for 30 min at 4 °C using a Sorvall LYNX 6000 ultracentrifuge (Thermo Scientific, Carlsbad, CA, USA) with an intermediate washing step in PBS (IIET, Wroclaw, Poland). The obtained MV pellets were resuspended in 150 µL of PBS and stored at −80 °C.

4.3. Analysis of MVs

The size distribution of MVs was measured with DLS (Malvern Zetasizer, Malvern, UK). The measurement was performed for 2 min at 25 °C. PBS was used to disperse the samples. Moreover, to confirm the size of the MVs, the samples were analyzed using transmission electron microscopy (TEM). The PBS-suspended MVs were placed on a carbon-coated copper grid (400 mesh) and incubated for 1 min, and the excess liquid was removed with filter paper. Next, the samples were stained with 2% uranyl acetate, dried, and examined with a transmission electron microscope (JEOL, Peabody, MA, USA) at 80 kV. The number of MVs was calculated using a BD Fortessa Flow Cytometer (BD Biosciences,

San Jose, CA, USA) and fluorescent counting beads (CountBright™ Absolute Counting Beads for flow cytometry, Thermo Scientific, Carlsbad, CA, USA). Prior to analysis, 10 µL of the MV sample was diluted in PBS to a final volume of 300 µL, after which 50 µL of counting beads were added. The threshold for the forward scatter (FSC) was set at 200. To determine the number of MVs in the samples, 5000 counting beads were collected using a BD Fortessa Flow Cytometer (BD Biosciences, San Jose, CA, USA). The data were analyzed using the BD FACSDiva Software (BD Biosciences, San Jose, CA, USA). The number of MVs was calculated according to the CountBright™ Absolute Counting Beads manufacturer's instructions, using the ratio of MV events and the number of counting bead events. The protein concentration of MVs was determined with a Bradford assay (Thermo Scientific, Carlsbad, CA, USA) according to the vendor's instructions. The MV samples or the BSA standard were briefly incubated with the Bradford reagent for 5 min on a 96-well plate. The absorbance was measured with a Synergy H4 plate reader (Biotek, Winooski, VT, USA) at 595 nm.

4.4. Flow Cytometry Analysis of HATMSC2 Cells and HATMSC2-MVs

HATMSC2 cells were detached using the trypsin/EDTA solution and incubated with PE-conjugated antibodies specific for the human CD73 (clone AD2), CD90 (clone 5E10), CD105 (clone 266), HLA ABC (clone G46-2.6), HLA DR (clone G46-6) (BD Biosciences, San Jose, CA, USA), and FITC-conjugated CD45 antibody (clone 2D1) (BD Biosciences, San Jose, CA, USA) and with the appropriate isotype controls (BD Biosciences, San Jose, CA, USA) for 30 min at 4 °C. Afterwards, the labeled cells were washed with PBS (IIET, Wroclaw, Poland) and analyzed using a FACSCalibur flow cytometer (BD Biosciences, San Jose, CA, USA). The obtained data were processed using the CellQuest software (BD Biosciences, San Jose, CA, USA). The histograms were created using Flowing Software 2. The surface markers of the MVs were analyzed using a BD Fortessa Flow Cytometer (BD Biosciences, San Jose, CA, USA) after staining with specific fluorophore-conjugated antibodies. MVs suspended in PBS were incubated with PE-conjugated antibodies specific for human CD73, CD90, and CD105, HLA ABC, HLA DR, and FITC-conjugated antibody for CD45 and with the appropriate isotype controls for 30 min at 4 °C. The percentage of positive MVs was calculated using the BD FACSDiva Software (BD Biosciences, San Jose, CA, USA).

4.5. Internalization of MVs

ES-2 and OAW-42 cells were seeded into a Lab-Tek II Chambered # 1.5 Coverglass system (Nalge Nunc International, Naperville, IL, USA) at a density of 15×10^3 cells per chamber. Fluorescence staining of the MVs was performed, as established in our recent study [45]. After washing with PBS, the MVs were resuspended in the DMEM + 10% FBS and OptiMEM GlutaMax + 3% FBS media (mixed in equal proportions), and added to the cells at a ratio of 5:1 (5 MVs per cell) and 10:1 (10 MVs per cell). The cells were incubated with MVs for 24 h and washed twice with PBS prior to imaging. The internalization of the MVs into target cells was immediately analyzed at 37 °C using an Axio Observer inverted microscope equipped with a dry 63x objective (Zeiss, Gottingen, Germany). The labeled MVs were detected using an EGFP Filter set. Thirty Z-sections with a 0.6-µm interval were recorded simultaneously in the brightfield and fluorescence channel. Optical orthogonal sectioning was performed in order to visualize the internalization of the MVs. Images were obtained and processed using the Zen Blue Software (Zeiss, Gottingen, Germany). A similar analysis of EV internalization using fluorescence microscopy was previously described by Adamiak et. al. [47]. After 24 h of incubation with MVs, the cells were washed once with PBS, detached using the trypsin/EDTA solution, washed once more with PBS, and analyzed using flow cytometry with FACSCalibur (BD Biosciences, San Jose, CA, USA). The cells were detected using the FL1 channel (480 nm). The histograms were created using Flowing Software 2 (Perttu Terho, Turku Centre for Biotechnology, Finland).

4.6. Proliferation Activity

The proliferation activity of ES-2 and OAW-42 treated with HATMSC2-MVs was measured using the MTT assay. The cells were seeded on a 96-well plate at a concentration of 2×10^3 cells/well in the DMEM + 10% FBS and OptiMEM GlutaMax + 3% FBS media (mixed in equal proportions); MVs at a ratio of 1:1 (1 MV per cell), 5:1 (5 MVs per cell), 10:1 (10 MVs per cell), and 100:1 (100 MVs per cell) were added to the cells. ES-2 and OAW-42 cells without MVs were used as a control. After 4 h, 24 h, 48 h, and 72 h, the absorbance of the formazan dye produced by living cells was measured using a Wallac 1420 Victor2 Microplate Reader (Perkin Elmer, Waltham, MA, USA) at 570 nm. After 72 h of co-incubation with HATMSC2-MVs, the ovarian cancer cells were stained using Calcein AM (Thermo Fisher, Carlsbad, USA). 100 µL of Calcein AM (1 µM solution) were added to each well. The cells were incubated for 15 min at room temperature. Images were obtained using an Axio Observer inverted microscope equipped with a dry 10x objective (Zeiss, Gottingen, Germany). The labeled cells were detected using an Alexa Fluor 488 Filter set. The images were processed with the Zen Blue software (Zeiss, Gottingen, Germany).

4.7. Cell Cycle Analysis

The cell cycle analysis was performed based on previously published method [20,48]. The cells were seeded on 24-well plates at a concentration of 12×10^3 in the DMEM + 10% FBS and OptiMEM GlutaMax + 3% FBS media (mixed in equal proportions). MVs at a ratio of 1:1 (1 MV per cell), 5:1 (5 MVs per cell), 10:1 (10 MVs per cell), and 100:1 (100 MVs per cell) were added to the cells. ES-2 and OAW-42 cells without MVs were used as a control. After 72 h, the cells were detached using the trypsin/EDTA solution; the conditioned media were also collected and mixed with the respective cell suspension samples. The samples were centrifuged at 1400 rpm for 4 min at 4 °C. After the supernatant was removed, the cells were resuspended in ice-cold 70% ethanol and incubated for 30 min on ice at 4 °C. Afterwards, PBS Ca^{2+} Mg^{2+} + 2.5% FBS was added to the cells, and the samples were centrifuged at 1400 rpm for 5 min. This step was repeated twice. The cells were then resuspended in a solution of propidium iodide in PBS (50 µg/mL) and RNase (20 µg/mL) and incubated overnight at 4 °C. The cells were analyzed using a FACSCalibur flow cytometer (BD Biosciences, San Jose, CA, USA). The obtained data were analyzed using Flowing Software 2 (Perttu Terho, Turku Centre for Biotechnology, Finland).

4.8. Cell Viability and Apoptosis Analysis Using Flow Cytometry

In order to determine the effect of HATMSC2-MVs on the viability of the cells, an Annexin V Apoptosis Detection Kit (Thermo Scientific, Carlsbad, CA, USA) was used. ES-2 and OAW-42 cells were seeded in a 24-well plate at a density of 25×10^3 in the DMEM + 10% FBS and OptiMEM GlutaMax + 3% FBS media (mixed in equal proportions). Before the analysis, the cells were treated with MVs at a ratio of 1:1 (1 MV per cell), 5:1 (5 MVs per cell), 10:1 (10 MVs per cell), and 100:1 (100 MVs per cell) for 72 h. ES-2 and OAW-42 cells without MVs were used as a negative control. After incubation with MVs, the cells were stained with Annexin V and propidium iodide according to the manufacturer's recommendations. The cells were analyzed for live (Annexin V negative and propidium iodide negative), early apoptotic (Annexin V positive and propidium iodide negative), late apoptotic (Annexin V positive and propidium iodide positive), and necrotic cells (Annexin V negative and propidium iodide positive) using a FACSCalibur flow cytometer (BD Biosciences, San Jose, CA, USA). The analysis was performed using Flowing Software 2 (Perttu Terho, Turku Centre for Biotechnology, Finland).

4.9. Flow Cytometry Analysis of Ovarian Cancer Cell Lines

In order to determine the effect of HATMSC2-MVs on the phenotype of ovarian cancer cell lines, flow cytometry analysis was performed. ES-2 and OAW-42 cells were treated for 72 h with MVs at a ratio of 10:1. ES-2 and OAW-42 cells were seeded in a 6-well plate at a density of 6×10^4 per well in the DMEM + 10% FBS and OptiMEM GlutaMax + 3% FBS media (mixed in equal proportions). MVs were added to the cells at a ratio of 10:1. ES-2 and OAW-42 cells without MVs were used as a control. After 72 h, the cells were washed with PBS, and the culture medium was replaced with DMEM without FBS. Following a subsequent 24 h of culture in DMEM without FBS, the cells were detached using the trypsin/EDTA solution and incubated with PE-conjugated antibodies specific for the human CD34 (clone 8G12), CD44 (clone 515), CD133 (clone W6B3C1), CD73 (clone AD2), CD90 (clone 5E10), and CD105 (clone 266) molecules and the PerCP-Cy5.5—SSEA4 antibody (clone MC813-70) (all from BD Biosciences, San Jose, CA, USA) and with the appropriate isotype controls (BD Biosciences, San Jose, CA, USA) for 30 min at 4 °C. Afterwards, the labeled cells were washed with PBS (IIET, Wroclaw, Poland) and analyzed using a FACSCalibur flow cytometer (BD Biosciences, San Jose, CA, USA). The obtained data were processed using the CellQuest software (BD Biosciences, San Jose, CA, USA). The histograms were created using Flowing Software 2 (Perttu Terho, Turku Centre for Biotechnology, Finland).

4.10. Secretion Profiles of Ovarian Cancer Cell Lines

In order to determine the effect of HATMSC2-MVs on the secretion profiles of ovarian cancer cell lines, a C-Series Human Cytokine Antibody Array C1000 (RayBio®, Norcross, GA, USA) was used. ES-2 and OAW-42 cells were seeded in a 6-well plate at a density of 6×10^4 per well in the DMEM + 10% FBS and OptiMEM GlutaMax + 3% FBS media (mixed in equal proportions). MVs were added to the cells at a ratio of 100:1. The ES-2 and OAW-42 cells without MVs were used as a control. After 72 h, the cells were washed with PBS, and the culture medium was replaced with DMEM without FBS. Following the subsequent 24 h of culture in DMEM without FBS, the conditioned medium was collected and centrifuged for 10 min at $300 \times g$ to remove cellular debris, and the cells were used for flow cytometry analysis (see 4.9. Briefly, 2 mL of blocking buffer were applied onto the membrane and incubated for 30 min at room temperature. Next, 2 mL of the supernatant collected from the control and treated cells were incubated with the membrane overnight at 4 °C. Following a series of washes, a biotinylated antibody cocktail was applied onto the membrane and incubated for 2 h at room temperature. Unbound antibodies were removed with a series of washes, and the membrane was placed in HRP-streptavidin and incubated for 2 h at room temperature. Following a third series of washes, chemiluminescence was detected, and the bound proteins were visualized using an X-ray film. Signal intensities were compared using the ImageJ software (MosaicJ, Philippe Thevenaz): relative differences in the expression levels of each analyzed sample were measured and normalized to the intensities of the positive control using the Protein Array Analyzer plugin. The obtained data were analyzed automatically using the Microsoft® Excel-based Analysis Software Tool for Human Cytokine Antibody Array C1000. The results were calculated as a percentage of expression, with positive control set to 100% and negative control set to 0% (relative expression). The threshold was set to 10%. All results equal to or above 10% were considered as real expression.

4.11. Statistical Analysis

All statistical analyses were performed using GraphPad Prism version 7 (GraphPad Software Inc., San Diego, CA, USA). The data were compared using the one-way ANOVA test with Dunnett's multiple comparison. All results are presented as mean ± SEM values.

Author Contributions: Conceptualization, A.K. (Aleksandra Klimczak) and A.S.; methodology, A.S., A.B.-P., A.K. (Agnieszka Krawczenko), M.P., O.D. and A.K. (Aleksandra Klimczak); formal analysis, A.S., A.B.-P. and A.K. (Aleksandra Klimczak); investigation, A.S., A.B.-P., A.K. (Agnieszka Krawczenko) and O.D.; data curation, A.S., A.B.-P. and A.K. (Aleksandra Klimczak); visualization, A.S. and O.D.; supervision, A.K. (Aleksandra Klimczak); funding acquisition, A.K. (Aleksandra Klimczak); writing—original draft preparation, A.S. and A.B.-P.; writing—review and editing, A.K. (Aleksandra Klimczak). All authors have read and agreed to the published version of the manuscript.

Funding: This research was funded with the internal funds of the Hirszfeld Institute of Immunology and Experimental Therapy PAS in Poland. No. 501-20.

Acknowledgments: The authors are grateful to Sylwia Nowak and Krzysztof Pawlik from the Hirszfeld Institute of Immunology and Experimental Therapy, Polish Academy of Sciences, for their support in analyzing the MVs using transmission electron microscopy.

Conflicts of Interest: The authors declare no conflict of interest.

Abbreviations

ATMSC	Adipose tissue-derived mesenchymal stem cell
BM-MSC	Bone marrow -derived mesenchymal stem cell
CSC	Cancer stem cells
DMEM	Dulbecco's modified Eagle's medium
EGF	Epidermal growth factor
FBS	Fetal bovine serum
FGF	Fibroblast growth factor
FITC	Fluorescein isothiocyanate
GRO	Growth- regulated oncogene, CXCL1 chemokine
HATMSC	Human adipose tissue mesenchymal stem cell line
IL	Interleukin
MCP-1	Macrophage chemoattractant protein-1, CCL2 chemokine
MVs	Microvesicles
MTT	(3-(4,5-Dimetylthiazol-2-yl)-2,5-Diphenyltetrazolium Bromide
PE	Phycoerythrin
RANTES	Regulated on Activation, Normal T Cell Expressed and Secreted, CCL5 chemokine
SSEA4	Stage Specific Embryonic Antigen 4
UC-MSC	Umbilical cord -derived mesenchymal stem cell
VEGF	Vascular endothelial growth factor

References

1. Al-Alem, L.F.; Pandya, U.M.; Baker, A.T.; Bellio, C.; Zarrella, B.D.; Clark, J.; DiGloria, C.M.; Rueda, B.R. Ovarian cancer stem cells: What progress have we made? *Int. J. Biochem. Cell Biol.* **2019**, *107*, 92–103. [CrossRef] [PubMed]
2. Cortez, A.J.; Tudrej, P.; Kujawa, K.A.; Lisowska, K.M. Advances in ovarian cancer therapy. *Cancer Chemother. Pharmacol.* **2018**, *81*, 17–38. [CrossRef] [PubMed]
3. Bregenzer, M.E.; Horst, E.N.; Mehta, P.; Novak, C.M.; Repetto, T.; Mehta, G. The Role of Cancer Stem Cells and Mechanical Forces in Ovarian Cancer Metastasis. *Cancers* **2019**, *11*, 1008. [CrossRef] [PubMed]
4. Keating, A. Mesenchymal stromal cells. *Curr. Opin. Hematol.* **2006**, *13*, 419–425. [CrossRef] [PubMed]
5. Klimczak, A.; Kozlowska, U. Mesenchymal Stromal Cells and Tissue-Specific Progenitor Cells: Their Role in Tissue Homeostasis. *Stem Cells Int.* **2016**, *2016*, 4285215. [CrossRef] [PubMed]
6. Kozlowska, U.; Krawczenko, A.; Futoma, K.; Jurek, T.; Rorat, M.; Patrzalek, D.; Klimczak, A. Similarities and differences between mesenchymal stem/progenitor cells derived from various human tissues. *World J. Stem Cells* **2019**, *11*, 347–374. [CrossRef]
7. Hass, R.; Kasper, C.; Bohm, S.; Jacobs, R. Different populations and sources of human mesenchymal stem cells (MSC): A comparison of adult and neonatal tissue-derived MSC. *Cell Commun. Signal.* **2011**, *9*, 12. [CrossRef]
8. Varderidou-Minasian, S.; Lorenowicz, M.J. Mesenchymal stromal/stem cell-derived extracellular vesicles in tissue repair: Challenges and opportunities. *Theranostics* **2020**, *10*, 5979–5997. [CrossRef]
9. Camussi, G.; Deregibus, M.C.; Bruno, S.; Cantaluppi, V.; Biancone, L. Exosomes/microvesicles as a mechanism of cell-to-cell communication. *Kidney Int.* **2010**, *78*, 838–848. [CrossRef]
10. Nawaz, M.; Fatima, F.; Vallabhaneni, K.C.; Penfornis, P.; Valadi, H.; Ekstrom, K.; Kholia, S.; Whitt, J.D.; Fernandes, J.D.; Pochampally, R.; et al. Extracellular Vesicles: Evolving Factors in Stem Cell Biology. *Stem Cells Int.* **2016**, *2016*, 1073140. [CrossRef]
11. Bobis-Wozowicz, S.; Kmiotek, K.; Sekula, M.; Kedracka-Krok, S.; Kamycka, E.; Adamiak, M.; Jankowska, U.; Madetko-Talowska, A.; Sarna, M.; Bik-Multanowski, M.; et al. Human Induced Pluripotent Stem Cell-Derived Microvesicles Transmit RNAs and Proteins to Recipient Mature Heart Cells Modulating Cell Fate and Behavior. *Stem Cells* **2015**, *33*, 2748–2761. [CrossRef] [PubMed]

12. Albini, A.; Sporn, M.B. The tumour microenvironment as a target for chemoprevention. *Nat. Rev. Cancer* **2007**, *7*, 139–147. [CrossRef] [PubMed]
13. Du, T.; Ju, G.; Wu, S.; Cheng, Z.; Cheng, J.; Zou, X.; Zhang, G.; Miao, S.; Liu, G.; Zhu, Y. Microvesicles derived from human Wharton's jelly mesenchymal stem cells promote human renal cancer cell growth and aggressiveness through induction of hepatocyte growth factor. *PLoS ONE* **2014**, *9*, e96836. [CrossRef] [PubMed]
14. Reza, A.; Choi, Y.J.; Yasuda, H.; Kim, J.H. Human adipose mesenchymal stem cell-derived exosomal-miRNAs are critical factors for inducing anti-proliferation signalling to A2780 and SKOV-3 ovarian cancer cells. *Sci. Rep.* **2016**, *6*, 38498. [CrossRef]
15. Lindoso, R.S.; Collino, F.; Vieyra, A. Extracellular vesicles as regulators of tumor fate: Crosstalk among cancer stem cells, tumor cells and mesenchymal stem cells. *Stem Cell Investig.* **2017**, *4*, 75. [CrossRef]
16. Kraskiewicz, H.; Paprocka, M.; Bielawska-Pohl, A.; Krawczenko, A.; Panek, K.; Kaczynska, J.; Szyposzynska, A.; Psurski, M.; Kuropka, P.; Klimczak, A. Can supernatant from immortalized adipose tissue MSC replace cell therapy? An in vitro study in chronic wounds model. *Stem Cell Res. Ther.* **2020**, *11*, 29. [CrossRef]
17. Whiteside, T.L. Exosome and mesenchymal stem cell cross-talk in the tumor microenvironment. *Semin. Immunol.* **2018**, *35*, 69–79. [CrossRef]
18. Bruno, S.; Collino, F.; Deregibus, M.C.; Grange, C.; Tetta, C.; Camussi, G. Microvesicles derived from human bone marrow mesenchymal stem cells inhibit tumor growth. *Stem Cells Dev.* **2013**, *22*, 758–771. [CrossRef]
19. Dong, L.; Pu, Y.; Zhang, L.; Qi, Q.; Xu, L.; Li, W.; Wei, C.; Wang, X.; Zhou, S.; Zhu, J.; et al. Human umbilical cord mesenchymal stem cell-derived extracellular vesicles promote lung adenocarcinoma growth by transferring miR-410. *Cell Death Dis.* **2018**, *9*, 218. [CrossRef]
20. Kalamegam, G.; Sait, K.H.W.; Ahmed, F.; Kadam, R.; Pushparaj, P.N.; Anfinan, N.; Rasool, M.; Jamal, M.S.; Abu-Elmagd, M.; Al-Qahtani, M. Human Wharton's Jelly Stem Cell (hWJSC) Extracts Inhibit Ovarian Cancer Cell Lines OVCAR3 and SKOV3 in vitro by Inducing Cell Cycle Arrest and Apoptosis. *Front. Oncol.* **2018**, *8*, 592. [CrossRef]
21. Khalil, C.; Moussa, M.; Azar, A.; Tawk, J.; Habbouche, J.; Salameh, R.; Ibrahim, A.; Alaaeddine, N. Anti-proliferative effects of mesenchymal stem cells (MSCs) derived from multiple sources on ovarian cancer cell lines: An in-vitro experimental study. *J. Ovarian Res.* **2019**, *12*, 70. [CrossRef] [PubMed]
22. Lisio, M.A.; Fu, L.; Goyeneche, A.; Gao, Z.H.; Telleria, C. High-Grade Serous Ovarian Cancer: Basic Sciences, Clinical and Therapeutic Standpoints. *Int. J. Mol. Sci.* **2019**, *20*, 952. [CrossRef] [PubMed]
23. Stronach, E.A.; Cunnea, P.; Turner, C.; Guney, T.; Aiyappa, R.; Jeyapalan, S.; de Sousa, C.H.; Browne, A.; Magdy, N.; Studd, J.B.; et al. The role of interleukin-8 (IL-8) and IL-8 receptors in platinum response in high grade serous ovarian carcinoma. *Oncotarget* **2015**, *6*, 31593–31603. [CrossRef]
24. Browne, A.; Sriraksa, R.; Guney, T.; Rama, N.; Van Noorden, S.; Curry, E.; Gabra, H.; Stronach, E.; El-Bahrawy, M. Differential expression of IL-8 and IL-8 receptors in benign, borderline and malignant ovarian epithelial tumours. *Cytokine* **2013**, *64*, 413–421. [CrossRef] [PubMed]
25. Matte, I.; Lane, D.; Laplante, C.; Rancourt, C.; Piche, A. Profiling of cytokines in human epithelial ovarian cancer ascites. *Am. J. Cancer Res.* **2012**, *2*, 566–580. [PubMed]
26. Coward, J.; Kulbe, H.; Chakravarty, P.; Leader, D.; Vassileva, V.; Leinster, D.A.; Thompson, R.; Schioppa, T.; Nemeth, J.; Vermeulen, J.; et al. Interleukin-6 as a therapeutic target in human ovarian cancer. *Clin. Cancer Res.* **2011**, *17*, 6083–6096. [CrossRef]
27. Huang, S.; Robinson, J.B.; Deguzman, A.; Bucana, C.D.; Fidler, I.J. Blockade of nuclear factor-kappaB signaling inhibits angiogenesis and tumorigenicity of human ovarian cancer cells by suppressing expression of vascular endothelial growth factor and interleukin 8. *Cancer Res.* **2000**, *60*, 5334–5339.
28. Yung, M.M.; Tang, H.W.; Cai, P.C.; Leung, T.H.; Ngu, S.F.; Chan, K.K.; Xu, D.; Yang, H.; Ngan, H.Y.; Chan, D.W. GRO-alpha and IL-8 enhance ovarian cancer metastatic potential via the CXCR2-mediated TAK1/NFkappaB signaling cascade. *Theranostics* **2018**, *8*, 1270–1285. [CrossRef]
29. Long, H.; Xie, R.; Xiang, T.; Zhao, Z.; Lin, S.; Liang, Z.; Chen, Z.; Zhu, B. Autocrine CCL5 signaling promotes invasion and migration of CD133+ ovarian cancer stem-like cells via NF-kappaB-mediated MMP-9 upregulation. *Stem Cells* **2012**, *30*, 2309–2319. [CrossRef]

30. Furukawa, S.; Soeda, S.; Kiko, Y.; Suzuki, O.; Hashimoto, Y.; Watanabe, T.; Nishiyama, H.; Tasaki, K.; Hojo, H.; Abe, M.; et al. MCP-1 promotes invasion and adhesion of human ovarian cancer cells. *Anticancer Res.* **2013**, *33*, 4785–4790.
31. Heilmann, T.; Vondung, F.; Borzikowsky, C.; Szymczak, S.; Kruger, S.; Alkatout, I.; Wenners, A.; Bauer, M.; Klapper, W.; Rocken, C.; et al. Heterogeneous intracellular TRAIL-receptor distribution predicts poor outcome in breast cancer patients. *J. Mol. Med.* **2019**, *97*, 1155–1167. [CrossRef] [PubMed]
32. Abdollahi, T. Potential for TRAIL as a therapeutic agent in ovarian cancer. *Vitam. Horm.* **2004**, *67*, 347–364. [PubMed]
33. Braga Lda, C.; Alvares da Silva Ramos, A.P.; Traiman, P.; Silva, L.M.; Lopes da Silva-Filho, A. TRAIL-R3-related apoptosis: Epigenetic and expression analyses in women with ovarian neoplasia. *Gynecol. Oncol.* **2012**, *126*, 268–273. [CrossRef] [PubMed]
34. Ke, C.; Hou, H.; Li, J.; Su, K.; Huang, C.; Lin, Y.; Lu, Z.; Du, Z.; Tan, W.; Yuan, Z. Extracellular Vesicle Delivery of TRAIL Eradicates Resistant Tumor Growth in Combination with CDK Inhibition by Dinaciclib. *Cancers* **2020**, *12*, 1157. [CrossRef]
35. Kalamegam, G.; Sait, K.H.W.; Anfinan, N.; Kadam, R.; Ahmed, F.; Rasool, M.; Naseer, M.I.; Pushparaj, P.N.; Al-Qahtani, M. Cytokines secreted by human Wharton's jelly stem cells inhibit the proliferation of ovarian cancer (OVCAR3) cells in vitro. *Oncol. Lett.* **2019**, *17*, 4521–4531. [CrossRef]
36. Lewis, A.M.; Varghese, S.; Xu, H.; Alexander, H.R. Interleukin-1 and cancer progression: The emerging role of interleukin-1 receptor antagonist as a novel therapeutic agent in cancer treatment. *J. Transl. Med.* **2006**, *4*, 48. [CrossRef]
37. Green, D.S.; Husain, S.R.; Johnson, C.L.; Sato, Y.; Han, J.; Joshi, B.; Hewitt, S.M.; Puri, R.K.; Zoon, K.C. Combination immunotherapy with IL-4 Pseudomonas exotoxin and IFN-alpha and IFN-gamma mediate antitumor effects in vitro and in a mouse model of human ovarian cancer. *Immunotherapy* **2019**, *11*, 483–496. [CrossRef]
38. Tudrej, P.; Olbryt, M.; Zembala-Nozynska, E.; Kujawa, K.A.; Cortez, A.J.; Fiszer-Kierzkowska, A.; Piglowski, W.; Nikiel, B.; Glowala-Kosinska, M.; Bartkowska-Chrobok, A.; et al. Establishment and Characterization of the Novel High-Grade Serous Ovarian Cancer Cell Line OVPA8. *Int. J. Mol. Sci.* **2018**, *19*, 2080. [CrossRef]
39. Bai, S.; Zhu, W.; Coffman, L.; Vlad, A.; Schwartz, L.E.; Elishaev, E.; Drapkin, R.; Buckanovich, R.J. CD105 Is Expressed in Ovarian Cancer Precursor Lesions and Is Required for Metastasis to the Ovary. *Cancers* **2019**, *11*, 1710. [CrossRef]
40. Chen, W.C.; Hsu, H.P.; Li, C.Y.; Yang, Y.J.; Hung, Y.H.; Cho, C.Y.; Wang, C.Y.; Weng, T.Y.; Lai, M.D. Cancer stem cell marker CD90 inhibits ovarian cancer formation via beta3 integrin. *Int. J. Oncol.* **2016**, *49*, 1881–1889. [CrossRef]
41. Lupia, M.; Angiolini, F.; Bertalot, G.; Freddi, S.; Sachsenmeier, K.F.; Chisci, E.; Kutryb-Zajac, B.; Confalonieri, S.; Smolenski, R.T.; Giovannoni, R.; et al. CD73 Regulates Stemness and Epithelial-Mesenchymal Transition in Ovarian Cancer-Initiating Cells. *Stem Cell Rep.* **2018**, *10*, 1412–1425. [CrossRef] [PubMed]
42. Turcotte, M.; Spring, K.; Pommey, S.; Chouinard, G.; Cousineau, I.; George, J.; Chen, G.M.; Gendoo, D.M.; Haibe-Kains, B.; Karn, T.; et al. CD73 is associated with poor prognosis in high-grade serous ovarian cancer. *Cancer Res.* **2015**, *75*, 4494–4503. [CrossRef] [PubMed]
43. Zhang, J.; Yuan, B.; Zhang, H.; Li, H. Human epithelial ovarian cancer cells expressing CD105, CD44 and CD106 surface markers exhibit increased invasive capacity and drug resistance. *Oncol. Lett.* **2019**, *17*, 5351–5360. [CrossRef] [PubMed]
44. Christodoulou, I.; Goulielmaki, M.; Devetzi, M.; Panagiotidis, M.; Koliakos, G.; Zoumpourlis, V. Mesenchymal stem cells in preclinical cancer cytotherapy: A systematic review. *Stem Cell Res. Ther.* **2018**, *9*, 336. [CrossRef] [PubMed]
45. Krawczenko, A.; Bielawska-Pohl, A.; Paprocka, M.; Kraskiewicz, H.; Szyposzynska, A.; Wojdat, E.; Klimczak, A. Microvesicles from Human Immortalized Cell Lines of Endothelial Progenitor Cells and Mesenchymal Stem/Stromal Cells of Adipose Tissue Origin as Carriers of Bioactive Factors Facilitating Angiogenesis. *Stem Cells Int.* **2020**, *2020*, 1289380. [CrossRef] [PubMed]
46. Witwer, K.W.; Buzas, E.I.; Bemis, L.T.; Bora, A.; Lasser, C.; Lotvall, J.; Nolte-'t Hoen, E.N.; Piper, M.G.; Sivaraman, S.; Skog, J.; et al. Standardization of sample collection, isolation and analysis methods in extracellular vesicle research. *J. Extracell. Vesicles* **2013**, *2*. [CrossRef]

47. Adamiak, M.; Cheng, G.; Bobis-Wozowicz, S.; Zhao, L.; Kedracka-Krok, S.; Samanta, A.; Karnas, E.; Xuan, Y.T.; Skupien-Rabian, B.; Chen, X.; et al. Induced Pluripotent Stem Cell (iPSC)-Derived Extracellular Vesicles Are Safer and More Effective for Cardiac Repair Than iPSCs. *Circ. Res.* **2018**, *122*, 296–309. [CrossRef]
48. Matuszyk, J.; Cebrat, M.; Kalas, W.; Strzadala, L. HA1004, an inhibitor of serine/threonine protein kinases, restores the sensitivity of thymic lymphomas to Ca^{2+}-mediated apoptosis through a protein kinase A-independent mechanism. *Int. Immunopharmacol.* **2002**, *2*, 435–442. [CrossRef]

Publisher's Note: MDPI stays neutral with regard to jurisdictional claims in published maps and institutional affiliations.

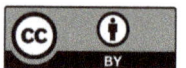

© 2020 by the authors. Licensee MDPI, Basel, Switzerland. This article is an open access article distributed under the terms and conditions of the Creative Commons Attribution (CC BY) license (http://creativecommons.org/licenses/by/4.0/).

MDPI
St. Alban-Anlage 66
4052 Basel
Switzerland
Tel. +41 61 683 77 34
Fax +41 61 302 89 18
www.mdpi.com

International Journal of Molecular Sciences Editorial Office
E-mail: ijms@mdpi.com
www.mdpi.com/journal/ijms